Neuroergonomics: A Cognitive Neuroscience Approach

Neuroergonomics: A Cognitive Neuroscience Approach

Editor: Thomson Andrew

AMERICAN
MEDICAL PUBLISHERS
www.americanmedicalpublishers.com

AMERICAN
MEDICAL PUBLISHERS
www.americanmedicalpublishers.com

Cataloging-in-Publication Data

Neuroergonomics : a cognitive neuroscience approach / edited by Thomson Andrew.
p. cm.
Includes bibliographical references and index.
ISBN 979-8-88740-306-9
1. Neuroergonomics. 2. Cognitive neuroscience. 3. Human engineering. 4. Neurology. I. Andrew, Thomson.
QP360.7 .N48 2023
612.802 85--dc23

American Medical Publishers,
41 Flatbush Avenue,
1st Floor, New York,
NY 11217, USA

ISBN 979-8-88740-306-9 (Hardback)

Contents

Preface

This book was inspired by the evolution of our times; to answer the curiosity of inquisitive minds. Many developments have occurred across the globe in the recent past which has transformed the progress in the field.

Neuroergonomics is an emerging science that is defined as the study of the human brain and behavior at work. It integrates two scientific disciplines, namely, neuroscience and ergonomics. Neuroscience is concerned with study of the structure and function of the brain while ergonomics deals with understanding the interactions among human and other elements of a system. Ergonomics also focuses on the optimization of this interaction. The objective of combining these two disciplines is to enhance the performance and expand the capabilities at workplace by providing new training methods. Functional neuroimaging, neurostimulation, and psychophysiology are the three principal approaches used in neuroergonomics. Some of the areas of study within this field are working memory, motor control, mental workload, visual attention and human-automation interaction. This book includes some of the vital pieces of work being conducted across the world, on various topics related to neuroergonomics. It brings forth some of the most innovative concepts and elucidates a cognitive neuroscience approach to this field. This book is a vital tool for all researching and studying in this field.

This book was developed from a mere concept to drafts to chapters and finally compiled together as a complete text to benefit the readers across all nations. To ensure the quality of the content we instilled two significant steps in our procedure. The first was to appoint an editorial team that would verify the data and statistics provided in the book and also select the most appropriate and valuable contributions from the plentiful contributions we received from authors worldwide. The next step was to appoint an expert of the topic as the Editor-in-Chief, who would head the project and finally make the necessary amendments and modifications to make the text reader-friendly. I was then commissioned to examine all the material to present the topics in the most comprehensible and productive format.

I would like to take this opportunity to thank all the contributing authors who were supportive enough to contribute their time and knowledge to this project. I also wish to convey my regards to my family who have been extremely supportive during the entire project.

Editor

1

Acute Supramaximal Exercise Increases the Brain Oxygenation in Relation to Cognitive Workload

Cem Seref Bediz[1,2], Adile Oniz[2], Cagdas Guducu[2], Enise Ural Demirci[1], Hilmi Ogut[2], Erkan Gunay[2,3], Caner Cetinkaya[3] and Murat Ozgoren[2]*

[1] Department of Physiology, Faculty of Medicine, Dokuz Eylul University, Izmir, Turkey, [2] Department of Biophysics, Faculty of Medicine, Dokuz Eylul University, Izmir, Turkey, [3] School of Sport Sciences and Technology, Dokuz Eylul University, Izmir, Turkey

***Correspondence:**
Cem Seref Bediz
cem.bediz@deu.edu.tr

Single bout of exercise can improve the performance on cognitive tasks. However, cognitive responses may be controversial due to different type, intensity, and duration of exercise. In addition, the mechanism of the effect of acute exercise on brain is still unclear. This study was aimed to investigate the effects of supramaximal exercise on cognitive tasks by means of brain oxygenation monitoring. The brain oxygenation of Prefrontal cortex (PFC) was measured on 35 healthy male volunteers via functional near infrared spectroscopy (fNIRS) system. Subjects performed 2-Back test before and after the supramaximal exercise wingate anerobic test (WAnT) lasting 30-s on cycle ergometer. The PFC oxygenation change evaluation revealed that PFC oxygenation rise during post-exercise 2-Back task was considerably higher than those in pre-exercise 2-Back task. In order to describe the relationship between oxygenation change and exercise performance, subjects were divided into two groups as high performers (HP) and low performers (LP) according to their peak power values (PP) obtained from the supramaximal test. The oxy-hemoglobin (oxy-Hb) values were compared between pre- and post-exercise conditions within subjects and also between subjects according to peak power. When performers were compared, in the HP group, the oxy-Hb values in post-exercise 2-Back test were significantly higher than those in pre-exercise 2-Back test. HP had significantly higher post-exercise oxy-Hb change (Δ) than those of LP. In addition, PP of the total group were significantly correlated with Δoxy-Hb.The key findings of the present study revealed that acute supramaximal exercise has an impact on the brain oxygenation during a cognitive task. Also, the higher the anerobic PP describes the larger the oxy-Hb response in post-exercise cognitive task. The current study also demonstrated a significant correlation between peak power (exercise load) and post-exercise hemodynamic responses (oxy-, deoxy- and total-Hb). The magnitude of this impact might be related with the physical performance capacities of the individuals. This can become a valuable parameter for future studies on human factor.

Keywords: PFC, human factor, fNIRS, cognition and exercise, N-back test

INTRODUCTION

Individuals usually feel a mental arousal and define an increase in their cognitive abilities after exercise. The relation between exercise and cognitive function has been investigated in several decades. It has been proposed that exercise durations, exercise intensity and the differences in cognitive tasks could cause some contradicting results in previous studies (Ando et al., 2011; Endo et al., 2013; Schmit et al., 2015). Despite the large variations of the reported results, there is meta-analytic evidence that describes significant beneficial effects of acute exercise on cognition in the general population (Lambourne and Tomporowski, 2010; McMorris and Hale, 2012). The positive effects of erobic exercise on various cognitive tasks have been reported mostly. However there are rarely any reports about the effect of anerobic exercise (*i.e., the protocol in the current study*), characterized as short term and highly intensive effort, on cognition. The specific mechanisms by which exercise affects cognitive functions remain largely unclear (Rupp and Perrey, 2008). One of the mechanisms proposed is the relationship between prefrontal cortex (PFC) oxygenation and cognitive function. With the development of imaging methods, it has been possible to show the brain oxygenation during or post exercise conditions. Most of the studies demonstrate an increment in oxygenation of PFC following exercise (Rupp and Perrey, 2008; Jung et al., 2015).

In the literature, effects of exercise on cognitive performance were investigated during exercise and after exercise period. It is largely accepted that the metabolic activity in brain increases during cognitive tasks. The consumption of energy in the neurons depending on the metabolic activity increase leads an increase in the cerebral blood flow to meet the increased demand of oxygen and glucose. For this reason, the increment in brain oxygenation is accepted to be/as the physiological indicator for cognitive workload. Near infrared spectroscopy (NIRS) is a non-invasive measurement based sensitive method that indicates cerebral hemodynamic response (Ozgoren et al., 2012) to cognitive tasks by means of changing levels of oxy- and deoxy-HB (Albinet et al., 2014). Some studies reported a relationship between cerebral oxygenation level and cognitive test scores (Ayaz et al., 2007, 2012; McMorris et al., 2011; McMorris and Hale, 2012). Additionally, Li et al. (2005) and Gateau et al. (2015), describe a higher dorsolateral PFC activation during working memory task by using functional near infrared spectroscopy (fNIRS). Inadequate increase in cerebral oxygenation during cognitive task defined as an indicator of cerebral fatigue (Nybo and Rasmussen, 2007; Mandrick et al., 2013; Mehta and Parasuraman, 2014). Dietrich (2003) reported that, aside from cerebral fatigue, the hypo-frontality may occur due to the challenge of source allocation between the areas responsible for physical and cognitive workload.

We hypothesized that the brain oxygenation during cognitive task after the acute supramaximal exercise is higher than the pre-exercise cognitive task. We also expected a higher behavioral performance after the acute supramaximal exercise. This study aimed to evaluate the hemodynamic and behavioral changes of cognitive processes following an acute (anerobic) supramaximal exercise.

TABLE 1 | Ages, heights, body weights, peak powers and maximal heart rates (Max-HR) of low performers (LP) and high performers (HP) groups were presented as mean ± SD.

	Age (yrs)	Height (m)	Weight (kg)	Peak Power (Watts)	Max-HR (beats/min)
HP (*n* = 18)	21.0 ± 2.6	165.9 ± 22.5	72.7 ± 9.6	800.7 ± 77.3	165.4 ± 22.8
LP (*n* = 17)	20.5 ± 2.1	168.9 ± 11.5	71.4 ± 11.1	634.3 ± 89.3	168.9 ± 11.5

MATERIALS AND METHODS

Participants and Experimental Design

Thirty-five male healthy and physically active subjects (1.78 ± 0.07 cm height and 72.1 ± 10.3 kg weight) aged between 18 and 23 years participated to the study (**Table 1**). All subjects were informed about the procedures and signed a written consent. Experiments were conducted in two visits. In first visit, the subjects were informed and became familiar to both exercise and N-Back test protocols. Within 3 days, subjects re-visited the laboratory to perform a short term-supramaximal acute exercise and cognitive tasks (2-Back tests) before and after exercise (**Figure 1**). Brain oxygenation was continuously measured via fNIRS during cognitive tasks and exercise. In order to evaluate the performance dependent results, an average peak power value was calculated for all subjects. Subjects who had higher power values than the average (751 Watt) was considered as high performers (HP), (*N* = 17 subjects) while who had lower power values than average were considered as low performers (LP), (*N* = 18 subjects). There were no statistically significant differences in terms of age, weight and height between the HP and LP groups. The Ethics Committee of Dokuz Eylul University approved all procedures and experimental design.

Cognitive Task Procedure

Cognitive performance was evaluated by N-Back test before and after exercise. N-Back test, which mainly evaluates the working memory as well as sustained attention, was administrated to evaluate working memory and inhibitory control of irrelevant information (Jonides et al., 1997; Jaeggi et al., 2010). N-Back test was developed in OpenGL by using C programming language, has been administered to the participants by a laptop. A pseudorandom sequence of 120 letters consisting "K, Q, H, X, M, F, R, and B" were displayed on the center of the screen, one by one. Participants were asked to press the button on a response pad only if a letter on the screen was the same as the letter shown "*n*" steps earlier. In the present study "2-Back" condition was employed. The probability of each letter to be same as the two-step earlier letter was 30%. Each letter was presented on the computer screen for 500 ms and the inter-stimulus interval was set to vary between 1500 and

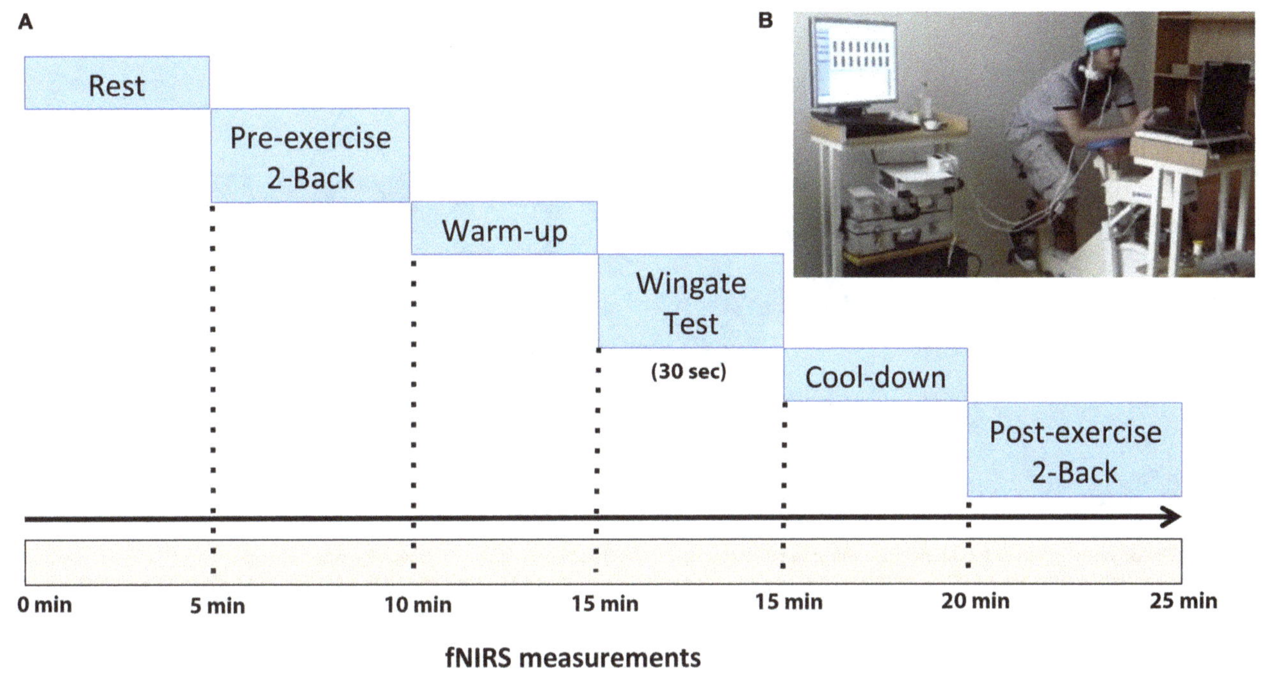

FIGURE 1 | (A) The demonstration of experimental design for the current study. **(B)** Participant seated at cycle ergometer during whole paradigm.

2000 ms. All tests were completed within 5 min. A brief training session, including a practice sequence of 15 letters, was given to all participants before the actual test to familiarize the subjects to the protocols. In order to evaluate working memory; reaction time for all stimuli total reaction time (TRT) and reaction time for the correct answers (CART), number of correct answers (CA), wrong answers (WA), and missed answers (M) have been obtained and measured. Nexus-10 bio-amplifier, which was equipped with appropriate sensors, was used to monitor the appearance of stimuli on the screen and participant responses in order to measure exact reaction times.

Exercise Procedure

Wingate Anerobic test (WAnT) protocol was applied as the supramaximal exercise. WAnT is an exhaustive exercise for assessment of anerobic performance (Dotan and Bar-Or, 1983). WAnT is also accepted as a standardized anerobic exercise model for evaluating physiological responses to supramaximal exercise under controlled conditions (Weinstein et al., 1998). Following a warm up on the bicycle for 5 min at intensity about 50 watts, all subjects performed WAnT on a mechanically braked cycle ergometer with an optical pedal counter (Monark 824E, Sweden). Two unloaded 5-s sprints were performed during warm up. Following the warm up, subjects were instructed to pedal as fast as possible for 30 s against a resistance of 80 g/kg body mass. The subjects were verbally encouraged to maintain high pedaling rate throughout the WAnT. Pedal revolutions were monitored and recorded at 1-s intervals. Power outputs were calculated as described in Weinstein et al. (1998). The highest power output in the first 5 s of the test was used to represent the peak power (PP; PP = Distance × Load/ Time).

fNIRS Recordings

The continuous wave (CW) fNIR system used in the present study (Imager 100, fNIR Devices LLC, MD, USA). System was connected to a flexible sensor pad, Sensor pad contained four light sources with built in peak wavelengths at 730 nm and 850 nm and 10 detectors designed to scan cortical areas underlying the forehead. The forehead area was cleaned with alcohol swap and scrubbing cream (NuPrep, USA). After the cleansing process the sensor was placed to the forehead region and covered by an elastic bandage specifically designed to hold it tightly across the head. Furthermore, a black head bandage was placed on top to eliminate the possible ambient light effects.

This system records two wavelengths and dark current for each of the 16 voxels, totaling 48 measurements for each sampling period (Ayaz et al., 2011, 2013). With a fixed source-detector separation of 2.5 cm, this configuration generates a total of 16 measurement locations (voxels) per wavelength. Data acquisition and visualization were conducted using COBI Studio software (Ayaz and Onaral, 2005). The fNIR device calculates relative changes to baseline values of oxy-hemoglobin (oxy-Hb) and deoxyhemoglobin (deoxy-Hb) molecules by means of a CW spectroscopy system that applies light to tissue at constant amplitude. The mathematical basis of CW-type measurements uses the modified Beer Lambert Law (Cope and Delpy, 1988). In the present study baseline condition was started at the beginning of the each task and lasted 20 s. The summation

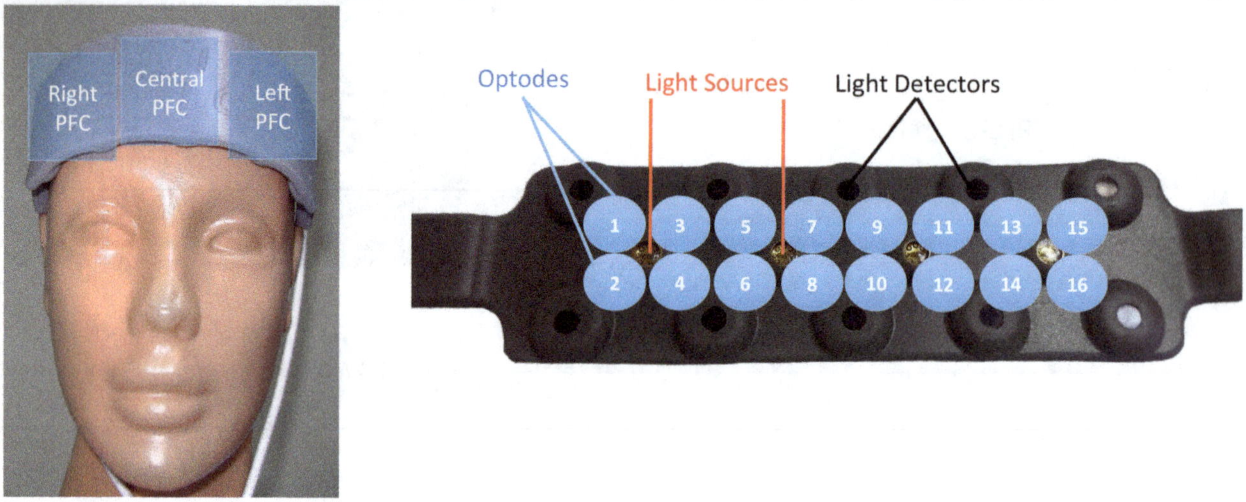

FIGURE 2 | The demonstration of functional near infrared spectroscopy (fNIRS) sensor pad. Brain oxygenation was measured from 16 locations over the forehead area via fNIRS sensor (left side). The sensor pad has 4 light sources, 10 light detectors and 16 optodes (right side). Optodes that are located on the leftmost side of the forehead namely 1, 2, 3 and 4 denotes left prefrontal cortex (PFC), optodes that are centrally located as 7, 8, 9 and 10 denotes central PFC, and optodes that are located on the rightmost side as 13, 14, 15 and 16 denotes right PFC.

of oxy-Hb and deoxy-Hb values was described as total-Hb. Moreover, Δoxy-Hb and Δdeoxy-Hb parameters were used to describe the value differences (oxygenation change; i.e., rise or fall) between average values of two different sessions (i.e. $\Delta OxyHb = OxyHb_{\text{post}} - OxyHb_{\text{pre}}$) for both oxy-Hb and deoxy-Hb.

fNIRS Analysis

The raw intensity measurements at 730, and 850 nm were Butterworth low-pass filtered with MATLAB program (MATLAB and Statistics Toolbox, 2007). Butterworth filter was designed to eliminate possible respiration and heart rate signals and unwanted high frequency noise (Huppert et al., 2009). The artifact removal process has been made according to Ayaz et al. (2012). The PFC oxygenation data retrieved via fNIRS were examined in right, left and central PFC areas and defined as region of interest (ROI; **Figure 2**). Optodes that are located on the leftmost side of the forehead namely 1, 2, 3 and 4 combined to denote left PFC, optodes that are centrally located as 7, 8, 9 and 10 combined to denote central PFC, and optodes that are located on the rightmost side as 13, 14, 15 and 16 combined to denote right PFC. fNIRS signals were calculated and averaged over the whole pre- and post-exercise 2-Back sessions (Endo et al., 2013).

Statistical Analysis

Shapiro-Wilk and Kolmogorov-Smirnov tests were used to control the normality of the data. All of the data were distributed normally. Age, height and weight differences between groups were tested via independent groups *t*-test, and the results were given in **Table 1**. We performed statistical analysis on combined channels as ROI wise.

A two-way group (LP vs. HP) and time (pre vs. post exercise) analysis of variance (ANOVA) was performed on fNIRS data and behavioral data. Moreover, oxy- and deoxy-Hb change were calculated as mentioned before (i.e., ΔOxyHb), and used for the statistical analysis. An independent group *t*-test was performed to test group differences (LP vs. HP) on oxy-, deoxy- and total-Hb changes. Also, the correlations between peak power and oxy-Hb, deoxy-Hb, and total-Hb changes were investigated via Spearman's rank order correlations test.

RESULTS

fNIRS Findings

In the present study, 35 healthy subjects were recruited. In order to evaluate the performance dependent results, pre and post exercise PFC oxygenation levels during 2-Back tests were compared for both HP and LP groups with two-way mixed ANOVA. The oxy-Hb, deoxy-Hb, and total-Hb values of the groups were demonstrated for pre- and post-exercise 2-Back sessions were demonstrated in **Table 2**. Also the demonstration of oxy-Hb and deoxy-Hb levels in central PFC area during pre- and post-exercise 2-Back tests were given for whole group averages in **Figure 3**. All of the figures represent the group averages during related task (pre- and post-exercise 2-back).

For oxygenation related analysis; pre- and post-exercise 2-Back tests oxy-Hb values were selected as within-subject factor and peak power was selected as between-subject factor. According to these analyses, oxygenation in post-exercise 2-Back test was higher than the oxygenation in pre-exercise 2-Back test for all three ROI of PFC [$F_{(1,33)} = 51.82, p < 0.001, \eta = 0.61$ for left; $F_{(1,33)} = 78.42, p < 0.001, \eta = 0.70$ for central; $F_{(1,33)} = 54.25$, $p < 0.001$ $\eta = 0.61$ for right]. For right PFC area there was

TABLE 2 | Pre- and post-exercise 2-back oxy-, deoxy, and total-Hb levels (mean ± SD) are given for total, LP and HP group in central prefrontal cortex (PFC) area.

	Pre-exercise 2-Back			Post-exercise 2-Back		
	Oxy-Hb (μMolar)	Deoxy-Hb (μMolar)	Total-Hb (μMolar)	Oxy-Hb (μMolar)	Deoxy-Hb (μMolar)	Total-Hb (μMolar)
Total Group	3.11 (± 3.41)	− 0.99 (± 0.94)	3.01 (± 3.71)	7.32 (± 4.85)***	0.84 (± 2.42)*	8.15 (± 6.56)***
HP	3.30 (± 3.62)	0.11 (± 0.94)	3.42 (± 4.04)	9.18 (± 4.90)***	1.84 (± 2.74)*	11.03 (± 6.88)***
LP	2.92 (± 3.30)	−0.30 (± 0.93)	2.62 (± 3.44)	5.54 (± 3.30)***	−0.11 (± 1.64)	5.43 (± 5.06)**

The significant differences related to comparisons of oxygenation, deoxygenation and total-Hb between pre- and post-exercise 2-Back session are marked with "" (where "*" denotes p < 0.05, "**" denotes p < 0.01, and "***" denotes p < 0.001).*

not any interaction so, the pairwise comparisons were used. According to pairwise comparisons there was not any significant difference between groups, but there were significant differences between pre and post oxygenation levels in right PFC ($p < 0.001$). Because of the significant interaction in left and central PFC areas between within group effects (Pre/Post) and between group effects (HP/LP) in terms of two-way ANOVA results, between group analyses could not be evaluated (McDonald, 2009). Further analyses were made to clarify the statistical significance via within group paired samples t-test analysis. Paired samples t-test was conducted separately for each group and post-exercise 2-Back test oxy-Hb levels were found significantly higher than the pre-exercise 2-Back test oxy-Hb level for both group [for HP group: in left PFC, $T_{(16)} = -5.99$, $p < 0.001$; in central PFC, $T_{(16)} = -8.12, p < 0.001$; for LP group: in left PFC, $T_{(17)} = -3.89$, $p < 0.001$; in central PFC, $T_{(17)} = -4.13, p < 0.001$].

Moreover, deoxy-Hb related analyses were conducted. For the analyses; pre- and post-exercise 2-Back tests deoxy-Hb values were selected as within-subject factor and peak power was selected as between-subject factor. According to these analyses, deoxy-Hb values were significantly higher in post-exercise 2-Back test than the deoxy-Hb values in pre-exercise 2-Back test for all three ROI of PFC [$F_{(1,33)} = 9.56$, $p < 0.01$, $\eta = 0.23$ for left PFC; $F_{(1,33)} = 7.03$, $p < 0.05$, $\eta = 0.17$ for central PFC; $F_{(1,33)} = 11.59$, $p < 0.01$ $\eta = 0.26$ for right PFC]. For right and left PFC areas there was not any interaction so, the pairwise comparisons were used. According to pairwise comparisons there was not any significant difference between groups, but there were significant differences between pre and post deoxygenation levels in left and right PFC ($p < 0.01$ for both). Because of the significant interaction in central PFC area between within group effects (Pre/Post) and between group effects (HP/LP) in terms of two-way ANOVA results, between group analyses could not be evaluated (McDonald, 2009). Further analysis was made to clarify the statistical significance via within group paired samples t-test analysis. Paired samples t-test was conducted separately for each group and post-exercise 2-Back test deoxy-Hb levels were found significantly higher than the pre-exercise 2-Back test deoxy-Hb level for HP group in central PFC area [$T_{(16)} = -2.67, p < 0.05$] and there was not any significance for LP group in central PFC area.

Also total-Hb was significantly higher in post-exercise 2-Back test for all three interested ROI of PFC [$F_{(1,33)} = 38.55, p < 0.001$, $\eta = 0.54$ for left PFC; $F_{(1,33)} = 47.20, p < 0.001, \eta = 0.59$ for central PFC; $F_{(1,33)} = 42.15$, $p < 0.001$ $\eta = 0.56$ for right PFC]. For right and left PFC areas there was not any interaction so, the pairwise comparisons were used. According to pairwise comparisons there was not any significant difference between groups, but there were significant differences between pre and post total-Hb levels in left and right PFC ($p < 0.001$ for both). Because of the

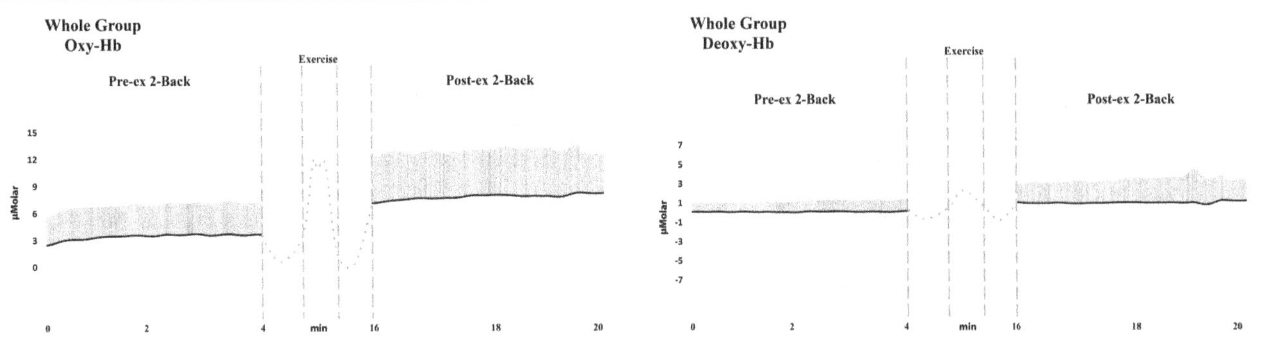

FIGURE 3 | The demonstration of oxy- and deoxy-Hb average levels in central PFC area during pre- and post-exercise 2-Back tests for the whole group. Standard deviations are also marked in line with average as vertical lines (Note that only positive deflection is displayed for the sake of simplicity). Left panel indicated oxy-Hb and right panel indicated deoxy-Hb results. Vertical scale denotes the strength of fNIRS signal in μMolar units, which is normalized to baseline. Horizontal scale denotes the time scale in minutes. Vertical dashed lines denote pre-, during and post- exercise onsets and durations. The dotted lines represent the periods of warm-up and cool-down.

TABLE 3 | Post- and pre-exercise oxy-Hb, deoxy-Hb, and total-Hb changes (Δoxy-Hb, Δdeoxy-Hb, and Δtotal-Hb) are given for LP and HP groups in all PFC area (mean ± SD).

	ΔOxy-Hb (μMolar)			ΔDeoxy-Hb (μMolar)			ΔTotal-Hb (μMolar)		
	Left	Central	Right	Left	Central	Right	Left	Central	Right
HP	5.66 (± 3.89)*	5.88 (± 2.98)**	4.87 (± 3.48)	1.89 (± 1.91)	2.32 (± 2.13)*	1.26 (± 1.18)	7.10 (± 5.59)*	7.61 (± 5.03)**	5.74 (± 4.52)
LP	2.71 (± 2.94)	2.62 (± 2.69)	3.25 (± 3.48)	1.62 (± 1.67)	1.16 (± 0.89)	1.65 (± 1.56)	3.60 (± 4.58)	2.81 (± 3.90)	4.42 (± 4.72)

Significances between groups are marked with "" (where "*" denotes $p < 0.05$, "**" denotes $p < 0.01$).*

significant interaction in central PFC area between within group effects (Pre/Post) and between group effects (HP/LP) in terms of two-way ANOVA results, between group analyses could not be evaluated (McDonald, 2009). Further analyses were made to clarify the statistical significance via within group paired samples t-test analysis. Paired samples t-test was conducted separately for each group and post-exercise 2-Back test total-Hb levels were found significantly higher than the pre-exercise 2-Back test total-Hb level for HP group [in central PFC, $T_{(16)} = -6.24$, $p < 0.001$], and for LP group [in central PFC, $T_{(17)} = -3.06$, $p < 0.01$].

In addition to these findings, the changes of oxy-Hb, deoxy-Hb, and total-Hb were compared between HP and LP groups via independent samples t-test (**Table 3**). While comparing the oxygenation changes (Δoxy-Hb) of the LP and HP group, PFC oxygenation rise in central PFC ($p < 0.01$) and left PFC ($p < 0.05$) areas were found significantly higher in HP group. While comparing the deoxygenation changes (Δdeoxy-Hb) of pre- and post-exercise 2-Back tests, HP group's PFC deoxygenation changes in central PFC area was found significantly higher ($p < 0.05$). While comparing the total-Hb changes (Δtotal-Hb) of pre- and post-exercise 2-Back tests, HP group's PFC total-Hb change in central PFC ($p < 0.01$) and left PFC ($p < 0.05$) areas were found significantly higher. Moreover, the peak power values (PP) of the total group were significantly correlated with Δoxy-Hb, Δdeoxy-Hb, and Δtotal-Hb values for central PFC area ($r = 0.042$ $p < 0.01$; $r = 0.035$ $p < 0.02$; $r = 0.040$ $p < 0.01$, respectively). The demonstration of average oxy-Hb and deoxy-Hb levels in central PFC area during pre- and post-exercise 2-Back Tests for HP and LP group were given in **Figures 4, 5**.

Behavioral Findings

All subjects have successfully completed the whole procedure. 2-Back test scores (CA, WA, M, CART, TRT) were compared for total group and there were no significant differences between pre- and post-exercise 2-Back test scores. The same comparison was made for HP and LP groups and also there were no significant differences within (pre-exercise vs. post-exercise sessions) and between groups (**Table 4**). Though not statistically significant the reaction times, the correct answer CART were slightly progressed after the exercise.

DISCUSSION

Both physical benefits and cognitive improvements of the exercise have been frequently studied in the field. In the present study, the effects of anerobic exercise on brain oxygenation were investigated in relation to cognitive workload. The results revealed an increment in oxy-, deoxy-, and total-Hb levels on the post-exercise session of cognitive task. The increments in these parameters have been found to be statistically higher than the pre-exercise session of the cognitive task. In the related literature, it has been demonstrated that the oxy-Hb level increases in PFC during both physical exercise and cognitive task. Such rise has been linked to the increase in neural-metabolic activation (González-Alonso et al., 2004; Shibuya et al., 2004; Rupp and Perrey, 2008; Endo et al., 2013). In their study Tam and Zouridakis (2014) describes the oxy-Hb, deoxy-Hb, their summation (oxy-Hb + deoxy-Hb), and their difference (oxy-Hb—deoxy-Hb) measurements corresponding to the changes in oxygen delivery, oxygen extraction, total blood volume delivered, and total oxygenation, respectively. The increasing level of oxy- and deoxy-Hb is accepted as an indicator of an increase in blood flow (Endo et al., 2013). The present study revealed a rise in all oxy-Hb, deoxy-Hb, and total-Hb levels during both pre- and post-exercise cognitive tasks, which might be related to regional increase of cerebral blood flow. In this context, regional blood flow in PFC during post-exercise session of cognitive task could be considered higher than the pre-exercise session of cognitive task. Such increased hemodynamic responses may be an indicator for the additional effort during post-exercise cognitive task (Mandrick et al., 2013).

In the present study, a relationship between brain's hemodynamic responses and physical performance (under anerobic supramaximal exercise conditions) has been revealed. The participants were divided into two groups by means of PP mentioned as high- and low-performers in order to address the performance relationship. Despite the similar hemodynamic response patterns during pre-exercise session of cognitive task, different hemodynamic response patterns have been observed between groups during post-exercise sessions of cognitive task (**Figures 3, 4**). As the most striking difference the rise of oxy-Hb and total-Hb levels of HP group have been found statistically higher than those of LP group in central and left PFC areas. These findings may demonstrate that the rise of oxygen consumption and demand in PFC is higher in the HP group, as known as higher anerobic capacity, than the LP group. In this context, Drigny et al. (2014), reported that the brain oxygenation could change with training in obese patients. Also, Khan and Hillman (2014) reviewed the connection between training and its effects on brain oxygenation levels and suggested a relationship between erobic fitness and cognitive processes that can be demonstrated

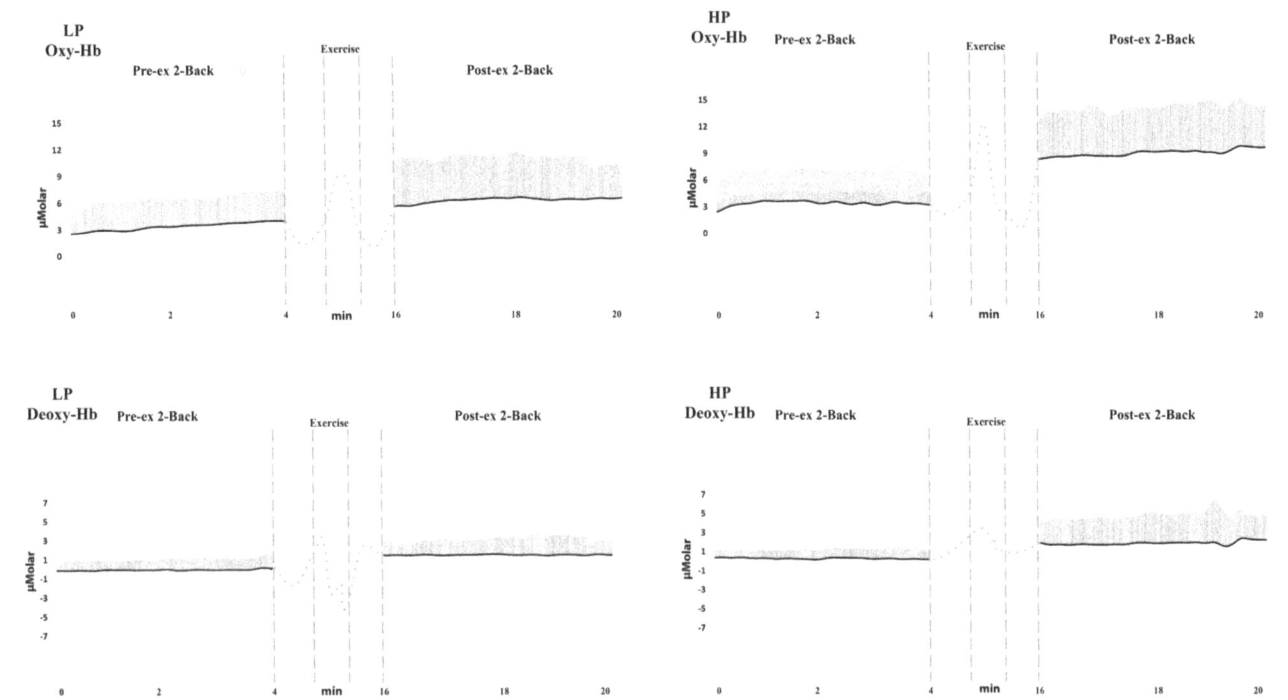

FIGURE 4 | The demonstration of oxy- and deoxy-Hb levels in central PFC area during pre- and post-exercise 2-Back tests for group averages. Standard deviations are also marked in line with average as vertical lines (Note that only positive deflection is displayed for the sake of simplicity). The four panels are divided into performers (low and high performance, left and right consequently) and oxy- and deoxy-Hb (upper and lower consequently). Left panel indicated oxy-Hb and right panel deoxy-Hb results. Vertical scale denotes the strength of fNIRS signal in µMolar units, which is normalized to baseline. Horizontal scale denotes the time scale in minutes Vertical dashed lines denote pre-, during and post- exercise onsets and durations. The dotted lines represent the periods of warm-up and cool-down.

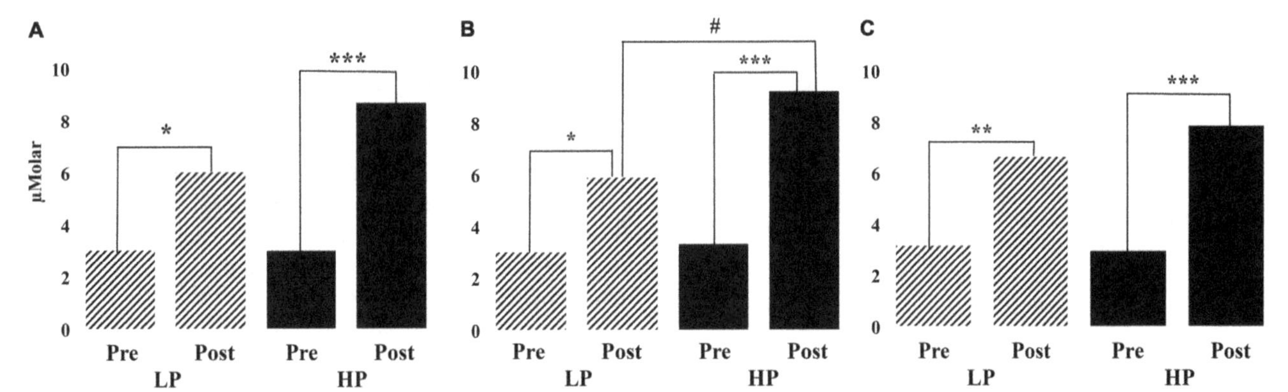

FIGURE 5 | The oxygenation values for pre- and post-exercise 2-Back sessions in left (A), center (B) and right (C) areas of PFC in high and low performance groups. Within group significances are marked with "*" (where "*" denotes $p < 0.05$, "**" denotes $p < 0.01$, and "***" denotes $p < 0.001$); between group significances are marked with "#" (where "#" denotes $p < 0.05$).

via different fMRI and EEG studies. A similar relationship was described between exercise and cognitive functions by Davenport et al. (2012). In the light of results of the present study, level of PFC oxygenation in physically better performing group during post-exercise cognitive task might be higher than the physically lower performing group during post-exercise cognitive tasks.

The current study also demonstrated a significant correlation between peak power (exercise load) and post-exercise change of hemodynamic responses (Δoxy-Hb, Δdeoxy-Hb, and Δtotal-Hb). This correlation also supports the aforementioned assumptions in which the higher performers have higher PFC oxygenation. This can become a valuable parameter for future studies on human factor by means of physical/cognitive

TABLE 4 | The demonstration of correct answers, wrong answers, missed answers; correct answers reaction time, and total reaction time (mean ± SD) for high (HP) and low performers (LP) group during pre- and post-exercise 2-Back sessions.

	Pre exercise 2-Back Session					Post exercise 2-Back Session				
	Correct answers	Wrong answers	Missed answers	Correct answers reaction time (ms)	Total reaction time (ms)	Correct answers	Wrong answers	Missed answers	Correct answers reaction time (ms)	Total reaction time (ms)
Total Group	25.49 (±5.65)	6.37 (±4.56)	10.34 (±5.57)	582.90 (±143.03)	596.60 (±147.39)	25.82 (±6.56)	7.97 (±4.61)	10.17 (±6.56)	576.60 (±186.63)	578.90 (±175.68)
HP	26.0 (±4.23)	6.12 (±4.21)	10.0 (±4.23)	561.76 (±148.61)	575.88 (±154.12)	26.29 (±6.12)	8.12 (±4.61)	9.71 (±6.12)	544.11 (±192.66)	551.17 (±181.71)
LP	25.0 (±6.56)	6.61 (±4.73)	10.67 (±6.45)	602.78 (±130.25)	616.11 (±133.46)	25.39 (±6.75)	7.83 (±4.48)	10.61 (±6.75)	607.22 (±169.70)	605.0 (±160.32)

load. Formerly using a different paradigm, our group has demonstrated the centrofrontal shift of the active brain areas due to cognitive load (Bayazıt et al., 2009). In that study, the cognitive load—such as conflict resolution—displayed a physical drive from the posterior areas towards frontal areas with an increased demand on the frontal regions. Similarly, in the current study, the high peak power task is not solely a motor one but also requires a multitude of cognitive activities. In order to cope with the higher motor (and cognitive) load, the brain has to perform increased levels of concentration, attention, coordination, environment monitoring, and reactive and interactive motor control. The frontal areas are the primary areas for these and similar executive and complex skills. Further clarification is needed in this context to describe the effect of physical fitness on brain oxygenation by means of new study designs and larger size groups.

The effects of acute exercise on cognitive functions have been investigated for decades. However, studies demonstrating the mechanisms of physical exercise on brain oxygenation in relation to cognitive performance via fNIRS are very limited and these mechanism are not well understood (Albinet et al., 2014; Drigny et al., 2014; Dupuy et al., 2015). In previous studies, the participants' performance for decision-making, mental processing speed, selective attention, and reaction time was investigated (Aks, 1998; Arcelin and Brisswalter, 1999; Emery et al., 2001). Moreover, Brisswalter et al. (2002) and Tomporowski (2003) reported that the cognitive performance could be improved by acute exercise. Interestingly, previous studies revealed different findings depending on the type of the exercise, while intense and exhausting exercise causes fatigue (Brisswalter et al., 2002), and light exercise (Varner and Ellis, 1998) causes cognitive performance impairment. Besides, some studies reported a decrease in cognitive functions related with the fatigue caused by the intensity or duration of the exercise (Mehta and Parasuraman, 2014). The physiological basis of this decrement could also be originated from the natural challenge between PFC area related with cognition and motor area related to motion, which causes a hypo-frontality (Dietrich, 2003). The experimental setup of the current study employed a high load but very short (30-sec) anerobic exercise, and such exercise model could cause higher oxygenation responses in PFC similar as erobic exercise models. As mentioned before, the behavioral results displayed only a small but non-significant increase in WA and slight but not significant increase in the CA after the exercise. Our results did not provide a strong support for neither an improvement nor decrement in cognitive scores after acute exercise.

In the related literature, Stroop test was frequently employed as a cognitive task, and generally the improvement of the total test time was accepted as an indicator of improved cognitive functions (Hyodo et al., 2012; Endo et al., 2013). In the present study we employed the 2-Back test as a cognitive task, and evaluated the whole parameters (CA, WA, MA, CART, TRT), but not the total test time. Therefore 2-Back test might not be the right tool as an indicator of the improved cognitive functions. Also the rise of PFC oxygenation could not fully mean an improvement in cognitive function during the post-exercise session. Another plausible explanation might be that the participants had to work harder "neurally" (indicated by increased oxy-Hb levels) to maintain the cognitive performance during post-exercise session.

In another view, some studies reported an improvement of cognitive functions after the moderate exercise (Potter and Keeling, 2005; Coles and Tomporowski, 2008). However, a recent meta-analysis (McMorris et al., 2011) raised an issue. Those authors examined the effect of acute, moderate intensity exercise on working memory tasks and found that speed and accuracy of processing were differentially affected. In particular, the positive effects of acute exercise seem to be disproportionately influential on executive control processes (i.e., planning, coordination, inhibition, mental flexibility, working memory) relative to tasks of recall and alertness (Chang et al., 2012; McMorris and Hale, 2012). N-Back task used in the current study indeed involves working memory, alertness, planning, and inhibition strategies. Therefore a possible explanation could be that there might be an increase in the cognitive (i.e., executive control process) functions due to prolonged total blood flow capacity increase in the brain metabolic capacity (both oxygen and glucose should be increased) but somehow 2-Back test might not be tough enough to elucidate such improvement. Another explanation could be that the increased metabolic activity in brain might be the mean of more neural effort to maintain the performance, not the indicator of cognitive improvement.

The findings of current literature are not sufficient to explain positive effects of exercise intensity on cognitive functioning (Soga et al., 2015). This study employed a short-term high intensity and all-out exercise model. Following this anerobic exercise, 2-Back test was administered and its results showed a non-significant enhancement in cognitive scores. The different effects of anerobic and erobic exercise on cognitive scores could cause the insignificant differences in test results despite the increase in brain oxygenation. Also the variation in cognitive tests that administered could lead such insignificant results. Finally, the administration time of post-exercise tests could affect the cognitive scores. Soga et al. (2015) reported that there is no clear information in literature about cool-down periods following exercise and administration time of cognitive test. In addition, they (Soga et al., 2015) underlined the importance of assessing both time and heart rate variables post-exercise before administering the cognitive tests for future studies.

In the related literature, it has been suggested that the increment in PFC oxygenation has a positive effect on PFC functions which uses erobic exercise (Endo et al., 2013). Our study has no statistically significant behavioral results to demonstrate such positive effects on PFC functioning. Though the current study used anerobic exercise model, the results (hemodynamic responses) are in line with the studies which consists erobic exercise model (Ando et al., 2011; Endo et al., 2013; Byun et al., 2014). The obtained changes in oxygenation levels are compatible with results of previous studies. But no statistical differences were found in cognitive performance parameters, which were positively affected by erobic exercise. The major dividing line between the erobic and anerobic exercise are the duration and intensity parameters. And these erobic definitions are mostly related to the body and muscle metabolism. As far as we know there is no certain study that has specifically displayed the dividing line between erobic and anerobic capacity in regard to brain only. This might be pointing to the fact that the relationship of the body metabolic capacity and the dynamic patterns might be different than of the brain's.

There are findings demonstrating that cognitive functions, especially following an intense exercise, could be impaired or not augmented. Soga et al. (2015) reported that exercise has different effects on working memory and inhibitory control components. In our study, despite the PFC oxygenation increment, no statistical differences were found between 2-Back test scores. The different effect mechanisms, exercise intensity, and administration time of cognitive tests could be the reason for this insignificancy. In future studies, with an experimental design employing both erobic and anerobic exercises, the hemodynamic and cognitive performance changes can be demonstrated.

Current study may have a considerable limitation. Heart rate may not recover linearly during post exercise (erobic or anerobic), it is likely that cerebral oxygenation, which is regulated by autonomic responses also change drastically from exhaustion to 1 min post recovery to 5 min post recovery. Therefore even though the oxygenation recordings were done post 5 min plus period we may have a bias in the aspect of fluctuations within the 5 min average periods.

CONCLUSION

In summary, acute supramaximal exercise increased the oxy-Hb, deoxy-Hb and total-Hb levels during post-exercise session of 2-Back test. This would indicate that the functions of PFC would increase after acute exercise but the comparison between pre- and post-exercise sessions of 2-Back test scores did not point out any significant improvement. These results could not reveal any cognitive performance augmentation despite the increased PFC oxygenation. As aforementioned in the discussion, such post-exercise oxygenation increase in PFC may not be only derived from cognitive performance. To clarify the basis and effects of oxygenation rise further studies is required with an experimental design, which consist the cognitive tasks in all three phases (pre-, during-, post-exercise).

HP group, who has higher PP, outperformed LP group by means of oxy-, deoxy-, and total-Hb changes. Such difference rise a question if the short-term brain oxygenation responses might be affected by physical performance. The current study could provide a methodological approach for human factor studies that would require combining of behavioral and objective methods (fNIRS, etc).

AUTHOR CONTRIBUTIONS

The study was planned by CSB, AO, and MO, with experimental design by CSB, CG, EUD, EG, CC. Data was collected and analyzed by CG, EUD, HO, CC. Work was drafted by EUD, CC, EG, and HO. Important intellectual support was given by

CSB, AO, MO, EG, and CG throughout the project. All authors prepared the manuscript and approved the final version of the manuscript.

FUNDING

This study was funded partly via Dokuz Eylul University, Department of Scientific Research Projects coded by 2012.KB.SAG.081 and 2014.KB.SAG.012.

ACKNOWLEDGMENTS

Authors would appreciate the research group of Dokuz Eylul University Human Factor Labs. Also authors would like to thank to all volunteers to their attendance to the study and to Ipek Ergonul for editing and commenting of manuscript. The authors would like to thank Dr. Pembe Keskinoglu for her contributions and comments to the statistical analyses.

REFERENCES

Aks, D. J. (1998). Influence of exercise on visual search: implications for mediating cognitive mechanisms. *Percept. Mot. Skills* 87, 771–783. doi: 10.2466/pms.1998.87.3.771

Albinet, C. T., Mandrick, K., Bernard, P. L., Perrey, S., and Blain, H. (2014). Improved cerebral oxygenation response and executive performance as a function of cardiorespiratory fitness in older women: a fNIRS study. *Front. Aging Neurosci.* 6:272. doi: 10.3389/fnagi.2014.00272

Ando, S., Kokubu, M., Yamada, Y., and Kimura, M. (2011). Does cerebral oxygenation affect cognitive function during exercise? *Eur. J. Appl. Physiol.* 111, 1973–1982. doi: 10.1007/s00421-011-1827-1

Arcelin, R., and Brisswalter, J. (1999). Performance stability in simultaneous tasks of pedalling and reaction time. *Percept. Mot. Skills* 88, 1193–1199. doi: 10.2466/pms.88.3.1193-1199

Ayaz, H., Izzetoglu, M., Bunce, S., Heiman-Patterson, T., and Onaral, B. (2007). "Detecting cognitive activity related hemodynamic signal for brain computer interface using functional near infrared spectroscopy," in *Neural Engineering, 2007. CNE '07. 3rd International IEEE/EMBS Conference on* (Kohala Coast, HI: IEEE), 342–345.

Ayaz, H., and Onaral, B. (2005). *Analytical Software and Stimulus-Presentation Platform to Utilize, Visualize and Analyze Near-Infrared Spectroscopy Measures.* Philadelphia, PA: Master's Degree thesis, Drexel University.

Ayaz, H., Onaral, B., Izzetoglu, K., Shewokis, P. A., McKendrick, R., and Parasuraman, R. (2013). Continuous monitoring of brain dynamics with functional near infrared spectroscopy as a tool for neuroergonomic research: empirical examples and a technological development. *Front. Hum. Neurosci.* 7:871. doi: 10.3389/fnhum.2013.00871

Ayaz, H., Shewokis, P. A., Bunce, S., Izzetoglu, K., Willems, B., and Onaral, B. (2012). Optical brain monitoring for operator training and mental workload assessment. *Neuroimage* 59, 36–47. doi: 10.1016/j.neuroimage.2011.06.023

Ayaz, H., Shewokis, P. A., Bunce, S., and Onaral, B. (2011). "An optical brain computer interface for environmental control," in *Engineering in Medicine and Biology Society, EMBC, 2011 Annual International Conference of the IEEE* (Boston, MA: IEEE), 6327–6330.

Bayazıt, O., Öniz, A., Hahn, C., Güntürkün, O., and Özgören, M. (2009). Dichotic listening revisited: trial-by-trial ERP analyses reveal intra- and interhemispheric differences. *Neuropsychologia* 47, 536–545. doi: 10.1016/j.neuropsychologia.2008.10.002

Brisswalter, J., Collardeau, M., and René, A. (2002). Effects of acute physical exercise characteristics on cognitive performance. *Sports Med.* 32, 555–566. doi: 10.2165/00007256-200232090-00002

Byun, K., Hyodo, K., Suwabe, K., Ochi, G., Sakairi, Y., Kato, M., et al. (2014). Positive effect of acute mild exercise on executive function via arousal-related prefrontal activations: an fNIRS study. *Neuroimage* 98, 336–345. doi: 10.1016/j.neuroimage.2014.04.067

Chang, Y. K., Labban, J. D., Gapin, J. I., and Etnier, J. L. (2012). The effects of acute exercise on cognitive performance: a meta-analysis. *Brain Res.* 1453, 87–101. doi: 10.1016/j.brainres.2012.02.068

Coles, K., and Tomporowski, P. D. (2008). Effects of acute exercise on executive processing, short-term and long-term memory. *J. Sports Sci.* 26, 333–344. doi: 10.1080/02640410701591417

Cope, M., and Delpy, D. T. (1988). System for long-term measurement of cerebral blood and tissue oxygenation on newborn infants by near infra-red transillumination. *Med. Biol. Eng. Comput.* 26, 289–294. doi: 10.1007/bf02447083

Davenport, M. H., Hogan, D. B., Eskes, G. A., Longman, R. S., and Poulin, M. J. (2012). Cerebrovascular reserve: the link between fitness and cognitive function? *Exerc. Sport Sci. Rev.* 1, 153–158. doi: 10.1097/JES.0b013e3182553430

Dietrich, A. (2003). Functional neuroanatomy of altered states of consciousness: the transient hypofrontality hypothesis. *Conscious. Cogn.* 12, 231–256. doi: 10.1016/s1053-8100(02)00046-6

Dotan, R., and Bar-Or, O. (1983). Load optimization for the Wingate Anaerobic test. *Eur. J. Appl. Physiol. Occup. Physiol.* 51, 409–417. doi: 10.1007/bf00429077

Drigny, J., Gremeaux, V., Dupuy, O., Gayda, M., Bherer, L., Juneau, M., et al. (2014). Effect of interval training on cognitive functioning and cerebral oxygenation in obese patients: a pilot study. *J. Rehabil. Med.* 46, 1050–1054. doi: 10.2340/16501977-1905

Dupuy, O., Gauthier, C. J., Fraser, S. A., Desjardins-Crèpeau, L., Desjardins, M., Mekary, S., et al. (2015). Higher levels of cardiovascular fitness are associated with better executive function and prefrontal oxygenation in younger and older women. *Front. Hum. Neurosci.* 9:66. doi: 10.3389/fnhum.2015.00066

Emery, C. F., Honn, V. J., Frid, D. J., Lebowitz, K. R., and Diaz, P. T. (2001). Acute effects of exercise on cognition in patients with chronic obstructive pulmonary disease. *Am. J. Respir. Crit. Care Med.* 164, 1624–1627. doi: 10.1164/ajrccm.164.9.2104137

Endo, K., Matsukawa, K., Liang, N., Nakatsuka, C., Tsuchimochi, H., Okamura, H., et al. (2013). Dynamic exercise improves cognitive function in association with increased prefrontal oxygenation. *J. Physiol. Sci.* 63, 287–298. doi: 10.1007/s12576-013-0267-6

Gateau, T., Durantin, G., Lancelot, F., Scannella, S., and Dehais, F. (2015). Real-time state estimation in a flight simulator using fNIRS. *PLoS One* 10:e0121279. doi: 10.1371/journal.pone.0121279

González-Alonso, J., Dalsgaard, M. K., Osada, T., Volianitis, S., Dawson, E. A., Yoshiga, C. C., et al. (2004). Brain and central haemodynamics and oxygenation during maximal exercise in humans: brain circulation and metabolism in exercise. *J. Physiol.* 557, 331–342. doi: 10.1113/jphysiol.2004.060574

Huppert, T. J., Diamond, S. G., Franceschini, M. A., and Boas, D. A. (2009). HomER: a review of time-series analysis methods for near-infrared spectroscopy of the brain. *Appl. Opt.* 48, D280–D298. doi: 10.1364/ao.48.00d280

Hyodo, K., Dan, I., Suwabe, K., Kyutoku, Y., Yamada, Y., Akahori, M., et al. (2012). Acute moderate exercise enhances compensatory brain activation in older adults. *Neurobiol. Aging* 33, 2621–2632. doi: 10.1016/j.neurobiolaging.2011.12.022

Jaeggi, S. M., Buschkuehl, M., Perrig, W. J., and Meier, B. (2010). The concurrent validity of the N-back task as a working memory measure. *Memory* 18, 394–412. doi: 10.1080/09658211003702171

Jonides, J., Schumacher, E. H., Smith, E. E., Lauber, E. J., Awh, E., Minoshima, S., et al. (1997). Verbal working memory load affects regional brain activation as measured by PET. *J. Cogn. Neurosci.* 9, 462–475. doi: 10.1162/jocn.1997.9.4.462

Jung, R., Moser, M., Baucsek, S., Dern, S., and Schneider, S. (2015). Activation patterns of different brain areas during incremental exercise measured by near-infrared spectroscopy. *Exp. Brain Res.* 233, 1175–1180. doi: 10.1007/s00221-015-4201-4

Khan, N. A., and Hillman, C. H. (2014). The relation of childhood physical activity and aerobic fitness to brain function and cognition: a review. *Pediatr. Exerc. Sci.* 26, 138–146. doi: 10.1123/pes.2013-0125

Lambourne, K., and Tomporowski, P. (2010). The effect of exercise-induced arousal on cognitive task performance: a meta-regression analysis. *Brain Res.* 1341, 12–24. doi: 10.1016/j.brainres.2010.03.091

Li, C., Gong, H., Zeng, S., and Luo, Q. (2005). "Verbal working memory load affects prefrontal cortices activation: evidence from a functional NIRS study in humans," in *Proceedings of SPIE - The International Society for Optical Engineering 5696*, San Jose, CA ed. V. V. Tuchin, 33–40.

Mandrick, K., Derosiere, G., Dray, G., Coulon, D., Micallef, J.-P., and Perrey, S. (2013). Prefrontal cortex activity during motor tasks with additional mental load requiring attentional demand: a near-infrared spectroscopy study. *Neurosci. Res.* 76, 156–162. doi: 10.1016/j.neures.2013.04.006

MATLAB and Statistics Toolbox. (2007). Natick, Massachusetts, United States: The MathWorks, Inc.

McDonald, J. H. (2009). *Handbook of Biological Statistics.* Baltimore: Sparky House Publishing.

McMorris, T., and Hale, B. J. (2012). Differential effects of differing intensities of acute exercise on speed and accuracy of cognition: a meta-analytical investigation. *Brain Cogn.* 80, 338–351. doi: 10.1016/j.bandc.2012.09.001

McMorris, T., Sproule, J., Turner, A., and Hale, B. J. (2011). Acute, intermediate intensity exercise and speed and accuracy in working memory tasks: a meta-analytical comparison of effects. *Physiol. Behav.* 102, 421–428. doi: 10.1016/j.physbeh.2010.12.007

Mehta, R. K., and Parasuraman, R. (2014). Effects of mental fatigue on the development of physical fatigue: a neuroergonomic approach. *Hum. Factors* 56, 645–656. doi: 10.1177/0018720813507279

Nybo, L., and Rasmussen, P. (2007). Inadequate cerebral oxygen delivery and central fatigue during strenuous exercise. *Exerc. Sport Sci. Rev.* 35, 110–118. doi: 10.1097/jes.0b013e3180a031ec

Ozgoren, M., Tetik, M., Izzetoglu, K., Oniz, A., and Onaral, B. (2012). "Effect of body position on NIRS based hemodynamic measures from prefrontal cortex," in *Advances in Brain Inspired Cognitive Systems Lecture Notes in Computer Science*, eds H. Zhang, A. Hussain, D. Liu and Z. Wang (Berlin, Heidelberg: Springer), 138–146.

Potter, D., and Keeling, D. (2005). Effects of moderate exercise and circadian rhythms on human memory. *J. Sport Exerc. Psychol.* 27, 117–125.

Rupp, T., and Perrey, S. (2008). Prefrontal cortex oxygenation and neuromuscular responses to exhaustive exercise. *Eur. J. Appl. Physiol.* 102, 153–163. doi: 10.1007/s00421-007-0595-4

Schmit, C., Davranche, K., Easthope, C. S., Colson, S. S., Brisswalter, J., and Radel, R. (2015). Pushing to the limits: the dynamics of cognitive control during exhausting exercise. *Neuropsychologia* 68, 71–81. doi: 10.1016/j.neuropsychologia.2015.01.006

Shibuya, K.-I., Tanaka, J., Kuboyama, N., and Ogaki, T. (2004). Cerebral oxygenation during intermittent supramaximal exercise. *Respir. Physiol. Neurobiol.* 140, 165–172. doi: 10.1016/j.resp.2003.11.004

Soga, K., Shishido, T., and Nagatomi, R. (2015). Executive function during and after acute moderate aerobic exercise in adolescents. *Psychol. Sport Exerc.* 16, 7–17. doi: 10.1016/j.psychsport.2014.08.010

Tam, N. D., and Zouridakis, G. (2014). Temporal decoupling of oxy- and deoxy-hemoglobin hemodynamic responses detected by functional near-infrared spectroscopy (fNIRS). *J. Biomed. Eng. Med. Imaging* 1, 18–28. doi: 10.14738/jbemi.12.146

Tomporowski, P. D. (2003). Effects of acute bouts of exercise on cognition. *Acta Psychol. (Amst)* 112, 297–324. doi: 10.1016/s0001-6918(02)00134-8

Varner, L. J., and Ellis, H. C. (1998). Cognitive activity and physiological arousal: processes that mediate mood-congruent memory. *Mem. Cognit.* 26, 939–950. doi: 10.3758/bf03201174

Weinstein, Y., Bediz, C., Dotan, R., and Falk, B. (1998). Reliability of peak-lactate, heart rate and plasma volume following the Wingate test. *Med. Sci. Sports Exerc.* 30, 1456–1460. doi: 10.1097/00005768-199809000-00017

2

Processing Functional Near Infrared Spectroscopy Signal with a Kalman Filter to Assess Working Memory during Simulated Flight

Gautier Durantin [1,2,3], Sébastien Scannella [1], Thibault Gateau [1], Arnaud Delorme [2,3] and Frédéric Dehais [1]*

[1] Département Conception et Conduite des Véhicules Aéronautiques et Spatiaux, Institut Supérieur de l'Aéronautique et de l'Espace (ISAE-Supaéro), Toulouse, France, [2] Centre de Recherche Cerveau et Cognition, Université Toulouse III - Paul Sabatier, Toulouse, France, [3] Centre National de la Recherche Scientifique, Centre de Recherche Cerveau et Cognition, Toulouse, France

***Correspondence:**
Gautier Durantin
gautier.durantin@isae.fr

Working memory (WM) is a key executive function for operating aircraft, especially when pilots have to recall series of air traffic control instructions. There is a need to implement tools to monitor WM as its limitation may jeopardize flight safety. An innovative way to address this issue is to adopt a Neuroergonomics approach that merges knowledge and methods from Human Factors, System Engineering, and Neuroscience. A challenge of great importance for Neuroergonomics is to implement efficient brain imaging techniques to measure the brain at work and to design Brain Computer Interfaces (BCI). We used functional near infrared spectroscopy as it has been already successfully tested to measure WM capacity in complex environment with air traffic controllers (ATC), pilots, or unmanned vehicle operators. However, the extraction of relevant features from the raw signal in ecological environment is still a critical issue due to the complexity of implementing real-time signal processing techniques without a priori knowledge. We proposed to implement the Kalman filtering approach, a signal processing technique that is efficient when the dynamics of the signal can be modeled. We based our approach on the Boynton model of hemodynamic response. We conducted a first experiment with nine participants involving a basic WM task to estimate the noise covariances of the Kalman filter. We then conducted a more ecological experiment in our flight simulator with 18 pilots who interacted with ATC instructions (two levels of difficulty). The data was processed with the same Kalman filter settings implemented in the first experiment. This filter was benchmarked with a classical pass-band IIR filter and a Moving Average Convergence Divergence (MACD) filter. Statistical analysis revealed that the Kalman filter was the most efficient to separate the two levels of load, by increasing the observed effect size in prefrontal areas involved in WM. In addition, the use of a Kalman filter increased the performance of the classification of WM levels based on brain signal. The results suggest that Kalman filter is a suitable approach for real-time improvement of near infrared spectroscopy signal in ecological situations and the development of BCI.

Keywords: fNIRS, Kalman filtering, Neuroergonomics, working memory, SVM

1. INTRODUCTION

The development of passive Brain Computer Interfaces (BCI) is a key topic of research in Neuroergonomics. In contrast with active ones, Passive BCI (Cutrell and Tan, 2008) allows the use of unintentionally produced brain activity to derive various cognitive states (Blankertz et al., 2010) such as excessive mental workload. Such states inference provides an interesting insight as they aim at dynamically adapting the nature of the human-system interactions to overcome cognitive limitations (Zander and Kothe, 2011; Brouwer et al., 2013). In the field of BCI design to enhance user performance, there is a growing interest for functional near infrared spectroscopy (fNIRS) based BCI (Coyle et al., 2004; Derosière et al., 2014; Strait et al., 2014). This brain imaging device uses near infrared light absorption properties to estimate local variations of cortical hemodynamics. It uses a modified Beer-Lambert law to link light transmittance through brain tissues to variations in local concentrations in oxygenated hemoglobin (HbO_2) and deoxygenated hemoglobin (HHb) (Villringer and Obrig, 2002). fNIRS has a good spatial resolution (around 1 cm^2) and interesting signal-to-noise ratio. Moreover, this technique has the advantage to be easy and fast to set over the participant's head with a short calibration process (Naseer and Hong, 2015). However, the processing of fNIRS signal faces a lack of methodological consensus and thus still represents a great challenge (Bashashati et al., 2007). The extraction of the relevant activity from brain signals requires complex techniques (van Erp et al., 2012), and most efficient ones often rely on long calibration times [e.g., in subspace artifact removal techniques (von Bünau et al., 2009), adaptive filtering (Zheng et al., 2002)]. The complexity of these methods limits their applicability for Neuroergonomics purpose, as the signal has to be useable in real-time.

Most BCI designs rely on classical linear bandpass filtering techniques such as Infinite Impulse Response (IIR) (Naseer and Hong, 2015), although current research focuses on the investigation of alternative signal processing techniques, such as the Moving Average Convergence Divergence (MACD) filter (Durantin et al., 2014b; Gateau et al., 2015). On this basis, the improvement of signal quality in real-world conditions as suggested in the Neuroergonomics approach, makes Kalman filtering an ideal candidate. This signal processing and estimation technique relies both on the measurements performed on a system and on a modeling of its dynamics to improve signal quality (Kalman, 1960). The use of a Kalman filter including a physiological model of brain function to improve signal usability has been previously applied to EEG (Georgiadis et al., 2005; Callan et al., 2015) or fMRI (Diamond et al., 2005). However, concerning fNIRS, this technique has been limited to the estimation of model parameters (Abdelnour and Huppert, 2009) or the correction of motion artifacts (Izzetoglu et al., 2010), therefore not requiring the use of a physiological model of hemodynamic response to stimulation.

One of the greatest challenges regarding Kalman filter design is the tuning of its parameters, i.e., to evaluate the level of measurement noise (R) affecting the signal and the state noise (Q) in the model (Diamond et al., 2005). The value of the ratio Q/R greatly influences the behavior of the Kalman filter. Indeed, a Kalman filter with a low value of Q/R will put confidence in the dynamical model, whereas a Kalman filter with a high value of Q/R will put confidence in the measurements. In practice, the value of this ratio often has to be chosen empirically (Abdelnour and Huppert, 2009; Callan et al., 2015), as there exists no efficient way to evaluate it. Consequently, the dynamics of the Kalman filter may not be adapted to the data needed to be improved. The challenge of this study was to design a Kalman filter suitable for fNIRS that includes a physiological model of hemodynamic response (Boynton et al., 1996). By applying this filter to fNIRS data collected during both controlled and ecological experiments, we also aimed at testing the improvements such a filter could bring to fNIRS signal toward the implementation of a passive BCI. To that end, we first designed a Kalman filter relying on a model of the hemodynamic response (Boynton et al., 1996) to improve signal quality. We then conducted a first experiment with a prefrontal fNIRS, involving a digit sequence memorization task used to measure Working Memory (WM) storage and update capacity. Provided that the development of a signal improvement technique usable in realistic operational settings was the objective of this study, this basic task was chosen as WM is a key executive function to operate complex systems (Causse et al., 2011). Data collected during the first experiment were used to select the value of the filter parameter Q/R using an optimization procedure. Finally, the improvement of the signal by the optimal Kalman filter was evaluated with formal classification during an ecological experiment which involved pilots performing a realistic WM task (i.e., recalling air traffic instructions) in a flight simulator.

2. KALMAN FILTER DESIGN

The functional model used to design the Kalman filter for fNIRS signal was inspired by the Hemodynamic Response Function (HRF) proposed by Boynton et al. (1996). This function is simple enough to be represented by a low order state-space model. This model assumes a third order impulsional response to stimulation, and has the following transfer function :

$$HRF(p) = \frac{\tau^3 e^{-\delta p}}{(p+\tau)^3} \tag{1}$$

As shown in Equation (1), the response shape depends on two parameters : δ represents the pure delay between stimulation and the start of HbO_2 increase ; τ influences the time-to-peak delay. Typical values that were chosen here were extracted from Boynton et al. (1996), and are $\delta = 2\,s$ and $\tau = 1.5\,s$. This choice leads to a time-to-peak delay from pulse stimulation of around $5\,s$ (Handwerker et al., 2004). Then, the Kalman filter principle requires the addition to the model of a state noise w (defined as the amount of noise affecting the model, i.e., the amount of errors in it) and of a measurement noise v (defined as the amount of noise affecting the measures). As shown on **Figure 1**, we chose to represent the state noise as a perturbation affecting the stimulus (i.e., the input of the model). This choice led us to consider that state noise represents a stimulus perception (or internalization) bias.

The perception bias perturbing the stimulus is noted b. In the nominal model, Kalman filter assumptions impose that $b = w$, where w is the state noise following a gaussian centered distribution. This model, in addition to the choice of a Q/R value (where Q is the variance of the state noise, and R is the variance of the measurement noise), allowed us to design a *Kalman filter* for fNIRS signal improvement. The inputs of the Kalman filter were the stimuli onsets and the fNIRS raw signal.

One of the main limitations of this approach is the fact that the stimulus perception bias has to be centered (i.e., $b = 0$ on average), which can be erroneous when the subject sustainably disengages from the task and doesn't pay attention to the stimuli. To take this element into account, we built a second model, which is an augmentation of the nominal model, and in which $\dot{b} = w$. Thus, as the first derivative of b follows the gaussian centered distribution, it is still possible to design a Kalman filter, without assuming that b is null on average. This augmented model, along with the value of Q/R, allowed the computation of the *augmented Kalman filter* for fNIRS signal processing. For both filters, the value of the ratio Q/R was fixed according to an optimization process (see next section).

3. FIRST STEP : SETTING THE FILTER PARAMETERS

3.1. Material and Methods

Nine healthy participants from the Institut Superieur de l'Aeronautique et de l'Espace (ISAE ; Mean age = 21.6; $SD = 1.5$; eight males, eight right handed) participated in the experiment. The volunteers performed a computer-based digit sequence memorization task, while fNIRS measurements of the prefrontal cortex were recorded. Data were recorded using a Biopac® fNIR100 device, composed of 16 optodes placed on the forehead (see **Figure 2**). Each optode of the device records hemodynamics at a frequency of 2 Hz in term of oxygenated hemoglobin (HbO_2) and deoxygenated hemoglobin (HHb) level variations in comparison to a baseline.

Each trial of the experiment consisted in the memorization of a sequence of 5, 7, or 9 randomly chosen digits. The size of the sequence defined a level of difficulty. **Figure 3** summarizes the time sequence of a trial. During each trial, the subjects were asked to look at a fixation cross at the center of the screen. The digit sequence was presented through the loudspeakers of the computer using prerecorded audio tracks, at a rate of one digit per second. After the presentation of the last digit, the fixation cross was replaced by three crosses, indicating that the subjects had 8 *s* to type the memorized sequence on the keyboard. Between two consecutive trials, the subjects looked passively at the fixation cross at the center of the screen for 6 to 9 *s* (the inter-trial interval was chosen randomly to avoid task periodicity). The experiment consisted of 27 trials (nine trials for each of the three levels of difficulty), presented in a randomized order.

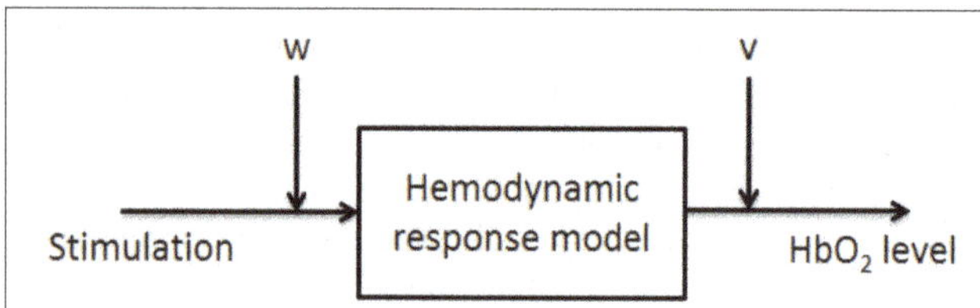

FIGURE 1 | Proposed approach for Kalman filtering of fNIRS. The state noise is considered as a perturbation of the input of the system.

3.2. Data Processing

Data were processed using Matlab®. Two different types of Kalman filters were applied to the data, the *nominal Kalman filter* (in which we assumed that the stimulus perception bias is null on average) and the *augmented Kalman filter* (without this assumption). The inputs for both filters were the stimuli onsets and the raw fNIRS data. For each filter, the value of the Q/R ratio chosen for the Kalman filter tuning ranged from 10^{-5} to 10^5, in order to look for the optimal results. Simultaneously, we also applied the MACD filter (Durantin et al., 2014b) to raw data in order to compare Kalman results with classical filtering.

For each trial, we computed the HbO_2 peak response (noted ΔHbO_2), i.e., the difference between the maximum value of HbO_2 in the 30 s following the trial onset and the value of HbO_2 at onset time. We similarly computed the HHb peak response (noted ΔHHb).

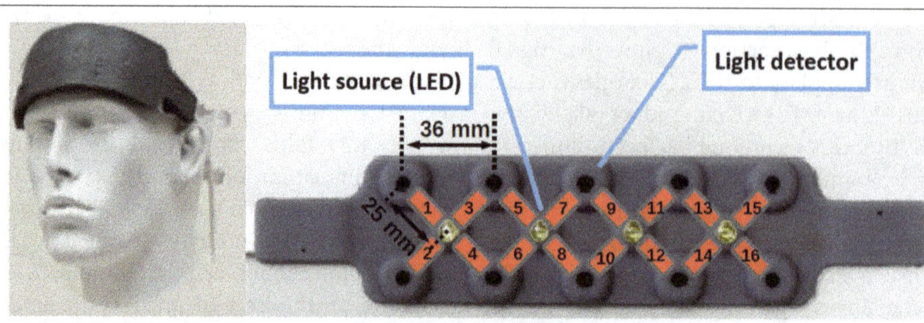

FIGURE 2 | fNIRS device optodes location. The device is composed of four light sources and 10 light detectors. The association of one light source and one light detector composes the optodes. The disposition of the sources and detectors leads to 16 optodes over the prefrontal cortex.

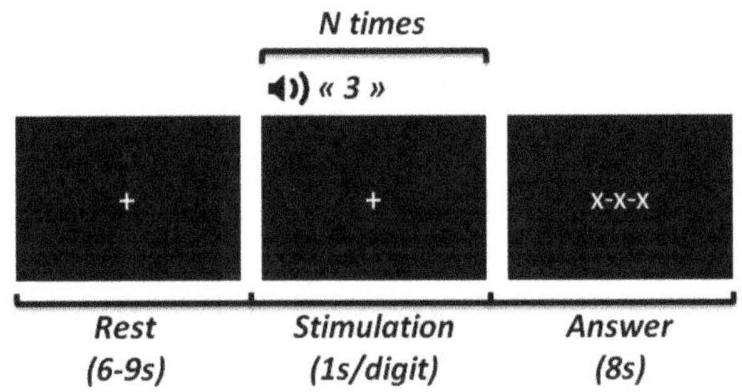

FIGURE 3 | Time course of one trial of the experiment. The experiment consisted of a total of 27 trials (three for each level of difficulty), presented in a random order. N = digit sequence size (5, 7, or 9).

Preliminary, the potential good values for Q/R (i.e., those leading to improvement in the signal) were isolated by computing an *Effect Size Index* (ESI, illustrated on **Figure 4**. For each filter (MACD, nominal Kalman or augmented Kalman with a given Q/R value) and each digit sequence size N, we computed the mean (μ_N) and standard deviation (σ_N) of the level of ΔHbO_2 or ΔHHb measured at each optode. We used these values to compute a confidence interval corresponding to one standard deviation as $[\mu_N - \sigma_N; \mu_N + \sigma_N]$. The *ESI* was defined as the gap between the confidence intervals of each condition (negative if the confidence intervals are overlapping), i.e.,

$$ESI = ((\mu_7 - \sigma_7) - (\mu_5 + \sigma_5)) + ((\mu_9 - \sigma_9) - (\mu_7 + \sigma_7))$$

We then proceeded to visual inspection to find the best values for Q/R ratio, by finding the parameters leading to higher ESI values. Each set of data was finally tested using a Two-way analysis of variance ANOVA, with two factors (16 optodes, three levels of difficulty), performed using STATISTICA® software. The strength of the statistical effect of the difficulty level, evaluated using the partial η^2, was used to compare the results of the different filters.

3.3. Results

As shown on **Figure 5**, the optimal results were obtained for HbO_2 at optode 2 recording mainly from the left inferior frontal gyrus, when using the nominal Kalman filter with $Q/R = 3.98$ or the augmented Kalman filter with $Q/R = 0.50$. **Table 1** summarizes the effect sizes obtained for each of the signal processing techniques tested (those effects showed an increase in the level of ΔHbO_2 with growing sequence sizes).

The frequency and phase responses (Bode diagram) of the nominal Kalman filter ($Q/R = 3.98$) and of the augmented Kalman filter ($Q/R = 0.50$) are given on **Figure 6**. As the two filters exhibit similar Bode diagrams (and therefore similar filtering properties), we retained only the augmented Kalman filter for testing on new data.

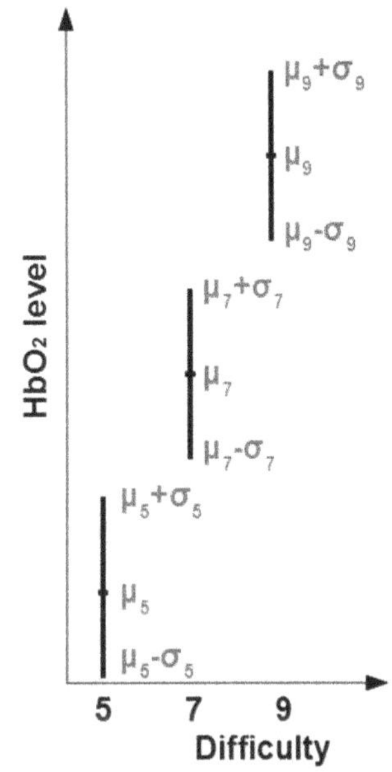

FIGURE 4 | Illustration of the computation of the Effect Size Index (ESI) for HbO_2. We computed the mean (μ) and standard deviation (σ) of the level of HbO_2 across subjects for each difficulty. For a difficulty N, a confidence interval corresponding to one standard deviation was computed as $[\mu_N - \sigma_N; \mu_N + \sigma_N]$. The corresponding ESI was computed as the sum of the gaps between the confidence intervals (negative if the confidence intervals are overlapping).

TABLE 1 | Effect sizes obtained for the effect of difficulty over all the subjects for the level of ΔHbO_2 measured at optode 2, depending on the type of filter used for signal processing.

Filter type	Q/R ratio	partial η^2
MACD		0.21
Nominal Kalman	3.98	0.32
Augmented Kalman	0.50	0.34

4. SECOND STEP : TESTING THE APPLICABILITY OF THE FILTER IN ECOLOGICAL CONDITIONS

4.1. Material and Methods

Data used for testing the Kalman filter were extracted from a second experiment involving a digit sequence memorization in a realistic flight simulator (see **Figure 7** for an illustration of the setup). The experiment was similar to Gateau et al. (2015), and included 18 healthy subjects (Mean age = 27.1; $SD = 6.4$; six women). Pilots heard prerecorded Air Traffic Controller (ATC) messages and were asked to dial the corresponding flight parameters in the Flight Control Unit (FCU) using the four knobs (i.e., speed, heading, altitude, and vertical speed knobs) of the FCU. The ATC messages were delivered at 78 dB SPL trough a Sennheiser® headset. We defined two levels of difficulty depending on the complexity of the message:

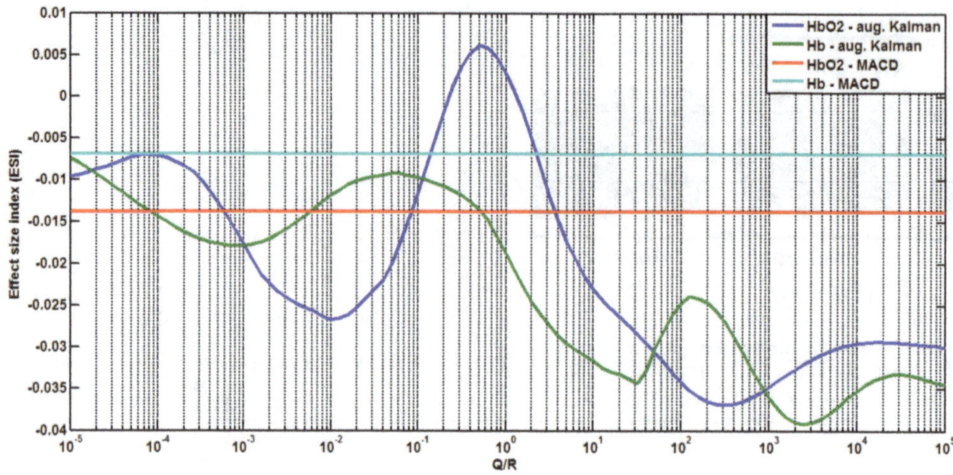

FIGURE 5 | Estimated Effect Size Index (ESI) for the augmented Kalman filter (for *HHb* –in green– and HbO_2 –in dark blue–) in function of the value of Q/R, compared to the ESI of the MACD filter (in red for HbO_2, in light blue for *HHb*). The index is estimated using the data from optode 2.

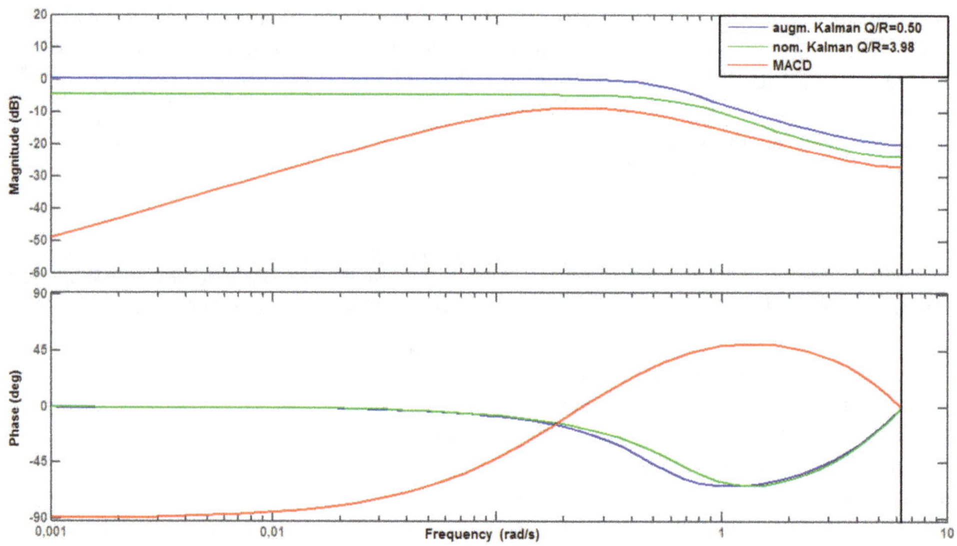

FIGURE 6 | Bode diagrams (frequency response, phase response) of the MACD filter, the nominal, and augmented Kalman filters.

- Low Load trial difficulty: only one major value per trial was used to set each flight parameter (e.g., 15 for "speed 150, heading 150, altitude 1500, vertical speed +1500").
- High Load trial difficulty: each flight parameter value was different from the previous one and composed of different digits to maximize the complexity (e.g., "speed 164, heading 235, altitude 8700, vertical speed −1600").

The task consisted in 20 repetitions of each difficulty for a total of 40 trials. Each ATC message started with the airplane call sign (i.e., "Supaero 32"), followed by the sequence of flight parameters. It ended with the message "over." The subjects were instructed to set the parameters strictly only after they heard the "over" message. A practice session was conducted for each subject before the actual experiments to allow them to become familiar with the experiment and the interface. After each message, the pilots had 18 seconds to enter the flight parameters. Trials were separated by 11 to 13 s of rest. During the experiment, hemodynamics of the prefrontal cortex were recorded using the same device than in the first experiment.

4.2. Data Processing and Classification

The raw HbO_2 data measured at each optode were filtered using three types of filter. First, we used the MACD filter and the augmented Kalman filter retained from the optimization phase ($Q/R = 0.50$). We also used a classical IIR Butterworth bandpass filter (0.02 Hz $< f < 0.1$ Hz), in order to compare the results to classical filtering. The statistical effect sizes of the level of ΔHbO_2 (computed in the same way than in the first experiment)

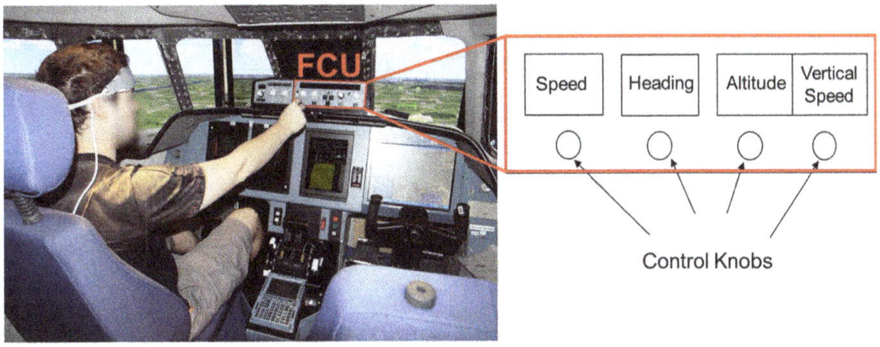

FIGURE 7 | Pilot's interaction with the auto flight system. The participants controlled the aircraft simulator of ISAE from the left seat. The red rectangle corresponds to the FCU (Flight Control Unit) dedicated to set the autopilot using the four control knobs, accordingly to ATC (Air Traffic Control) clearances (speed, heading, altitude, and vertical speed selection). Adapted from Gateau et al. (2015).

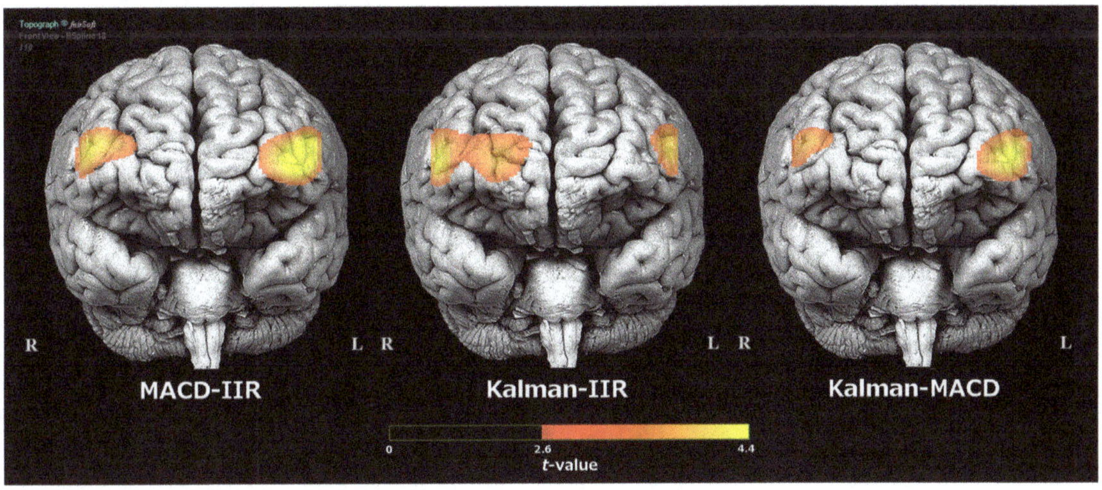

FIGURE 8 | Comparison of the *t*-maps for the contrast *High load - Low load* on the level of *HbO_2* over the prefrontal cortex obtained in function of the type of filter used for signal processing (classical IIR, MACD, or Kalman). The topographical view was extracted from fNIRSoft® and the threshold was fixed at the statistical significance level with $\alpha = 0.01$, to account for multiple comparisons.

were evaluated using repeated measures ANOVA performed with STATISTICA®. The performance of the different filters were compared in terms of partial η^2. In addition, we computed the statistical t-maps representing the differences in the contrasts between high and low load conditions in terms of level of HbO_2 for each type of filters. This computation was done using Matlab and plotted using the topograph tool from fNIRSoft®.

The improvement of the signal depending on the type of filter used for processing was also evaluated by performing formal classification on the data. This analysis was performed using the Statistics and Machine Learning toolbox from Matlab. The ΔHbO_2 values extracted from each optode were used to train and test a Linear Support Vector Machine (SVM) classifier through a 10-fold cross validation process : for each subject, data from all trials were randomly divided in 10. The difficulty (high or low load) of the trials of each 10% of data was predicted by a SVM classifier that was previously trained on the 90% remaining data. The predicted labels were then examined to evaluate the *Accuracy* (probability of good classification), *Sensitivity* (probability of good classification for high load trials), and *Specificity* (probability of good classification for low load trials) of the classifier.

4.3. Results

The partial η^2 obtained for each type of filters are given in **Table 2** (for each optode and across all the optodes). The results show that the use of MACD elicits a better statistical effect size than the classical IIR filter. Similarly, the use of Kalman filter yields better results than both MACD and IIR filters. This result is true not only when filtering data from optode 2, but present notably at all optodes located in the bilateral dorsolateral areas of the prefrontal cortex (optodes 1, 2, 3, 4 and 13, 14 ,15, 16).

The effect of trial difficulty on the level of HbO_2 measured over the prefrontal cortex is shown on **Figure 8**. On this figure, we observe that both the MACD and Kalman filter over classical IIR

TABLE 2 | Effect sizes (partial η^2) obtained for the effect of difficulty over all the subjects for the level of HbO_2 measured for each optodes (plus main effect size over all optodes), depending on the type of filter used for signal processing.

Optode number	1	2	3	4	5	6	7	8	
IIR	0.34	0.36	**0.48**	0.35	0.15	0.32	0.32	0.00	
MACD	**0.51**	**0.44**	**0.50**	**0.53**	0.24	0.26	0.15	0.01	
Augmented Kalman ($Q/R = 0.50$)	**0.64**	**0.55**	**0.57**	**0.55**	0.38	0.36	0.39	0.15	
Optode number	**9**	**10**	**11**	**12**	**13**	**14**	**15**	**16**	**All**
IIR	0.29	0.26	0.32	0.11	**0.41**	0.34	0.33	0.30	0.36
MACD	0.15	0.01	0.31	0.12	**0.50**	0.25	0.39	0.38	0.33
Augmented Kalman ($Q/R = 0.50$)	**0.42**	0.35	**0.53**	0.39	**0.55**	**0.55**	**0.52**	**0.49**	**0.52**

The effect sizes corresponding to a significant effect ($p < 0.05$) after correction for multiple comparisons are reported in bold font.

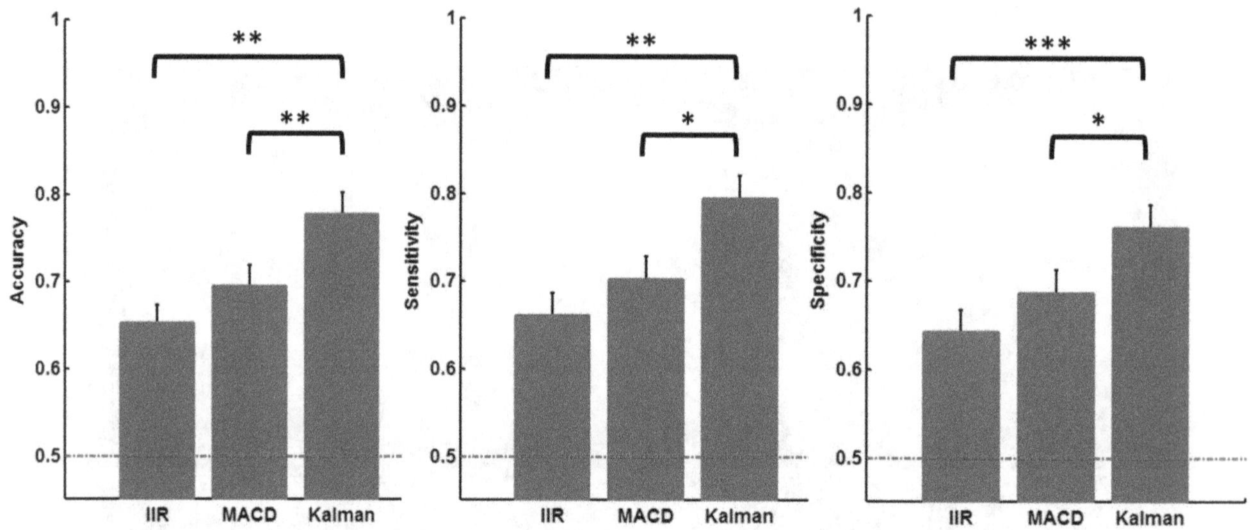

FIGURE 9 | Accuracy, sensitivity, and specificity obtained from the 10-fold cross-validation procedure for each type of filter. The dashed red line represents chance level (50%). The error bars represent the standard error of the mean across subjects, and statistical significance after correction for multiple comparisons is indicated by stars (*$p < 0.05$; **$p < 0.01$; ***$p < 0.001$).

filter improve the discriminability between the two conditions in the lateral areas of the prefrontal cortex.

Ultimately, the cross-validation procedure performed on the data to classify low-load vs. high-load trials are presented in **Figure 9** in terms of accuracy, sensitivity, and specificity. The classification results were all significantly better than chance, although Kalman filter led to statistically better results than IIR and MACD filters. Using Kalman filtering, the classification accuracy reached 77.8%, with a sensitivity of 79.4% and a specificity of 76%.

5. DISCUSSION

The objective of the study was to design a Kalman filter to improve fNIRS signal for Neuroergonomics applications. In particular, the main challenge concerned the tuning of the parameters Q and R (Diamond et al., 2005), representing the state noise and measurement noise variances. Based on a simple model of the hemodynamic response to neuronal stimulation (Boynton et al., 1996), we designed a Kalman filter model taking into account both the measurement noise and the stimulus perception bias that can occur in periods of disengagement or when the level of attention varies. During an optimization process, we showed that it was possible to find values for the parameters which leads to better statistical results ($Q/R = 0.50$) with an augmented model. Interestingly, the relatively low value of the Q/R ratio in the second model suggests that the Kalman filter put more confidence in the dynamical model of hemodynamics response than in fNIRS data. The higher optimal value obtained for this ratio when using the first choice of model ($Q/R = 3.98$) suggests this model was less consistent with the actual hemodynamics characteristics.

We applied the optimal results found in the first experiment on new data from an ecological experiment in a flight simulator, and showed that the optimal Kalman filter tuning could be applied generically. This filter led to higher effect sizes when looking at the effect of task difficulty in both tasks, compared to classical filters (see **Figure 8**). It is argued that the use of a dynamical physiological model by the Kalman filter implies less variability across trials and subjects, therefore explaining the greater stability of the results obtained with this filter. These results suggest that this filter would be suitable to improve the discriminability between the two conditions toward the implementation of a BCI to assist the operator, and would support the use of Kalman filtering to improve fNIRS signal (Izzetoglu et al., 2010). In particular, the Kalman filter helped us perform better during the SVM-based classification procedure between low-load and high-load trials, which confirms its contribution to the improvement of the signal. In addition, the experiment also confirmed that the MACD filter brings good results compared to classical IIR filtering, as it was previously demonstrated (Durantin et al., 2014b; Gateau et al., 2015). Although the discriminability obtained with this filter is not as good as the one obtained with the Kalman filter, it presents the advantage of not requiring any information on the stimulus onsets.

Interestingly, the optimal results for the first experiment were found at optode 2 recording mainly from the left inferior frontal gyrus. More generally, when applying the optimal Kalman filter in the second experiment, the WM solicitation elicited an activation of bilateral areas in the inferior and middle frontal gyri, part of the dorsolateral prefrontal cortex (see **Figure 8** and **Table 2**). This result is in agreement with previous fNIRS studies that have found these regions are sensitive to WM solicitation (Ayaz et al., 2012; Durantin et al., 2014a). Therefore, the improvement of the fNIRS signal collected in this region suggests that this filter could be applied to any experiment recruiting the same functional areas. In particular, the optimization process carried in this study would avoid the need of a calibration phase or of a convergence phase (in case of adaptive filtering) to improve signal quality. However, further investigation is still needed to assess whether this filter could be used with the same model and tuning in experiments recruiting different brain areas. Similarly, further investigation is also needed to assess the usability of these filters in ecological conditions that would differ from a simulated flight (e.g., with higher levels of light variations or motion artifacts).

Nevertheless, some modifications of the model could lead to better usability and performance of the Kalman filter. For instance, the use of a stimulus onset detection technique such as the detection technique based on the MACD filter (Durantin et al., 2014b; Gateau et al., 2015) could replace the stimulus onsets input of the Kalman filter, therefore reducing the complexity of the filter. In addition, it would be interesting to compare the results of the current Kalman model relying on a simple modeling of the hemodynamic response to more complex physiological models (e.g., Buxton et al., 2004). Finally, using an adaptive Q/R gain or realizing an optimization process for each subject instead of using a generic filter could also yield better results, although it would add complexity and a calibration phase to the procedure.

Altogether, the promising results of the study stand in favor of the use of Kalman filtering as a signal improvement technique for fNIRS signals with applications in Neuroergonomics. In particular, the improved signal would be available in real-time and without a calibration phase, and would allow better classification of WM levels in ecological settings.

AUTHOR CONTRIBUTIONS

All the authors contributed to the experiment design, results discussion, and paper redaction. Data collection was made by GD, TG, and SS. Signal processing tools (Kalman filter, MACD), were developed by GD.

ACKNOWLEDGMENTS

This research was supported by the Midi-Pyrénées region and Pôle de Recherche et d'Enseignement Supérieur (Neurocockpit project), and the AXA research fund (Neuroergonomics for flight safety). The work was approved by the Inserm Committee of Ethics Evaluation (Comité d'Évaluation Éthique de l'Inserm - CEEI/IRB00003888).

REFERENCES

Abdelnour, A. F., and Huppert, T. (2009). Real-time imaging of human brain function by near-infrared spectroscopy using an adaptive general linear model. *Neuroimage* 46, 133–143. doi: 10.1016/j.neuroimage.2009.01.033

Ayaz, H., Shewokis, P. A., Bunce, S., Izzetoglu, K., Willems, B., and Onaral, B. (2012). Optical brain monitoring for operator training and mental workload assessment. *Neuroimage* 59, 36–47. doi: 10.1016/j.neuroimage.2011.06.023

Bashashati, A., Fatourechi, M., Ward, R. K., and Birch, G. E. (2007). A survey of signal processing algorithms in brain–computer interfaces based on electrical brain signals. *J. Neural Eng.* 4, R32. doi: 10.1088/1741-2560/4/2/R03

Blankertz, B., Tangermann, M., Vidaurre, C., Fazli, S., Sannelli, C., Haufe, S., et al. (2010). The berlin brain–computer interface: non-medical uses of bci technology. *Front. Neurosci.* 4:198. doi: 10.3389/fnins.2010.00198

Boynton, G. M., Engel, S. A., Glover, G. H., and Heeger, D. J. (1996). Linear systems analysis of functional magnetic resonance imaging in human v1. *J. Neurosci.* 16, 4207–4221.

Brouwer, A.-M., van Erp, J., Heylen, D., Jensen, O., and Poel, M. (2013). "Effortless passive BCIs for healthy users," in *Universal Access in Human-Computer Interaction. Design Methods, Tools, and Interaction Techniques for eInclusion*, eds C. Stephanidis and M. Antona (Berlin: Springer), 615–622.

Buxton, R. B., Uludağ, K., Dubowitz, D. J., and Liu, T. T. (2004). Modeling the hemodynamic response to brain activation. *Neuroimage* 23, S220–S233. doi: 10.1016/j.neuroimage.2004.07.013

Callan, D. E., Durantin, G., and Terzibas, C. (2015). Classification of single-trial auditory events using dry-wireless eeg during real and motion simulated flight. *Front. Syst. Neurosci.* 9:11. doi: 10.3389/fnsys.2015.00011

Causse, M., Dehais, F., and Pastor, J. (2011). Executive functions and pilot characteristics predict flight simulator performance in general aviation pilots. *Int. J. Aviat. Psychol.* 21, 217–234. doi: 10.1080/10508414.2011.582441

Coyle, S., Ward, T., Markham, C., and McDarby, G. (2004). On the suitability of near-infrared (nir) systems for next-generation brain–computer interfaces. *Physiol. Meas.* 25, 815. doi: 10.1088/0967-3334/25/4/003

Cutrell, E., and Tan, D. (2008). "Bci for passive input in hci," in *Proceedings of CHI*, Vol. 8 (Florence: Citeseer), 1–3.

Derosière, G., Dalhoumi, S., Perrey, S., Dray, G., and Ward, T. (2014). Towards a near infrared spectroscopy-based estimation of operator attentional state. *PLoS ONE* 9:e92045. doi: 10.1371/journal.pone.0092045

Diamond, S. G., Huppert, T. J., Kolehmainen, V., Franceschini, M. A., Kaipio, J. P., Arridge, S. R., et al. (2005). "Physiological system identification with the Kalman filter in diffuse optical tomography," in *Medical Image Computing and Computer-Assisted Intervention–MICCAI 2005*, eds J. S. Duncan and G. Gerig (Charlestown, MA: Springer), 649–656.

Durantin, G., Gagnon, J.-F., Tremblay, S., and Dehais, F. (2014a). Using near infrared spectroscopy and heart rate variability to detect mental overload. *Behav. Brain Res.* 259, 16–23. doi: 10.1016/j.bbr.2013.10.042

Durantin, G., Scannella, S., Gateau, T., Delorme, A., and Dehais, F. (2014b). "Moving average convergence divergence filter preprocessing for real-time event-related peak activity onset detection: application to fnirs signals," in *Engineering in Medicine and Biology Society, 2014. EMBS 2014. 36th Annual International Conference of the IEEE* (Chicago, IL: IEEE).

Gateau, T., Durantin, G., Lancelot, F., Scannella, S., and Dehais, F. (2015). Real-time state estimation in a flight simulator using fnirs. *PLoS ONE* 10:e0121279. doi: 10.1371/journal.pone.0121279

Georgiadis, S. D., Ranta-aho, P. O., Tarvainen, M. P., and Karjalainen, P. A. (2005). Single-trial dynamical estimation of event-related potentials: a Kalman filter-based approach. *Biomed. Eng. IEEE Trans.* 52, 1397–1406. doi: 10.1109/TBME.2005.851506

Handwerker, D. A., Ollinger, J. M., and D'Esposito, M. (2004). Variation of bold hemodynamic responses across subjects and brain regions and their effects on statistical analyses. *Neuroimage* 21, 1639–1651. doi: 10.1016/j.neuroimage.2003.11.029

Izzetoglu, M., Chitrapu, P., Bunce, S., and Onaral, B. (2010). Motion artifact cancellation in nir spectroscopy using discrete Kalman filtering. *Biomed. Eng. Online* 9:16. doi: 10.1186/1475-925X-9-16

Kalman, R. E. (1960). A new approach to linear filtering and prediction problems. *J. Fluids Eng.* 82, 35–45. doi: 10.1115/1.3662552

Naseer, N., and Hong, K.-S. (2015). fnirs-based brain-computer interfaces: a review. *Front. Hum. Neurosci.* 9:3. doi: 10.3389/fnhum.2015.00003

Strait, M., and Scheutz, M. (2014). What we can and cannot do with near infrared spectroscopy. *Front. Neurosci.* 8:117. doi: 10.3389/fnins.2014.00117

van Erp, J. B. F., Lotte, F., and Tangermann, M. (2012). Brain-computer interfaces: beyond medical applications. *Computer* 45, 26–34. doi: 10.1109/MC.2012.107

Villringer, A., and Obrig, H. (2002). "Near-infrared spectroscopy and imaging," in *Brain Mapping; The Methods*, eds A. W. Toga and J. C. Mazziotta (San Diego, CA: Academic Press), 141–158. doi: 10.1016/B978-012693019-1/50008-3

von Bünau, P., Meinecke, F. C., Király, F. C., and Müller, K.-R. (2009). Finding stationary subspaces in multivariate time series. *Phys. Rev. Lett.* 103:214101. doi: 10.1103/PhysRevLett.103.214101

Zander, T. O., and Kothe, C. (2011). Towards passive brain–computer interfaces: applying brain–computer interface technology to human–machine systems in general. *J. Neural Eng.* 8:025005. doi: 10.1088/1741-2560/8/2/025005

Zheng, Y., Martindale, J., Johnston, D., Jones, M., Berwick, J., and Mayhew, J. (2002). A model of the hemodynamic response and oxygen delivery to brain. *Neuroimage* 16, 617–637. doi: 10.1006/nimg.2002.1078

3

Benefits of Instructed Responding in Manual Assembly Tasks: An ERP Approach

Pavle Mijović[1], Vanja Ković[2], Maarten De Vos[3], Ivan Mačužić[1], Branislav Jeremić[1] and Ivan Gligorijević[1]*

[1] *Department for Production Engineering, Faculty of Engineering, University of Kragujevac, Kragujevac, Serbia,* [2] *Laboratory for Neurocognition and Applied Cognition, Department for Psychology, Faculty of Philosophy, University of Belgrade, Belgrade, Serbia,* [3] *Department of Engineering, The Institute of Biomedical Engineering, University of Oxford, Oxford, UK*

***Correspondence:**
Pavle Mijović
p.mijovic@kg.ac.rs

The majority of neuroergonomics studies are focused mainly on investigating the interaction between operators and automated systems. Far less attention has been dedicated to the investigation of brain processes in more traditional workplaces, such as manual assembly, which are still ubiquitous in industry. The present study investigates whether assembly workers' attention can be enhanced if they are instructed with which hand to initiate the assembly operation, as opposed to the case when they can commence the operation with whichever hand they prefer. For this aim, we replicated a specific workplace, where 17 participants in the study simulated a manual assembly operation of the rubber hoses that are used in vehicle hydraulic brake systems, while wearing wireless electroencephalography (EEG). The specific EEG feature of interest for this study was the P300 components' amplitude of the event-related potential (ERP), as it has previously been shown that it is positively related to human attention. The behavioral attention-related modality of reaction times (RTs) was also recorded. Participants were presented with two distinct tasks during the simulated operation, which were counterbalanced across participants. In the first task, digits were used as indicators for the operation initiation (Numbers task), where participants could freely choose with which hand they would commence the action upon seeing the digit. In the second task, participants were presented with arrows, which served as instructed operation initiators (Arrows task), and they were instructed to start each operation with the hand that corresponded to the arrow direction. The results of this study showed that the P300 amplitude was significantly higher in the instructed condition. Interestingly, the RTs did not differ across any task conditions. This, together with the other findings of this study, suggests that attention levels can be increased using instructed responses without compromising work performance or operators' well-being, paving the way for future applications in manual assembly task design.

Keywords: neuroergonomics, wireless electroencepholagraphy, event-related potentials, P300, attention, manual assembly

INTRODUCTION

The importance of studying the human brain processes while executing everyday complex tasks in naturalistic environments was pinpointed by Parasuraman (2003), through a new direction in human factors and ergonomics (HF/E) research. This novel direction was tentatively named neuroergonomics (Parasuraman, 2003; Parasuraman and Rizzo, 2006; Parasuraman, 2011). Although Parasuraman and Wilson (2008) modestly stated that neuroergonomics should not be thought of as revolutionary, but rather as another step in HFE research, the growing body of neuroergonomics research refutes this statement. In fact, ever advancing technology has facilitated neuroergonomics research and only 12 years from its inception it has become one of the principal directions in HFE research. Ultimately, understanding brain processes in naturalistic environments can lead to improvement of existing industrial processes design and to creation of safer and more efficient working conditions (Parasuraman, 2003), consequently improving the operators' overall well-being.

Neuroergonomics has had significant success in evaluating brain activity in its interaction with automated systems, through the studies of mental workload, dual-task performance (Ayaz et al., 2013) and operators' vigilance (Warm and Parasuraman, 2006; Warm et al., 2009). Additionally, it has gone a step further with the development of state-of-the-art neuroadaptive systems facilitating the mutual interaction between an automated system and operators, in the sense that both human and the system can initiate a change in the level of automation when needed (Scerbo, 2006; Mehta and Parasuraman, 2013). On the one hand, this trend is understandable as industry, over several decades, has tried to reach the "lights-out manufacturing" concept (Tompkins et al., 2010), i.e., completely automated factories which can operate without the direct presence of human operators in the production processes. In that case, human supervisory control of automated systems becomes essential (Sheridan and Parasuraman, 2005), as human operators would be solely responsible for controlling the automated production systems (Warm et al., 2008). On the other hand, although automation is becoming ubiquitous in industry and everyday life (Parasuraman and Wilson, 2008), the "lights-out" concept is still rather futuristic and there is still a need for human manual operations in production processes. This is especially notable in assembly tasks and processes where costs related to process automation are generally not justifiable (Tang et al., 2003).

For these reasons, it is evident that neuroergonomics studies should pay additional attention to more traditional workplaces, through investigation of concurrent physical and cognitive work. This approach has received far less attention in neuroergonomic studies (for review see Mehta and Parasuraman, 2013). For example, in the car manufacturing industries the majority of processes are automated, however human operators play a crucial role in the final car cockpit and interior assembly, i.e., final assembly (Michalos et al., 2010). Typically, manual assembly tasks require a large number of repetitions and are monotonous in nature, thus leading to hypo-vigilance of operators (Spath et al., 2012). In turn, operators have difficulty in sustaining the desired level of attention during the task, and therefore, the risk of work-related injuries, material damage or even accidents is increased (Kletz, 2001). Therefore, employing existing neuroimaging techniques to understand the way the brain processes various stimuli in this class of tasks could be beneficial, as the task design could be optimized in such a way as to obtain and maintain sufficient operator attention, thereby avoiding possibly hazardous situations.

An extensive review of neuroimaging techniques applicable to neuroergonomics research has been recently published by Mehta and Parasuraman (2013). Although functional near infrared spectroscopy (fNIRS) presents a convenient technique for the neuroergonomics research in naturalistic setting due to its light weight and portability (Ayaz et al., 2010, 2012; Mehta and Parasuraman, 2013), it suffers from low temporal resolution and its use in dynamic everyday environments is still somewhat limited (Gramann et al., 2011). On the other hand, Electroencephalography (EEG) and therefrom derived event related potentials (ERPs) belong to the neuroimaging techniques that directly measure brain activity (Gramann et al., 2011; Mehta and Parasuraman, 2013) and both EEG and ERPs possesses high temporal resolution (down to the order of milliseconds) making them suitable for real-time investigation of brain dynamics in complex environments (Gramann et al., 2011). Even though Parasuraman (1990) proposed the introduction of ERPs in ergonomics research, until recently the traditional EEG recording suffered from long wiring between the electrode cap and amplifier unit, which engenders the artifacts that degrades signal quality (Debener et al., 2012). Additionally, EEG recordings usually required shielded, dimly lit and sound attenuated rooms, which was one of the main precondition for its recording, thus limiting its use in naturalistic environments (Gramann et al., 2011). However, these problems were recently overcome by the development of wearable EEG systems, empowering its use in everyday and applied settings (Debener et al., 2012; De Vos et al., 2014; Wascher et al., 2014; Mijović et al., 2016). Consequently, operators' brain dynamics can nowadays be successfully investigated with wearable EEG in faithfully replicated workplaces, by simulating the work activity (Wascher et al., 2014; Mijović et al., 2016). This can provide insight in how the brain responds to complex industrial tasks and these findings can contribute to more efficient task designs.

The aim of this article is the investigation of assemblers' mental states, by utilizing ERPs in a realistically replicated workplace. Neuroergonomics implies that overt performance measurements are unreliable (Parasuraman, 2003), since they do not provide the possibility for timely investigation of the underlying covert cognitive processes during everyday tasks. To get better insights into the temporal course of the underlying attention processes engaged in manual assembly operation, we selected two tasks in which we triggered goal-directed actions of workers by presenting them with either digits (in one) or arrows (in the other task) prior to initiating the operation. In this way we wanted to elicit the P300 ERP component (also called P3 or P3b), which is represented by the positive ERP voltage deflection that usually appears between 300 and 500 ms after appearance of the task-relevant stimuli (Polich and Kok, 1995; Verleger et al., 2005). The P300 component is often used to identify the depth of cognitive information processing and its amplitude and latency are considered to be related to the human attention level (Johnson, 1988; Polich, 2007; De Vos et al., 2014).

The P300 complex is the most prominent over the midline scalp sites (Polich, 2007) and it is among the most prominent ERP components (Verleger et al., 2014), making it one of the most studied components of human ERP. However, there is still a lack of consensus regarding what brain functions the P300 component represents (the arguments are briefly summarized in Verleger et al., 2014). One influential view is that the P300 component can be explained through the context updating hypothesis that was proposed by Donchin (1981) and which governs that the P3 reflects the updating of working memory that is related to task-relevant and unexpected events. The context updating theory assumes that the mental process that elicit the P3 component reflects a revision of the model of the environment rather than serving to organize a response to the eliciting stimulus (Verleger et al., 2005). In other words, it is assumed that following an initial sensory processing, an attention-related process evaluates the presentation of the previous event in working memory and if a new stimulus in a train of standard stimuli is detected, the attention-related process updates, which is followed by production of the P300 component (Polich, 2007). However, we have also witnessed arguments against the context updating theory (Verleger et al., 2005, 2014). In fact, Verleger et al. (2005) proposed a new hypothesis in which they argued that the P300 component is related both to stimuli processing and organizing the response. In order to prove this hypothesis, Verleger et al. (2005) compared the P3 amplitude in stimulus- and response-locked ERPs and they found that both P3 amplitudes were comparable. Therefore, it was confirmed that P300 amplitude does not reflect just the simple reaction to stimulus change. Rather, P300 reflects a process that mediates between perceptual analysis and response (Verleger et al., 2005), i.e., it is related to the organization of the response and it depends on the stimulus-response links (Verleger et al., 2014).

Based on these findings, the present study investigated whether and how the neural correlates of goal-directed actions would differ if the operators were requested to initiate the simulated assembly operation spontaneously (upon seeing a digit), as opposed to the condition where participants were instructed with which hand to commence the operation (upon seeing an arrow). In the spontaneous condition (the Numbers task), we adopted the stimuli from the original SART paradigm that is a simple "go/no-go" task, which consists of consecutively presenting digits from "1" to "9" and participants are required to give a speedy response on all stimuli, with the exception of digit "3" (Robertson et al., 1997). The main difference between the original SART and the Numbers paradigm (used in our study) is that the digits in Numbers are randomized. Further, in the original SART paradigm it is requested that participants provide the speedy response with the index finger upon the stimulus presentation. However, this would impede the simulation of the real working operation, since it would require an additional, task-unrelated operation from participants. Instead, in the Numbers paradigm, participants were instructed to initiate the assembly operation as soon as the visual (target) stimulus appeared on the screen, with whichever hand they felt more comfortable (the assembly operation is explained in detail in Section "Simulated Assembly Operation"). For the instructed responding (the Arrows) task, we adopted the stimuli and procedures from Donkers and van Boxtel (2004). The Arrows task is essentially a choice reaction task, where the arrows pointing to the left and right appear on the screen; white arrows represent the target ("go") condition, while red arrows represent the "no-go" stimulus. The main difference between the Numbers and Arrows tasks was that in the Numbers task participants could freely choose the hand with which they would initiate the assembly operation, while in the Arrows task, participants were instructed to commence each operation with the hand that corresponds to the direction in which the white arrow on the screen was pointing. An important notion is that not only the simple stimulus difference between the tasks was varied (digit vs. arrow), but also the informational value of those stimuli: the Arrows task arguably requires stimulus-response mapping, which in turn requires more cognitive evaluation, consequently inducing higher-level attentional processing than in the simple "go/no-go" task. In both the task specific and spontaneous condition, the visual stimuli (digits and arrows) appeared in the center of a screen that was placed in front of the participants.

We expected attention, when assessed through the P300 amplitude, to be more enhanced in the instructed responding (Arrows) task, compared to the one where participants could initiate the assembly operation upon seeing the task unspecific cue (Numbers task). Further, we wanted to investigate whether the difference in the task condition would also influence the reaction times (RTs), as the performance of the participants is also important, since this study simulates the naturalistic assembly task replicated from the industry. In other words, we wanted to investigate whether the participants would be slower in the case when they are instructed with which hand they should start the assembly operation, as compared to the condition when they can spontaneously initiate the assembly operation with whichever hand they prefer.

MATERIALS AND METHODS

Participants

Seventeen healthy subjects, from which one was left-handed, aged between 19 and 21 years volunteered as participants in the study. Due to abnormalities in the recording three subjects were excluded from further analysis, leaving a total of 14 participants. The study was restricted to male participants, both to exclude possible inter-gender differences and to replicate the selected job task more faithfully, since in the company that supported our research only males occupy the specific workplace under study.

Participants did not report any past or present neurological or psychiatric conditions and were free of medication and psychoactive substances. They were instructed not to take any alcoholic drinks prior to, nor on the day of, participation in the study. All participants had normal or corrected-to-normal vision. They agreed to participate in the study and signed informed consent after reading the experiment summary in accordance with the *Declaration of Helsinki*. The Ethical Committee of the University of Kragujevac approved the study and procedures for the participants.

Replication of the Workplace

As we stated in the introduction, reliable EEG recording still relies on wet electrodes, limiting on-site industrial EEG recording. For that reason, we simulated the production process of the rubber hoses, which are used in hydraulic brake systems in the automotive industry, in a faithfully replicated workplace (**Figure 1**). Full-scale replica of the specific workplace was created at the laboratory of University of Kragujevac, in consultation with the car sub-component manufacturing company. In order to create a naturalistic environment, all major elements from the real factory settings have been included while preserving respective spatial ratios and replicating ambient conditions.

The laboratory was air-conditioned and microclimate conditions controlled, keeping the ambient temperature at 24 ± 1°C while the measured relative air humidity value was between 40% and 60%. The luminance at the real workplace was also replicated from the industrial settings, using the same lighting and maintaining the luminance value at 810 lx. Finally, the noise trace was obtained by recording sounds in the vicinity of the original production facility, using cardiodid condenser microphone AT2020USB (Audio-technica, Japan), and this was replayed during the experiments with an SW-HF 5.1 6000 surround multimedia speaker (Genius, Taiwan). The ambient (light, noise) and microclimate (temperature, humidity) condition values were obtained using multifunctional environmental meter device PCE-EM882 (PCE instruments, UK).

The experimental setup used in this study was similar to previously reported studies (Mijović et al., 2015a,b, 2016), while the experimental task and procedure were modified. For clarity, we will repeat the detailed experimental setup here.

Simulated Assembly Operation

In the production process, an operator carries out a crimping operation in order to join a metal extension to a rubber hose. This

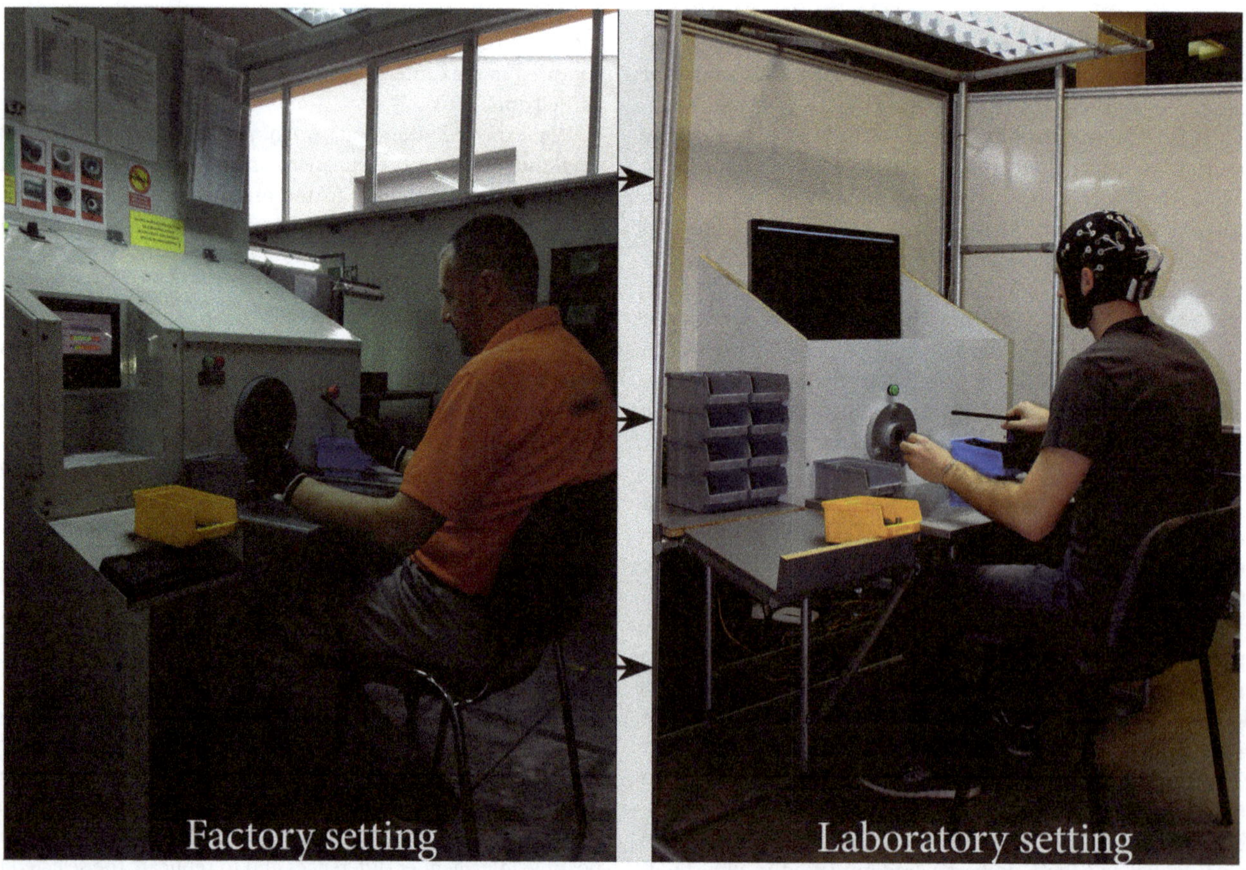

FIGURE 1 | Left image—Real workplace (replicated from our industrial partner); Right image—Replicated workplace.

single operation, carried out in a sitting position, consists of eight simple steps (actions). Step-by-step simulated operation, carried out by participants in the replicated working environment, is graphically presented in **Figure 2A** and explained in detail further in the text.

The major production steps can be summarized as follows (**Figure 2A**): first, the information to initiate the simulated assembly operation is presented to the participant, in the form of visual stimulus (step 1, explained in detail in Section "Experimental Procedure"), upon which he is instructed to instantly initiate the operation by taking the metal part (step 2) and the rubber hose (step 3). Following this, participants should place the metal part on the hose (step 4) and place both inside the crimping machine (step 5). Once the rubber hose and metal part are correctly placed inside the opening, the industrial green lamp lights and presents a visual cue to the participant, informing him that the part has been correctly placed. Participant then proceed by promptly pressing the pedal, which initiates the improvised machine and replicates the real machines' crimping sound with a duration of 3500 ms (step 6). The real crimping operation that would happen upon pressing the pedal was avoided, preserving its major aspects from operator's perspective—the sound it produces and the cessation of which indicates the end of machine operation, analogously to the real case. Upon completion of the simulated crimping process, the participant removes the component and places it in the box with completed parts (step 7). Finally, following these steps, the participant sits still, waiting for the subsequent stimulus (step 8) indicating the next-in-line operation.

Although the assembly task consists of eight sub-actions, the whole operation lasts less than 10 s and a single operator

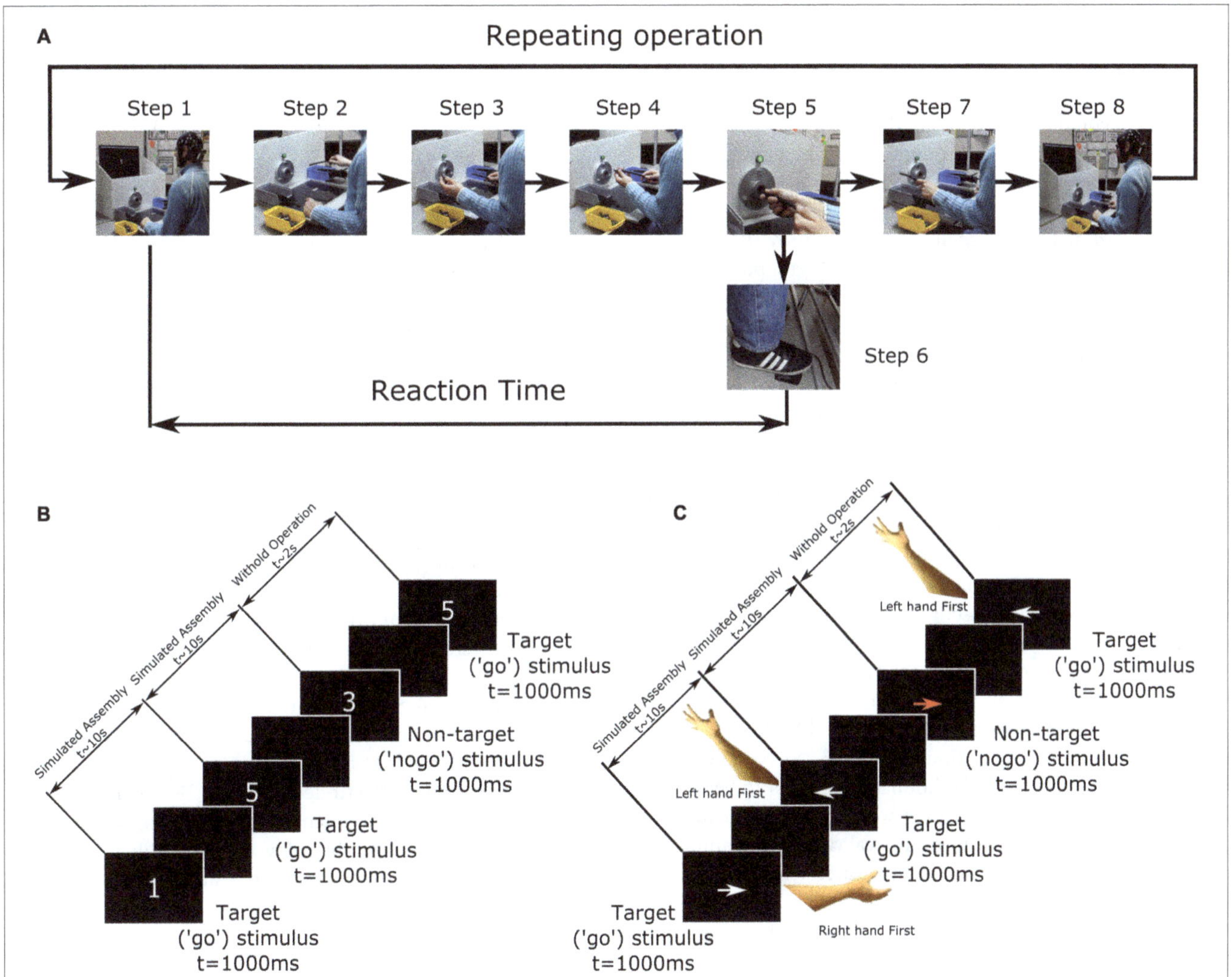

FIGURE 2 | (A) Step by step representation of the simulated working process. Step 1—Stimulus presentation; Step 2—Taking the rubber hose; Step 3—Taking the metal part; Step 4—Placing metal part on the rubber hose; Step 5—Insertion of the uncompleted part inside the improvised machine opening; Step 6—Pressing the pedal in order to initiate the simulated crimping operation; Step 7—Placing the completed into the box with completed parts; Step 8—Waiting for the successive stimulus presentation. **(B)** Graphical representation of the Numbers Task. **(C)** Graphical Representation of the Arrows task.

completes between 2500–3000 elements during a work shift. Hence, this workplace represents a typical example of a repetitive, monotonous operational task in industrial assembly settings.

Preparation

Each participant arrived to the laboratory at 9:00 a.m. Upon carefully reading the experiment summary and signing the informed consent for participation in the study, participants started the training session in order to gain familiarity with the task. Due to its simplicity, they were given 15 min for practicing, following which they confirmed their readiness to start the experiment. Finally, an EEG cap and amplifier were mounted on the participant's head (as explained in the Section "EEG Recording") and the recording started around 9:30 a.m.

Experimental Procedure

During the experiment, at least two experimenters were constantly present in the laboratory in order to assure that experimental procedures were strictly followed. The experimenters were seated behind an opaque board (so that participants could not see them during the task) and they observed the participants through a red-blue-green (RGB) camera that recorded the entire experiment.

Participants were seated in a comfortable chair in front of an improvised workplace including the improvised machine (**Figure 1**). In order to extract the ERP component from continuous EEG recording, a single functional modification in the simulated assembly task was made. Simultaneously with the simulated assembly process, the participants were subjected to either the Numbers (**Figure 2B**) or Arrows (**Figure 2C**) task to prompt initiation of the assembly operation. Both tasks were presented on the 24" screen from a distance of approximately 100 cm in a balanced order across participants (with a 15 min break between the tasks). The screen was height adjustable and the center of the screen was set to be level with participants' eyes. Upon presentation of the stimuli on the screen, the participants were instructed to complete the previously explained assembly operation (also graphically presented in **Figure 2A**).

All the stimuli were presented for 1000 ms on a black screen background. In both tasks the appearance of the stimuli was randomized, with the condition that forbade the two consecutive appearance of the "no-go" stimuli (digit "3" in Numbers, and red arrow in Arrows task). Additionally, in the Numbers tasks, five randomly allocated digit sizes were presented to increase the demands for processing the numerical value and to minimize the possibility that subjects would set a search template for some perceptual feature of the "no-go" trial (the digit "3"). Digit font sizes were 60, 80, 100, 120 and 140 in Arial text font (similar to Dockree et al., 2005). The main difference between the tasks is that in the Arrows tasks the participants were instructed to initiate the simulated operation with the right hand (step 2) if the white arrow was pointing to the right, or with the left hand (step 3) if pointing left (as depicted on **Figure 2C**), while in the Numbers task, the participants could freely choose between step 2 or step 3 (from the **Figure 2A**) upon seeing the digit. Each task consisted of 500 stimuli, where the probability of appearance of the "no-go" stimuli was set at 10% (50 in total), while the "go" stimuli were presented 450 times. The inter-stimulus interval (ISI) between two consecutive "go" stimuli was on average 11,240 ms (STD = 410 ms), while between "no-go" and following "go" stimuli the average ISI was 3210 ms (STD = 120 ms). The duration of the each task was around one and a half hours, upon which participants had a 15 min break, before starting the second task. Thus, the whole experiment lasted around 3 h and 15 min.

The task specifications were programmed in Simulation and Neuroscience Application Platform (SNAP)[1], developed by the Swartz Center for Computational Neuroscience (SCCN). As explained in Bigdely-Shamlo et al. (2013) and Gramann et al. (2014), SNAP is a python-based experiment control framework that is able to send markers as strings to Lab Streaming Layer (LSL)[2]. LSL is a real-time data collection and distribution system that allows multiple continuous data streams as well as discrete marker timestamps to be acquired simultaneously in an eXtensible Data Format (XDF)[3]. This data collection method provides synchronous, precise recording of multi-channel, multi-stream data that is heterogeneous in both type and sampling rate (Bigdely-Shamlo et al., 2013; Gramann et al., 2014), and is obtained via a local area network (LAN).

EEG Recording

EEG data acquisition was performed using the SMARTING (mBrainTrain, Serbia) wireless EEG system, with a sampling frequency of 500 Hz and 24-bit data resolution. The small and lightweight EEG amplifier (85 × 51 × 12 mm, 60gr) is tightly connected to a 24-channel electrode cap (Easycap, Germany) at the occipital site of the participant's head, using an elastic band. The connection between the EEG amplifier and recording computer was obtained using a Bluetooth connection, and the data were streamed to the described LSL recorder. The design of the cap-amplifier unit ensured minimal isolated movement of individual electrodes, cables, or the amplifier, which strongly reduced electromagnetic interference and movement artifacts. Further, the small dimensions of the recording system provided full mobility and comfort to the participants, as movement constraints were not imposed. The electrode cap contained sintered Ag/AgCl electrodes that were placed based on the international 10–20 System: Fp1, Fp2, Fz, F7, F8, FC1, FC2, Cz, C3, C4, T7, T8, CPz, CP1, CP2, CP5, CP6, TP9, TP10, Pz, P3, P4, O1 and O2. The electrodes were referenced to FCz and the ground electrode was AFz. Before initiation of the experiments, the experimental procedure imposed that the electrode impedances must be below the 5 kΩ value, which was confirmed by the device acquisition software.

ERP Processing

EEG signal processing was performed offline using EEGLAB (Delorme and Makeig, 2004) and MATLAB (Mathworks Inc.,

[1]https://github.com/sccn/SNAP
[2]https://code.google.com/p/labstreaminglayer/
[3]https://code.google.com/p/xdf/

Natick, MA, USA). EEG data were first bandpass filtered in the 1–35 Hz range, following which the signals were re-referenced to the average of the mastoid channels (Tp9 and Tp10). Further, an extended infomax Independent Component Analysis (ICA) was used to semi-automatically attenuate contributions from eye blink and (sometimes) muscle artifacts (as explained in Viola et al., 2009; De Vos et al., 2010, 2011). After this data preprocessing, ERP epochs were extracted from −200 to 800 ms with respect to timestamp values of "go" and "no-go" stimuli indicated by the SNAP software. Baseline values were corrected by subtracting mean values for the period from −200 to 0 ms from the stimuli. The identified electrode sites of interest for the ERP analysis in this study were Fz, Cz, CPz and Pz, as the P300 component is most prominent over the central and parieto-central scalp locations (Picton, 1992).

For the "no-go" condition we extracted and averaged the ERPs across the trials. For the "go" condition, the ERPs that preceded the "no-go" condition were calculated. Following these steps, the grand average (GA) ERPs across participants were formed. Further, the P300 amplitude was calculated for both "go" and "no-go" conditions and for each experimental condition, using mean amplitude measure (Luck, 2005) in the time window from 350 to 450 ms, with regard to the time stamps of the stimuli. Finally, the statistical analysis on the obtained results was carried out.

Reaction Times

As already stated in Section "Experimental Procedure", our experimental design did not allow subjects to react with the button press upon seeing the visual "go" stimulus. Therefore, the RT could not be measured in the traditional fashion, as the time elapsed between the stimulus presentation and the response by the participants (usually executed with the right index finger). Instead, the RTs here were measured as the time elapsed between the stimulus presentation (step 1) and the pedal press (step 6 from the Section "Preparation", also depicted on the **Figure 2A**). The pedal used in our study was actually a modified mouse button and it was connected to the recording computer via USB connection. As LSL is capable of real-time recording of the timestamps of the mouse button press, it enabled us to gather precise information regarding the time when pedal was pressed. This allows the calculation of RTs, as the difference between timestamps from stimulus presentation (operation initiation) and the beginning of the machine simulated crimping process.

Error Processing

Errors of omission were classified as the errors occurring when participants did not respond to the appearance of the "go" stimuli. The commission errors processing was challenging, since our task did not require a speeded button press and therefore, the errors of commission were difficult to interpret. In fact, the most obvious classification of commission errors would be when participants completely execute the simulated operation upon appearance of the "no-go" stimuli. However, it is important to note that participants sometimes made slight movements upon appearance of the "no-go" stimuli (in sense that they showed intention to initiate the action) and then they inhibited the response upon realization that it was a "no-go" stimulus. This kind of error we classified as near-misses. The identification of the near misses and commission errors was conducted initially by the experimenters in the room and subsequently confirmed in an off-line analysis, by replaying the videos recorded with the RGB camera during the experiment.

Statistical Analysis

The statistical analysis was performed using IBM SPSS software. The ERPs used for statistical analysis included all ERPs related to the "no-go" condition and 50 ERPs related to "go" preceding the "no-go" condition. The 4 × 2 × 2 × 2 repeated measures analysis of variance (ANOVA) was conducted with Site (Fz, Cz, CPz and Pz), Task (Arrows vs. Numbers) and Condition ("go/no-go") as within subject factors and Order of presentation (first vs. second) as between-subject factor. Additionally, a 2 × 2 ANOVA comparing RTs across Task (Arrows vs. Numbers) as within subject factors and Order of presentation (first vs. second) as between subject factor was conducted. Finally, we carried out a 2 × 2 ANOVA comparing near misses across Task (Arrows vs. Numbers) as within subject factors and Order of presentation (first vs. second) as between subject factor. Greenhouse-Geissser corrections (FG) were applied where necessary. Since the participants did not make any omission errors and only seven commission errors occurred across the participants they were exempted from further statistical analysis.

RESULTS

Behavioral Results

Reaction Times

The 2 × 2 ANOVA comparing RTs across Task (Arrow vs. SART) condition as within subject factor and Order of presentation (first vs. second) as between subject factor revealed neither significant main effects, nor interaction effects.

Errors

As stated in the "Materials and Methods" Section (Section "Statistical Analysis"), the participants did not make any omission errors and the low number of omission errors were not statistically analyzed. However, regarding near-misses, the ANOVA revealed only a significant effect of task ($F_{(1,8)} = 11.9$, $p < 0.01$, $\eta = 0.60$) with more near-misses occurring in the Numbers compared to the Arrows task.

ERP Results

The GA ERPs for each task (Arrows and Numbers), each condition ("go/no-go") and each electrode site under study (Fz, Cz, CPz and Pz) are depicted in **Figure 3**.

The 4 × 2 × 2 × 2 ANOVA revealed that the ERPs differed depending on the condition (Go/No-Go: $F_{(1,12)} = 5.99, p < 0.05$, $\eta = 0.33$), the task (Task: $F_{(1,12)} = 17.06$, $p < 0.001$, $\eta = 0.59$), the order of presentation (Order of presentation: $F_{(1,12)} = 15.635$, $p < 0.01$, $\eta = 0.57$) and across the scalp (Site: $F_{(1.48,17.75)} = 5.352$,

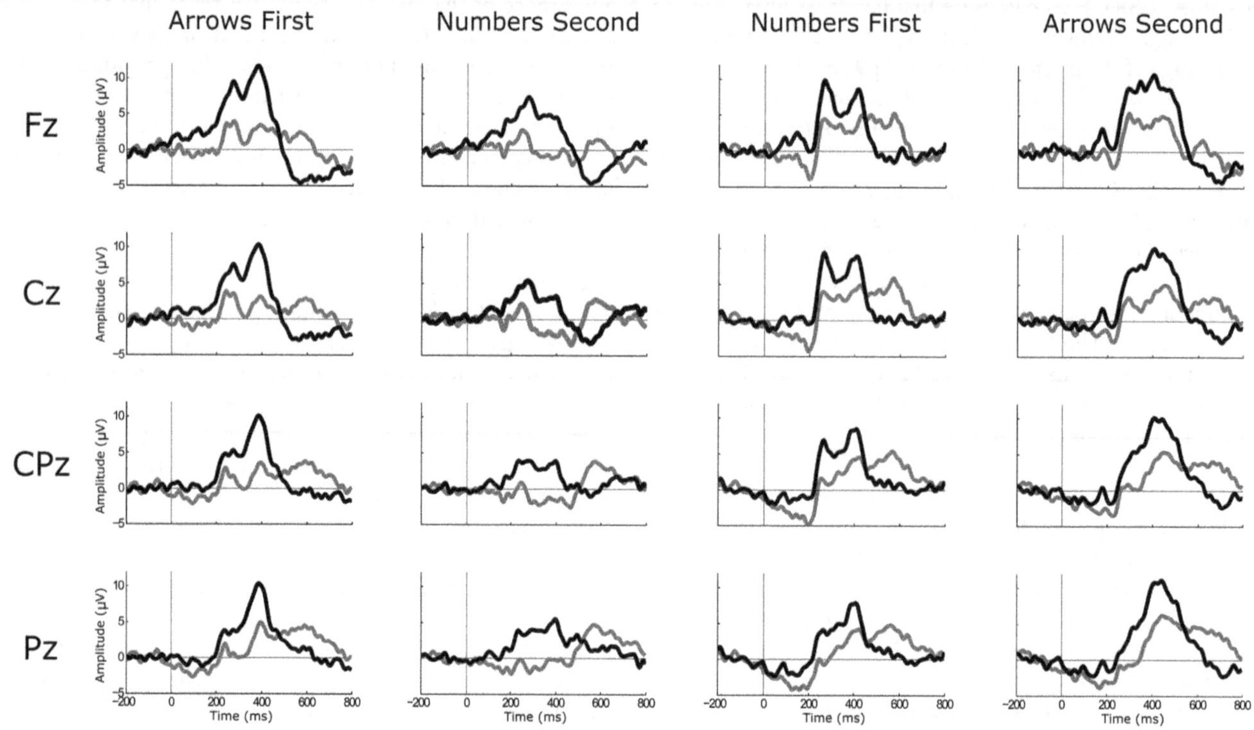

FIGURE 3 | Graphical representation of the grand average (GA) event-related potentials (ERPs) for each task and each electrode location under study. The black line represents the "go" condition, while the gray line depicts the GA ERPs for the "no-go" condition.

$p < 0.05$, $\eta = 0.31$). Namely, the P300 amplitudes elicited for "go" trials were higher than for "no-go" trials ($M = 5.73$, $SD = 1.47$; $M = 2.25$, $SD = 1.41$, respectively). Further, the Arrow task produced higher amplitudes in comparison to Numbers ($M = 5.24$, $SD = 1.11$; $M = 2.73$, $SD = 1.46$, respectively). The P300 amplitudes elicited with regard to the Order of presentation demonstrated higher amplitudes for whichever task was presented first in comparison to second task ($M = 5.11$, $SD = 1.31$; $M = 2.86$, $SD = 1.54$, respectively). Finally, amplitudes elicited at Pz were significantly higher than the amplitudes at the other three sites and amplitudes at CPz site were higher than at Cz and Fz sites at the $p < 0.05$ level. All the other comparisons were significant in the same direction apart from the Fz-Cz difference.

Figure 4 depicts the GA ERPs elicited over all four electrode sites under study for the "go" condition.

The P300 amplitude differences for all four sites and depending on the task representation order are presented in **Figure 5**.

DISCUSSION

The present study investigated whether operators' attention is enhanced when they are instructed with which hand to initiate the manual assembly operation, as compared to spontaneous and free choice of preferred hand. The attention was assessed through the P300 amplitude, as it is widely accepted that the P300 amplitude is positively related to the human level of attention (Ford et al., 1994; Polich, 2007; De Vos et al., 2014). For this aim we simulated a manual assembly operation, where we provided the participants with two distinct psychological tasks (Numbers and Arrows) simultaneously with the simulated operation.

The P300 components' amplitude was significantly higher in magnitude for the frequent "go" (target), than for the infrequent "no-go" condition (as presented on the **Figure 3**). This finding is in contrast to the majority of previously reported studies where an infrequent target condition elicits a higher magnitude of the P300 amplitude, since the participants are usually required to note the occurrence of infrequent targets by button press or by silent counting (Strüber and Polich, 2002). On the other hand, in our task target stimuli were the frequent ones, as the continuity of operation in manual assembly is essential, while the participants were instructed just to sit still and with no actions during the infrequent "no-go" condition. As such, it is not surprising that the lower magnitude of the P300 amplitude were elicited in infrequent non-target condition, as passive stimulus processing induces smaller P300 amplitudes than active tasks (Polich, 2007). This was also supported by the results from the study of Potts et al. (2004), where they reported that the P300 amplitude was larger in frequent "go" condition as compared to rare non-target condition in the task where the ratio between "go" and "no-go" condition was 80/20. Moreover, it was found that the ISI between target stimuli influences the P300 amplitude, in the sense that a short ISI leads to decreased amplitude, while relatively long ISIs elicit the

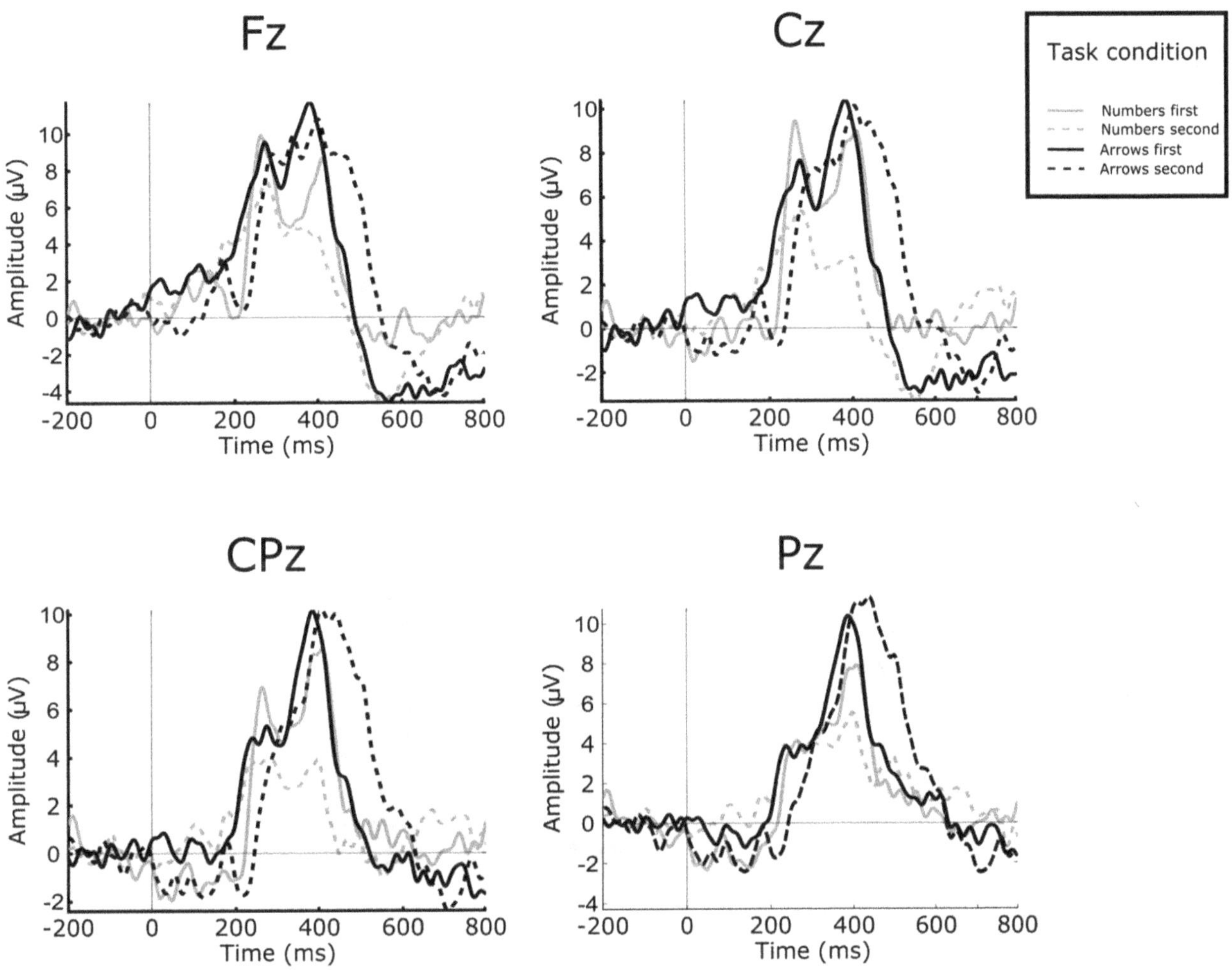

FIGURE 4 | The GA ERPs elicited for "go" condition in all four experimental conditions. ERPs elicited for The Numbers task are represented with the gray color, while the ERPs elicited in the Arrows task are depicted with the black color. The full line represents that the task was presented as a first task and the dashed line if the task was presented as second task.

higher P300 amplitude, which is the case even in the single-stimulus paradigm (Strüber and Polich, 2002; Polich, 2007). This was the case also in our study, since the ISI was relatively long (approximately 11 s) and we believe that it was suitable for eliciting the P300 amplitude even in the frequent target condition.

The main finding of the present study is that the P300 amplitude was considerably higher in magnitude when participants were instructed with which hand to initiate the simulated assembly operation, as compared to the case when participants could freely choose the preferred hand for the operation initiation. This may not be surprising, since in the choice reaction task (Arrows) participants were subjected to slightly higher demands of the incoming stimuli evaluation, as they were un-aware of the direction in which the white arrow stimuli would point. On the other hand, the digit stimulus carries considerably lower information, as participants are required just to make distinction whether it is a "go" or "no-go" stimulus and to perform their action accordingly, i.e., the participants may stop evaluating the content of the stimuli after some time. Therefore, the response selection requirements during the Arrows task are substantially higher than in Numbers task, which may lead to increased P300 amplitude in the condition which required instructed responding from the participants (Verleger et al., 2005, 2014). Following this finding, it may be proposed that the workers on repetitive and monotonous assembly tasks should not receive information solely on whether they should initiate the operation or not, but it should be beneficial if they receive information that carries slightly higher cognitive demands. In fact, the task that consisted of the stimuli with the higher cognitive demands induced the higher P300 amplitude, which may be related to the attention of the worker for the task in hand. An important notion, however, is that there is possibility that the P300 amplitude in this study does not reflect solely the attention level of a worker, but it also may be influenced by the different cognitive demands of the tasks. For that reason, it is important to further investigate whether the P300 amplitude was influenced by the presented

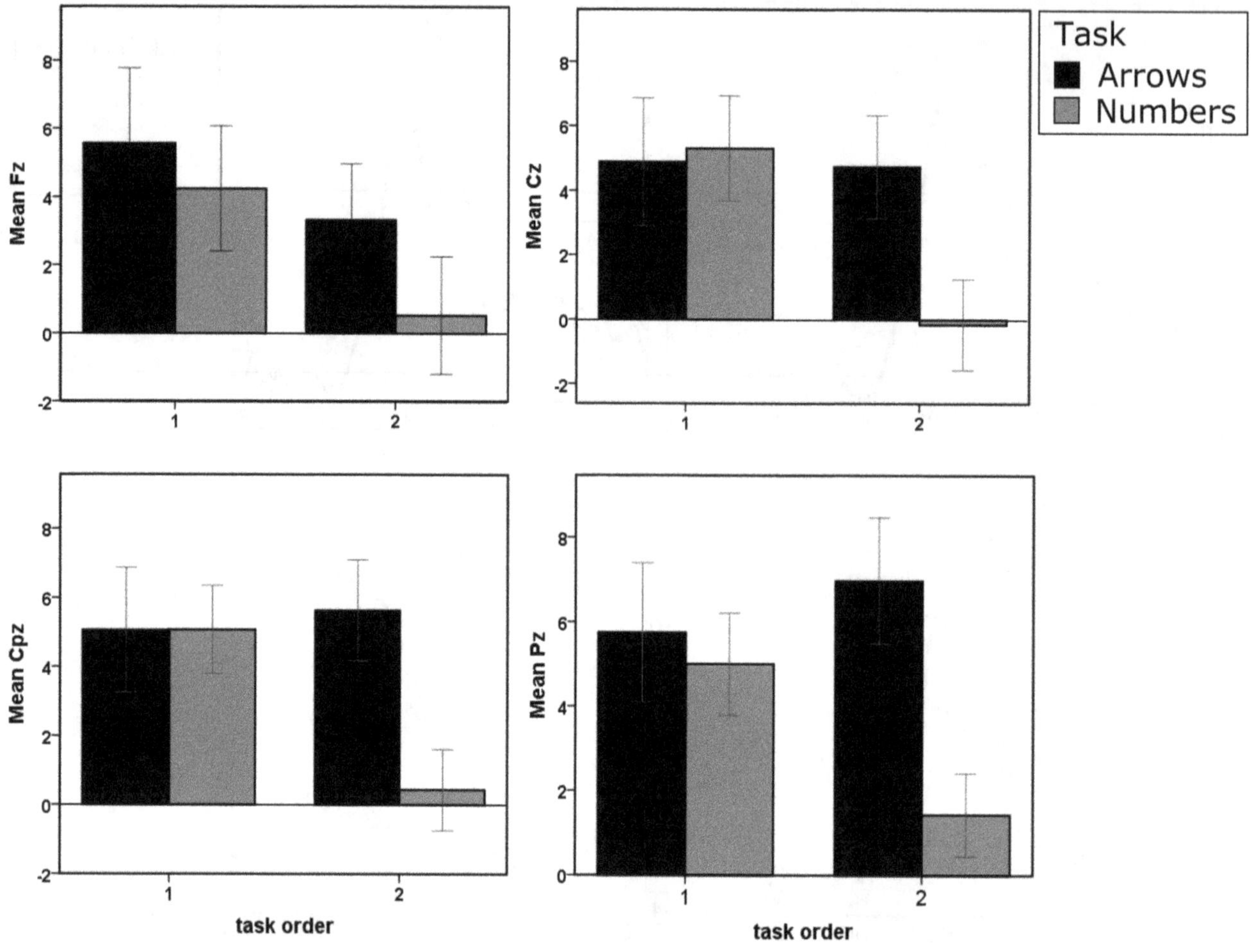

FIGURE 5 | The amplitude values for all four electrode sites and for all experimental conditions. The black color depicts the Arrows task, while the Numbers task is represented with the gray color. The error bars represents ±2 SE.

task demands, or it was solely related to the attention of the workers.

Interestingly, although it was expected that the RTs could differ between the two tasks, this was not the case in our study. One of the possible reasons for the absence of the response time effect could be the methodology used for the RTs calculation. In fact, the time period for RT calculation is much longer than in the conventional studies, where a speeded response from the participants is expected. Apart from that, the RT calculation includes several coordinated hand movements before the foot switch is pressed. All of these could induce a large variation within and between subject conditions, which may induce inaccuracy of the RT methodology used in this study. Further, with regard to behavioral measurements, the number of commission errors was relatively low and did not differ between the tasks. However, there was significantly higher amount of near-misses in the Numbers than in the Arrows task. The fact that there was larger number of near-misses in the Numbers task may be expected, as the Arrows task imposes a higher workload on the participants, due to the higher response selection requirements, and as it was previously reported, the errors and mental workload are related according to a U-shaped curve (Desmond and Hoyes, 1996).

Although we showed that the Arrows task produced a higher P300 amplitude than the Numbers task, one could argue about the selection of the tasks, as the stimulus type between task conditions significantly differed (digits vs. arrows). The main reason for not investigating the difference between instructed and non-instructed condition with the same type of stimuli was the avoidance of the interference effect (Pashler, 1994). In fact, if only stimuli from Numbers task were used and dedicated the directions to specific digits in the hand instructing task (e.g., odd numbers means left and even numbers right hand first), it would be highly likely that the memory would strongly influence the attention processing. On the other hand, if we only used the Arrows stimuli type, an undesired bias would be included in the condition when participants could initiate the operation with their preferred hand. An additional concern is whether the two distinct psychological tests trigger different attentional resources, given that they are composed of different stimulus types and that the Arrows task alternates the response hand, while in the Numbers task participants could respond with whichever hand they preferred. The answer to this doubt could be found in premotor theory of attention (Rizzolatti et al., 1994), which states that attention orienting processes are triggered during uni-manual response preparation and that the orienting processes are assumed to be equivalent to the processes elicited during instructed endogenous shifts of spatial attention (Eimer et al., 2005). Moreover, Ranzini et al. (2009) also used the tasks with Arabic digits and Arrows and they demonstrated that processes evoked by these cues are alike and that the volitional and non-volitional attentional shifts rely on the same fronto-parietal brain networks. Thus, both Numbers and Arrows tasks should evoke the same cognitive resources of attention, which gives legitimacy to the choice of the tasks used in this study.

One of the limitations of the present study is that it was conducted in a simulated working environment, instead of a real factory setting. The main reason for this was usage of the wet-electrode EEG recording system, which is still uncomfortable for application in actual industrial environments. Nevertheless, we replicated both the spatial dimensions and ambient conditions and performed the wearable EEG study, demonstrating its applicability for the investigation of covert cognitive processes in naturalistic environments for HF/E studies. Another limitation is that, simultaneously with the simulated operation, we used two distinct psychological tests, with the aim of eliciting the P300 ERP component. Although it could be argued that psychological tests could interfere with the simulated operation, an important notion is that the assembly workers should be provided with timely information regarding the performed operation (Stork and Schubö, 2010). Therefore, we believe that this modification did not significantly differ from the actual assembly operation in industrial environments. Moreover, in naturalistic settings it is usually hard to isolate and analyze the specific cognitive process, since they should first be evoked and co-occurring cognitive factors should be isolated (Bulling and Zander, 2014). Thus, this modification in the information presentation to the participants was necessary in order to elicit the anticipated P300 ERP component during the simulated assembly operation. Unfortunately, the present study is unable to compare brain responses between self-paced (as in this specific workplace) and externally paced work routines that we used in our study. This issue should be addressed in future studies.

The present study demonstrated that wearable EEG recording could be beneficial for task design in HF/E studies. Future studies should investigate whether the reported findings also hold for similar job positions, which are monotonous and repetitive in nature but require continuous focus of the worker on the industrial task (e.g., quality control tasks). Although the present study utilized wearable EEG in a faithfully replicated workplace environment, it seems that it is just a matter of time until EEG systems will be willingly accepted for everyday use (van Erp et al., 2012; Mihajlovic et al., 2015). This could even lead to the application of passive brain-computer interfaces, which could be used for real-time assessment of the cognitive user states in industrial environments (Zander and Kothe, 2011). Nevertheless, the fact that it is nowadays possible to investigate brain dynamics during natural movements (without imposing movements constraints) of the recorded individual brings us a step closer to the guiding principle of the neuroergonomics, that is, to investigate how the brain carries out the complex tasks of everyday life and not just simplified and artificial tasks in the laboratory settings (Parasuraman and Rizzo, 2006).

CONCLUSION

Comparing monotonous ("go/no-go") Numbers task to the choice-reaction (Arrows) task, which instructs the participants with which hand to commence the assembly operation, the present study indicates that the latter is more suitable to preserve participants' attention during the initiation of externally-paced assembly task. This finding was achieved through investigation of the ERP waveform, where it was found that the P300 amplitude, which is related to the level of attention, was enhanced in the task that instructed the participants with which hand to initiate the simulated assembly operation. This study demonstrated the potential benefits of introducing the EEG measurements in the industrial task design, as from the presented results it may be concluded that in in monotonous assembly tasks, instructed responding, or a similar method of engagement, should be imposed on operators, since it is indicated that additional engagement enhances the worker's attention.

AUTHOR CONTRIBUTIONS

Study design and protocols were created by PM, VK, MDeV, BJ, IM and IG. Data acquisition was performed by PM and IG. Data analysis was performed by PM, VK, MDeV, IM and IG. The data interpretation was performed by PM, VK, BJ, IM and IG. The manuscript was written by PM and VK and critical editing was performed by MDeV, BJ, IM and IG. Final approval of the version was obtained from all co-authors. All co-authors agree on all aspects of the work and ensure that questions related to the accuracy and integrity of any part of the submitted work are appropriately investigated and resolved.

ACKNOWLEDGMENTS

This research is financed under EU—FP7 Marie Curie Actions Initial Training Networks—FP7-PEOPLE-2011-ITN, project name "Innovation Through Human Factors in Risk Analysis and Management (InnHF)", project number: 289837. We would further like to acknowledge company "Gomma Line" (Serbia), for their assistance and advisory during the experimental setup phase. We would like to acknowledge Nora Balfe from Center for Innovative Human Systems (CIHS), Trinity College Dublin, Department for Psychology, for the critical comments of the manuscript.

REFERENCES

Ayaz, H., Onaral, B., Izzetoglu, K., Shewokis, P. A., McKendrick, R., and Parasuraman, R. (2013). Continuous monitoring of brain dynamics with functional near infrared spectroscopy as a tool for neuroergonomic research: empirical examples and a technological development. *Front. Hum. Neurosci.* 7:871. doi: 10.3389/fnhum.2013.00871

Ayaz, H., Shewokis, P. A., Bunce, S., Izzetoglu, K., Willems, B., and Onaral, B. (2012). Optical brain monitoring for operator training and mental workload assessment. *Neuroimage* 59, 36–47. doi: 10.1016/j.neuroimage.2011.06.023

Ayaz, H., Willems, B., Bunce, B., Shewokis, P. A., Izzetoglu, K., Hah, S., et al. (2010). "Cognitive workload assessment of air traffic controllers using optical brain imaging sensors," in *Advances in Understanding Human Performance: Neuroergonomics, Human Factors Design and Special Populations*, eds T. Marek, W. Karwowski, and V. Rice (Boca Raton, FL: CRC press), 21–31.

Bigdely-Shamlo, N., Kreutz-Delgado, K., Robbins, K., Miyakoshi, M., Westerfield, M., Bel-Bahar, T., et al. (2013). "Hierarchical event descriptor (HED) tags for analysis of event-related EEG studies," in *Global Conference on Signal and Information Processing (GlobalSIP)*, Austin, TX, 1–4.

Bulling, A., and Zander, T. O. (2014). Cognition-aware computing. *IEEE Perv. Comp.* 13, 80–83. doi: 10.1109/mprv.2014.42

De Vos, M., De Lathauwer, L., and Van Huffel, S. (2011). Spatially constrained ICA algorithm with an application in EEG processing. *Sign. Process.* 91, 1963–1972. doi: 10.1016/j.sigpro.2011.02.019

De Vos, M., Gandras, K., and Debener, S. (2014). Towards a truly mobile auditory brain-computer interface: exploring the P300 to take away. *Int. J. Psychophysiol.* 91, 46–53. doi: 10.1016/j.ijpsycho.2013.08.010

De Vos, M., Riès, S., Vanderperren, K., Vanrumste, B., Alario, F. X., van Huffel, S., et al. (2010). Removal of muscle artifacts from EEG recordings of spoken language production. *Neuroinformatics* 8, 135–150. doi: 10.1007/s12021-010-9071-0

Debener, S., Minow, F., Emkes, R., Gandras, K., and de Vos, M. (2012). How about taking a low-cost, small and wireless EEG for a walk? *Psychophysiology* 49, 1617–1621. doi: 10.1111/j.1469-8986.2012.01471.x

Delorme, A., and Makeig, S. (2004). EEGLAB: an open source toolbox for analysis of single-trial EEG dynamics including independent component analysis. *J. Neurosci. Methods* 134, 9–21. doi: 10.1016/j.jneumeth.2003.10.009

Desmond, P. A., and Hoyes, T. W. (1996). Workload variation, intrinsic risk and utility in a simulated air traffic control task: evidence for compensatory effects. *Saf. Sci.* 22, 87–101. doi: 10.1016/0925-7535(96)00008-2

Dockree, P. M., Kelly, S. P., Robertson, I. H., Reilly, R. B., and Foxe, J. J. (2005). Neurophysiological markers of alert responding during goal-directed behavior: a high-density electrical mapping study. *Neuroimage* 27, 587–601. doi: 10.1016/j.neuroimage.2005.05.044

Donchin, E. (1981). Surprise!... surprise? *Psychophysiology* 18, 493–513. doi: 10.1111/j.1469-8986.1981.tb01815.x

Donkers, F. C., and van Boxtel, G. J. (2004). The N2 in go/no-go tasks reflects conflict monitoring not response inhibition. *Brain Cogn.* 56, 165–176. doi: 10.1016/j.bandc.2004.04.005

Eimer, M., Forster, B., Van Velzen, J., and Prabhu, G. (2005). Covert manual response preparation triggers attentional shifts: ERP evidence for the premotor theory of attention. *Neuropsychologia* 43, 957–966. doi: 10.1016/j.neuropsychologia.2004.08.011

Ford, J. M., Sullivan, E. V., Marsh, L., White, P. M., Lim, K. O., and Pfefferbaum, A. (1994). The relationship between P300 amplitude and regional gray matter volumes depends upon the attentional system engaged. *Electroencephalogr. Clin. Neurophysiol.* 90, 214–228. doi: 10.1016/0013-4694(94)90093-0

Gramann, K., Ferris, D. P., Gwin, J., and Makeig, S. (2014). Imaging natural cognition in action. *Int. J. Psychophysiol.* 91, 22–29. doi: 10.1016/j.ijpsycho.2013.09.003

Gramann, K., Gwin, J. T., Ferris, D. P., Oie, K., Jung, T. P., Lin, C. T., et al. (2011). Cognition in action: imaging brain/body dynamics in mobile humans. *Rev. Neurosci.* 22, 593–608. doi: 10.1515/RNS.2011.047

Johnson, R. (1988). "The amplitude of the P300 component of the event-related potential: review and synthesis," in *Advances in Psychophysiology: A Research Annual*, (Vol. 3), eds P. Ackles, J. R. Jennings and M. G. H. Coles (Greenwich, CT.: JAI press), 69–137.

Kletz, T. A. (2001). *An Engineer's View of Human Error.* (Vol. 3), Rugby: Institution of Chemical Engineers.

Luck, S. J. (2005). *An Introduction to the Event-Related Potential Technique.* Cambridge, MA: MIT Press.

Mehta, R. K., and Parasuraman, R. (2013). Neuroergonomics: a review of applications to physical and cognitive work. *Front. Hum. Neurosci.* 7:889. doi: 10.3389/fnhum.2013.00889

Michalos, G., Makris, S., Papakostas, N., Mourtzis, D., and Chryssolouris, G. (2010). Automotive assembly technologies review: challenges and outlook for a flexible and adaptive approach. *CIRP J. Manuf. Sci. Tech.* 2, 81–91. doi: 10.1016/j.cirpj.2009.12.001

Mihajlovic, V., Grundlehner, B., Vullers, R., and Penders, J. (2015). Wearable, wireless EEG Solutions in daily life applications: what are we missing? *IEEE J. Biomed. Health Inform.* 19, 6–21. doi: 10.1109/jbhi.2014.2328317

Mijović, P., Ković, V., De Vos, M., Mačužić, I., Todorović, P., Jeremić, B., et al. (2016). Towards continuous and real-time attention monitoring at work: reaction times versus brain response. *Ergonomics* doi: 10.1080/00140139.2016.1142121 [Epub ahead of print].

Mijović, P., Ković, V., Mačužić, I., Jeremić, B., Todorović, P., Milovanović, M., et al. (2015a). "Do micro-breaks increase the attention level of an assembly worker? An ERP study," in *Proceedings of 6th International Conference of Applied Human Factors and Ergonomics (AHFE 2015)*, Las Vegas, NV.

Mijović, P., Milovanović, M., Minović, M., Mačužić, I., Ković, V., and Gligorijević, I. (2015b). "Towards creation of implicit HCI model for prediction and prevention of operators' error," in *Human-Computer Interaction: Interaction Technologies*, ed. M. Kurosu (Cham: Springer International Publishing), 341–352.

Parasuraman, R. (1990). "Event-related brain potentials and human factors research," in *Event-Related Brain Potentials: Basic Issues and Applications*, eds J. Rohbaugh, R. Parasuraman, and R. Johnson (New York, NY: Oxford University Press), 279–300.

Parasuraman, R. (2003). Neuroergonomics: research and practice. *Theor. Issues Ergon. Sci.* 4, 5–20. doi: 10.1080/14639220210199753

Parasuraman, R. (2011). Neuroergonomics brain, cognition and performance at work. *Curr. Dir. Psychol. Sci.* 20, 181–186. doi: 10.1177/0963721411409176

Parasuraman, R., and Rizzo, M. (Eds.) (2006). *Neuroergonomics: The Brain at Work.* New York, NY: Oxford University Press.

Parasuraman, R., and Wilson, G. F. (2008). Putting the brain to work: neuroergonomics past, present and future. *Hum. Factors* 50, 468–474. doi: 10.1518/001872008x288349

Pashler, H. (1994). Dual-task interference in simple tasks: data and theory. *Psych. Bull.* 116, 220–244. doi: 10.1037/0033-2909.116.2.220

Picton, T. W. (1992). The P300 wave of the human event-related potential. *J. Clin. Neurophysiol.* 9, 456–479. doi: 10.1097/00004691-199210000-00002

Polich, J. (2007). Updating P300: an integrative theory of P3a and P3b. *Clin. Neurophysiol.* 118, 2128–2148. doi: 10.1016/j.clinph.2007.04.019

Polich, J., and Kok, A. (1995). Cognitive and biological determinants of P300: an integrative review. *Biol. Psychol.* 41, 103–146. doi: 10.1016/0301-0511(95)05130-9

Potts, G. F., Patel, S. H., and Azzam, P. N. (2004). Impact of instructed relevance on the visual ERP. *Int. J. Psychophysiol.* 52, 197–209. doi: 10.1016/j.ijpsycho.2003.10.005

Ranzini, M., Dehaene, S., Piazza, M., and Hubbard, E. M. (2009). Neural mechanisms of attentional shifts due to irrelevant spatial and numerical cues. *Neuropsychologia* 47, 2615–2624. doi: 10.1016/j.neuropsychologia.2009.05.011

Rizzolatti, G., Riggio, L., and Sheliga, B. M. (1994). Space and selective attention. *Atten. Perform. XV* 15, 231–265.

Robertson, I. H., Manly, T., Andrade, J., Baddeley, B. T., and Yiend, J. (1997). Oops!': performance correlates of everyday attentional failures in traumatic brain injured and normal subjects. *Neuropsychologia* 35, 747–758. doi: 10.1016/s0028-3932(97)00015-8

Scerbo, M. (2006). "Adaptive automation," in *Neuroergonomics: The Brain at Work*, eds R. Parasuraman and M. Rizzo (New York, NY: Oxford University Press), 239–252.

Sheridan, T. B., and Parasuraman, R. (2005). Human-automation interaction. *Rev. Hum. Fact. Ergon.* 1, 89–129. doi: 10.1518/155723405783703082

Spath, D., Braun, M., and Meinken, K. (2012). "Human factors in manufacturing," in *Handbook of Human Factors and Ergonomics*, ed. G. Salvendy (New Jersey, NJ: John Wiley & Sons), 1643–1666.

Stork, S., and Schubö, A. (2010). Human cognition in manual assembly: theories and applications. *Adv. Eng. Inform.* 24, 320–328. doi: 10.1016/j.aei.2010.05.010

Strüber, D., and Polich, J. (2002). P300 and slow wave from oddball and single-stimulus visual tasks: inter-stimulus interval effects. *Int. J. Psychophysiol.* 45, 187–196. doi: 10.1016/s0167-8760(02)00071-5

Tang, A., Owen, C., Biocca, F., and Mou, W. (2003). "Comparative effectiveness of augmented reality in object assembly," in *Proceedings of the SIGCHI Conference on Human Factors in Computing Systems.* (New York, NY: ACM), 73–80.

Tompkins, J. A., White, J. A., Bozer, Y. A., and Tanchoco, J. M. A. (2010). *Facilities Planning.* New Jersey, NJ: John Wiley & Sons.

van Erp, J. B., Lotte, F., and Tangermann, M. (2012). Brain-computer interfaces: beyond medical applications. *IEEE Comput.* 45, 26–34. doi: 10.1109/mc.2012.107

Verleger, R., Baur, N., Metzner, M. F., and Śmigasiewicz, K. (2014). The hard oddball: effects of difficult response selection on stimulus-related P3 and on response-related negative potentials. *Psychophysiology* 51, 1089–1100. doi: 10.1111/psyp.12262

Verleger, R., Ja śkowski, P., and Wascher, E. (2005). Evidence for an integrative role of P3b in linking reaction to perception. *J. Psychophysiol.* 19, 165–181. doi: 10.1027/0269-8803.19.3.165

Viola, F. C., Thorne, J., Edmonds, B., Schneider, T., Eichele, T., and Debener, S. (2009). Semi-automatic identification of independent components representing EEG artifact. *Clin. Neurophysiol.* 120, 868–877. doi: 10.1016/j.clinph.2009.01.015

Warm, J. S., Matthews, G., and Parasuraman, R. (2009). Cerebral hemodynamics and vigilance performance. *Mil. Psych.* 21, S75–S100. doi: 10.1080/08995600802554706

Warm, J. S., and Parasuraman, R. (2006). "Cerebral hemodynamics and vigilance," in *Neuroergonomics: The Brain at Work*, eds R. Parasuraman and M. Rizzo (New York, NY: Oxford University Press), 146–158.

Warm, J. S., Parasuraman, R., and Matthews, G. (2008). Vigilance requires hard mental work and is stressful. *Hum. Factors* 50, 433–441. doi: 10.1518/001872008x312152

Wascher, E., Heppner, H., and Hoffmann, S. (2014). Towards the measurement of event-related EEG activity in real-life working environments. *Int. J. Psychophysiol.* 91, 3–9. doi: 10.1016/j.ijpsycho.2013.10.006

Zander, T. O., and Kothe, C. (2011). Towards passive brain-computer interfaces: applying brain-computer interface technology to human-machine systems in general. *J. Neural Eng.* 8:025005. doi: 10.1088/1741-2560/8/2/025005

4

Transcranial Direct Current Stimulation Modulates Neuronal Activity and Learning in Pilot Training

Jaehoon Choe[1], *Brian A. Coffman*[1,2,3], *Dylan T. Bergstedt*[1,4], *Matthias D. Ziegler*[1,5] and *Matthew E. Phillips*[1*]

[1] HRL Laboratories LLC, Malibu, CA, USA, [2] Department of Psychiatry, The University of Pittsburgh, Pittsburgh, PA, USA, [3] Psychology Clinical Neuroscience Center, The University of New Mexico, Albuquerque, NM, USA, [4] Department of Sports Medicine, Pepperdine University, Malibu, CA, USA, [5] Advanced Technologies Laboratories, Lockheed Martin, Arlington, VA, USA

***Correspondence:**
Matthew E. Phillips
mephillips@hrl.com

Skill acquisition requires distributed learning both within (online) and across (offline) days to consolidate experiences into newly learned abilities. In particular, piloting an aircraft requires skills developed from extensive training and practice. Here, we tested the hypothesis that transcranial direct current stimulation (tDCS) can modulate neuronal function to improve skill learning and performance during flight simulator training of aircraft landing procedures. Thirty-two right-handed participants consented to participate in four consecutive daily sessions of flight simulation training and received sham or anodal high-definition-tDCS to the right dorsolateral prefrontal cortex (DLPFC) or left motor cortex (M1) in a randomized, double-blind experiment. Continuous electroencephalography (EEG) and functional near infrared spectroscopy (fNIRS) were collected during flight simulation, n-back working memory, and resting-state assessments. tDCS of the right DLPFC increased midline-frontal theta-band activity in flight and n-back working memory training, confirming tDCS-related modulation of brain processes involved in executive function. This modulation corresponded to a significantly different online and offline learning rates for working memory accuracy and decreased inter-subject behavioral variability in flight and n-back tasks in the DLPFC stimulation group. Additionally, tDCS of left M1 increased parietal alpha power during flight tasks and tDCS to the right DLPFC increased midline frontal theta-band power during n-back and flight tasks. These results demonstrate a modulation of group variance in skill acquisition through an increasing in learned skill consistency in cognitive and real-world tasks with tDCS. Further, tDCS performance improvements corresponded to changes in electrophysiological and blood-oxygenation activity of the DLPFC and motor cortices, providing a stronger link between modulated neuronal function and behavior.

Keywords: tDCS, EEG, fNIRS, DLPFC, M1, flight simulation, skill learning

INTRODUCTION

There has recently been a rapid increase in the number of published studies in the field of neuromodulation due to the availability of non-invasive stimulation technologies such as transcranial direct current stimulation (tDCS). New tools for training enhancement are emerging which target specific, basic cognitive functions, with the goal of increasing performance in high-level, real-world tasks, such as pilot training. For example, Clark et al. (2012) demonstrated enhanced concealed image detection training with tDCS. Others have observed enhanced skill learning with tDCS in spatial and verbal working memories (Martin et al., 2014; Richmond et al., 2014), language acquisition (Flöel et al., 2008) and motor skills development (Banissy and Muggleton, 2013; Reis et al., 2015; Rumpf et al., 2015). For a review of tDCS enhancements (see Coffman et al., 2014).

Computerized cognitive training methods have been only moderately successful in enhancing performance (Ball et al., 2002). However, computerized procedural training (flight simulation) has been an important part of airplane pilot training since the mid 1970's. Commercial and military pilot training programs now utilize flight simulation extensively for training basic flight and combat skills (Bell and Waag, 1998; Rosenkopf and Tushman, 1998). Research on the effectiveness of flight simulator training has historically been limited by the high cost of full flight simulators, and occurs in the context of ongoing pilot training programs, rather than unbiased third-party research programs (Hays et al., 1992; Rosenkopf and Tushman, 1998). The field has recently overcome this limitation by the commercialization of relatively low-cost flight simulator devices available for purchase and use in standard research environments. These personal computer-based flight simulators are also used in various contexts for flight training (Koonce and Bramble, 1998), lending ecological validity to simulator studies.

Piloting an airplane is a demanding task requiring skillful execution of learned procedures. This has been observed as a correlation between flight simulator performance and measures of reasoning and working memory in general aviation pilots (Causse et al., 2011), and a concurrent decline in working memory and flight errors (Dismukes, 2008; Engle, 2010). Furthermore, neurophysiological markers of both short-term (e.g., fatigue) and long-term (e.g., expertise) cognitive functions correlate with behavioral performance (Ayaz et al., 2013; Borghini et al., 2014). Pilot skill development requires a synthesis of multiple cognitive faculties, many of which are enhanced by tDCS and include: dexterity (Boggio et al., 2006), mental arithmetic (Hauser et al., 2013), cognitive flexibility (Chrysikou et al., 2013), visuo-spatial reasoning (Heimrath et al., 2012), and working memory (Gill and Hamilton, 2014)—an important predictor of flight situation awareness in novices (Sohn and Doane, 2004).

Working memory is linked primarily with brain activity in the dorsolateral prefrontal cortex (DLPFC) (Courtney et al., 1996; Braver et al., 1997; Curtis and D'Esposito, 2003), an area often targeted by non-invasive brain stimulation in cognitive research. Most researchers agree that tDCS of DLPFC has substantial effects on working memory (for a review see Coffman et al., 2014); however, Horvath et al. (2015) recently reported disconfirming evidence for this hypothesis in a meta-analysis of selected studies investigating the cognitive effects of tDCS. In this meta-analysis, tDCS did not have a significant effect on any cognitive measure. However, their approach may be confounded by calculation of effect sizes based only on post-stimulation scores, rather than accounting for pre-stimulation differences between groups. Chhatbar and Feng (2015) illustrated this issue in their response paper, where they show substantial effects of tDCS when calculating effect sizes from pre-post difference scores rather than post-stimulation scores alone.

The focality of stimulation is also a critical component of tDCS-driven behavioral changes, and this aspect of experimental design is difficult to capture in meta-study. Large pad-type electrodes used in previous studies have comparatively poor focality and target current intensity as compared to the multiple electrode montage approach (Dmochowski et al., 2011). Finite elements modeling work with MRI-derived brain models performed by various groups demonstrate optimization of currents to the brain that improve focality and intensity to areas of interest by 80 and 98%, respectively (Bikson et al., 2009; Datta et al., 2011, 2012; Dmochowski et al., 2011; Faria et al., 2011; Edwards et al., 2013). The importance of this modeling work is underscored by clinical investigations that show differences in targeting and stimulation intensity results in marked differences in behavioral output and stimulation efficacy (Valle et al., 2009; Moliadze et al., 2010; Mendonca et al., 2011). Finally, Santarnecchi et al. (2015) have suggested that the impact of tDCS on target brain structures is dependent on not only the placement of electrodes and current density, but also the current state of activity in those brain areas. This crucial point is often overlooked in tDCS research, and investigators should carefully consider the cognitive task performed during stimulation to maximize the desired effect.

Despite recent controversy over the effects of tDCS on working memory, tDCS applied to specific brain regions has been reported to improve behavioral performance in a diverse array of cognitive categories: attention (Coffman et al., 2014), reaction time (Teo et al., 2011), object recognition (Clark et al., 2012), memory (Manenti et al., 2013), creativity (Chrysikou et al., 2013), and motor skill acquisition (Nitsche et al., 2003). In addition to acute improvement of various performance measures, some laboratories have also observed persistence of cognitive enhancement even after the electrical current is removed (Snowball et al., 2013; Lefebvre et al., 2014). These results indicate that, in some cases, stimulation need only be applied initially or periodically to achieve continual performance gains. Although the modulation of procedural learning through enhancement of working memory has remained an open question in the field, non-invasive brain stimulation methods are potential vehicles to enhance learning and performance and nootropic benefits for commercial and military applications (Clark et al., 2012; Phillips and Ziegler, 2014).

The application of neuroimaging techniques, such as functional near-infrared spectroscopy (fNIRS) and electroencephalography (EEG), allow the precise measurement of spatial and dynamic functional brain activity. The development of these non-invasive, low overhead and high-resolution tools have given investigators the ability to observe the activity of the human brain *in vivo* with an unprecedented degree of control (Been et al., 2007; McKendrick et al., 2015).

EEG results confirm tDCS-related modulation of brain processes involved in working memory, as evidenced by increased midline frontal theta-band oscillatory brain activity (MFT) during a working memory task (Miller et al., 2015). MFT is most commonly measured during maintenance of information in working memory, and reflects theta coupling between the DLPFC and anterior cingulate cortex (Sauseng et al., 2004). MFT is positively correlated with attentional demands during mental calculation (Ishii et al., 2014) and working memory load (Jensen and Tesche, 2002), and theta-band synchrony between frontal and parietal areas is directly related to individual working memory capacity (Palva et al., 2010). Further evidence supporting the functional relationship comes from studies temporarily disrupting the DLPFC with transcranial magnetic stimulation—leading to performance decrements in working memory tasks (Grafman et al., 1994; Pascual-Leone and Hallett, 1994). Other frequency bands have also been implicated in working memory and attentional control. For example, tonic increases (and phasic decreases) in parietal alpha-band power reflects greater perceptual involvement for tasks requiring attention to the environment (Klimesch, 1999), suggesting a role of alpha in perception. Furthermore, Sauseng et al. (2009) showed that alpha band activity over sensorimotor areas indicates greater excitability in that region, as measured with transcranial magnetic stimulation. Therefore, stimulation of either M1 or DLPFC could increase tonic alpha band activity in this study compared to sham by enhancing sensorimotor excitability and/or perceptual involvement.

Other imaging studies, employing fNIRS have found significant correlations between cognitive performance and blood oxygenation in the DLPFC (Yanagisawa et al., 2010; McKendrick et al., 2014). fNIRS is an non-invasive imaging technique that measures the relative concentrations of oxygenated (Hboxy) and deoxygenated (Hbdeoxy) hemoglobin to infer neuronal activity. fNIRS relies on differences in the near infrared absorption spectra of oxygenated and deoxygenated hemoglobin along with a neuro-vascular hemodynamic response function to relate relative chances in localized cerebral blood flow to neuronal activity (Villringer et al., 1993).

Hbdeoxy and total hemoglobin concentrations (Hbtot) are linked to levels of cognitive workload in the anterior prefrontal cortex (PFC) (Ayaz et al., 2012). For example, using a Scarborough adaptation of the Tower of London task, Ruocco et al. (2014) found that difficult problems were associated with greater Hboxy concentrations in the DLPFC relative to a baseline condition. The study also found that participants who scored higher in deliberation, or careful thinking, before acting, showed greater activation in this same region, regardless of task difficulty. The magnitude of Hbtot and Hbdeoxy concentration changes in specific brain regions has been used as a proxy for mental workload and expertise. Hbtot levels increase in the PFC during difficult trials in the N-back task, suggesting greater recruitment of neural resources (Herff et al., 2013). In addition, during a complex flight task, Hbtot levels decrease in the PFC over a 9-day learning period with progression from beginner to intermediate and finally advanced levels of performance (Ayaz et al., 2012). Furthermore, blood oxygenation level-dependent (BOLD) responses, which correlate with Hboxy, Hbdeoxy and Hbtot concentrations (Cui et al., 2011), decrease with improvements in response time, suggesting more efficient activation of PFC (Holland et al., 2011). Decreases in hemoglobin concentrations exist in the motor system (Hbdeoxy—Wolf et al., 2007), and in prefrontal cortex where they were correlated with reward value (Hboxy and Hbtot—DiStasio and Francis, 2013).

Although reported effects of primary motor cortex (M1) stimulation on skill acquisition and procedural learning have been promising, these methods have primarily been investigated in standard psychological and motor tasks including the serial reaction time task (Nitsche et al., 2003), the tower of London task (Dockery et al., 2009); and sequential visual isometric pinch task (Reis et al., 2009). Increasing evidence for the application of tDCS to enhance real-world skills has been reported for vehicle control (Beeli et al., 2008; Sakai et al., 2014), golf (Zhu et al., 2015), threat detection in image analysis (Falcone et al., 2012), air traffic control (Nelson et al., 2014). tDCS has also decreased resumption lag after interruption (Blumberg et al., 2014), and maintained vigilance (McIntire et al., 2014) in real-world tasks.

Critical for the acquisition of these real-work skills are both online and offline learning. Online learning is the change in behavioral performance across trials within an experimental session and is analogous to encoding (Reis et al., 2009). Offline learning is the change in performance, between sequential experimental sessions, from the last trial of the n-1th session to the first trial of the nth session, and is analogous to consolidation (Robertson et al., 2004). The modulation of online and offline learning rate for practical, real-world skill acquisition with tDCS of M1 or DLFPC stimulation have remained unexplored.

Here, we investigated changes in skill acquisition and learning rates with tDCS applied to either DLPFC or M1 during custom pilot training exercises developed and administered with a commercially available flight simulator (X-Plane). These results were recently reported in a poster presentation at the Society for Neuroscience Meeting (Choe et al., 2015). We measured task-evoked changes in functional activity using fNIRS and EEG as subjects learned to complete flight simulator and N-back training exercises at increasing levels of expertise across four daily consecutive sessions. We hypothesized that stimulation of DLPFC over the course of flight simulation and N-back training would alter group variability in skill learning, MFT power, and Hboxy and Hbtot concentrations in the DLPFC. Furthermore, we hypothesized that tDCS of M1 will alter tonic alpha-band power over parietal cortex.

MATERIALS AND METHODS

Participants

Thirty-two right-hand dominant, healthy adult HRL Laboratories employees (31 males) participated in this study.

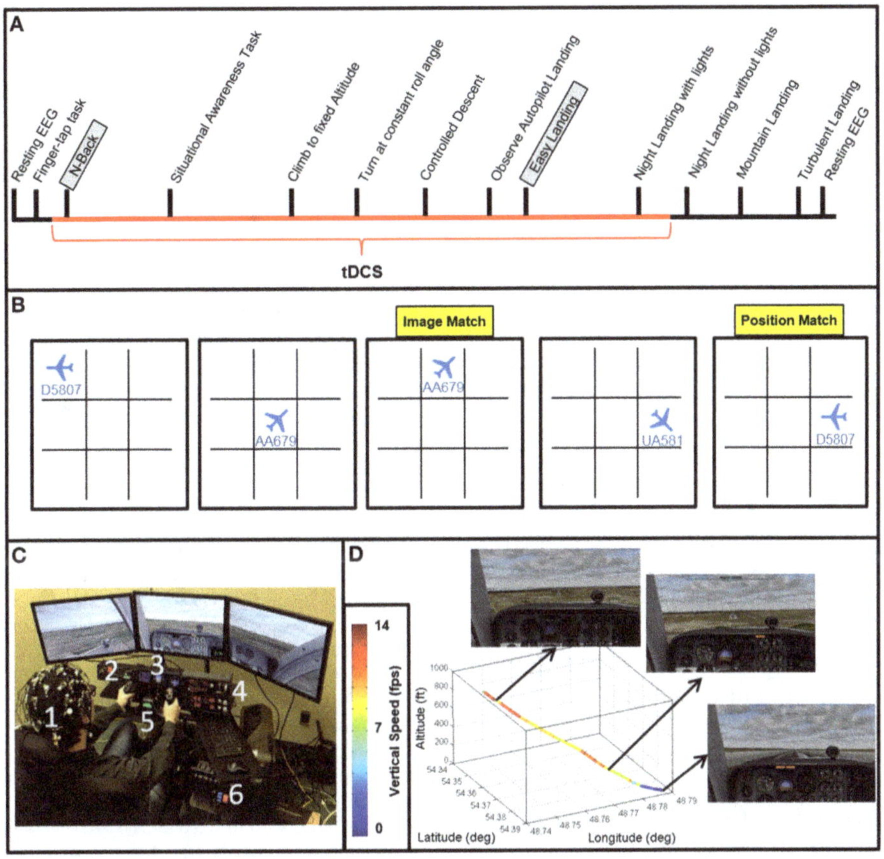

FIGURE 1 | Experimental design. (A) Experiment timeline depicting the relative timing of each task (see **Table 1** for descriptions of each task). The N-Back and Easy Landing tasks are highlighted, and the duration of tDCS is depicted in red. **(B)** An example of 6 trials of the N-Back task is shown. 1-back orientation and location match trials are highlighted in yellow. **(C)** The flight simulator, neuroimaging (EEG and FNIRS) and tDCS setup is shown with on a subject (1). Flight simulator equipment includes three-panel display, a radio panel (2), an instrument panel (3) with (from left to right) compass, altimeter, airspeed indicator, vertical speed indicator, and turn/slip indicator, a multi-panel (4) with (from left to right) autopilot settings, auto throttle switch, flaps switch, and elevator trim wheel, yoke (5), and throttle quadrant system (6). **(D)** Autopilot flight path for the Easy Landing task is shown in 3 dimensions, color-coded by vertical speed. Screenshots for initial descent, approach, and landing are also shown.

Their ages ranged from 21 to 64 (mean ± STD = 38 ± 13). Participants were randomly assigned to one of four groups: DLPFC stim ($n = 7$, age = 35 ± 11), DLPFC sham ($n = 7$, age = 42 ± 13), M1 stim ($n = 10$, age = 41 ± 16), or M1 sham ($n = 8$, age = 31 ± 5). HRL Laboratories employees are a vulnerable class of subjects for this study. In order to manage the risk of any undue influence, coercion, or confidentiality breach we only allowed individuals who are not directly supervised by the investigators of this study to volunteer, and only performed experiments during normal business hours (9 a.m.–5 p.m.) to mitigate any possibility for recourse or reward for participation in performance evaluation or job advancement. To maintain confidentiality, each subject was assigned a unique number, known only to the investigators of the study and subject identities were not shared. This design is in line with the recommendations of Meyers (1979) on student and employees as a vulnerable population of subjects and complies with DHHS: protected human subject 45 CFR 46; FDA: informed consent 21 CFR 50. Inclusion criteria were: (1) normal or corrected-to-normal vision, (2) no prior history of epileptic seizures or known neurological disorders, and (3) no females who are pregnant or are likely to become pregnant during the course of the study. All participants provided written informed consent to participate in the experiment. JC, MDZ, and MEP are listed as inventors in patent applications on brain stimulation methods.

Materials

Flight Simulator

Flight simulation tasks were designed and administered with the XForce Dream Simulator package (X-Force PC) and the X-plane 10 Flight Simulator software (Laminar Research). A depiction of the XForce Dream Simulator package can be seen in **Figure 1C**, and included a yoke, a radio panel, an instrument panel with compass, attitude indicator, altimeter, airspeed indicator, vertical speed indicator, and turn/slip indicator, a multi-panel with autopilot settings, auto throttle switch, flaps switch, and elevator trim wheel, and a throttle quadrant system. This flight simulator included an adjustable seat for maximum comfort for the subject. Three monitors were placed at an optimal distance from the subject to avoid any eyestrain. Custom scenarios were designed using the simulator software development kit following a model of flight training (Williams, 2012, see **Table 1**).

Neuroimaging

We recorded continuous EEG and fNIRS data during flight simulation training, N-back, finger tapping, situational awareness, and resting-state assessments. Horizontal and vertical electro-oculogram (EOG) was also recorded. EEG was collected using a 32-channel acti32Champ system, with electrodes placed in a custom, 10-10 based arrangement to accommodate tDCS electrodes (StarStim Neuroelectrics) and fNIRS illuminators/receivers (NIRSport NIRX) within custom headcaps (BrainVision). EEG caps were selected for each subject based on individual head size and aligned to Cz. Conductive gel (Signagel) was applied onto each EEG electrode and ultrasound gel (Aquasonic clear) was applied to each fNIRS source and detector. fNIRS was recorded with dual-wavelength continuous-wave (CW) near infrared (NIR) diffuse tomographic measurements at 760 and 850 nm. A total of 20 fNIRS channels (source-detector pairs) were recorded over the left M1 (10 channels) and right DLPFC (10 channels, see **Figure 2**). The distance between source-detector pairs was <3.5 cm (see **Figure 2**). EEG data were collected at 500 Hz, and fNIRS data were collected at 8 Hz. Locations of EEG electrodes and fNIRS channels can be seen in **Figure 2**.

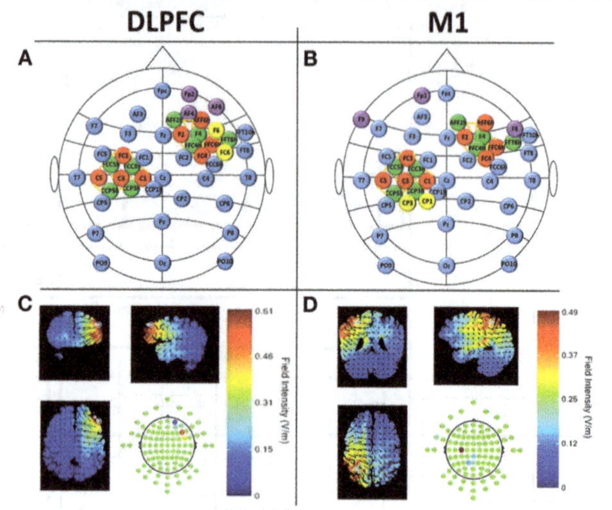

FIGURE 2 | Neuroimaging and tDCS experimental setup for DLPFC (A,C) and M1 stimulation (B,D). (A,B) EEG locations are denoted in blue and follow the 10–20 locations where possible. fNIRS sources (red) and detectors (green) are shown over the left-M1 and right DLPFC with channels depicted as orange lines (M1 channels: FC3-FCC5h, FC3-FCC3h, C5-FCC5h, C3-FCC5h, C3-FCC3h, C1-FCC3h, C5-CCP5h, C3-CCP5h, C3-CCP3h, C1-CCP3h; DLPFC channels: AFF6h-AFF2h, AFF6h-F4, F2-AFF2h, F2-F2, F2-FFC4h, FFC6h-F4, FFC6h-FFT8h, FFC6h-FFC4h, FC4-FFC4h, FC4-F4) tDCS electrodes are denoted in purple (cathodes) and yellow (anodes) and follow the current values specified in Section Neuroimaging CandDBal prefrontal cortex (DLPFC [e confidence bound was >4x the size of the positive confidence bound]). Predicted electric field intensities from the maximum focality montages from the Male 1 model in the Soterix HD Targets software (Soterix Medical).

tDCS

Sham or actual tDCS was applied with the Starstim system (Neuroelectrics) following the finger tapping task (see **Figure 1A**). The total current applied was 2 mA, with scalp current density of 0.04 A/m^2 for active tDCS (for 60 min), or 0.1 mA (0.002 A/m^2) for sham tDCS (for 1 min). Currents were applied with a 1 min ramp-in at initiation and a 1 min ramp-out at termination. Sham stimulation was used as a control condition to induce the physical sensation associated with tDCS (e.g., tingling) without directly stimulating the brain areas located below the electrodes (Coffman et al., 2012b). Silver/silver chloride electrodes were each 3.14 cm^2 in size (total anode area = 6.28 cm^2; total cathode area = 9.42 cm^2). During stimulation the impedance value was limited to 20 kΩ for operation of the device; actual impedance values typically were below 10 kΩ and impedances were observed to be stable throughout the duration of the experiment. tDCS channel impedances were continually monitored at 1 HZ. To achieve maximum focality for the targeted brain regions of interest, electrode placements were derived using HD Targets (Soterix Medical) with stimulation targets in the left M1 (right posterior field orientation model) and right DLPFC (left anterior field orientation model) and possible electrode locations were defined using standard 10-10 electrode locations (see **Figure 2**). HD Targets uses a MRI-derived finite element brain model that provides predictions for current flow and alignment for multiple interacting electrodes; this model was used to calculate maximal focality and intensity for regions of interest. For M1 stimulation, this resulted in current values of: CP1 = 1244 μA, CP3 = 745 μA, FP1 = −417 μA, F8 = −448 μA, and F9 = −1124 μA. For DLPFC stimulation, current values were F6 = 1511 μA, FC6 = 482 μA, AF8 = −271 μA, AF4 = −283 μA, and FP2 = −1439 μA (see **Figure 2**). The predicted field intensities at the target locations were 0.56 V/m (DLPFC) and 0.45 V/m (M1). Groups are denoted as: DLPFC stim, DLFPC sham, M1 stim, and M1 sham.

Procedures

All participants performed flight simulation training, N-back, finger tapping, situational awareness, and resting-state assessments once per day for four consecutive daily sessions (see **Figure 1**). Resting-state brain activity was collected for 1 min both before and after the experiment. During resting scans, subjects observed autopilot flight (level flight at 5000 ft. altitude) and were instructed to keep their eyes open and observe the visual scene while keeping their hands in their laps. Following the pre-experiment resting-state assessment, motor reference scans were taken during a simple motor sequence task in which subjects were instructed to touch each fingertip with the thumb of the right hand in sequence/cycle, continuously for 30 s (**Figure 1A**, finger-tapping task). We analyzed neuroimaging data recorded during the finger-tapping task as a confirmatory

TABLE 1 | Experimental task schedule performed on each of the four consecutive experimental sessions.

Task	# of trials	Task instruction/Description	Average duration (minutes)
Survey	1	Setup and Explanation (day 1) Learn the basic controls via explanation	1
Rest	1	Eyes open, hand resting on yoke Observe straight and level autopilot flight	1
Finger tap	1	Using right hand, touch thumb to each finger in sequence	0.5
N-back	6	Adaptive threshold (at 80% accuracy) N-back on 3 × 3 grid of visual orientation of aircraft, flight number and spatial location (3 × 3 grid)	10
Situational awareness	4	Memorize gauge cluster images with 15 s distractor task and 30 s. for recall	10
Climb to fixed altitude	1	Adjust altitude from 5000 to 6000 ft. and back to 5000 ft. Maintain vertical speed at <1000 ft./min with level roll	5
Turn at constant roll angle	1	Change bearing/azimuth from 90° to 180° and back to 90° with a maximum roll angle of 20°	5
Descend @ constant Rate	1	Adjust altitude from 3000 to 1000 ft. at a 800 ft./min rate of descent	5
Autopilot landing (observe)	1	Observe the autopilot approach on the "Easy Landing" runway in perfect weather and high visibility	2
Easy landing	5	Control all aspects of landing in perfect weather and high visibility	10
Nighttime landing	2	Control all aspects of landing in perfect weather at night, with runway lights (low visibility)	4
No-lights landing	2	Control all aspects in approach with zero visibility	4
Hard landing (Mountains)	1	Difficult visual-only approach over terrain where the runway is initially obstructed from view over a mountain range	6
Hard landing (Turbulence)	1	Control all aspects of landing with turbulence value is set to level 1 out of 10 (instead of 0), with high visibility	2

measure (see Supplementary Figures S4, S5), where sensorimotor network activity was expected to be evident in EEG as increased power in the beta band, and reduced power in the alpha band, compared to baseline, and in fNIRS as an increase in deoxygenated hemoglobin beneath M1 sensors.

Participants then performed the N-back task followed by a series of basic flight training exercises including a situational awareness task, climbing to fix altitude, turning at a constant roll angle, and a controlled descent. Follow these fight control tasks participants performed a series of landing task including the "easy landing" task, nighttime landing, nighttime landing without runway lights, a landing in mountainous terrain, and a landing in turbulent weather (**Figure 1A**). Results for the situational awareness, free flight, climb to fixed altitude, heading change at constant roll angle, descent at constant vertical speed, nighttime landing, no-lights landing, mountain, and turbulence landing task are the subject of subsequent manuscripts.

N-Back

The Brain Workshop N-back task was implemented in this study (Paul Hoskinson, V.4.8.8 http://brainworkshop.sourceforge.net/). Participants monitored position and image for N-back matches without audio feedback. Custom N-back images were used, showing airplanes in eight different orientations with 1 of 3 possible flight numbers (24 total image possibilities, see **Figure 1B**). Subjects completed six blocks of 20 trials each day. Every subject began the N-Back task at the 1-back level, and was instructed at the beginning of each block to focus on a central fixation point. Subjects were free to move their eyes during the task. Upon reaching an upper threshold of accuracy within a given block (>80%), the task difficulty was increased (N + 1) using an adaptive threshold paradigm (Jaeggi et al., 2008). Upon reaching a lower threshold of accuracy (<20%), the task difficulty was decreased (N − 1). Each time this occurred, the changes were explained to the subjects between blocks. At the completion of each block, subjects were allowed to review the rules and ask clarifying questions about the tasks.

Autopilot Landing Observation

Subjects viewed a replay video of the autopilot executing an "optimal" landing from ~800 ft. altitude onto a runway. Initial aircraft position was aligned with the runway and aircraft was already maintaining proper vertical speed for ideal glide slope. This scenario presents a wide, long, flat runway with no visual obstructions and no landscape features that interfere with landing the aircraft. Subjects were instructed not to manipulate controls or control the simulation in any way, but were told to pay close attention to the flight parameters through the instrumentation, as well as the visual field displayed by the simulator as the aircraft proceeded with landing. Particular emphasis was placed on two key parameters: azimuth (20°) for runway alignment, and vertical speed (~700–800 ft./min) for appropriate glide slope. Attention was also drawn to the final control input to landing (pitch up at ground contact), and subjects were instructed to minimize landing force (G-force) as a top priority. Once the autopilot landing was viewed in its entirety, subjects were given the opportunity to ask questions about the landings. Most subjects asked very few, if any questions, typically on the first trial day.

Easy Landing Task

Subjects were instructed to complete the landing task as shown by the autopilot under daylight conditions and 100% visibility. Subjects attempted landing under these conditions a total of 5 times per day. As the subject attempted replication of the autopilot landing, the experimenter made observations in three categories: (1) Vertical speed maintenance; (2) Runway alignment; and (3) Final approach dynamics (pitch angle at touchdown). Any large deviations from the autopilot in any of these modalities were noted, then provided as feedback to the subject after the plane had touched down and the simulator paused. When given, feedback was ~1–2 min in length and conducted in an informal manner. The time duration of feedback also shortened throughout training as the subject made fewer errors. Following feedback, the subject was offered opportunity to ask any questions regarding landing technique, then the scenario was restarted. If subjects passed beyond the terminal end of the runway, the attempt was ended and the landing listed as "missed landing." This counted against the number of subject attempts (i.e., attempts were not repeated due to missed landing). Feedback methods and handling of missed landings was identical for all landing task.

Data Analysis

EEG

EEG data were preprocessed using EEGLAB (Delorme and Makeig, 2004) by applying a 0.5 Hz high-pass filter (Butterworth, 12 dB/oct) and removing bad channels (max = 19%). Adaptive Mixture Independent Components Analysis (AMICA) (Delorme et al., 2012) was then used to detect and remove artifacts associated with eye blinks, vertical and horizontal electrooculogram, electrocardiogram, and tDCS-related voltage fluctuation. Following artifact rejection using AMICA, data were back-reconstructed and channels removed prior to AMICA decomposition were interpolated back into the data by spherical interpolation. Blocks corresponding to N-back, resting-state, and Easy Landing tasks were then segmented from the data.

Frequency decomposition was performed using FieldTrip (Oostenveld et al., 2011) by first segmenting data for each task into sequential 1-s epochs. Data were then windowed using a hanning taper, and frequency content of each trial was assessed at 1 Hz increments from 4 to 7 Hz (theta-band) or 8–12 Hz (alpha-band) using Fast Fourier Transform (multitaper method). After frequency decomposition, epochs with average theta or alpha power greater than two standard deviations from the mean were rejected, and remaining epochs were averaged for each participant, training day, and task. Data missing due to equipment issues (i.e., amplifier battery failure: $N = 4$, stimulus trigger errors: $N = 1$, or excessive noise/artifact during recording which could not be removed with AMICA: $N = 7$) were replaced with the mean for that participant group and training day prior to statistical analysis. We verified sensorimotor network activity during the finger-tapping task on the first day of flight simulator training (prior to tDCS) within baseline-subtracted beta and alpha band power maps, calculated across all subjects (Supplementary Figures S4, S5).

Participants receiving tDCS were compared with sham tDCS participants at each of the 4 days of training using independent-samples t-tests, which separately tested differences in alpha-band and theta-band activity at each sensor. Additionally, day 1 was compared to day 4 within each tDCS group and sensor using paired t-tests to assess training-related effects on alpha-band and theta-band activity. Statistical tests were corrected for multiple comparisons using cluster-based permutation tests (500 repetitions, data point $\alpha = 0.05$, cluster-level $\alpha = 0.05$, minimum spatial extent = 2 channels). Results from these comparisons are reported separately for each cluster of significant differences between groups/conditions. We calculated mean alpha/theta band power within clusters for use in examining relationships between task-related EEG and fNIRS/behavioral data.

We also examined correlations between behavioral measures, fNIRS beta values, and mean theta/alpha power across clusters identified during cluster-based permutation tests comparing days 1 to 4. fNIRS beta values were unavailable for 7 subjects (4 active M1 subjects and 3 sham M1 subjects) because time stamps could not be parsed from the fNIRS data files; therefore, the number of participants used in this analysis were: M1 stim = 6, M1 sham = 5, DLPFC sham = 7, and DLPFC stim = 7. These correlations were examined only within the stimulation groups where significant clusters were identified. To investigate relationships between midline frontal theta-band activity (Midline frontal theta-band activity was calculated as the mean theta power across electrodes Fz and FC1, the electrodes nearest to medial prefrontal cortex) and behavioral measures in the easy landing and N-Back task, Pearson correlation statistics were examined. We compared midline frontal theta-band activity in the easy landing task with autopilot displacement, g-force at landing, vertical speed at landing, roll at landing, pitch at landing, or online/offline learning rates for number of control inputs, autopilot displacement, vertical speed deviance from autopilot, or vertical speed variance. In the N-Back task, we compared midline frontal theta-band activity with average N level achieved and online/offline learning rates. Correlations were examined separately for DLPFC and M1 groups, stim and sham groups, and days of training. Because of the large number of correlation statistics examined, we used a conservative alpha of 0.001 to determine statistical significance. We additionally report statistics with a relaxed alpha of 0.05; however, these effects will be considered trends in this analysis.

In addition to cluster-based permutation tests across all channels, 3-way split-plot ANOVA was used to compare midline frontal theta-band activity between tDCS conditions (stim and sham), days of training (day 1, 2, 3, and 4), and training block (Block 1, 2, 3, 4, and 5) for the N-back and easy landing tasks. Huynh-Feldt epsilon was used to correct degrees of freedom for assumptions of sphericity, and Fishers Least Significant Difference corrections of alpha were used for simple-effects/pairwise comparisons (Maxwell and Delaney, 2004).

fNIRS

fNIRS data was processed within the nirsLAB analysis package (NIRx Medical Technologies, Glen Head, NY; Xu et al., 2014). The Gratzer Spectrum was used to measure the absorbance

TABLE 2 | Average ± standard deviation of day 1, day 4, and day 4–day 1 Hboxy, Hbdeoxy, and Hbtot concentrations across subjects and channels for M1 and the DLPFC.

			Easy landing			N-Back		
			Day 1	Day 4	Day 4–Day 1	Day 1	Day 4	Day 4–Day 1
DLPFC Stim	M1	Oxy	−0.00060 ± 0.0018	−0.0019 ± 0.0013	**−0.0013 (8)**	0.00059 ± 0.0010	−0.00041 ± 0.00076	−0.00099
		Deoxy	−0.00037 ± 0.00051	0.00012 ± 0.0011	**0.0005 (4)**	−0.00017 ± 0.00012	0.00021 ± 0.00074	0.00039
		Total	−0.00098 ± 0.0017	−0.0017 ± 0.0012	**−0.00077 (8)**	0.00041 ± 0.0010	−0.00019 ± 0.00043	−0.00061
	DLPFC	Oxy	0.0030 ± 0.0022	0.00055 ± 0.0014	**−0.0024 (8)**	0.0021 ± 0.0014	0.00048 ± 0.00091	−0.0016
		Deoxy	−0.00024 ± 0.00058	−0.00034 ± 0.00041	−0.000095	−0.00018 ± 0.00019	−0.00014 ± 0.00021	0.000041
		Total	0.0027 ± 0.0013	0.00021 ± 0.0014	−0.0025	0.0019 ± 0.0014	0.00034 ± 0.00088	0.0016
DLPFC Sham	M1	Oxy	−0.0018 ± 0.0020	−0.0018 ± 0.0019	**−0.0000082 (10)**	−0.000094 ± 0.0012	−0.000033 ± 0.00098	**0.000062 (10)**
		Deoxy	−0.00022 ± 0.00063	0.000065 ± 0.0011	**0.00028 (4)**	−0.000099 ± 0.00053	−0.00011 ± 0.00022	**−0.00001 (4)**
		Total	−0.0020 ± 0.0019	−0.0017 ± 0.0012	**0.00028 (10)**	−0.00019 ± 0.00077	−0.00014 ± 0.00086	**0.000052 (10)**
	DLPFC	Oxy	−0.000033 ± 0.0018	−0.00046 ± 0.0014	**−0.00043 (1)**	0.00067 ± 0.0012	0.00035 ± 0.0012	**−0.00032 (4)**
		Deoxy	−0.00056 ± 0.00043	−0.00053 ± 0.00021	0.000035	−0.00034 ± 0.00020	−0.00036 ± 0.00013	**−0.000017 (8)**
		Total	−0.00059 ± 0.0019	−0.00099 ± 0.0013	**−0.0004 (4)**	0.00032 ± 0.0012	−0.000015 ± 0.0012	**−0.00034 (4)**
M1 Stim	M1	Oxy	0.00024 ± 0.0031	−0.000084 ± 0.0015	**−0.00032 (4)**	0.0013 ± 0.0017	0.00045 ± 0.00088	−0.00084
		Deoxy	−0.00019 ± 0.0014	−0.00049 ± 0.00028	**−0.0003 (5)**	−0.00048 ± 0.00045	−0.00027 ± 0.00031	0.00021
		Total	0.000043 ± 0.0039	−0.00057 ± 0.0014	−0.00062	0.00080 ± 0.0016	0.00017 ± 0.00085	−0.00063
	DLPFC	Oxy	0.00050 ± 0.0026	−0.00060 ± 0.00055	−0.0011	0.00015 ± 0.00051	−0.00031 ± 0.00036	**−0.00046**
		Deoxy	−0.000045 ± 0.00092	−0.00017 ± 0.00020	−0.00012	−0.00027 ± 0.00030	−0.00012 ± 0.000088	0.00015
		Total	0.00046 ± 0.0035	−0.000766 ± 0.00056	−0.0012	−0.00012 ± 0.00078	−0.00043 ± 0.00035	**−0.00031**
M1 Sham	M1	Oxy	−0.00097 ± 0.0010	−0.00080 ± 0.00085	**0.00017 (10)**	0.00022 ± 0.0012	0.00047 ± 0.0016	0.00025
		Deoxy	−0.00017 ± 0.00020	−0.00013 ± 0.00021	**0.000032 (8)**	−0.00015 ± 0.00016	−0.00018 ± 0.00020	−0.000031
		Total	−0.0011 ± 0.00091	−0.00093 ± 0.00089	**0.0002**	0.000074 ± 0.0012	0.00029 ± 0.0017	0.00022
	DLPFC	Oxy	−0.00041 ± 0.00087	−0.00054 ± 0.0019	−0.00013	0.00011 ± 0.00030	−0.00030 ± 0.00034	−0.00041
		Deoxy	−0.000019 ± 0.00038	0.00084 ± 0.0013	0.00086	−0.000087 ± 0.00019	0.00026 ± 0.00071	0.00035
		Total	−0.00043 ± 0.0011	0.00030 ± 0.0032	0.00073	0.000022 ± 0.00029	−0.000043 ± 0.00041	−0.000065

All values are presented are in mM concentration units. Bold numbers indicate a significant difference between days 4 and 1 as determined by a SPM (see Materials and Methods Section fNIRS).

spectra of Hbdeoxy and Hboxy, with average wavelengths of 760 and 850 nm, respectively. The corresponding molar extinction coefficients ε are ε_{Hboxy} [1097.0 781.0] cm-1/M and $\varepsilon_{Hbdeoxy}$ = [645.5 1669.0] cm-1/M, (nirsLAB, NIRx Medical Technologies). The differential path lengths were 5.98 for Hboxy and 7.15 for Hbdeoxy (Essenpreis et al., 1993). In the Beer-Lambert law calculation, the distance between source-detector pair was =< 3.5 cm, and the exact distances were computed within NIRSLab according to the corresponding distances on the headcap.

Hbdeoxy, Hboxy and Hbtot concentration time series were band-pass filter from 0.01 to 0.2 Hz (finite impulse response with least-squares error minimization), to remove slow drifts in the signal and respiratory and cardiac rhythms. Inter-trail data was removed from the time series, and the average baseline concentration values were subtracted from the task-evoked concentration measurements.

The average concentration value of Hbtot, Hboxy, and Hbdeoxy were computed separately for each channel, subject, task, and day. Concentration values were averages within days, across all 20 trails of each of the 6 blocks in the N-back, and all 5 trials of the easy landing task. Individual channel concentration values were then averaged across channels within regions (M1 and DLPFC) and across subjects within each group. Day1 group-averaged concentration values were then subtracted from Day 4 concentrations to compute the change in concentrations across the duration of the experiment.

Statistical significance of group-averaged concentrations changes from days 1 to 4 was determined using Statistical Parametric Mapping (SPM version 8). SPM was performed based on a general linear model of the canonical hemodynamic response function, with a discrete cosine transformation used for temporal filtering. A t-statistic-thresholded, baseline-subtracted Beta image was generated for each subject for baseline-subtracted, task-evoked Hbtot, Hboxy, and Hbdeoxy concentrations for days 1 and 4 (corrected for multiple comparisons across channels using the Bonferroni correction: # channels = 20, $p < 0.0025$). Paired t-statistic maps (subtracting the day 1 from day 4 betas) were generated from baseline-subtracted, trial/block-averaged (within day $n = 5$

Easy landing, $n = 6$ N-back) task betas obtained from individual subjects. If a t-statistic exceeded the corrected p-value threshold of 0.0025 the days 4–1 concentration values were determined to be significant (**Table 2**—denoted by bolded values).

Channel-wise statistical analysis was performed on all channels for measurements of Hboxy, Hbdeoxy, and Hbtot days 4–1 concentrations in easy landing and N-back for all subjects. Significance was determined if the trial-wise average exceeded 3.5 standard deviations from the null hypothesis of no concentration change (Bonferroni corrected, two-sided, Fischer's test $p < 0.00035$).

Behavioral Performance

N-Back

Raw percent accuracy values for each subject and for each block were scaled according to the information content required for each back condition. A 100% score on a 1-back trial requires both an image match: 9 possible plane orientations, 4 possible flight numbers, and a position match: 9 possible

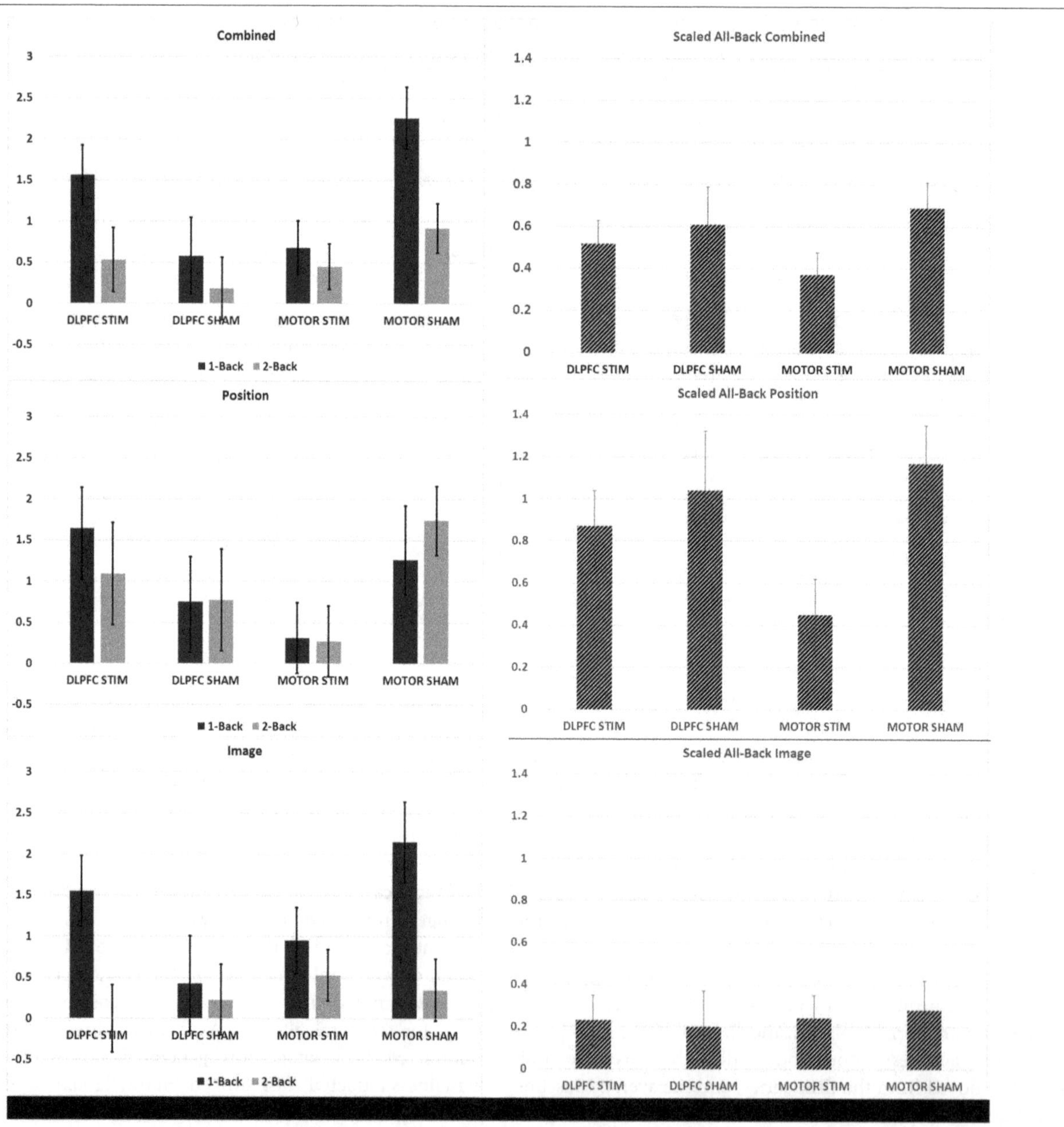

FIGURE 3 | N-back learning rates across experimental groups. The average group-learning rate is shown for each group in 1 and 2 back trials (left) and for all back trials (right column scaled by information content see Section N-Back). Learning rates computed by combining across position and image match trials **(top row)**, for position trails **(middle row)** and image trials **(bottom row)** are shown.

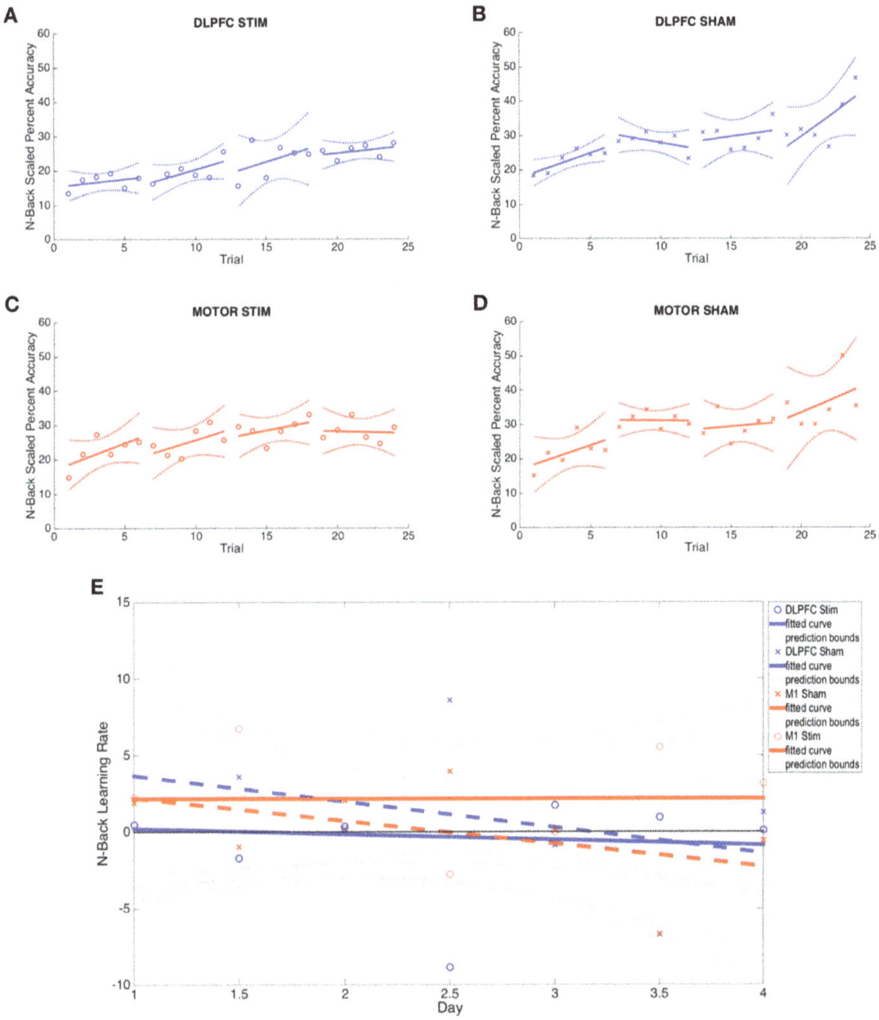

FIGURE 4 | N-back results across all four experimental groups. (A–D) The average percent correct is plotted across all 4 days (6 trials per day) for each group. Percent correct values are scaled based on the required information for a 100% correct response (see Section N-Back). **(E)** Online and offline N-back learning rates are plotted for each experimental group across the duration of the experiment. Whole numbers on the x-axis represent the average online learning rate (slope of scaled percent correct linear regression for each subject across 6 blocks within a day and ½ numbers of the x-axis represent offline learning rates (slope of the percent correct on the last trials of the N-1 day to the first trial of the Nth day).

spatial location, a 100% score on 2-back doubles the required information kept in working memory, and a 100% score on a 3-back trial triples this value. The normalization weights used for the 1–, 2–, and 3–back raw accuracy values were therefore 0.33, 0.66, and 1.0. Alternative normalization schemes (e.g., bit-wise maximum information and log-scaling) did not generate substantial differences in the outcome metrics. Learning rates were determined by the slope (±standard deviation) of a linear regression over block-wise group-averaged scaled percent accuracy: (1) across all 4 days (overall learning rate), (2) within each day independently (online learning rate), and (3) between the accuracy of the first trial of the nth day and the last trial of the n-1th day (offline learning rate) (Reis et al., 2009). Meta-learning rate was determined from the slope of the linear regression over the combined online/offline learning rate time series (the rate of change in the learning rates over time). The average number of trials for each group to reach the 2 and 3 back levels in the adaptive N-back task and the average streak (number of consecutive trials) at 2 and 3 back were calculated for each group. Learning rates were compared using one-sample against zero or paired, two-tailed t-tests (both $\alpha = 0.05$) were noted.

Easy landing

G-force assessment. Flight parameters were sampled from the simulator at 10 Hz, including altitude (above ground level), longitude, and latitude. The derivative of the vertical speed of the aircraft at runway touchdown determined the landing impact g-force (acceleration divided by 9.8 m/s^2). Smaller g-force landings reflected improved skill with the landing task as subjects were asked to minimize this value to the best of their ability for each trial. The impact g-force is a "one-shot" assessment of landing skill at the most difficult and critical phase of the landing task, while ignoring other factors of landing performance (e.g., approach, glide slope, alignment, aircraft attitude). Online, offline, and meta learning rates are negative indicating a reduction in the applied G-force at landing (Supplementary Table S2, **Figure 4**).

Flight path deviation. Latitude, longitude, and altitude were transformed into Cartesian (X-Y-Z) coordinates and the Euclidean distance between coordinates of subject and autopilot were computed over the flight path $\Sigma\text{sqrt}(x^2+y^2+z^2)$ using a moving window average to resample and align the flight paths. The Euclidean distances for each sample were then summed in order to provide the total deviation from the autopilot flight path. Unlike G-force, this metric takes into account the entire approach, including all flight maneuvers leading up to the final descent and touchdown. This measure, however, does not take into account proficiency with aircraft controls or avionics; it merely assesses the ability of the subject to adhere to the reference flight path. Subjects were instructed to replicate the flight path of the autopilot landing observation. With this metric, a better landing would have lower deviation values (Supplementary Table S2, **Figure 5**).

Vertical speed deviation. The vertical speed of the subject throughout the landing trial was subtracted from the vertical speed of the autopilot landing at each time step and summed as in the flight path deviation. The vertical speed profile of the aircraft is stereotypic for an excellent landing and this parameter is visible on the aircraft's instruments. Subjects could therefore be reasonably expected to match the vertical speed of their aircraft with that of the example shown during autopilot

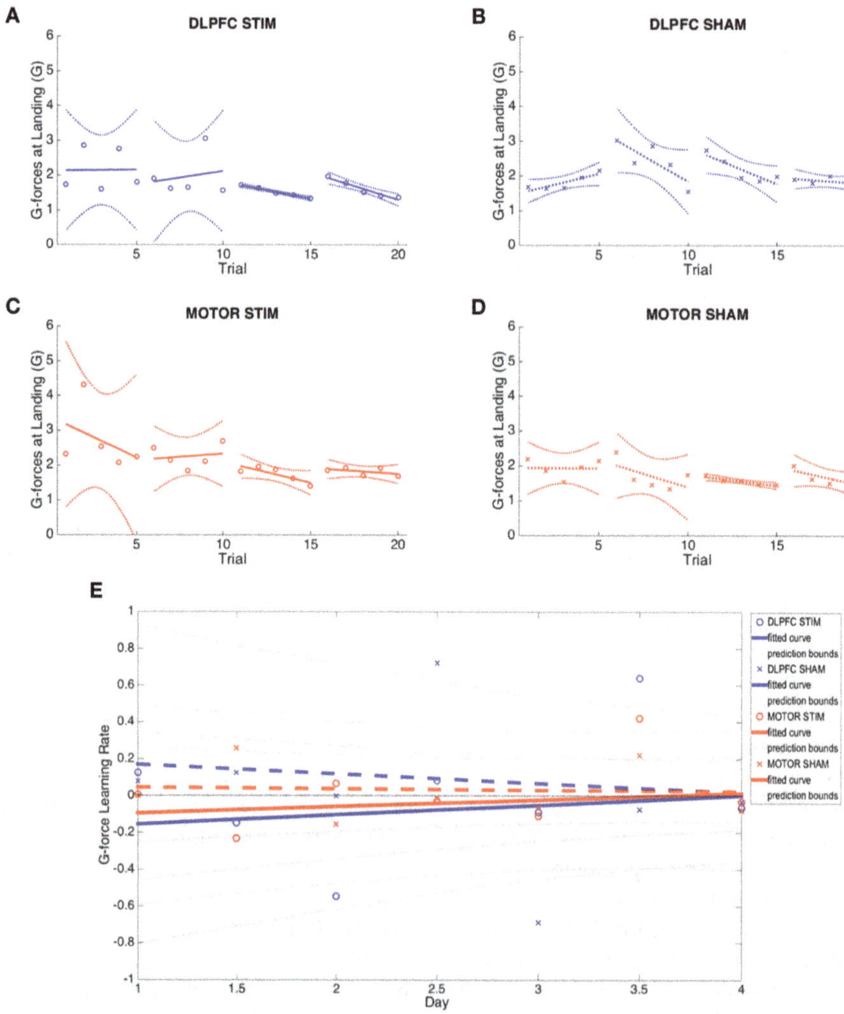

FIGURE 5 | G-force at moment of landing results across all four experimental groups. (A–D) Average g-force at moment of landing across all 4 days is plotted for each group. Note reduction in between-subject variance in days 3 and 4 of the DLPFC stim group. **(E)** Online and offline g-force learning rates are plotted for each experimental group across the duration of the experiment. Whole numbers on the x-axis represent the average online learning rate (slope of scaled percent correct linear regression for each subject across 6 blocks within a day) and ½ numbers on the x-axis represent offline learning rate (slope of the percent correct on the last trials of the N-1 day to the first trial of the Nth day). Smaller G-force indicates improved performance.

observation (vertical speed maintained at 600 ft./min for majority of approach, see **Figure 1D**). Replication of the autopilot-derived demonstration flight should result in lower overall vertical speed deviation values as performance improves (Supplementary Table S2, **Figure 5**).

Vertical speed variance. The amount of vertical speed variation throughout the landing approach was summed across trials to represent the degree to which a subject could maintain a steady, continuous descent. This measure does not penalize the subject for deviating from the ideal flight path, it merely assesses the degree to which the subject can maintain a smooth descent with little variation. This removes the goal-directed aspect of flight parameter maintenance while focusing on the motor aspect of flight parameter maintenance. As a means of comparison, the autopilot flight data only changes vertical speed in the final 5 s before landing, which minimizes this variance in the autopilot. In the ideal scenario, vertical speed stays constant, with only slight changes necessary for the final phase of landing; therefore, smaller variances indicate superior flight performance (Supplementary Table S2, **Figure 6**).

Control input measure. The number of control inputs was computed over landing trials by identifying the number of sign-changes in the vertical speed parameter throughout the landing period. This metric identifies to what extent subjects could maintain a consistent vertical speed profile (negative vertical speed indicates descent, positive ascent). Since maintaining vertical speed with minimal control input adjustment does not require specific planning of actions or prediction of flight path, it was hypothesized to be a primarily motor-processing focused measure. The number of sign-changes in the vertical speed variable was summed between start and end of the landing. As a means of comparison, the autopilot had 1 major control input at the nose flair ~1 s. before touchdown.

Outlier rejection

For each metric, trial-wise data were examined for outliers across subjects across all groups. If any trial exceeded three standard deviations from the mean, it was determined an outlier and removed from analysis. Outlier rejection was performed on a trial-wise basis for all computed metrics.

Group variance analysis

For each metric, the variance in the average online learning rate was computed as the change in the group's average accuracy treating each subject's performance in a trial as a repeated sample within days. For the n-back task, the metric used was the scaled percent accuracy across 6 trials per day. For the easy landing task, flight metrics, performed over the course of 5 landing trials per day. This measure is the variance in the online learning rate linear regression (Reis et al., 2009). Significant differences in learning rate variance was assessed with a two-sample *F*-test for equal variances. The null hypothesis that two independent samples of two subject pools come from a single normal distribution with the same variance was tested against the alternative that they come from two normal distributions with different variances. F-stat criticality was computed by generating a F cumulative distribution function appropriate to the variance ratio and degrees of freedom of sample pools. The resulting critical values are asymmetric and can be used at either tail. We were then able to determine the distance between computed F and $F = 1$ (null hypothesis). Across days, Bartlett's test was performed to test the hypothesis of equal population variance across groups. This test was performed on the average subject metrics (across trials within days) to preserve sample independence. Reported *p*-values represent the probability of observing the given result by chance if the null hypothesis were true (Snedecor and Cochran, 1989).

RESULTS

Finger-Tapping Task

As expected, the finger-tapping task induced beta band oscillatory activity and increased the concentration of Hbdeoxy over sensorimotor cortex, and reduced alpha band activity over frontal and parietal cortex compared to baseline (Supplementary Figures S4, S5). Power in the beta band was greatest over left sensorimotor cortex, contralateral to the hand used during the finger-tapping task.

N-Back Task

Behavioral Results

DLPFC stimulation

The DLPFC stim group showed significant overall learning in five separate learning rate measures, compared to two significant learning rates observed for the DLPFC sham simulation group (one-sample, two-tailed *t*-test, see **Figures 3, 4**, and Supplementary Table S1). Significant overall learning was observed for the DLPFC stim group collectively across all trial types (combining image and position match trials—denoted as "combined trials," and for position match trails) aggregating across all 1/2/3 back trials (scaled according to the methods in Section N-Back). Significant overall learning was also observed for the DLPFC stim group in 1-Back combined, position, and image trials. Significant overall learning was observed for the DLPFC sham group for combined and position trials, across all backs (see **Figure 3**). Meta-learning regressions did not show statistically significant changes in learning rates between stim and sham groups.

Neither the initial nor the final behavioral performance were significantly different between DLPFC stimulation and sham groups (Supplementary Table S1). The average trial duration to reach 2-/3-back was not significantly different between stimulation and sham groups. In addition, the average number of trials to reach 2-/3- back and the average 2-/3- back streak durations were not statistically different between groups. Significant differences in online, offline, and combined learning rates were not observed between stimulation and sham groups (see Supplementary Table S1, **Figure 4E**).

The variance in the DLPFC stim group's learning rate was significantly less than the variance of the DLPFC sham group. Examined across days, the DLPFC stim group had significantly reduced variance compared to the DLPFC sham group on

Day 3 of experimentation [$Chi_{(1)} = 5.77$, $p < 0.02$, see **Figures 4A,B**]. Examined at the trial-level, the reduced variance reached statistical significance in >33% of individual N-back trials comparing DLPFC stim with DLPFC sham, and no trials showed greater variance in the DLPFC sham group [Day 1 Trial 2: $F_{(6, 6)} = 0.21$; Day 1 Trial 4: $F_{(6, 6)} = 0.18$; Day 1 Trial 6: $F_{(6, 6)} = 0.23$; Day 2 Trial 5: $F_{(6, 6)} = 0.095$; Day 3 Trial 1: $F_{(5, 5)} = 0.069$; Day 3 Trial 2: $F_{(5, 5)} = 0.17$; Day 3 Trial 6: $F_{(5, 5)} = 0.15$; Day 4 Trial 6: $F_{(5, 4)} = 0.021$; $p < 0.05$]. These results support the hypothesis that tDCS of the right DLPFC would reduce the variability in individual learning rates in a cognitive task.

M1 stimulation

The M1 stim group showed significant overall learning in five separate learning rate measures, compared to six significant overall learning rates observed for the M1 sham stimulation group. Significant overall learning was observed for the M1 stim group for combined, image and position trails aggregating across all 1/2/3 back trials. Significant overall learning was also observed for M1 stim in 1-Back combined and image trails. Significant overall learning was observed for the M1 sham group for combined trails, aggregating across all backs and for 1 and 2-Back trials as well as for position trails (all and 2-Backs) and 2-Back image trials (see **Figure 3**). Meta-learning regressions did not show statistically significant changes in learning rates between stim and sham groups.

As with the DLPFC groups, initial and final behavioral performance between stimulation and sham groups was not significantly different (Supplementary Table S1). The average duration to reach 2-/3-back was not significantly different between stimulation and sham groups. In addition, the average number of trials to reach 2-/3- back and the average 2-/3- back streak durations were not statistically different between groups. Significant differences in online, offline, and combined learning rates were not observed between stimulation and sham groups (see Supplementary Table S1 and **Figures 3, 4E**).

Unlike the results observed for DLPFC stimulation, M1 stimulation resulted in minimal differences in learning rate variance between stimulation and sham groups. Only 1 trial showed reduced M1 stim variance compared to M1 sham variation, while there were 3/24 trials that indicated smaller M1 sham variance when compared with the values from the M1 stim group. Examined across days, no trials shows significant differences in variance under Bartlett's Test.

FNIRS Results

DLPFC stimulation

Hboxy. Exclusion criterion for individual FNIRS channels were greater than 0.001 mM fluctuations between the maximum and minimum measured concentrations during baseline. We did not observe any concentration fluctuations above this cutoff threshold for any of the 20 FNIRS channels (10 above the DLPFC and 10 above the M1 cortex) across all 4 days of recording for the 25 subjects analyses (7 DLPFC stim, 7 DLPFC sham, 6 M1 stim, 5 M1 sham). Subjects were not included ($n = 3$ in M1 stim, and $N = 3$ in M1 sham) if event time stamps could not be identified robustly within the fNIRS data files.

Average Hboxy concentrations across subjects and channels significantly increased between day 1 and day 4 in M1 channels, and significantly decreased in DLPFC channels for the DLPFC sham group and (see **Table 2**, **Figure 7**). Individual channel analysis showed no significant change in Hboxy concentrations from days 1 to 4.

Hbdeoxy. Average Hbdeoxy concentrations across subjects and channels significantly decreased between day 1 and day 4 in M1 and DLPFC channels for the DLPFC sham group (see **Table 2**).

Hbtot. Like Hboxy, average Hbtot concentrations across subjects and channels significantly increased between day 1 and day 4 in M1 channels for the DLPFC sham group, and significantly decreased in DLPFC channels for the DLPFC sham group (see **Table 2**). Individual channel analysis showed no significant change in Hbtot concentrations from days 1 to 4.

M1 stimulation

Hboxy. The average Hboxy concentration across subjects and channels within the DLPFC channels significantly decreased between days 1 and 4 in the M1 stim group (see **Table 2**). Individual channel analysis shows no significant change in Hboxy concentrations from day 1 to 4.

Hbtot. The average Hbtot concentration across subjects and channels within the DLPFC channels significantly decreased between day 1 and 4 in the M1 stim group (see **Table 2**). Individual channel analysis shows no significant change in Hbtot concentrations from days 1 to 4.

EEG Results

Theta (4–7 Hz)

DLPFC stimulation. In each day, significant differences in theta-band power were found between DLPFC stim and sham tDCS groups in frontal/central electrodes (**Table 3**). In days 1–3, right frontotemporal theta power was higher in DLPFC stim participants, compared to sham. Statistical differences were distributed over midline frontal electrodes in day 4. Comparison of days 1 and 4 revealed a significant increase in midline frontal theta-band power in stim, but not sham participants (see **Figure 8A** and **Table 3**). Split-plot ANOVA comparing MFT in the N-back task revealed a trend-level main effect of tDCS group, with DLPFC stim participants showing a greater effect than DLPFC sham participants [$F_{(1, 12)} = 4.65$, $p = 0.052$]. There was no main effect of training or interaction between tDCS group and day of training ($p > 0.1$).

M1 stimulation. For M1 stimulation, broadly-distributed differences in theta-band power were seen between stim and sham participants during N-Back performance on days 1 and 3, which were mostly left-lateralized, and were strongest near the site of stimulation (**Table 3**). Importantly, no differences between days 1 and 4 were seen for M1 stim or sham participants in the N-Back (see **Table 3** and **Figure 8A**). Split-plot ANOVA

TABLE 3 | Cluster statistics for comparisons of alpha- and theta-band power during the N-back task.

	Electrodes	t^*	p^{**}
THETA (4–7 Hz)			
DLPFC stimulation *Actual vs. Sham* Day 1 Cluster 1	E5, FT8, T8, FC2, CP2, CP6	2.89	0.020
Day 2 Cluster 1	FT8, FC2, E11, CP2, CP6, PO10	3.15	0.006
Day 3 Cluster 1	FT8, E11, T8, CP6	3.11	0.020
Day 4 Cluster 1	AF3, F3, Fz	3.21	0.038
Day 4 vs. Day 1 Actual Cluster 1	FC1, Cz, E19	3.23	0.020
M1 stimulation *Actual vs. Sham* Day 1 Cluster 1	FC5, FC1, T7, Cz, C4, T8, E19, CP2, P7, Pz, P8, PO10	2.82	0.004
Day 3 Cluster 1	E5, T8, Cz, CP5, CP2, CP6, P7, Pz	2.27	0.020
Cluster 2	E5, FC2, C4, CP6	2.35	0.028
ALPHA (8–12 Hz)			
DLPFC stimulation *Actual vs. Sham* Day 2 Cluster 1	E5, FT8, E11, T8	2.85	0.008
Cluster 2	AF3, F7, F3	2.69	0.042
Day 4 Cluster 1	Pz, P8, Oz	2.74	0.048
Day 4 vs. Day 1 Actual Cluster 1	FC5, T7, CP5, P7	−3.12	0.032
M1 stimulation *Actual vs. Sham* Day 1 Cluster 1	F3, Fz, FC5, FC1, FC2, Cz	2.88	0.014
Day 3 Cluster 1	FC5, T7, CP5, P7	2.66	0.034

Reported t-values are the average t-statistic across all electrodes in a given cluster.
**Reported p-values are corrected for multiple comparisons using cluster-based permutation tests.*

comparing MFT revealed a significant main effect of day of training [$F_{(3, 48)} = 3.23$, $p = 0.048$]; however no significant or trend-level pairwise comparisons were found, There was no main effect of tDCS group or interaction between group and day of training.

Alpha (8–12 Hz)

DLPFC stimulation. Alpha-band power differences between DLPFC stim and sham groups were found in days 2 and 4 (**Table 3**). In day 2, frontal alpha power was greater in DLPFC stim than sham participants. In day 4, differences existed in parietal and occipital electrode sites, with DLPFC stim greater than sham. Differences between day 1 and 4 were found only for the DLPFC stim group, characterized by reduced alpha power at left temporoparietal sites (see **Table 3** and **Figure 8B**).

M1 stimulation. Greater alpha-band power was found for M1 stim compared to sham participants in days 1 and 3 (**Table 3**). These differences were distributed over frontal, central, and parietal electrode sites, mostly near the site of stimulation. No differences in alpha power were found in the comparison of days 1 and 4, for either M1 stim or M1 sham (see **Table 3** and **Figure 8B**).

EEG/fNIRS/behavioral correlations

We did not find any significant correlations between MFT or alpha power in the N-Back task and behavioral measures (i.e., average N level achieved and online/offline learning rates, p's > 0.05). No correlations were identified between fNIRS beta values and either MFT or alpha power in the N-Back task for any group (p's > 0.1).

Easy Landing Task

G-Force

DLPFC stimulation

tDCS to DLPFC reduced the variability (standard deviation) of the third and fourth day online learning rates compared to sham (DLPFC stim: day 3 = 0.355, day 4 = 0.583; DLPFC sham: day 3 = 0.846, day 4 = 0.637, see **Figure 5**). First trial comparisons of variance between DLPFC stim and DLPFC sham groups in day 3 showed statistically significant changes in between-subject variance [$F_{(4, 5)} = 0.046$, $p < 0.02$]. There were no significant differences in variance for first trials of day 1 and day 2 ($p > 0.1$). Trial 1 of day 4 also did not show significant changes in variance ($p > 0.1$). Examined across days, Bartlett's comparisons of variance between DLPFC stim and DLPFC sham groups in day 3 showed statistically significant changes in between-subject variance [$Chi_{(1)} = 7.33$, $p < 0.01$]. There were no significant differences in variance for days 1, 2, or 4 ($p > 0.1$). These results support the hypothesis that tDCS of the right DLPFC would reduce the variability in individual learning rates in the easy landing task.

Learning rates were determined by computing the rates at which performance improved (i.e., reduction of G Force over time, see **Figures 5A–D**). Meta-learning regressions did not show statistically significant changes in learning rates between stim and sham groups. The DLPFC stim group exhibited positive meta-learning rates (DLPFC stim = 0.052 ± 0.090), where the DLPFC sham group, by contrast, showed overall negative meta-learning (DLPFC sham = −0.051 ± 0.106), but this between-group difference did not reach statistical significance due to large within -group variance ($p > 0.1$; **Figure 5E**).

There were also no statistically significant differences in offline learning rates (p's > 0.1), but DLPFC stim showed a relatively strong offline learning between day 1 and 2 (−0.149 ± 0.52) compared to sham (0.124 ± 0.990).

The number of missed landings (did not land before or during the runway) was not different across groups over days (DLPFC stim: day 1: 2.9%, day 2: 2.9%, day 3: 0%, day 4: 0%; DLPFC sham:

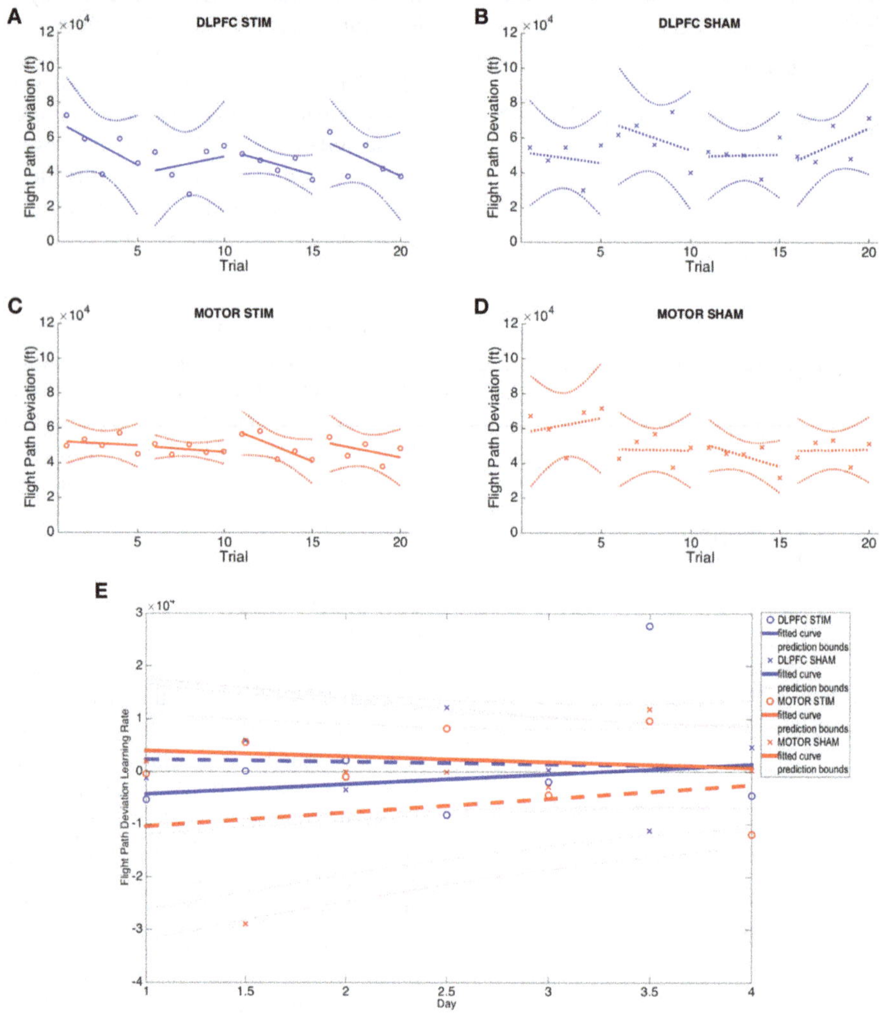

FIGURE 6 | Flight path deviation results across all four experimental groups. (A–D) Average flight path deviation of subjects from ideal autopilot-guided glide slope is shown for each group. **(E)** Online and offline flight path deviation learning rates are plotted for each experimental group across the duration of the experiment. Whole numbers on the x-axis represent the average online learning rate (slope of scaled percent correct linear regression for each subject across 6 blocks within a day) and ½ numbers on the x-axis represent offline learning rate (slope of the percent correct on the last trials of the N-1 day to the first trial of the Nth day). Reduced flight path deviation indicates improved performance.

day 1: 2.9%, day 2: 14.3%, day 3: 5.7%, day 4: 0%). Missed landings typically occurred on the first trial of the day.

M1 stimulation

tDCS to M1 resulted in no significant changes in inter-subject variance when compared to the M1 sham group across days (Bartlett's Test, *p*'s > 0.1). M1 sham appeared to have unusually low variance during day 2 (**Figure 3D**), and this was determined to be a statistically significant reduction of variance when compared to the M1 stim group for three of the five trials of Day 2 [$F_{(8,\,7)} = 6.32$, $F_{(8,\,7)} = 3.86$, $F_{(8,\,7)} = 5.07$; $p < 0.05$]. However, this reduction in variance only applied to Day 2 and in single trials only in Day 1 and 3. All trials on Day 4 had no significant change between M1 stim and sham variances. There were no statistically significant changes in learning rates between stim and sham groups (Supplementary Table S2). As with DLPFC stim group, there were also no statistically significant differences in offline learning rates (*p*'s > 0.1), but M1 stim showed a relatively strong offline learning between day 1 and 2 (−0.235 ± 0.676) compared to sham (0.258 ± 1.330).

Initial starting (day 1 average), group averaged (across all days and the final (day 4 average) G-forces were not significantly different between experimental and control groups (paired *t*-test $p > 0.1$), which are similar to the results found with the N-back task. Though performance improved in both sham and stimulation cohorts (reduced overall G-force), the ultimate performance of each subject group was similar. It is probable that the landing task was effectively learned over the course of four training days, and subjects reached a G-force performance ceiling.

The number of missed landings were not different across groups over days (M1 stim: day 1: 10%, day 2: 10%, day 3: 2.0%, day 4: 0%; M1 sham: day 1: 0%, day 2: 0%, day 3: 0%, day 4: 2.5%).

3D Autopilot Displacement

No group (DLPFC stim/sham nor M1 stim/sham) exhibited statistically significant learning (i.e., reduction of flight path displacement over time), as inter-subject variability was very high for this metric (**Figures 6A–D**). All groups showed inconsistent positive and negative learning slopes, and though the M1 stim group had negative online learning slopes for all 4 days, none of these reached statistical significance (p's>0.1). When comparing group variances for 3D autopilot displacement over experiment days, the M1 stim group showed greater variance compared with the M1 sham group during Day 1 [$Chi_{(1)} = 8.46$, $p < 0.01$]. The variance for the M1 stim group, however, was significantly lower than that of DLPFC stim group for 3 trials across 3 days of training [Day 1, Trial 1: $F_{(5, 9)} = 5.1032$; Day 2, Trial 4: $F_{(6, 9)} = 6.03$; Day 3 Trial 2: $F_{(6, 7)} = 3.99$; $p < 0.05$]. Interestingly, this was also true for M1 sham vs. DLPFC stim [Day 1, Trial 1: $F_{(5, 7)} = 13.67$; Day 2 Trial 4: $F_{(6, 7)} = 4.74$; $p < 0.001$]. No other variance comparisons yielded statistically significant results (Supplementary Table S2, **Figure 6**). While the combined learning intercept for the M1 sham group was negative (-13140 ± 13300, $p < 0.05$) this resulted from an isolated day 1/2 offline learning rate with a large standard deviation (-29011 ± 41147).

Vertical Speed Variance

The M1 stim group exhibited the lowest average values of vertical speed variance on the final day of training (4.955 ± 0.433; Supplementary Figure S2C). This is similar to the M1 sham (Supplementary Figure S2D) value of 5.051 ± 0.502 and an improvement over DLPFC groups (5.684 ± 0.690 and 5.647 ± 0.718, for stim and sham groups, respectively, but this does not reach significance under 2-way ANOVA ($p > 0.1$; Supplementary Figures S2A,B). This appears to be derived from the relatively higher online/offline learning rates in both M1 groups as compared with the DLPFC groups, though the overall rates were not statistically significant. ANCOVA, covarying the learning rates of vertical speed variance with group identity, performed on this data shows that the slopes appear identical ($p > 0.9$ vs. null hypothesis) but the initial performance (intercept) approaches significance ($p < 0.07$).

Online, offline and meta-learning rates were largely flat, and training effects were not observes within any group (p's < 0.1 level (Supplementary Table S2, Supplementary Figure S2). Because vertical speed variation is primarily a motor-centric task, it may be subject to a different learning curve that was not specifically measured during this study.

Autopilot Vertical Speed Deviation

M1 sham showed significant overall offline learning, with smaller deviations of vertical speed on Day 4 as compared with Day 1 (-12.21 ± 2.51, $p < 0.05$, Supplementary Figure S3D). DLPFC sham (Supplementary Figure S3B) also had a negative slope indicating reduced deviation from ideal vertical speeds, but this was not statistically significant (-69.71 ± 952.145, $p > 0.05$). However, both of these offline learning effects were washed out when combined into overall learning rates across the 4 days (M1 sham: -5.98 ± 20.26; DLPFC sham: -17.09 ± 25.80). Overall performance did not significantly change over the course of the 4 days, and initial/final performance were not significantly different across groups (p's > 0.1; Supplementary Figure S3E).

Unlike tests of G-force and flight path deviation, F-tests do not show any significant difference for inter-subject variance during 1st trial comparisons across all groups (p's > 0.1).

Number of Control Inputs

Variance between subjects for both DLPFC groups appeared larger than that of both M1 groups (Supplementary Figure S1). However, no meta, online, offline, or combined learning rates reach significance, and no significant changes were observed between groups (see Supplementary Table S2 and Supplementary Figure S1).

fNIRS Results

DLPFC Stimulation

Hboxy

Average Hboxy concentrations across subjects and channels significantly decreased between days 1 and 4 in M1 channels for the DLPFC stim and DLPFC sham groups, and decreased between days 1 and 4 in DLPFC channels for the DLPFC stim group (see **Table 2**, **Figure 7**).

Furthermore, individual channel analysis revealed that only two subjects (S7 in the DLPFC stim group, and S7 in the DLPFC sham group) showered a significant change in Hboxy concentrations from days 1 to 4 (−0.01 mM decrease at DLPFC channel: source AFF6h to detector F4 in DLPFC stim subject 7, and 0.02 mM increase at DLPFC channel: source FC4 to detector FFC4h in DLPFC sham subject 7, see **Figure 2** for channel locations). Within the DLPFC stim group, of all 70 channels measured across subjects in the DLPFC region (10 channels per subject, 7 subjects per group) 65 showed a decrease in Hboxy concentration from days 1 to 4 (compared to 40/70, 33/60, 325/50 for DLPFC sham, M1 stim, and M1 sham respectively).

Hbdeoxy

The average Hbdeoxy concentration across subjects and channels within M1 significantly increased between day 1 and day 4 in the DLPFC stim and DLPFC sham groups (see **Table 2**). Individual channel analysis shows no significant change in Hbdeoxy concentrations from days 1 to 4.

Hbtot

Average Hbtot concentrations across subjects and channels significantly decreased between days 1 and 4 in M1 channels for DLPFC stim and in the DLPFC channels for the DLPFC sham, and increased in M1 channels for the DLPFC sham group (see **Table 2**). Individual channel analysis revealed that only one subject (S7 in the DLPFC stim group) showed a significant change in Hbtot concentrations from days 1 to 4 (−0.01 mM decrease at DLPFC channel: source AFF6h to detector F4, see **Figure 2**). Within the DLPFC stim group 64/70 channels in the DLPFC region showed a decrease in Hbtot concentration from

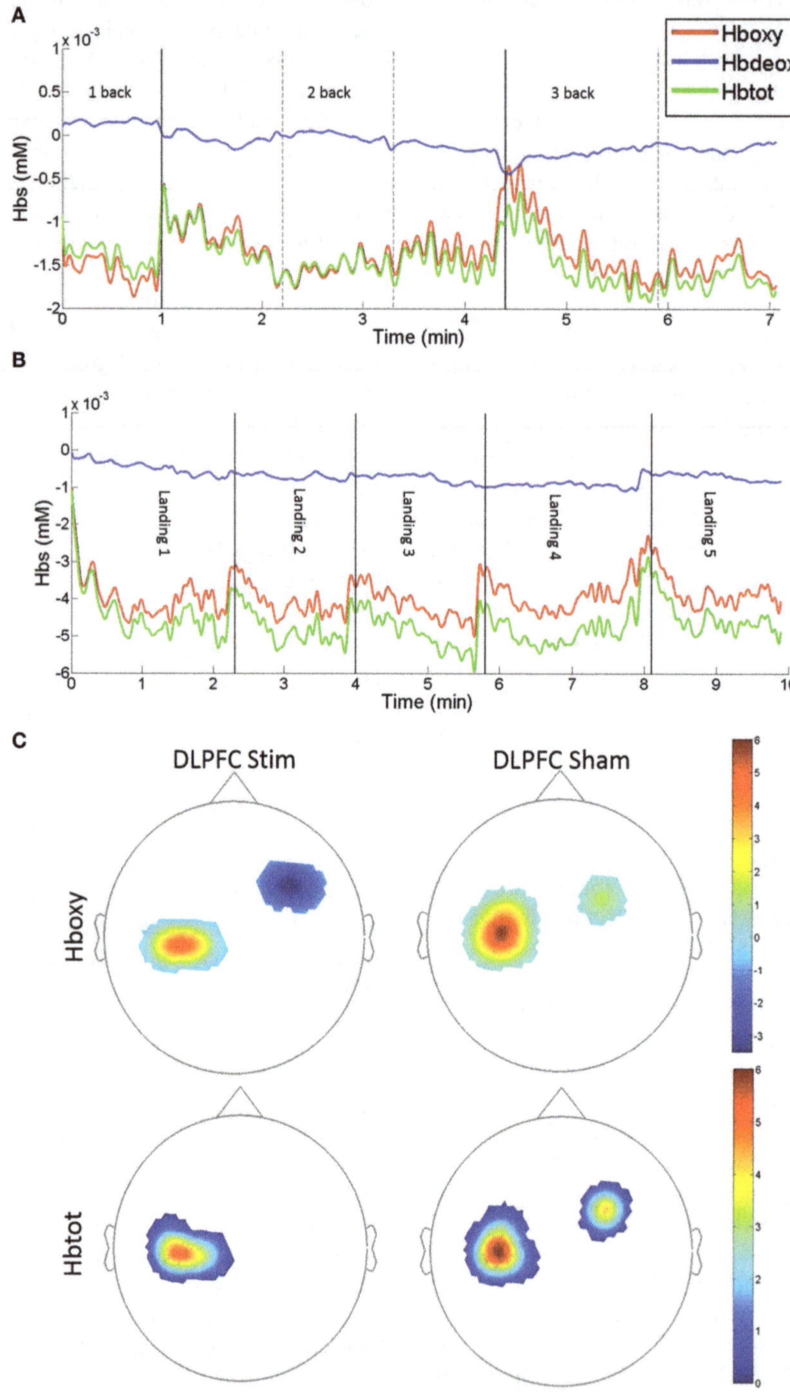

FIGURE 7 | Example fNIRS Hboxy, Hbdeoxy, and Hbtot concentration time-series and group average t-statistic beta maps. (A) N-back concentration time series for DLPFC sham subject #S6 recorded on day 1. Traces denote DLPFC channel #10: source: FC4, detector: F4. **(B)** Easy landing blocked concentration time series for DLPFC stim subject #S1 recorded on day 1. Traces denote DLPFC channel #5: source FFC6h, detector: F4 [vertical solid and dotted lines denote blocks, solid lines indicate 1/2 and 2/3-back block types in **(A)**, and easy landing trials in **(B)**]. An upward displacement in Hboxy and Hbtot concentrations can be seen during pauses between subsequent blocks. **(C)** fNIRS t-statistic beta maps of Day 4 vs. Day 1 Hboxy (top) and Hbtot (bottom) in the Easy landing task. Images are the averages for the DLPFC stim (left) and DLPFC sham (right) groups (Bonferroni corrected $p < 0.0025$, see **Table 2** for the corresponding concentration changes averaged over all channels within M1 and DLPFC).

days 1 to 4 (compared to 37/70, 34/60, 32/50 for DLPFC sham, M1 stim, and M1 sham respectively).

M1 Stimulation

Hboxy

Average Hboxy concentrations across subjects and channels significantly decreased between days 1 and 4 in M1 channels for the M1 stim group, and increased within M1 channels for the M1 sham group (see **Table 2**). Individual channel analysis shows no significant change in Hboxy concentrations from days 1 to 4.

Hbdeoxy

Average Hbdeoxy concentrations across subjects and channels significantly decreased between days 1 and 4 in M1 channels for the M1 stim group, and increased within M1 channels for the M1 sham group (see **Table 2**). Individual channel analysis shows no significant change in Hbdeoxy concentrations from days 1 to 4.

Hbtot

The average Hbtot concentration across subjects and channels significantly increased between days 1 and 4 in M1 channels for the M1 sham group (see **Table 2**). Individual channel analysis shows no significant change in Hbtot concentrations from days 1 to 4.

EEG

Theta (4–7 Hz)

DLPFC stimulation

In each day, significant differences in theta-band power were found between DLPFC stim and sham groups in frontal/central electrodes (**Table 4**). In days 1 and 3, right frontotemporal theta power was higher in DLPFC stim participants. Statistical differences were more broadly distributed in days 2 and 4, encompassing bilateral frontotemporal and midline frontal electrode sites. Comparison of days 1 and 4 revealed a significant increase in midline frontal theta-band power in DLPFC stim, but not DLPFC sham participants (see **Figure 8A** and **Table 4**). Split-plot ANOVA comparing MFT in the easy landing task revealed a significant main effect, with DLPFC stim greater than DLPFC sham [$F_{(1,\,12)} = 4.86, p = 0.048$]. Additionally, an interaction was found between group and day of training [$F_{(3,\,36)} = 4.54, p = 0.014$]. Simple-effects comparisons revealed increased MFT in stim compared to sham for only day 4 [day 4: $F_{(1,\,12)} = 6.47, p = 0.026$]. Simple-effect of day within the DLPFC stim group reached trend-level significance [$F_{(3,\,16)} = 3.15, p = 0.087$].

M1 stimulation

Theta-band differences between M1 groups during the easy landing task were found only in day 3, and were restricted to central/parietal electrodes (**Table 4**). Broadly-distributed differences in theta-band power were seen between days 1 and 4 in M1 stim participants, but not M1 sham participants (see **Table 4** and **Figure 8A**). No main effects or interactions were found in ANOVA comparing MFT in the easy landing task between M1 groups.

TABLE 4 | Cluster statistics for comparisons of alpha- and theta-band power during the Easy Landing task.

	Electrodes	t^*	p^{**}
THETA (4–7 Hz)			
DLPFC stimulation *Actual vs. Sham* Day 1 Cluster 1	E5, FT8, C4, CP6	2.58	0.024
Day 2 Cluster 1	AF3, F3, E5, FT8, FC1, FC2, E11, T7, Cz, C4, T8, E19, CP2, CP6	3.51	0.020
Day 3 Cluster 1	FT8, E11, T8, CP6	2.99	0.008
Day 4 Cluster 1	AF3, F3, FT8, FC1, FC2, E11, Cz, C4, T8, CP5, CP2, CP6, Pz, P8, Oz	3.81	0.002
Day 4 vs. Day 1 Actual Cluster 1	AF3, F3	3.23	0.044
M1 stimulation *Actual vs. Sham* Day 3 Cluster 1	Cz, CP2, CP5, P7, Pz	2.72	0.030
Day 4 vs. Day 1 Actual Cluster 1	F7, E5, FC5, FC1, T7, C4, CP5, E19, CP2, CP6, P7, Pz, P8, Oz, PO10	3.28	0.002
ALPHA (8–12 Hz)			
DLPFC stimulation *Actual vs. Sham* Day 1 Cluster 1	CP2, CP6, Pz, Oz	2.85	0.030
Day 4 Cluster 1	E5, FT8, Fz, FC2, E11, C4, T8	2.73	0.026
Cluster 2	FT8, E11, T8	3.56	0.040
Cluster 3	AF3, F3, Fz	2.94	0.048
M1 stimulation *Actual vs. Sham* Day 1 Cluster 1	F3, E5, Fz, FC5, FC1, FC2, C4, CP2, CP5, CP6	2.85	0.014
Day 4 vs. Day 1 Actual Cluster 1	CP5, E19, Pz	2.89	0.034
Cluster 2	E11, T8	−2.62	0.050

*Reported t-values are the average t-statistic across all electrodes in a given cluster.
**Reported p-values are corrected for multiple comparisons using cluster-based permutation tests.

Alpha (8–12 Hz)

DLPFC stimulation

Significant differences in alpha-band power were found between DLPFC stim and sham groups in parietal/occipital electrodes (day 1) and frontal/central electrodes (day 3), with greater power in the DLPFC stim group (**Table 4**). No differences in alpha power were found in the comparison of day 1 and 4, for either DLPFC stim or sham groups (see **Table 4** and **Figure 8B**).

M1 stimulation

Alpha-band differences between M1 groups during the easy landing task were found only in day 1, and were broadly distributed over frontal, central, and parietal electrode sites

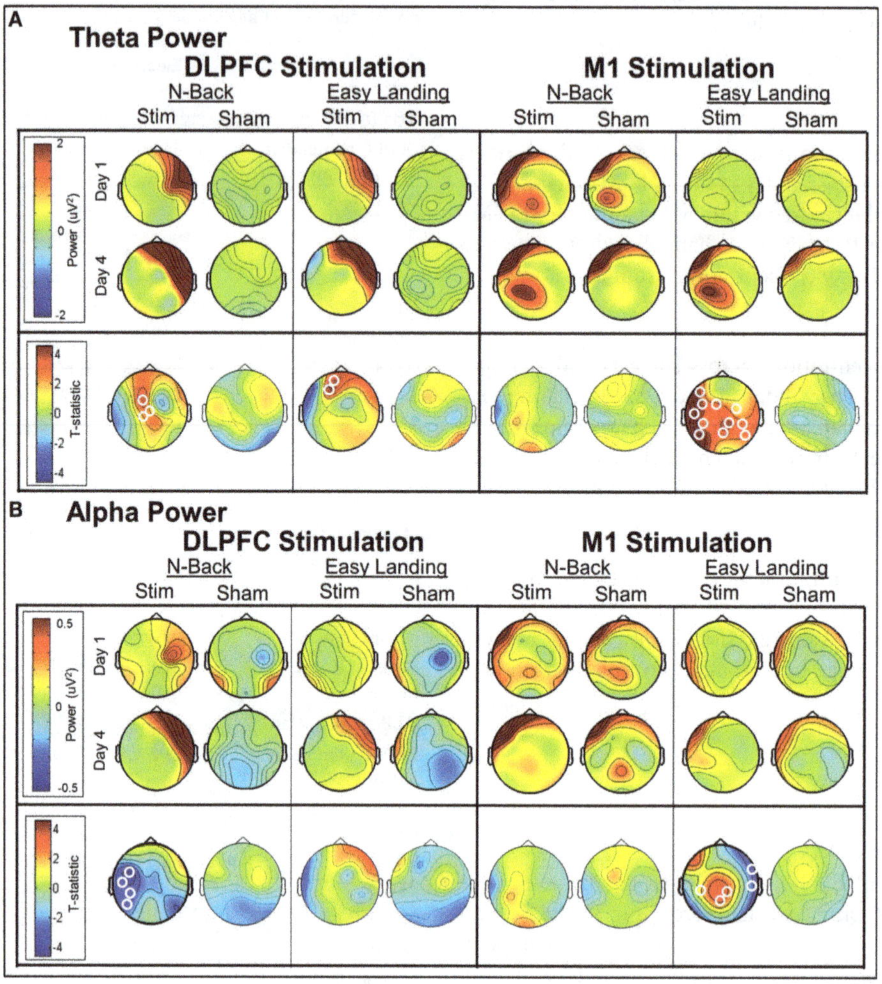

FIGURE 8 | Day 4 vs. day 1 average theta power (A) and alpha power (B) changes per group (t-statistic maps). Significant electrode clusters are depicted by white circles at electrode locations. Increases in midline frontal theta power were seen between days 1 and 4 in both tasks for all groups; however, cluster-level significance between days was found only for the DLPFC stim group. Decreased alpha power was found between days 1 and 4 for DLPFC stim in the N-Back task, where cluster-level significance was found in left temporoparietal electrodes. For M1 stimulation, cluster-level increases in central/parietal alpha and broadly-distributed theta power were found in the Easy Landing task.

(**Table 4**). Two separate clusters of significant differences in alpha-band power were seen between days 1 and 4 for M1 stim participants, but not M1 sham participants (see **Table 4** and **Figure 8B**). The first cluster revealed increased alpha power in the M1 stim group over parietal electrode sites. The second revealed decreased alpha power in right temporal electrodes.

EEG/fNIRS/behavioral correlations

There were positive correlations between change in MFT power (day 4 minus day 1) and both average Hbtot and average Hboxy beta values in DLPFC channels for M1 stim subjects. The direction of this correlation indicates that increased theta from days 1 to 4 is correlated with less reduction of Hboxy/Hbtot from days 1 to 4 in DLPFC fNIRS channels (**Table 5**). There were also strong negative correlations between change in alpha power and both average Hbtot and average Hboxy beta values in M1 channels for M1 stim subjects, indicating that increased parietal alpha power is correlated with reduced fNIRS beta values. No correlations were identified between theta/alpha power and fNIRS beta values for sham groups, there was no correlation between theta and fNIRS beta values at M1 channels, and there was no correlation between alpha power and fNIRS beta values at DLPFC channels (p's > 0.1).

DISCUSSION

Overview

In this study, we measured task-evoked changes in functional neural activity and the modulation of learning from tDCS to the right DLPFC or left M1. Simultaneous fNIRS and EEG measured changes in neural activity as subjects learned to complete flight simulator and n-back training exercises at increasing levels of expertise across four daily consecutive sessions. Assessment of

TABLE 5 | Significant correlations among EEG, fNIRS, and behavioral results in the Easy Landing task, for the M1 stim group.

	r	*p*
SIGNIFICANT EEG/BEHAVIOR CORRELATIONS		
Day 2	0.66	0.038
Online Learning		
MFT × Number of control inputs		
MFT × autopilot displacement	0.85	0.002
MFT × VSDFA	0.84	0.002
MFT × vertical speed variance	0.84	0.002
Offline learning	−0.85	0.002
MFT × autopilot displacement		
MFT × VSDFA	−0.85	0.002
MFT × vertical speed variance	−0.85	0.002
Day 4	−0.70	0.025
Online Learning		
Broadly-Distributed Theta Power × VSDFA		
Central/Parietal Alpha Power × VSDFA	−0.85	0.002
SIGNIFICANT EEG/fNIRS CORRELATIONS (DAY 4–DAY 1)		
MFT × Hbtot	0.82	0.045
MFT × Hboxy	0.81	0.051
Parietal Alpha Power × Hbtot	−0.95	0.005
Parietal Alpha Power × Hboxy	−0.94	0.005

VSDFA, Vertical Speed Deviance from Autopilot.

TABLE 6 | Summary of behavioral and neurophysiological results.

Group	N-Back	G-force	fNIRS	EEG
DLPFC Stim	- Variance	- Variance	- Hboxy and Hbtot in the DLPFC (flight only)	+ MFT power (N-back and flight)
M1 Stim				+ Parietal Alpha power (flight only)

behavioral performances were performed on n-back accuracy, flight metrics of landing performance, as well as for online and offline learning rates associated with practice and skill acquisition. We report that tDCS to the right DLPFC reduced the variability in online learning across individuals in the n-back task, and in g-force on the easy landing task. This was associated with decreased Hboxy and Hbtot in the DLFPC across days for the landing task, and increased MFT power in both the n-back and landing tasks. Additionally, tDCS to the left M1 increased tonic parietal alpha power, which was correlated with changes in Hboxy and Hbtot at M1 fNIRS channels.

Interpretation—Behavior

The observed reduction in group variability in online learning may be attributed to "convergence to the mean" (i.e., increasing online learning rates of low performing individuals and reducing online learning rates of high performing individuals). Subjects may have employed distinct cognitive and behavioral strategies, with correspondingly different brain networks, to complete and learn the n-back task across sessions. tDCS of the right DLPFC may have therefore facilitated the deployment and consolidation of a particular strategy in some subjects, and inhibited certain behaviors in others. The variance in the learning rates did not arise from individual differences of untrained performance, as initial and final performances were similar (see Section Behavioral Results). Furthermore, the results could indicate that all groups reached a ceiling of behavioral performance, or that our measures are under-powered to detect a change in performance statistically, or that a reduction in individual variability produced this observation.

The variability results reported for the easy-landing task were specific to DLPFC stim subjects for the g-force metric [a similar reduction in variance was not seen for the same data in the autopilot displacement (**Figure 6**), the number of control inputs (Supplementary Figure S1), the variability of vertical speed (Supplementary Figure S2), and the vertical speed deviation from autopilot (Supplementary Figure S3)]. Since both the initial and final g-force values were not significantly different across stim and sham groups, the reduction in DLPFC stim group variability implies a similar convergence to the mean phenomenon observed for n-back learning. tDCS of the DLPFC may therefore, facilitate the learning of a smoother landing procedure in subjects who would otherwise consolidated an incorrect landing procedure and increased landing g-forces in subsequent days. Likewise, tDCS of the DLPFC may have hindered some subjects who would have otherwise consolidated a superior landing procedure and decreased landing g-forces in subsequent days.

It should be noted that for the measure of 3D autopilot flight path deviation (Section 3D Autopilot Displacement), it was not readily apparent to subjects when the aircraft deviated from the prescribed flight path of the autopilot; there is no visual field indication that they are deviating from the glide slope, and the Flight Director instrument does not indicate degree of displacement from optimal glide slope. Additionally, for deviation from the autopilots vertical speed (Section Autopilot Vertical Speed Deviation) is possible that, because vertical speed was a peripheral skill required for landing (i.e., non-essential for a successful landing), subjects did not train to maintain a low vertical speed deviation from the reference glide path. As subjects needed only to maintain one constant vertical speed during the landing task, they may have reached maximal capacity to do so beginning from day 1. The combined learning rates and online learning metrics seem to support this view (see Supplementary Table S2, Supplementary Figure S3). Furthermore, low-G Force landings can be performed from a wide range of glide slopes, which can mask large deviations from the "ideal" flight path.

Interpretation—Neurophysiology

We observed an increase in MFT in the DLPFC stim group compared to the DLPFC sham group, as well as experience-related increase in MFT and decrease in central/parietal alpha in DLPFC stim, indicating increased working memory and attention (Klimesch et al., 1997; Jensen and Tesche, 2002; Ishii et al., 2014). Increased theta/alpha band activity in M1 stim compared to M1 sham near the site of stimulation may indicate greater motor cortex excitability (Sauseng et al., 2009). Furthermore, experience-related increases (day 4 vs. 1) in broad central/parietal theta/alpha in M1 stim during flight tasks implicate greater tactile/proprioceptive monitoring. For example, Baumeister et al. (2008) observed that increased parietal theta during goal-directed learning was associated with increased motor skill performance. Although MFT nor parietal alpha power increases were correlated with behavioral performance increases in this study, it is possible that increases in MFT or parietal alpha may be indirectly associated with cognitive performance enhancement. The significant correlations observed between MFT and online and offline learning of autopilot displacement, vertical speed variance and deviation in the M1 stim group support this hypothesis (**Table 5**).

We observed a decrease in Hboxy and Hbtot in DLPFC channels for the DLPFC stim group in the easy landing task (**Table 2** and results Hboxy and Hbtot). This evidence suggests that tDCS produced more efficient neural activation to consolidate the newly-learned procedural skills as has been previously reported (Wolf et al., 2007; Holland et al., 2011; Ayaz et al., 2012; DiStasio and Francis, 2013). Previous literature from McKendrick et al. (2015) suggest that some, but not all, of these changes may be related to the task performance enhancements associated with tDCS. However, changes in Hbtot concentration may also be related to task reward value (DiStasio and Francis, 2013), the recruitment of additional motor resources (Herff et al., 2013), or a behavioral ceiling effect where low-performing subjects were not able to advance to expert performance levels as shown by Ayaz et al. (2012). Although reward was not explicitly manipulated in the easy landing task, subject's motivations may have played a role based on their prior day's performance. Similarly, the motor resources required for the easy landing task may have changed as subjects learned more advanced motor programs to complete the task. Finally, a ceiling effect could explain the more efficient neural activation, and the trend in meta-learning for stim groups supports this theory (**Figure 5E**).

Hbtot and Hboxy were also significantly correlated with MFT from days 4 to 1 in the easy landing task in the M1 stim group. These results suggest that these separate neurophysiological measures are not totally independent. Future studies should examine the relationships between MFT, Hbtot, and behavioral performance in a larger cohort to determine whether these effects are truly concomitant.

Relation to Prior Investigations of tDCS in Real-World Tasks

To date, there have been few studies in which procedural/real world learning tasks have been tested with a tDCS intervention (Izzetoglu et al., 2014; Nelson et al., 2014), and even fewer with a significant motor component as the focus of performance/training enhancement (Zhu et al., 2015). However, tDCS enhancement of real-world skills has been reported for complex motor control tasks. For example, Beeli et al. (2008) reported that anodal tDCS to either the left or right DLPFC (10/20 EEG site F3 or F4) significantly improved the care of driving style as measures by following distance, average speed and number of errors. Similarly, Sakai et al. (2014) reported that anodal tDCS to the right DLPFC significantly improved car-following and lane-keeping performance in a driving simulator task across days. Finally, Zhu et al. (2015) reported that cathodal tDCS to the left DLPFC suppressed verbal working memory but improved motor learning. The results presented here support these findings, as we observed that tDCS to the right DLPFC reduced online learning variability in higher cognitive measures (e.g., affecting the g-force value of landing by judging multi-modal flight-data in a timely fashion, or n-back accuracy variance) more than those related motor planning or judgment (e.g., flight path deviation see **Table 6**).

Furthermore, real-world skill enhancement from right inferior frontal tDCS has been reported in a perceptual threat detection (Clark et al., 2012; Falcone et al., 2012), and tDCS of the DLPFC has been shown to increase regional cerebral blood oxygenation and behavioral performance in target detection in an air traffic control task (Nelson et al., 2014). The results presented here are indirectly related to these findings as the reduction in behavioral variance we observed from tDCS to the right DLPFC could be attributed to increase in spatial attention, vigilance, or perceptual discrimination (e.g., when to judge an n-back match or the correct time for a nose-flare maneuver during landing). We also observed that tDCS of the right DLPFC decreased Hboxy and Hbtot in DLFPC channels across days in the easy landing task. One possible explanation for the difference reported in cerebral blood oxygenation between the two studies concerns the disparate experimental designs employed. Here, all subjects returned for four consecutive days of testing, regardless of physiological or behavioral measures, whereas Nelson et al. (2014) had subjects return for days 2–4 only if performance and blood flow velocity declined over the course of the first 40-min session.

Relation to Prior Investigations of tDCS in Working Memory

Previous studies have reported evidence that working memory improvements are correlated with the administration of tDCS in diverse contexts (Grafman et al., 1994; Nitsche et al., 2003; Dockery et al., 2009; McKendrick et al., 2015). Specifically, tDCS over DLPFC was associated with acute increases in working memory accuracy (Stagg and Johansen-Berg, 2013; Chhatbar and Feng, 2015; De Putter et al., 2015; Santarnecchi et al., 2015). Although, we observed a reduction in learning rate variance from tDCS to the right DLPFC in the n-back task, but did not find an increase in working memory accuracy for tDCS of either the DLPFC or M1. This discrepancy may be attributed to the adaptive n-back design employed here, the long durations of experimental sessions, and a potential ceiling effect from repeated tDCS and n-back sessions across consecutive days. In addition, the application of tDCS began directly prior to the n-back task (see **Figure 1**) and the effects of stimulation may require more time to produce the reported improvements in n-back accuracy.

Limitations and Future Directions

A goal of this research was to determine if tDCS stimulation would improve training techniques for pilots in a flight simulator.

Such improvements could drastically reduce time and therefore the cost of training a pilot, as it would in any training environment. While our results show decreased variability in training, it is too early to confirm or deny any useful improvements to simulation training until an understanding of the sources and contributing factors to the observed behavioral variance is achieved.

Additional studies must be performed to further investigate n-back accuracy improvement with tDCS by comparing different stimulation montages, stimulation timing, and task paradigms. Because we were unable to parametrically manipulate these parameters in this study, we are unable to determine which of these factors may have led to null effects of tDCS on n-back accuracy. The baseline performance of individuals with differing initial skill levels in n-back and flight tasks are important, and measures of this were limited by the study design employed. In addition, the experimental design employed here (continuous, multiple tasks over 60 min duration) did not provide a sufficient means to control the endogenous brain state of subjects before and throughout the experimental session given the numerous tasks, and instructions and feedback required for subjects to perform them. Thus, subject's diverse experiences and resultant brain states throughout the session may be a significant factor in the interpretation of our findings. For example, the n-back task was performed near the beginning of the stimulation period, while the easy flight landing was performed near the end of the stimulation period. Future studies should examine relationships between tDCS effects and EEG microstates and/or brain metabolic activity.

Some of the null findings in this study were related to exceptionally high within-group variance. One potential method to examine within and across group behavioral variance is to categorize subjects by learning rate bins or perform a cluster analysis of tDCS responders and non-responders. Since the same tDCS protocol may have variable effects across individuals, possibly due to neuroanatomical and neurophysiological differences, and that the same tDCS protocol may produce different effects within an individual over time, due to changes resulting from neural plasticity, the absence of *post-hoc* categorization of subjects likely reduces the statistical power and interpretability of our results (e.g., Supplementary Table S2). Future studies may benefit from real-time assessments and individualized tDCS planning rather than a "one size fits all" approach. While a priori selection or *post-hoc* classification of subjects within experimental groups can control for differences in baseline performance levels, it is not realistic when transferring this technology into real-world training environments.

The high variability between subjects and the need for personalized training becomes more important when we recognize the subject pool for this experiment all fit the western, educated, industrialized, rich and democratic (WEIRD) population. Although this population of subjects for the experiment goal of pilot training was acceptable, we speculate that the inclusion of a wider demographic range of the world populous may produce an even larger variability in behavioral performance. Therefore, a systematic understanding of the sources and contributing factors to the observed behavioral variance is extremely important for the application of tDCS across a wider range of subjects.

CONCLUSIONS

The results presented here underscore the importance of developing the understanding to identify and optimize neurostimulation protocols. Our results suggest that the time course of both online and offline learning is critical for the observed changes in working memory and procedural flight performance. Repeated training sessions reveal time-dependent factors regarding the interaction between tDCS and the learning processes that remain unclear in the literature. Applying such interventions in the real-world will require a much larger investment than initially anticipated in order for the scientific community to measure and catalog the precise behavioral, learning, and neurophysiological changes resulting from each component of procedural skill acquisition. Because there appears to be a differential, region-based effect of neurostimulation interventions, it is critical to determine the optimal targets, stimulation parameters, timing relative to the target behaviors, and synchrony between innate learning processes and strategies and exogenous stimulation for maximally-effective augmentation.

AUTHOR CONTRIBUTIONS

JC, MZ, and MP designed the experiments; JC and DB performed the experiments; JC, BC, and MP analyzed the data; and JC, BC, and MP wrote the manuscript.

REFERENCES

Ayaz, H., Çakır, M. P., Ýzzetoğlu, K., Curtin, A., Shewokis, P., Bunce, S. C., et al. (2012). "Monitoring expertise development during simulated UAV piloting tasks using optical brain imaging," in *Aerospace Conference, 2012 IEEE* (Big Sky, MT: IEEE), 1–11.

Ayaz, H., Onaral, B., Izzetoglu, K., Shewokis, P. A., McKendrick, R., and Parasuraman, R. (2013). Continuous monitoring of brain dynamics with functional near infrared spectroscopy as a tool for neuroergonomic research: empirical examples and a technological development. *Front. Hum. Neurosci.* 7:871. doi: 10.3389/fnhum.2013.00871

Ball, K., Berch, D. B., Helmers, K. F., Jobe, J. B., Leveck, M. D., Marsiske, M., et al. (2002). Effects of cognitive training interventions with older adults: a randomized controlled trial. *JAMA* 288, 2271–2281. doi: 10.1001/jama.288.18.2271

Banissy, M. J., and Muggleton, N. G. (2013). Transcranial direct current stimulation in sports training: potential approaches. *Front. Hum. Neurosci.* 7:129. doi: 10.3389/fnhum.2013.00129

Baumeister, J., Reinecke, K., Liesen, H., and Weiss, M. (2008). Cortical activity of skilled performance in a complex sports related motor task. *Eur. J. Appl. Physiol.* 104, 625–631. doi: 10.1007/s00421-008-0811-x

Beeli, G., Koeneke, S., Gasser, K., and Jancke, L. (2008). Brain stimulation modulates driving behavior. *Behav. Brain Funct.* 4:34. doi: 10.1186/1744-9081-4-34

Been, G., Ngo, T. T., Miller, S. M., and Fitzgerald, P. B. (2007). The use of tDCS and CVS as methods of non-invasive brain stimulation. *Brain Res. Rev.* 56, 346–361. doi: 10.1016/j.brainresrev.2007.08.001

Bell, H. H., and Waag, W. L. (1998). Evaluating the effectiveness of flight simulators for training combat skills: a review. *Int. J. Aviat. Psychol.* 8, 223–242. doi: 10.1207/s15327108ijap0803_4

Bikson, M., Datta, A., and Elwassif, M. (2009). Establishing safety limits for transcranial direct current stimulation. *Clin. Neurophysiol.* 120, 1033–1034. doi: 10.1016/j.clinph.2009.03.018

Blumberg, E. J., Foroughi, C. K., Scheldrup, M. R., Peterson, M. S., Boehm-Davis, D. A., and Parasuraman, R. (2014). Reducing the disruptive effects of interruptions with noninvasive brain stimulation. *Hum. Factors.* 57, 1051–1062. doi: 10.1177/0018720814565189

Boggio, P. S., Castro, L. O., Savagim, E. A., Braite, R., Cruz, V. C., Rocha, R. R., et al. (2006). Enhancement of non-dominant hand motor function by anodal transcranial direct current stimulation. *Neurosci. Lett.* 404, 232–236. doi: 10.1016/j.neulet.2006.05.051

Borghini, G., Astolfi, L., Vecchiato, G., Mattia, D., and Babiloni, F. (2014). Measuring neurophysiological signals in aircraft pilots and car drivers for the assessment of mental workload, fatigue and drowsiness. *Neurosci. Biobehav. Rev.* 44, 58–75. doi: 10.1016/j.neubiorev.2012.10.003

Braver, T. S., Cohen, J. D., Nystrom, L. E., Jonides, J., Smith, E. E., and Noll, D. C. (1997). A parametric study of prefrontal cortex involvement in human working memory. *Neuroimage* 5, 49–62. doi: 10.1006/nimg.1996.0247

Causse, M., Dehais, F., and Pastor, J. (2011). Executive funcitons and pilot characteristics predict flight simulator performance in general aviation pilots. *Int. J. Aviat. Psychol.* 21, 217–234. doi: 10.1080/10508414.2011.582441

Chhatbar, P. Y., and Feng, W. (2015). Data synthesis in meta-analysis may conclude differently on cognitive effect from transcranial direct current stimulation. *Brain Stimul.* 8, 974–976. doi: 10.1016/j.brs.2015.06.001

Choe, J., Coffman, B. A., Ziegler, M. D., Bhattacharyya, R., and Phillips, M. E. (2015). "tDCS modulates neuronal activity, dynamics and improves procedural learning and skill acquisition," in *Socity for Neuroscience Meeting* (Chicago, IL).

Chrysikou, E. G., Hamilton, R. H., Coslett, H. B., Datta, A., Bikson, M., and Thompson-Schill, S. L. (2013). Noninvasive transcranial direct current stimulation over the left prefrontal cortex facilitates cognitive flexibility in tool use. *Cogn. Neurosci.* 4, 81–89. doi: 10.1080/17588928.2013.768221

Clark, V. P., Coffman, B. A., Mayer, A. R., Weisend, M. P., Lane, T. D., Calhoun, V. D., et al. (2012). TDCS guided using fMRI significantly accelerates learning to identify concealed objects. *Neuroimage* 59, 117–128. doi: 10.1016/j.neuroimage.2010.11.036

Coffman, B. A., Clark, V. P., and Parasuraman, R. (2014). Battery powered thought: enhancement of attention, learning, and memory in healthy adults using transcranial direct current stimulation. *Neuroimage* 85, 895–908. doi: 10.1016/j.neuroimage.2013.07.083

Coffman, B. A., Trumbo, M. C., Flores, R. A., Garcia, C. M., Van Der Merwe, A. J., Wassermann, E. M., et al. (2012b). Impact of tDCS on performance and learning of target detection: interaction with stimulus characteristics and experimental design. *Neuropsychologia* 50, 1594–1602. doi: 10.1016/j.neuropsychologia.2012.03.012

Courtney, S. M., Ungerleider, L. G., Keil, K., and Haxby, J. V. (1996). Object and spatial visual working memory activate separate neural systems in human cortex. *Cereb. Cortex* 6, 39–49. doi: 10.1093/cercor/6.1.39

Cui, X., Bray, S., Bryant, D. M., Glover, G. H., and Reiss, A. L. (2011). A quantitative comparison of NIRS and fMRI across multiple cognitive tasks. *Neuroimage* 54, 2808–2821. doi: 10.1016/j.neuroimage.2010.10.069

Curtis, C. E., and D'Esposito, M. (2003). Persistent activity in the prefrontal cortex during working memory. *Trends Cogn. Sci.* 7, 415–423. doi: 10.1016/S1364-6613(03)00197-9

Datta, A., Baker, J. M., Bikson, M., and Fridriksson, J. (2011). Individualized model predicts brain current flow during transcranial direct-current stimulation treatment in responsive stroke patient. *Brain Stimul.* 4, 169–174. doi: 10.1016/j.brs.2010.11.001

Datta, A., Truong, D., Minhas, P., Parra, L. C., and Bikson, M. (2012). Inter-individual variation during transcranial direct current stimulation and normalization of dose using MRI-derived computational models. *Front. Psychiatry* 3:91. doi: 10.3389/fpsyt.2012.00091

Delorme, A., and Makeig, S. (2004). EEGLAB: an open source toolbox for analysis of single-trial EEG dynamics including independent component analysis. *J. Neurosci. Methods* 134, 9–21. doi: 10.1016/j.jneumeth.2003.10.009

Delorme, A., Palmer, J., Onton, J., Oostenveld, R., and Makeig, S. (2012). Independent EEG sources are dipolar. *PLoS ONE* 7:e30135. doi: 10.1371/journal.pone.0030135

De Putter, L. M., Vanderhasselt, M. A., Baeken, C., De Raedt, R., and Koster, E. H. (2015). Combining tDCS and working memory training to down regulate state rumination: a single-session double blind sham-controlled trial. *Cognit. Ther. Res.* 39, 754–765. doi: 10.1007/s10608-015-9710-8

Dismukes, R. K. (2008). "Prospective memory in aviation and everyday settings," in *Prospective Memory: Cognitive, Neuroscience, Developmental, and Applied Perspectives*, eds M. Kliegel, M. McDaniel, and G. Einstein (Florence, KY: Psychology Press), 411–428.

DiStasio, M. M., and Francis, J. T. (2013). Use of frontal lobe hemodynamics as reinforcement signals to an adaptive controller. *PLoS ONE* 8:e69541. doi: 10.1371/journal.pone.0069541

Dmochowski, J. P., Datta, A., Bikson, M., Su, Y., and Parra, L. C. (2011). Optimized multi-electrode stimulation increases focality and intensity at target. *J. Neural Eng.* 8:046011. doi: 10.1088/1741-2560/8/4/046011

Dockery, C. A., Hueckel-Weng, R., Birbaumer, N., and Plewnia, C. (2009). Enhancement of planning ability by transcranial direct current stimulation. *J. Neurosci.* 29, 7271–7277. doi: 10.1523/JNEUROSCI.0065-09.2009

Edwards, D., Cortes, M., Datta, A., Minhas, P., Wassermann, E. M., and Bikson, M. (2013). Physiological and modeling evidence for focal transcranial electrical brain stimulation in humans: a basis for high-definition tDCS. *Neuroimage* 74, 266–275. doi: 10.1016/j.neuroimage.2013.01.042

Engle, R. W. (2010). Role of working-memory capacity in cognitive control. *Curr. Anthrop* 51, S17–S26. doi: 10.1086/650572

Essenpreis, M., Elwell, C. E., Cope, M., Van der Zee, P., Arridge, S. R., and Delpy, D. T. (1993). Spectral dependence of temporal point spread functions in human tissues. *Appl. Opt.* 32, 418–425. doi: 10.1364/AO.32.000418

Falcone, B., Coffman, B. A., Clark, V. P., and Parasuraman, R. (2012). Transcranial direct current stimulation augments perceptual sensitivity and 24-hour retention in a complex threat detection task. *PLoS ONE* 7:e34993. doi: 10.1371/journal.pone.0034993

Faria, P., Hallett, M., and Miranda, P. C. (2011). A finite element analysis of the effect of electrode area and inter-electrode distance on the spatial distribution of the current density in tDCS. *J. Neural Eng.* 8:066017. doi: 10.1088/1741-2560/8/6/066017

Flöel, A., Rösser, N., Michka, O., Knecht, S., and Breitenstein, C. (2008). Noninvasive brain stimulation improves language learning. *J. Cogn. Neurosci.* 20, 1415–1422. doi: 10.1162/jocn.2008.20098

Gill, J., and Hamilton, R. (2014). Transfer of working memory performance enhancement induced by transcranial direct current stimulation (tDCS)(P3. 220). *Neurology* 82(10 Suppl.), P3–P220.

Grafman, J., Pascual-Leone, A., Alway, D., Nichelli, P., Gomez-Tortosa, E., and Hallett, M. (1994). Induction of a recall deficit by rapidrate transcranial magnetic stimulation. *Neuroreport* 5, 1157–1160. doi: 10.1097/00001756-199405000-00034

Hauser, T. U., Rotzer, S., Grabner, R. H., Mérillat, S., and Jäncke, L. (2013). Enhancing performance in numerical magnitude processing and mental arithmetic using transcranial Direct Current Stimulation (tDCS). *Front. Hum. Neurosci.* 7:244. doi: 10.3389/fnhum.2013.00244

Hays, R., Jacobs, J., Prince, C., and Salas, E. (1992). Flight simulator training effectiveness: a meta-analysis. *Military Psychol.* 4, 63. doi: 10.1207/s15327876mp0402_1

Heimrath, K., Sandmann, P., Becke, A., Müller, N. G., and Zaehle, T. (2012). Behavioral and electrophysiological effects of transcranial direct current stimulation of the parietal cortex in a visuo-spatial working memory task. *Front. Psychiatry* 3:56. doi: 10.3389/fpsyt.2012.00056

Herff, C., Heger, D., Fortmann, O., Hennrich, J., Putze, F., and Schultz, T. (2013). Mental workload during n-back task—quantified in the prefrontal cortex using fNIRS. *Front. Hum. Neurosci.* 7:935. doi: 10.3389/fnhum.2013.00935

Holland, R., Leff, A. P., Josephs, O., Galea, J. M., Desikan, M., Price, C. J., et al. (2011). Speech facilitation by left inferior frontal cortex stimulation. *Curr. Biol.* 21, 1403–1407. doi: 10.1016/j.cub.2011.07.021

Horvath, J. C., Forte, J. D., and Carter, O. (2015). Quantitative review finds no evidence of cognitive effects in healthy populations from single-session transcranial direct current stimulation (tDCS). *Brain Stimul.* 8, 535–550. doi: 10.1016/j.brs.2015.01.400

Ishii, R., Canuet, L., Ishihara, T., Aoki, Y., Ikeda, S., Hata, M., et al. (2014). Frontal midline theta rhythm and gamma power changes during focused attention on mental calculation: an MEG beamformer analysis. *Front. Hum. Neurosci.* 8:406. doi: 10.3389/fnhum.2014.00406

Izzetoglu, K., Ayaz, H., Hing, J. T., Shewokis, P. A., Bunce, S. C., Oh, P., et al. (2014). "UAV operators workload assessment by optical brain imaging technology (fNIR)," in *Handbook of Unmanned Aerial Vehicles*, eds K. P. Valavanis and G. J. Vachtsevanos (Dordrecht: Springer Netherlands), 2475–2500.

Jaeggi, S. M., Buschkuehl, M., Jonides, J., and Perrig, W. J. (2008). Improving fluid intelligence with training on working memory. *Proc. Natl. Acad. Sci. U.S.A.* 105, 6829–6833. doi: 10.1073/pnas.0801268105

Jensen, O., and Tesche, C. D. (2002). Frontal theta activity in humans increases with memory load in a working memory task. *Eur. J. Neurosci.* 15, 1395–1399. doi: 10.1046/j.1460-9568.2002.01975.x

Klimesch, W. (1999). EEG alpha and theta oscillations reflect cognitive and memory performance: a review and analysis. *Brain Res. Rev.* 29, 169–195. doi: 10.1016/S0165-0173(98)00056-3

Klimesch, W., Doppelmayr, M., Pachinger, T., and Ripper, B. (1997). Brain oscillations and human memory: EEG correlates in the upper alpha and theta band. *Neurosci. Lett.* 238, 9–12. doi: 10.1016/S0304-3940(97)00771-4

Koonce, J. M., and Bramble, W. J. Jr. (1998). Personal computer-based flight training devices. *Int. J. Aviat. Psychol.* 8, 277–292. doi: 10.1207/s15327108ijap0803_7

Lefebvre, S., Thonnard, J. L., Laloux, P., Peeters, A., Jamart, J., and Vandermeeren, Y. (2014). Single session of dual-tDCS transiently improves precision grip and dexterity of the paretic hand after stroke. *Neurorehabil. Neural Repair.* 28, 100–110. doi: 10.1177/1545968313478485

Manenti, R., Brambilla, M., Petesi, M., Ferrari, C., and Cotelli, M. (2013). Enhancing verbal episodic memory in older and young subjects after non-invasive brain stimulation. *Front. Aging Neurosci.* 5:49. doi: 10.3389/fnagi.2013.00049

Martin, D. M., Liu, R., Alonzo, A., Green, M., and Loo, C. K. (2014). Use of transcranial direct current stimulation (tDCS) to enhance cognitive training: effect of timing of stimulation. *Exp. Brain Res.* 232, 3345–3351. doi: 10.1007/s00221-014-4022-x

Maxwell, S. E., and Delaney, H. D. (2004). *Designing Experiments and Analyzing Data: A Model Comparison Perspective*, Vol. 1. Florence, KY: Psychology Press.

McIntire, L. K., McKinley, R. A., Goodyear, C., and Nelson, J. (2014). A comparison of the effects of transcranial direct current stimulation and caffeine on vigilance and cognitive performance during extended wakefulness. *Brain Stimul.* 7, 499–507. doi: 10.1016/j.brs.2014.04.008

McKendrick, R., Ayaz, H., Olmstead, R., and Parasuraman, R. (2014). Enhancing dual-task performance with verbal and spatial working memory training: continuous monitoring of cerebral hemodynamics with NIRS. *Neuroimage* 85, 1014–1026. doi: 10.1016/j.neuroimage.2013.05.103

McKendrick, R., Parasuraman, R., and Ayaz, H. (2015). Wearable functional near infrared spectroscopy (fNIRS) and transcranial direct current stimulation (tDCS): expanding vistas for neurocognitive augmentation. *Front. Syst. Neurosci.* 9:27. doi: 10.3389/fnsys.2015.00027

Mendonca, M. E., Santana, M. B., Baptista, A. F., Datta, A., Bikson, M., Fregni, F., et al. (2011). Transcranial DC stimulation in fibromyalgia: optimized cortical target supported by high-resolution computational models. *J. Pain* 12, 610–617. doi: 10.1016/j.jpain.2010.12.015

Meyers, K. (1979). Drug company employees as research subjects: programs, problems, and ethics. *IRB* 1, 5–6. doi: 10.2307/3564165

Miller, J., Berger, B., and Sauseng, P. (2015). Anodal transcranial direct current stimulation (tDCS) increases frontal-midline theta activity in the human EEG: a preliminary investigation of non-invasive stimulation. *Neurosci. Lett.* 588, 114–119. doi: 10.1016/j.neulet.2015.01.014

Moliadze, V., Antal, A., and Paulus, W. (2010). Electrode-distance dependent after-effects of transcranial direct and random noise stimulation with extracephalic reference electrodes. *Clin. Neurophysiol.* 121, 2165–2171. doi: 10.1016/j.clinph.2010.04.033

Nelson, J. T., McKinley, R. A., Golob, E. J., Warm, J. S., and Parasuraman, R. (2014). Enhancing vigilance in operators with prefrontal cortex transcranial direct current stimulation (tDCS). *Neuroimage* 85, 909–917. doi: 10.1016/j.neuroimage.2012.11.061

Nitsche, M. A., Schauenburg, A., Lang, N., Liebetanz, D., Exner, C., Paulus, W., et al. (2003). Facilitation of implicit motor learning by weak transcranial direct current stimulation of the primary motor cortex in the human. *J. Cogn. Neurosci.* 15, 619–626. doi: 10.1162/089892903321662994

Oostenveld, R., Fries, P., Maris, E., and Schoffelen, J. M. (2011). FieldTrip: open source software for advanced analysis of MEG, EEG, and invasive electrophysiological data. *Comp. Intel Neurosci.* 2011:156869. doi: 10.1155/2011/156869

Palva, J. M., Monto, S., Kulashekhar, S., and Palva, S. (2010). Neuronal synchrony reveals working memory networks and predicts individual memory capacity. *Proc. Natl. Acad. Sci. U.S.A.* 107, 7580–7585. doi: 10.1073/pnas.09131 13107

Pascual-Leone, A., and Hallett, M. (1994). Induction of errors in a delayed response task by repetitive transcranial magnetic stimulation of the dorsolateral prefrontal cortex. *Neuroreport* 5, 2517–2520. doi: 10.1097/00001756-199412000-00028

Phillips, M. E., and Ziegler, M. D. (2014). A neurostimulation-based advanced training system for human performance augmentation. *Brain Stimul.* 7, e11–e12.2013 doi: 10.1016/j.brs.2014.01.041

Reis, J., Fischer, J. T., Prichard, G., Weiller, C., Cohen, L. G., and Fritsch, B. (2015). Time- but not sleep-dependent consolidation of tDCS-enhanced visuomotor skills. *Cereb. Cortex* 25, 109–117. doi: 10.1093/cercor/bht208

Reis, J., Schambra, H. M., Cohen, L. G., Buch, E. R., Fritsch, B., Zarahn, E., et al. (2009). Noninvasive cortical stimulation enhances motor skill acquisition over multiple days through an effect on consolidation. *Proc. Natl. Acad. Sci. U.S.A.* 106, 1590–1595. doi: 10.1073/pnas.0805413106

Richmond, L. L., Wolk, D., Chein, J., and Olson, I. R. (2014). Transcranial direct current stimulation enhances verbal working memory training performance over time and near transfer outcomes. *J. Cogn. Neurosci.* 26, 2443–2454. doi: 10.1162/jocn_a_00657

Robertson, E. M., Pascual-Leone, A., and Miall, R. C. (2004). Current concepts in procedural consolidation. *Nat. Rev. Neurosci.* 5, 576–582. doi: 10.1038/nrn1426

Rosenkopf, L., and Tushman, M. L. (1998). The coevolution of community networks and technology: lessons from the flight simulation industry. *Indust. Corp. Change* 7, 311–346. doi: 10.1093/icc/7.2.311

Rumpf, J. J., Hinselmann, K., Fricke, C., Weise, D., and Classen, J. (2015). P148. Timing of post-training transcranial direct current stimulation to enhance consolidation of motor sequence learning in older people. *Clin. Neurophysiol.* 126, e135–e136. doi: 10.1016/j.clinph.2015.04.219

Ruocco, A. C., Rodrigo, A. H., Lam, J., Di Domenico, S. I., Graves, B., and Ayaz, H. (2014). A problem-solving task specialized for functional neuroimaging: validation of the Scarborough adaptation of the Tower of London (S-TOL) using near-infrared spectroscopy. *Front. Hum. Neurosci.* 8:185. doi: 10.3389/fnhum.2014.00185

Sakai, H., Uchiyama, Y., Tanaka, S., Sugawara, S. K., and Sadato, N. (2014). Prefrontal transcranial direct current stimulation improves fundamental vehicle control abilities. *Behav. Brain Res.* 273, 57–62. doi: 10.1016/j.bbr.2014.07.036

Santarnecchi, E., Brem, A. K., Levenbaum, E., Thompson, T., Kadosh, R. C., and Pascual-Leone, A. (2015). Enhancing cognition using transcranial electrical stimulation. *Curr. Opin. Behav. Sci.* 4, 171–178. doi: 10.1016/j.cobeha.2015.06.003

Sauseng, P., Klimesch, W., Doppelmayr, M., Hanslmayr, S., Schabus, M., and Gruber, W. R. (2004). Theta coupling in the human electroencephalogram during a working memory task. *Neurosci. Lett.* 354, 123–126. doi: 10.1016/j.neulet.2003.10.002

Sauseng, P., Klimesch, W., Gerloff, C., and Hummel, F. C. (2009). Spontaneous locally restricted EEG alpha activity determines cortical excitability in the motor cortex. *Neuropsychologia* 47, 284–288. doi: 10.1016/j.neuropsychologia.2008.07.021

Snedecor, G. W., and Cochran, W. G. (1989). *Statistical Methods*, 8th *Edn*. Iowa City, IA: Iowa State University Press.

Snowball, A., Tachtsidis, I., Popescu, T., Thompson, J., Delazer, M., Zamarian, L., et al. (2013). Long-term enhancement of brain function and cognition using cognitive training and brain stimulation. *Curr. Biol.* 23, 987–992. doi: 10.1016/j.cub.2013.04.045

Sohn, Y. W., and Doane, S. M. (2004). Memory processes of flight situation awareness: interactive roles of working memory capacity, long-term working memory, and expertise. *Hum. Factors* 46, 461–475. doi: 10.1518/hfes.46.3.461.50392

Stagg, C. J., and Johansen-Berg, H. (2013). Studying the effects of transcranial direct-current stimulation in stroke recovery using magnetic resonance imaging. *Front. Hum. Neurosci.* 7:857. doi: 10.3389/fnhum.2013.00857

Teo, F., Hoy, K. E., Daskalakis, Z. J., and Fitzgerald, P. B. (2011). Investigating the role of current strength in tDCS modulation of working memory performance in healthy controls. *Front. Psychiatry* 2:45. doi: 10.3389/fpsyt.2011.00045

Valle, A., Roizenblatt, S., Botte, S., Zaghi, S., Riberto, M., Tufik, S., et al. (2009). Efficacy of anodal transcranial direct current stimulation (tDCS) for the treatment of fibromyalgia: results of a randomized, sham-controlled longitudinal clinical trial. *J. Pain Manag.* 2, 353–361.

Villringer, A., Planck, J., Hock, C., Schleinkofer, L., and Dirnagl, U. (1993). Near infrared spectroscopy (NIRS): a new tool to study hemodynamic changes during activation of brain function in human adults. *Neurosci. Lett.* 154, 101–104. doi: 10.1016/0304-3940(93)90181-J

Williams, B. (2012). *Scenario-Based Training with X-Plane and Microsoft Flight Simulator: Using PC-Based Flight Simulations Based on FAA-Industry Training Standards*. Hoboken, NJ: Wiley and Sons.

Wolf, M., Ferrari, M., and Quaresima, V. (2007). Progress of near-infrared spectroscopy and topography for brain and muscle clinical applications. *J. Biomed. Opt.* 12, 062104–062104. doi: 10.1117/1.2804899

Xu, Y., Graber, H., and Barbour, R. (2014). "nirsLAB: a computing environment for fNIRS neuroimaging data analysis," in *Biomedical Optics OSA Technical Digest (Online)* (Miami, FL: Optical Society of America), paper BM3A.1.

Yanagisawa, H., Dan, I., Tsuzuki, D., Kato, M., Okamoto, M., Kyutoku, Y., et al. (2010). Acute moderate exercise elicits increased dorsolateral prefrontal activation and improves cognitive performance with Stroop test. *Neuroimage* 50, 1702–1710. doi: 10.1016/j.neuroimage.2009.12.023

Zhu, F. F., Yeung, A. Y., Poolton, J. M., Lee, T. M., Leung, G. K., and Masters, R. S. (2015). Cathodal transcranial direct current stimulation over left dorsolateral prefrontal cortex area promotes implicit motor learning in a golf putting task. *Brain Stimul.* 8, 784–786. doi: 10.1016/j.brs.2015.02.005

5

Exploring Neuro-Physiological Correlates of Drivers' Mental Fatigue Caused by Sleep Deprivation Using Simultaneous EEG, ECG, and fNIRS Data

Sangtae Ahn [1†], Thien Nguyen [2†], Hyojung Jang [1], Jae G. Kim [2] and Sung C. Jun [1*]*

[1] *School of Electrical Engineering and Computer Science, Gwangju Institute of Science and Technology, Gwangju, South Korea,* [2] *Department of Biomedical Science and Engineering, Gwangju Institute of Science and Technology, Gwangju, South Korea*

***Correspondence:**
Jae G. Kim
jaekim@gist.ac.kr;
Sung C. Jun
scjun@gist.ac.kr

Investigations of the neuro-physiological correlates of mental loads, or states, have attracted significant attention recently, as it is particularly important to evaluate mental fatigue in drivers operating a motor vehicle. In this research, we collected multimodal EEG/ECG/EOG and fNIRS data simultaneously to develop algorithms to explore neuro-physiological correlates of drivers' mental states. Each subject performed simulated driving under two different conditions (well-rested and sleep-deprived) on different days. During the experiment, we used 68 electrodes for EEG/ECG/EOG and 8 channels for fNIRS recordings. We extracted the prominent features of each modality to distinguish between the well-rested and sleep-deprived conditions, and all multimodal features, except EOG, were combined to quantify mental fatigue during driving. Finally, a novel driving condition level (DCL) was proposed that distinguished clearly between the features of well-rested and sleep-deprived conditions. This proposed DCL measure may be applicable to real-time monitoring of the mental states of vehicle drivers. Further, the combination of methods based on each classifier yielded substantial improvements in the classification accuracy between these two conditions.

Keywords: EEG/ECG/EOG/fNIRS, neuro-physiological correlates, drivers' mental fatigue, sleep deprivation, simulated driving, multimodal integration, driving condition level

INTRODUCTION

Neuroergonomics is an emerging field that investigates human mental states and their workloads in order to improve the reliability of human performance, and ensure its stability in various environments (Parasuraman, 2003; Parasuraman and Rizzo, 2008). In neuroergonomics, both the fundamental principles of neuroscience and human factors are considered thoroughly, and neural behaviors have been investigated primarily when people are engaged in tasks in a work environment (Parasuraman and Wilson, 2008). Due to the implications for public safety, a major application of neuroergonomics is the assessment of driver fatigue. In general, driver fatigue is categorized as either mental or physical. Mental fatigue occurs because of gradual and cumulative mental effort (Grandjean, 1979) during driving, or sleep deprivation before driving (Durmer and Dinges, 2005). In contrast, physical fatigue represents reduced muscular strength and coordination. Physical fatigue may be countered by deliberate action; however, mental fatigue is difficult to resolve. Because of mental fatigue, drivers begin to doze involuntary, which often results in traffic accidents (Horne and Reyner, 1999; Connor et al., 2002; Herman et al., 2014).

One potential method that may be used to reduce traffic accidents is to measure inherent mental fatigue before or during driving, in order to predict a driver's mental condition and determine whether s/he can drive safely. Because driving requires complex cognitive processes and sustained concentration, predicting a driver's mental fatigue before or during driving could be effective in preventing traffic accidents. Thus, we attempted in this work to explore neuro-physiological correlates in two different conditions, one well-rested with a low risk of fatigue, and the other sleep-deprived with a high risk of fatigue.

Among many studies performed to evaluate drivers' fatigue in real-time, computer vision-based systems have been used widely. Bergasa et al. (2006) proposed a noninvasive system to monitor a driver's vigilance using several parameters, including percentage or duration of eye closure, blinking, and the frequency of nodding. By using a fuzzy classifier, the researchers then inferred the level of the drivers' fatigue. However, the reliability of the findings decreased when the drivers wore glasses or the surrounding brightness changed. To address these problems, D'Orazio et al. (2007) designed an experimental paradigm that incorporated conditions in which some subjects had different eye colors, wore glasses, and drove vehicles in light of varying intensities. Using the proposed visual framework, the authors obtained robust results. In addition, various visual cues that characterized eyelid, gaze, and head movements, as well as facial expressions were employed in a probabilistic model developed to predict fatigue (Ji et al., 2004) that yielded even more robust results. Recently, Wang et al. (2014) developed an online, closed-loop lapse detection system featuring a mobile wireless electroencephalograph (EEG), and were able to extract certain EEG signatures associated with fatigue.

To date, EEG has been found to be a promising indicator for investigations of driver fatigue (Lal and Craig, 2001). EEG data have shown that there is a significant increase in theta and delta activity, and a decrease in heart rate (HR) associated with fatigue (Lal and Craig, 2002). Further, in a subsequent study that considered three phases of fatigue (early, medium, and extreme), software was developed to monitor driving fatigue, and was validated with EEG data from 35 subjects engaged in a simulated driving task (Lal et al., 2003). Another study (Lin et al., 2005) estimated drowsiness and driver performance by correlating changes in log power spectra. To detect drowsiness, they constructed an individualized linear regression model to assess EEG dynamics continuously based on an independent component analysis. Because drowsiness is a crucial factor in driving, Lin and his colleagues investigated the effect of continuous arousing auditory feedback on sustained attention in a driving simulator (Lin et al., 2010). They found that spectral powers in alpha and theta bands were suppressed and lasted 30 s or longer after feedback. This finding was introduced to estimate classification accuracy; as a result, they achieved a classification accuracy of approximately 78% using the maximum likelihood classifier (Lin et al., 2013) and applied it to develop an online, closed-loop system for practical lapse detection in real environments (Wang et al., 2014).

Various other methods have been used to explore drivers' mental fatigue, such as a support vector machine (SVM) (Shen et al., 2008; Yeo et al., 2009), Bayesian network (Yang et al., 2010), wavelet analysis (Kar et al., 2010; Li and Chung, 2013), and others. In addition to EEG studies, electrocardiography (ECG) and electrooculography (EOG) have been used to determine neuro-physiological correlates of drivers' mental fatigue. One study (Patel et al., 2011) used neural network analysis and demonstrated that the variability in drivers' HRs differed significantly in alert and fatigued states. They investigated the power spectral density behaviors between the two states during long-term driving and reported that the neural network was 90% accurate in classifying mental state.

Eyelid-related features from EOG data also have been reported to be possible candidates to detect whether or not a driver is drowsy (Hu and Zheng, 2009). In this report, they used vertical and horizontal EOG channels to extract and validate eye blinks according to eyelid movement parameters, such as blink duration, speed, and amplitude. Three conditions (alert, sleepy, and very sleepy) were classified with high reliability using SVM. Simultaneous recording of EEG/ECG (Zhao et al., 2012) and the combination of multimodal features from EEG, EOG, and ECG data (Khushaba et al., 2011) demonstrated significant differences during long-term driving. In this study, the researchers developed an efficient, fuzzy mutual information-based wavelet packet transformation that combined EEG, EOG, and ECG features to detect drivers' drowsiness; this technique yielded a classification accuracy greater than 90%.

An emerging portable and noninvasive brain functional imaging technique, functional near infra-red spectroscopy (fNIRS), has been introduced to monitor cognitive workload or fatigue in simulated environments (Ayaz et al., 2012). fNIRS data from the prefrontal cortex were collected during a complex air-traffic control task that required the subjects to prevent collisions between aircraft in their sectors. As the number of aircraft in their sector increased, a concomitant increase in prefrontal cortex activation was observed, which suggests that fNIRS provides a sensitive index of cognitive workload. fNIRS also demonstrated changes in prefrontal activation during skill acquisition in both basic working memory tasks (McKendrick et al., 2014) and more complex piloting tasks (Harrison et al., 2014; Gateau et al., 2015).

A portable fNIRS device was developed for use in mobile neuroimaging of the prefrontal cortex (Ayaz et al., 2013). In a driving environment, Li et al. (2009) observed changes in cerebral oxygenation during prolonged simulated driving. Forty healthy subjects were divided randomly into two groups (driving vs. non-driving), and the driving group performed a simulated 3 h driving task. The authors found a relative increase in frontal cortex oxygenation in the driving group by comparison to the non-driving group, and oxygenation decreased gradually after the driving task. Considering real driving situations, Yoshino et al. (2013) investigated the changes in cerebral oxygen exchange during actual driving on an expressway. An fNIRS signal was recorded in the subjects' parietal and prefrontal cortices using an fNIRS device mounted in the vehicle. They found that the areas activated varied depending on the driving task, such as parking, acceleration, driving at constant speed, deceleration, and U-turns. Thus, the use of fNIRS may be an effective approach to evaluate brain activity in various driving environments.

Recently, hybrid approaches that combine two different modalities (Pfurtscheller et al., 2010) to improve performance and reduce classification error have been reported as promising for future brain-computer interfaces (BCI). One example of a hybrid BCI that incorporates both EEG electrical activity and fNIRS hemodynamic changes yielded improved classification performance in sensorimotor rhythm-based BCI systems (Fazli et al., 2012). The researchers calculated classification accuracies in the movements executed and motor imagery by estimating a meta-classifier. After the estimation of both classifiers (EEG and fNIRS), the combination of outputs of each classifier resulted in improved classification accuracy. Khan et al. (2014) decoded four movement directions (left, right, forward, and backward) using the mixed features of EEG and fNIRS, in which EEG features were used to classify left/right, and fNIRS features were used to classify forward/backward. In addition, hybrid BCI may be used as a brain switch that determines whether a certain task is active. Koo et al. (2015) employed a novel experimental paradigm to detect the occurrence of motor imagery in fNIRS data. Threshold-based detection with a feature value of the fNIRS data determined whether or not the action of a motor imagery task was attempted. The combination of EEG and fNIRS is also applicable to language studies (Wallois et al., 2012) and cortical current estimation (Morioka et al., 2014). Hybrid BCIs may provide a good opportunity to increase BCI performance by offering the synergistic effects of multimodal brain imaging techniques.

In this work, we recorded multimodal EEG/ECG/EOG and fNIRS data simultaneously in a driving simulator and combined their features to distinguish drivers with high- and low-risks of fatigue using neuro-physiological correlates and a classification method. Hemodynamic changes in the prefrontal cortex (Li et al., 2009; Ayaz et al., 2012, 2013; Yoshino et al., 2013; Harrison et al., 2014; McKendrick et al., 2014; Gateau et al., 2015) have been used to neuro-physiological correlates, and these activities were reported to play an important role in neuroergonomics, such as mental workload (Mandrick et al., 2013a), cognitive operation (Mandrick et al., 2013b), and emotional function (Doi et al., 2013). Furthermore, it is clear that EEG, ECG, and EOG are also promising indicators that may be used to investigate the neuro-physiological correlates of drivers' mental fatigue (Lal and Craig, 2001). Therefore, combining this hybrid system with prefrontal fNIRS may be a far more informative measure for identifying neuro-physiological correlates under varying driving conditions. To the best of our knowledge, this multimodal approach has been tested rarely to explore neuro-physiological correlates of drivers' mental fatigue.

Thus, the goal of this study was to determine modality-specific features of EEG, EOG, ECG, and fNIRS. These features were then used to distinguish between well-rested and sleep-deprived conditions, and resulted in a classifier that showed whether or not a driver was in an alert mental state. The use of a reasonable combination of these multimodal features may improve classification accuracy and its quantification may yield a real-time strategy to monitor drivers' mental fatigue.

MATERIALS AND METHODS

Experimental Procedure

Eleven healthy subjects (10 males, 1 female, aged 26.6 ± 1.4, range = 24–28) who had valid driver's licenses participated in a custom-built virtual driving simulation task, as depicted in **Figure 1A**. The subjects practiced repeatedly until they were familiar with the simulation system. The purposes of, and instructions for, the experiment were explained in advance, and all of the subjects signed an informed consent. Subjects received approximately $10 per h as compensation for their participation. Each subject performed simulated driving under two conditions (well-rested and sleep-deprived) on different days. Under the well-rested condition, subjects were instructed to sleep at least 7 h before the experiment, as sleeping seven or more hours is known to maintain healthy mental alertness (Kripke et al., 2002). In the sleep-deprived condition, the subjects were instructed to stay up all night in order to produce mental fatigue.

Driving tests in both conditions were performed before 9 a.m. In this experiment, we assumed that subjects would be significantly mentally fatigued after one night of sleep deprivation. To determine the degree of fatigue produced by sleep deprivation, a subjective questionnaire was administered to the subjects before the experiment to score their levels of fatigue, and the scores demonstrated clearly that the sleep-deprived subjects were substantially more fatigued than were the well-rested subjects. The subjects sat in a comfortable driver's seat and drove on an oval track for a minimum of 30 min. The maximum driving speed was set at 100 km/h in both conditions. The steering wheel vibrated whenever the vehicle collided with a crash barrier in order to prevent the drivers from falling asleep completely. A high-definition webcam (Logitech HD Pro C920) was used to record each subject's behavior in real-time. This experiment was approved by the Institutional Review Board at the Gwangju Institute of Science and Technology (20150615-HR-18-02-06).

Data Recording of EEG/ECG/EOG and fNIRS

Sixty-four EEG electrodes were attached to the drivers' scalps according to the 10–20 international position system. Horizontal and vertical EOGs were used and two ECG electrodes were attached to the left/right chest (Biosemi ActiveTwo System). These data were collected at a 512 Hz sampling rate using BCI2000 software (Schalk et al., 2004). Biosemi ActiView software monitored the stability and reliability of the EEG signal. After the experiment, bad channels that contained abnormal noise were identified by visual inspection and excluded from the analysis.

A custom-built fNIRS system (continuous wave, 10 Hz sampling rate) was used to record hemodynamic changes in the brain. This was an updated version of one described in a

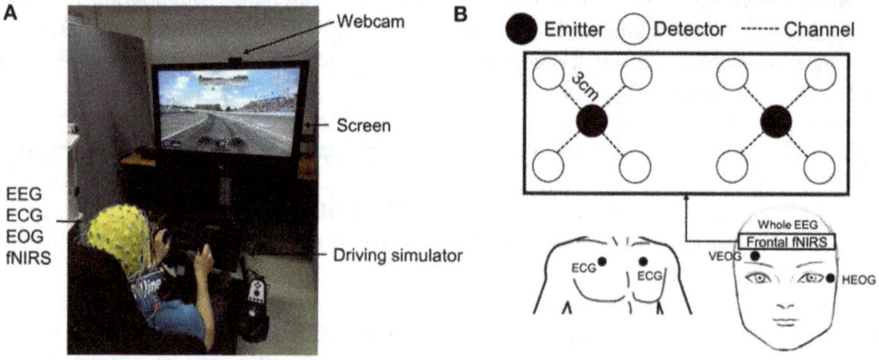

FIGURE 1 | Experimental setup for simulated driving. (A) Driving simulation environment with EEG/ECG/EOG/fNIRS measurements. **(B)** fNIRS setup in the prefrontal cortex. Two emitters and eight detectors (eight channels) were attached to the forehead. The distance between emitter and detector was 3 cm.

previous work (Kim et al., 2015). The system consists of probe and control circuits. The probe includes 2 LEDs (emitters) and 8 photodetectors (detectors). The LEDs emit near infrared (NIR) light at two wavelengths (735 and 850 nm). The emitter and four surrounding detectors were separated by 3 cm, as Homma et al. (1996) suggested that in soft tissues, NIR is able to attain a penetration depth equal to half of the emitter-detector separation. Therefore, with a 3.0 cm emitter-detector separation, our system should have been able to collect brain activity at a depth of 1.5 cm below the scalp. An emitter-detector pair form one fNIRS channel that measures hemodynamic changes midway between the emitter and the detector. Given a suitable geometric arrangement, many detectors may receive light from one emitter. This enabled us to design an 8-channel probe with 2 LEDs and 8 photodetectors. The 8-channel probe was attached to the prefrontal region to investigate the subjects' mental state, as illustrated in **Figure 1B** (Li et al., 2009; Sato et al., 2013). The control circuit receives a signal from the probe, amplifies it, and sends it to the computer via serial communication. Matlab-based software was programmed to record, process, and display the hemodynamic signals. Interference between EEG/EOG/ECG electrodes and fNIRS emitters has been observed and is believed to result from light leakage from the emitters, which may cause deterioration in the quality of electrical data (Koo et al., 2015). This interference was removed by blocking light leakage from the emitters and applying a simple pre-processing technique. Two desktop computers were used to record the EEG/ECG/EOG and fNIRS data simultaneously. Triggers for start and end times were sent to the BCI2000 software to synchronize the multimodal EEG/ECG/EOG and fNIRS data. The computer that recorded EEG/ECG/EOG data sent a start trigger, at which time the second computer began to record fNIRS data. The end time of the experiment was marked in the same way.

Data Analysis

Feature Extraction and Classification from EEG

After the experiment, the data collected were inspected visually and bad channels were rejected. The logistic infomax independent component analysis (Bell and Sejnowski, 1995) was used to remove EOG artifacts and the data were then band-pass filtered from 1 to 50 Hz. We analyzed data from the first 30 min only after the drivers began the task, because fatigue levels between well-rested and sleep-deprived subjects were likely to be quite different during the initial minutes of driving. From the real-time webcam video monitoring data, we observed that even some well-rested subjects became drowsy and quite bored after that length of time.

EEG data (30 min) were divided into 10 s (a trial) to yield a total of 180 trials for each driving condition. A power spectral density was computed for each trial using the EEGLAB library (Delorme and Makeig, 2004), and a relative power level (RPL) was computed in order to reduce session/subject variability (Ahn et al., 2013a,b, 2014; Cho et al., 2015). To calculate the RPL, we considered five spectral band ranges: delta (1–4 Hz), theta (4–8 Hz), alpha (8–13 Hz), beta (13–30 Hz), and gamma (30–50 Hz). Next, each band-power was normalized by the total power, defined as the sum over all band powers, after which we extracted the most informative RPL features between the two driving conditions. On the other hand, to discriminate between the well-rested and sleep-deprived conditions, pre-processed data (180 trials) from each driving condition (well-rested and sleep-deprived) were firstly divided into 2 groups (training and test) and according to time sequence; training and test groups were composed of 126 (70%) and 54 trials (30%), respectively. Then, to avoid temporal dependency between groups, last 6 trials (1 min) for each group were excluded; thus, for each of driving conditions, 120 and 48 trials for training and test were obtained, respectively. By this grouping, temporal dependency (adjacency) was included within groups, but was excluded between groups. This procedure was repeated 30 times by sliding temporal window of 1 min (6 trials) and then choosing training and test groups. Thereafter, each feature vector of the training and test data using RPL was fed into the classifier. The training group was used to construct a classifier based on Fisher's linear discriminant analysis (FLDA), and the test group was input to a constructed classifier in order to measure classification accuracy. A classifier was generated from the training data and the classification accuracy was estimated from the test data.

Finally, 30 classification accuracies were estimated to obtain an average accuracy.

Feature Extraction and Classification from ECG and EOG

The HRs of each subject were extracted using two ECG channels (left/right chest). During pre-processing, ECG data were band-pass filtered from 0.1 to 30 Hz and were detrended to remove the baseline shift. After detrending, a QRS-complex was observed to be the most prominent repeating peak in the ECG signal. The QRS-wave is used commonly to determine subjects' HRs or predict abnormalities in cardiac function. Specifically, the emergence of an R-peak indicated a subject's HR clearly and was extracted easily by adjusting a deterministic threshold of the ECG magnitude. Next, the number of R-peaks per minute was counted and used to determine HR per minute. HRs from the two ECG channels on the left and right chest were calculated for the entire 30 min and averaged to reduce possible detection error and bias. To classify mental state from the ECG data, we adopted the extraction of RR-peak interval features (de Chazal et al., 2004). After detection of the R-peak in each 10-s trial, the intervals between one R-peak and the next were averaged, and the procedure was repeated for all trials. In this way, 180 R-peak intervals were estimated as a feature set. The EOG signal was used to extract the rate of eye blinking in each 1-min trial, which has been reported to be associated well with a human's mental state (Schleicher et al., 2008): when the eye blinks, a clear, sharp wave is observed. After baseline drift removal was applied, a peak detection algorithm (Pettersson et al., 2013) was used with a given threshold of signal magnitude. Finally, the number of peaks per minute, which represented the eye-blinking rate, was used as the EOG feature.

Feature Extraction and Classification from fNIRS

We adopted the modified Beer-Lambert's law (mBLL) to retrieve relative concentration changes from the light intensities of the 8 detectors (Cope et al., 1988; Kocsis et al., 2006). The change in optical density at two wavelengths (735 and 850 nm) is related to changes in oxy-hemoglobin concentration (HbO) and deoxy-hemoglobin concentration (HbR). Data with abnormal noise were removed by visual inspection, and the remaining data were filtered with a 0.01 Hz high-pass filter to remove baseline drifts. Light intensities for 30 s after the initiation of the experiment were averaged and set as baseline intensities. HbO and HbR were estimated with the following equations:

$$\Delta HbO = \frac{log\frac{I_b^{\lambda 1}}{I_t^{\lambda 1}}\varepsilon_{HbR}^{\lambda 2} - log\frac{I_b^{\lambda 2}}{I_t^{\lambda 2}}\varepsilon_{HbR}^{\lambda 1}}{d \cdot DPF\left[\varepsilon_{HbO}^{\lambda 1}\varepsilon_{HbR}^{\lambda 2} - \varepsilon_{HbO}^{\lambda 2}\varepsilon_{HbR}^{\lambda 1}\right]}, \quad (1)$$

$$\Delta HbR = \frac{log\frac{I_b^{\lambda 2}}{I_t^{\lambda 2}}\varepsilon_{HbO}^{\lambda 1} - log\frac{I_b^{\lambda 1}}{I_t^{\lambda 1}}\varepsilon_{HbO}^{\lambda 2}}{d \cdot DPF\left[\varepsilon_{HbO}^{\lambda 1} \cdot \varepsilon_{HbR}^{\lambda 2} - \varepsilon_{HbO}^{\lambda 2} \cdot \varepsilon_{HbR}^{\lambda 1}\right]}, \quad (2)$$

where
I_b^{λ} : *baseline intensity* (λ_1 : 735 *nm* λ_2 : 850 *nm*)
I_t^{λ} : *transient intensity*
d: *emitter* – *detector separation*
$\varepsilon_{Hb}^{\lambda}$: *extinction coefficient*
DPF : *differential path length factor*

In continuous wave fNIRS, the differential path length factor (DPF) is unknown. However, it is similar for both wavelengths and is included conventionally in the unit of hemodynamic changes as a scaling factor. Thus, HbO and HbR have the same unit of mM/DPF, and the extinction coefficients are specific for HbO and HbR at each wavelength. Matcher et al. (1995) measured extinction coefficients of hemoglobin at different wavelengths as follows:

at wavelength λ_1= 735 nm,

$$\varepsilon_{HbO}^{\lambda 1} = 0.4646mM^{-1}cm^{-1} \text{ and } \varepsilon_{HbR}^{\lambda 1} = 1.2959mM^{-1}cm^{-1},$$

at wavelength λ_2= 850 nm,

$$\varepsilon_{HbO}^{\lambda 2} = 1.1596mM^{-1}cm^{-1} \text{ and } \varepsilon_{HbR}^{\lambda 2} = 0.7861mM^{-1}cm^{-1}.$$

Like EEG feature extraction, 10 s of data were defined as one trial, which yielded a total of 180 trials per condition. Next, relative concentration changes were estimated for each trial. To reduce the effects of fluctuations and noise, fNIRS data were smoothed using 10-s temporal windowing with a 50% overlap. Finally, the amplitudes of HbO and HbR were used as informative features for classification of the two driving conditions.

RESULTS

Relative Power Level from EEG

We investigated RPL values over five spectral bands—delta, theta, alpha, beta, and gamma—and found that the RPL values for delta, theta, and gamma did not differ statistically between the two driving conditions. However, alpha and beta RPL values differed clearly in the two conditions, as shown in **Figure 2A**. Grand-averaged topographies were described for each condition, and alpha RPL in the sleep-deprived condition was activated to a greater degree in the right centro-parietal region. Such an increase in alpha power has been reported in the literature as a notable marker in driving (Lal and Craig, 2001; Simon et al., 2011). A decrease in beta RPL over the fronto-central region was observed in the sleep-deprived condition. This decrease in beta power may indicate a lack of arousal, which is consistent with the results of several studies (Tanaka et al., 2012; Zhao et al., 2012).

Figure 2B shows the distributions of alpha and beta RPLs from subject S5 in a two-dimensional Cartesian coordinate space. We note that most subjects showed similar physiological behaviors, and S5's results were chosen as representative because they yielded the highest classification accuracy in the EEG, as shown in **Table 3**. For the purposes of consistency and comparison, the other results (ECG, fNIRS) from subject S5 are also illustrated in the subsequent sections. Each RPL was averaged spatially over significant regions, such as the centro-parietal for alpha and the fronto-central for beta. Each dot

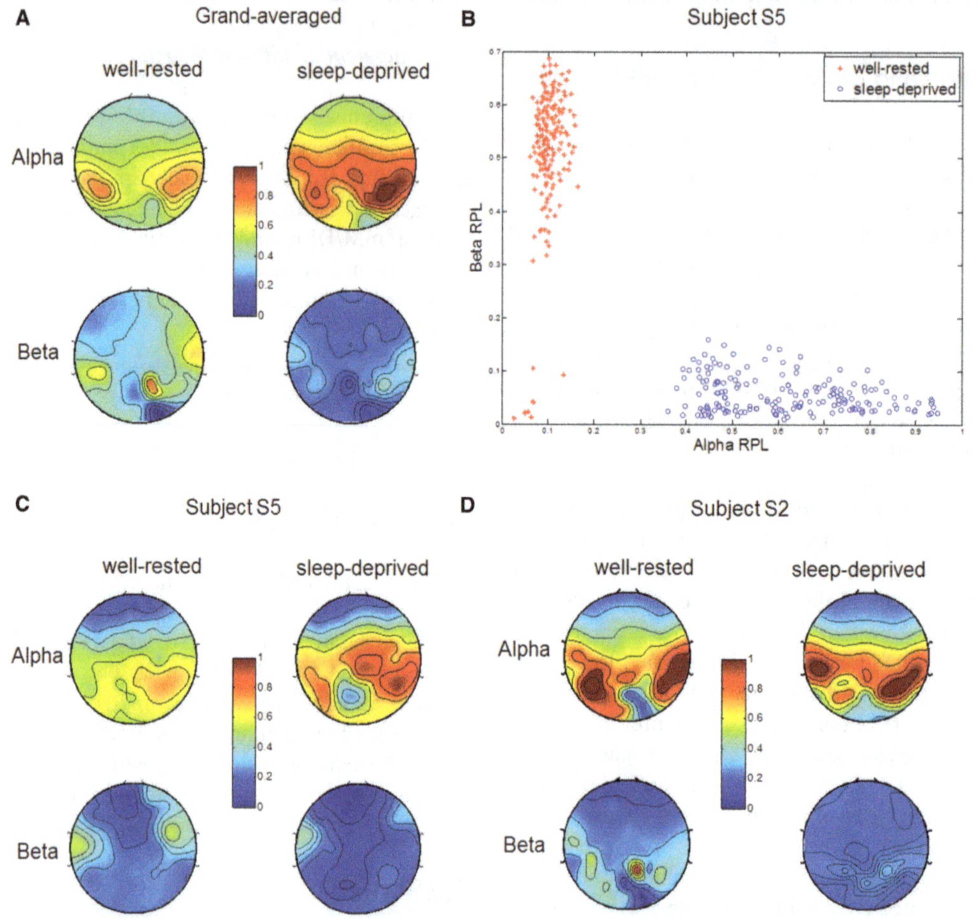

FIGURE 2 | Relative power levels from EEG in two different conditions. (A) Grand-averaged alpha and beta RPLs in well-rested and sleep-deprived conditions. Alpha and beta RPLs differed significantly in the right centro-parietal and frontal regions, respectively. **(B)** Scatter plot of alpha (x-axis) and beta (y-axis) RPLs in two driving conditions (red asterisk: well-rested, blue circle: sleep-deprived) for subject S5. **(C,D)** Indicate alpha and beta RPLs in the well-rested and sleep-deprived conditions, in which subject S5 had the highest and S2 had the lowest classification accuracy, respectively.

represents corresponding alpha (x-coordinate) and beta (y-coordinate) RPLs for one trial in each condition (well-rested and sleep-deprived). In the well-rested condition, most RPL dots were distributed in the upper left area in R^2 space, while they were distributed in the lower right area in the sleep-deprived condition. Thus, these features (centro-parietal alpha RPL and fronto-central beta RPL) in the dataset collected allowed us to achieve a discriminative classification between the two driving conditions quite well.

To investigate inter-subject variability (Ahn and Jun, 2015), we plotted RPL topographies in **Figures 2C,D**, respectively, for two subjects who achieved the highest (S5) and the lowest (S2) EEG classification accuracies (**Table 3**). As depicted in the figures, subject S5 showed a clear alpha RPL increase in the right centro-parietal region and beta RPL decrease in the fronto-central region in the sleep-deprived condition. In contrast, subject S2, who demonstrated the lowest classification accuracy, showed a slight alpha RPL increase and a beta RPL decrease in the sleep-deprived condition. Interestingly, this subject (S2) was likely to have been fatigued already, despite being in the well-rested condition before the experiment. Our investigation of this subject will be described in detail in the Discussion section.

Time Course of Relative Concentration Changes from fNIRS

The time course of the relative concentration changes of HbO and HbR were estimated through mBLL. **Figure 3** depicts the concentration changes at channels 1 and 5 for subject S5. Because all channels were attached to the prefrontal cortex, they all showed similar behaviors over time. Thus, for the purpose of illustration, we chose two representative channels (1 and 5). The concentration changes of HbO increased gradually over time in the well-rested condition and demonstrated the highest level at channels 1 and 5 between 20 and 30 min. Paying attention while driving a vehicle requires high oxygen consumption in the brain, which induces an increase in cerebral blood flow; this increase in cerebral oxygenation, as shown by an increase in HbO and decrease in HbR, indicates that the cerebral blood flow increased during

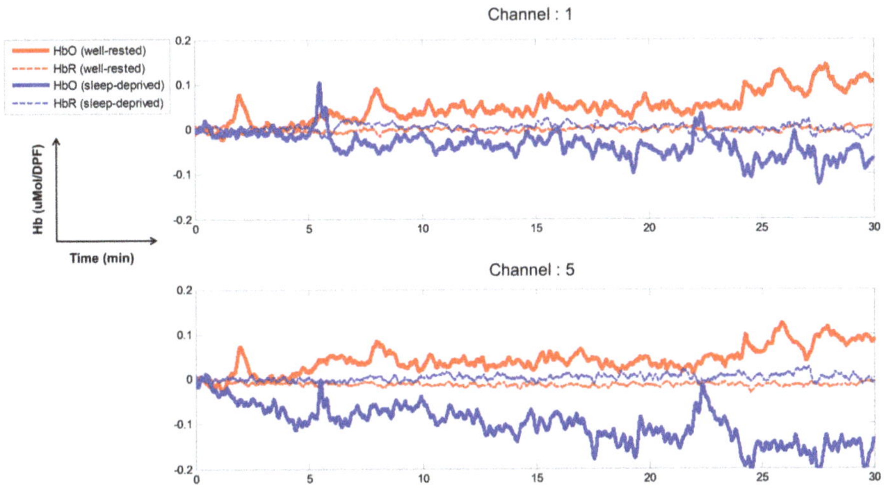

FIGURE 3 | Time course of relative concentration changes of HbO and HbR (channels 1 and 5). Solid, thick red and blue-colored lines indicate HbO for well-rested and sleep-deprived conditions, respectively. Dashed thin lines indicate HbR in the two conditions.

driving under the well-rested condition. On the other hand, concentration changes of HbO decreased slightly (Channel 1) or remained stable (Channel 5) compared to the baseline, and HbR concentration maintained baseline values while driving under the sleep-deprived condition. Less oxygen may be consumed when mentally fatigued, and therefore, brain activity is likely to be suppressed, resulting in less blood flow to the brain.

Reduced Heart Rate and Eye Blinking in the Sleep-Deprived Condition

The mean HRs of all subjects were calculated from ECG signals over the entire 30-min driving period (average of varied HRs), as tabulated in **Table 1** and depicted in **Figure 4A**. As shown in the table and figure, HRs in the sleep-deprived condition were significantly lower than were those in the well-rested condition for all subjects ($p < 0.01$, Wilcoxon signed-rank test). **Figure 4B** shows the HR of subject S5 over time (from initiation to 30 min of driving). HRs in the well-rested condition were higher than those in the sleep-deprived condition; however, the difference in the HR between the two conditions decreased gradually as driving time increased and became quite small at the end of the driving task (~30 min). We deduced from this time variance in the HR that even a well-rested driver began to feel fatigued after some duration of driving and was considerably fatigued by the end of the task.

Because of the EOG signal, we expected that subjects in the sleep-deprived condition would demonstrate a relatively higher rate of eye blinking than those in the well-rested condition. Instead, we observed (not shown here) that some subjects showed higher rates of eye blinking in the well-rested than in the sleep-deprived condition, although the differences were not statistically significant. From the video data, we found that these subjects closed and opened their eyes frequently to overcome drowsiness, and this action on their part may have affected seriously the rate of eye blinking derived from the EOG data.

Driving Condition Level and Relative Driving Condition Level

We attempted to demonstrate that it may be possible to evaluate neuro-physiological correlates of drivers' mental fatigue using the significant features found in EEG, ECG, and fNIRS data. To that end, we used the three factors extracted from multimodal signals in the previous sections: RPL (ratio of beta to alpha) from EEG, HbO from fNIRS, and the averaged HR from ECG. Each feature was normalized by scaling between 0 and 1 for equal contribution, as formulated in Equation (3). Each value of the EEG, ECG, and fNIRS was distributed well between those values. Significantly abnormal values—greater than 95% (mean $\pm$ 2$*\sigma$)—were considered outliers and were shrunk to their maximum or minimum values in the feature set. The summation of all three normalized factors was proposed as the driving condition level (DCL), as depicted in Equation (4). In addition, we estimated the relative difference in DCL between the well-rested and sleep-deprived conditions (rDCL), which represented the degree of the drivers' fatigue compared to that in the well-rested condition, as defined in Equation (5); a higher rDCL indicates greater fatigue.

$$norm(x) = \frac{x - \min(x)}{\max(x) - \min(x)}, \tag{3}$$

$$DCL = norm\left(\frac{beta\ RPL}{alpha\ RPL}\right) + norm(HbO) + norm(HR), \tag{4}$$

$$\left(0 \le \mathrm{norm}\left(\frac{beta\ RPL}{alpha\ RPL}\right) norm(HbO)norm(HR) \le 1,\ 0 \le \mathrm{DCL} \le 3\right)$$

$$rDCL\ (\%) = 100 - \frac{DCL_{sleep-deprived}}{DCL_{well-rested}} * 100, \tag{5}$$

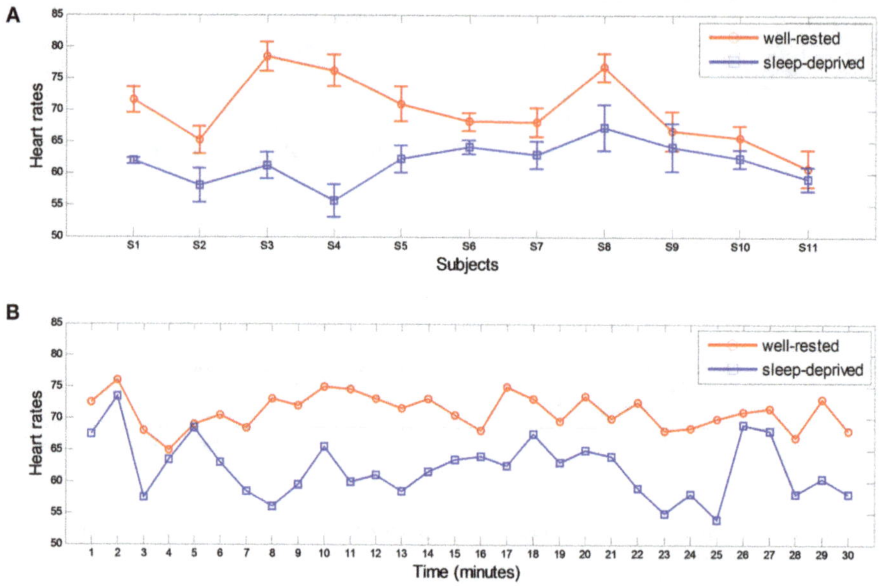

FIGURE 4 | Heart rates from ECG in two different conditions. (A) Averaged heart rates for all subjects in well-rested and sleep-deprived conditions. **(B)** Subject 5's HRs over time. Each HR was estimated every minute.

TABLE 1 | Averaged heart rates (HRs) in well-rested and sleep-deprived conditions.

Subject	S1	S2	S3	S4	S5	S6	S7	S8	S9	S10	S11	Mean	*p*-value
Well-rested	71.6 (2.0)	65.3 (2.2)	78.5 (2.3)	76.2 (2.5)	71 (2.8)	68.2 (1.4)	68.1 (2.3)	76.8 (2.2)	66.7 (3.1)	65.7 (1.9)	60.9 (2.9)	69.9 (3.3)	0.0009
Sleep-deprived	62 (0.5)	58.2 (2.7)	61.3 (2.1)	55.7 (2.6)	62.3 (2.2)	64.2 (1.1)	63 (2.2)	67.3 (3.7)	64.2 (3.8)	62.4 (1.4)	59.2 (1.9)	61.8 (3.5)	

Values in parentheses indicate standard deviations for each HR. The Wilcoxon signed-rank test was performed.

Using our proposed definition of DCL (Equation 4), DCL values were estimated in the two conditions for each subject. For all subjects, 30 min of multimodal data were used to estimate the values. DCL ranged from 0 to 3, with a smaller DCL indicating greater fatigue. These DCL values are tabulated in **Table 2**. Subject S8 showed the highest DCL value in the well-rested condition, while subject S4 showed the lowest DCL value in the sleep-deprived condition. We found that the two drivers' conditions (well-rested and sleep-deprived) differed significantly ($p < 0.01$, Wilcoxon signed rank test). In addition, rDCL, which represents the percentage of the fatigue in a drivers' mental condition, was introduced in this work. All rDCLs were consistently greater than 30%, except for those for two of 11 subjects (S7 and S9); thus, when rDCL is tuned more finely with more data, it may be used as a predictor of mental fatigue.

To investigate the drivers' mental fatigue over time, each DCL value (per a minute) was estimated by extracting features of RPL (beta over alpha), HbO, and averaged HR. **Figure 5** shows the DCL values of subject S5, in which the values decreased gradually over time in the well-rested condition, and remained consistent at approximately 1 in the sleep-deprived condition. Sleep-deprived subjects were quite fatigued already at the beginning of the driving task. From the questionnaire, we found a weak correlation ($r^2 = 0.42$) between rDCL values in the sleep-deprived condition and subjects' reported degree of sleepiness (1: rarely sleepy to 5: very sleepy). The average scores for sleepiness over all subjects were 1.4 and 4.1 in the well-rested and sleep-deprived conditions, respectively, while the average hours of sleep reported were 7.36 and 0 h, respectively.

Multimodal Integration to Determine Neuro-Physiological Correlates

In this work, we recorded simultaneous EEG/ECG/EOG and fNIRS signals for multimodal analysis. Multimodal integration is an efficient technique that yields important insights into brain processes (Uludağ and Roebroeck, 2014). Even though the EOG signals did not differ statistically in this work, they were used to eliminate eye movement artifacts in the EEG data. On the other hand, EEG/ECG and fNIRS data yielded clear features that discriminated between the driving conditions, and each feature from the three different modalities differed significantly between the well-rested and sleep-deprived conditions. Based on these features, DCL (summation of these normalized factors) was proposed to determine neuro-physiological correlates of drivers'

TABLE 2 | Driving condition level (DCL) in well-rested and sleep-deprived conditions.

Subject	S1	S2	S3	S4	S5	S6	S7	S8	S9	S10	S11	Mean
Well-rested	2.52	2.48	2.31	2.04	2.24	2.75	1.94	2.80	1.94	2.01	2	2.34
Sleep-deprived	1.47	1.17	1.44	1.07	1.11	1.73	1.42	1.88	1.54	1.19	1.21	1.39
rDCL (%)	41.7	52.8	37.7	47.5	50.2	37.1	26.7	32.9	21	40.8	39.5	40.7

Relative DCL (rDCL) indicates percentage of fatigue level by comparison to well-rested condition.

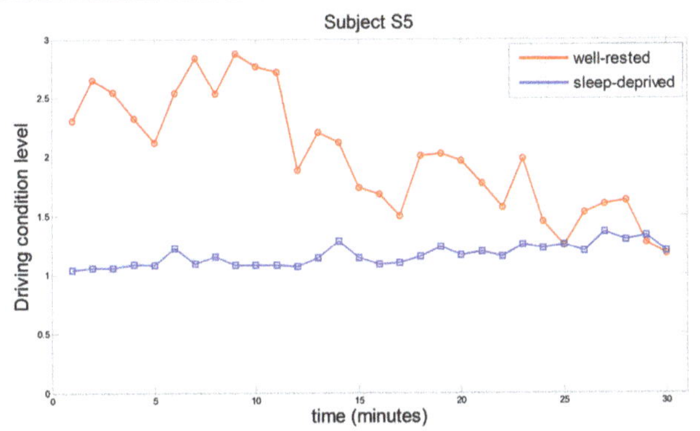

FIGURE 5 | Comparative driving condition level behavior in well-rested and sleep-deprived conditions while subject S5 was driving. Each point represents the averaged DCL value during one minute of driving. Red circles and blue squares represent the DCL in the well-rested and sleep-deprived conditions, respectively.

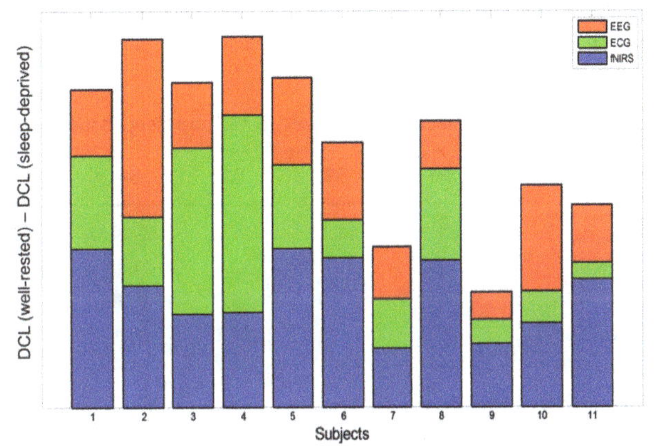

FIGURE 6 | DCL difference (subtraction of sleep-deprived from well-rested) for all subjects. Each color represents modality-specific contribution to DCL difference (red: EEG, green: ECG, blue: fNIRS). Summation of the three colored bars indicates the synergistic effect of multimodal data on classification between the two driving conditions.

mental fatigue in a quantitative manner. As a result, we observed that DCL may offer a reasonable method to discriminate well between the two driving conditions. To illustrate the individual contribution of each modality to the differences in DCL between the two driving conditions, the modality-specific contributions are shown for all subjects in **Figure 6**. Accumulation of the three colored bars indicates DCL differences in the multimodal data (EEG+ECG+fNIRS), which represent the synergistic effect of these data. As shown in this figure, subjects S2 and S4 demonstrated the greatest differences in DCL, while the DCL of subjects S7 and S9 differed the least between the two conditions. Because of the unbiased combination, the averaged contributions of each modality (EEG, ECG, and fNIRS) to the DCL differences were quite similar (0.46, 0.45, and 0.46, respectively).

Comparison of Hybrid Approaches Using EEG/ECG and fNIRS

To investigate the hybrid effect of the classification for the two different driving conditions, we compared various combinations of modalities with respect to the classifiers' outputs. For the combined classifiers in each modality, each classifier's outputs (EEG, ECG, and fNIRS) were regarded as features of the second classifier. Thereafter, the outputs of the second classifier represent the results of the combined classifiers. A flow diagram of this procedure is depicted in **Figure 7**.

Classification accuracies of single modalities (EEG, ECG, fNIRS) and all combinations of modalities (EEG+ECG, EEG+fNIRS, ECG+fNIRS, and EEG+ECG+fNIRS) at the classification level are summarized in **Table 3**. Most of the subjects (8 of 11) achieved improved performance in the combined EEG+ECG+fNIRS, and the average performance of this combination was greater than that of the others. A one-way ANOVA conducted on the seven different approaches indicated that there was a considerably significant difference [$F_{(6, 70)} = 4.38$, $p = 0.0008 < 0.10$]. Further, the EEG+ECG+fNIRS combinations differed significantly from the others ($p < 0.05$, Wilcoxon signed-rank test). Each level of significance is marked with asterisks in **Table 3**. Notably, subject S6 showed the greatest improvement (~30.5%) in the EEG+ECG+fNIRS combination compared to EEG only.

DISCUSSION

EEG Spectral Changes and Driving Conditions

To date, most researchers have investigated driving fatigue using EEG changes, which are promising indicators of this phenomenon (Lal and Craig, 2001), and EEG has the advantages of being portable, noninvasive, inexpensive, and safe to measure during driving. With EEG recording, Lal and Craig (2002) found substantial increases in delta, theta, and alpha activity in the transition to fatigue, which was

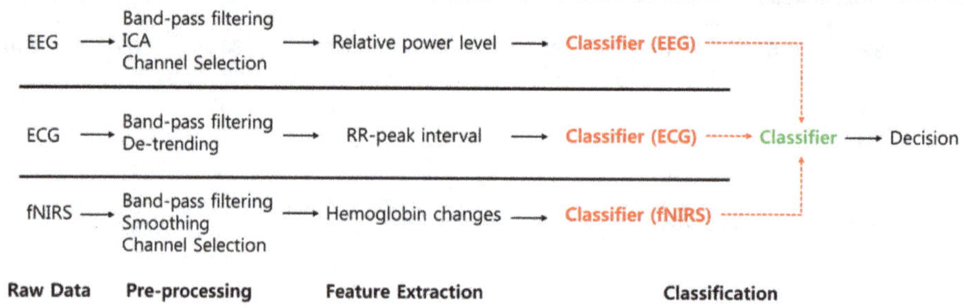

FIGURE 7 | Flow diagram for classifier combination. Each classifier's output is regarded to second classifier's input.

TABLE 3 | Classification accuracies in well-rested and sleep-deprived conditions.

Subject	S1	S2	S3	S4	S5	S6	S7	S8	S9	S10	S11	Mean
**EEG	61.3	52.1	58.9	54.4	70.8	55.2	68.9	64.3	61.0	52.2	58.1	59.7
**ECG	79.4	72.0	52.8	76.3	60.5	52.3	63.9	72.2	61.2	58.8	59.7	64.5
*fNIRS	68.4	**84.5**	55.6	65.9	76.8	80.8	**72.9**	61.5	52.6	57.7	58.3	66.8
**EEG+ECG	76.2	60.0	**74.3**	68.1	72.9	68.9	64.3	73.5	71.4	60.4	69.5	69.0
**EEG+fNIRS	83.3	63.3	66.7	65.5	72.7	63.3	63.3	70.0	73.3	60.3	70.0	68.3
**ECG+fNIRS	82.8	64.8	63.3	73.3	73.3	73.3	60.0	76.7	63.3	56.7	73.3	69.2
EEG+ECG+fNIRS	**84.5**	73.7	71.8	**77.9**	**78.1**	**85.7**	67.0	**83.8**	**74.6**	**62.4**	**75.2**	**75.9**

*The highest accuracies among seven approaches are displayed in bold. Asterisks indicate the level of signficance with the EEG+ECG+fNIRS combination (**$p < 0.01$: *$p < 0.05$).*

consistent with existing findings described in a review paper (Sahayadhas et al., 2012). Alpha activity is believed to be the most prominent indicator of driver fatigue. With this reasoning, Simon et al. (2011) verified alpha spindle activity based on a short-time Fourier transformation in real traffic conditions. Statistical analysis of these actual driving data revealed significant increases for all alpha spindle parameters, such as rate, duration, amplitude, and power, between the awake and drowsy states during 20 min of driving. Similarly, in the EEG recordings in this work, we observed a significant increase in alpha based on RPL. To reduce session and subject variability, a normalized alpha RPL was introduced and a significant alpha RPL difference was found in the centro-parietal region.

It is known that attention is also correlated with alpha power suppression. In our experiment, visual attention may be expected to be related closely to a simulated driving task. Such visual attention-related alpha power suppression may be observed normally in the occipital region, as reported in previous studies (Worden et al., 2000; Sauseng et al., 2005; Rihs et al., 2007). However, in our study, notable alpha suppression was observed in the centro-parietal region alone, which is consistent with results in previous studies of fatigue (Lal and Craig, 2001, 2002; Simon et al., 2011; Sahayadhas et al., 2012). For this reason, it is clear that a reduction in power in the alpha band was correlated with fatigue in this experiment. We observed beta RPL changes in the sleep-deprived condition, and beta power may be an additional indicator of mental fatigue. Tanaka et al. (2012) found that beta power densities decreased significantly after tiring cognitive tasks. They calculated EEG power spectra in each band and showed that beta waves decreased significantly in the fronto-central region with increased driving times. It also has been reported that beta rhythm is associated closely with increased alertness and arousal (Okogbaa et al., 1994), which is likely to be applicable to driving situations (Yeo et al., 2009; Yang et al., 2010; Zhao et al., 2012). In this work, we inferred that the lack of arousal and alertness caused by mental fatigue and sleep deprivation may result in a decreased beta rhythm during simulated driving.

Until now, most studies related to the detection of mental fatigue during driving have been experimental, and driving conditions have been divided according to the elapsed duration of driving. For example, data from the first 10 min have been considered to be the normal condition, while those from the last 10 min were specified as the fatigued condition (Li et al., 2009; Simon et al., 2011). Such an approach may not be appropriate, however, as some people may not develop fatigue even after 2–3 h of driving, especially professional drivers. Therefore, in order to discriminate between high- and low-risk conditions explicitly, each subject was both at high and low risk of fatigue before the driving tests, depending on how many hours they slept at night. Because sleep deprivation is well known to affect decision-making, attention, vigilance, human performance, and mental fatigue (Åkerstedt et al., 2004; Alhola and Polo-Kantola, 2007), it is appropriate to refer to sleep deprivation as analogous to fatigue. In addition, in our driving simulator, the steering wheel vibrated whenever the car crashed into a barrier to prevent drivers from actually falling asleep. Preventing the subjects from falling asleep may have suppressed activation in the delta and theta bands because these waves are associated closely with deep sleep (Maquet et al., 1997) and REM sleep (Jouvet, 1969), respectively.

Observations of Fatigue in the Well-Rested Condition

Before the experiment, all subjects with well-rested condition were instructed to sleep over 7 h to ensure that they were mentally alert and physically refreshed. However, several subjects experienced fatigue in the driving task nonetheless, due to various internal or external environmental factors, even though they reported that they had slept well the previous night. Subjects S7 and S9 had the lowest DCL values in the well-rested condition, as shown in **Table 2** and **Figure 6**. According to their questionnaires, these two subjects recorded a score of 2 in the sleepiness section (1: rarely sleepy to 5: very sleepy) prior to the experiment, yet they often nodded off during driving. Their behavior was recorded on the HD-Webcam, and showed clearly that they were drowsy. Furthermore, they reported scores of 4 and 5, respectively, on the sleepiness scale after the experiment. **Figure 8** represents the DCLs for these two subjects over time. As shown, their DCLs in the well-rested condition were similar to those in the sleep-deprived condition. The DCLs fluctuated in the well-rested condition, as shown by repeated increases and decreases. Moreover, these two subjects achieved low classification accuracies in a single modality, as shown in **Table 3**, although their accuracy improved when measured with mixed features. Clearly, we believe that these two subjects were likely to have been fatigued despite their assignment to the well-rested condition. In this work, we used the HD-webcam only to monitor the subjects, and did not measure or analyze behavioral data. Analyzing subjects' behavior in real-time, such as head or eye movements, may offer supporting evidence that some subjects slept well but experienced mental fatigue nonetheless. We will collect such behavioral data in the online mental fatigue monitoring system, which is currently under investigation.

Temporal Mismatch between EEG and fNIRS

Recently, many studies have tried to combine EEG and fNIRS to improve classification accuracy or increase the degrees of freedom in BCI systems (Fazli et al., 2012; Khan et al., 2014; Putze et al., 2014; Koo et al., 2015; Yin et al., 2015). However, the fNIRS system measures hemodynamic change, which is a delayed response compared to neuronal electrical activity, and it also has a relatively low temporal resolution (<10 Hz), both of which are critical drawbacks in fNIRS measurements. Because of their low temporal resolution, it is sometimes difficult to combine fNIRS data with other brain imaging data. Nevertheless, one of the most significant merits of the fNIRS system is its ability to measure oxygen consumption related to blood flow in the brain, similar to that in functional magnetic resonance imaging (fMRI), and fNIRS has been nicknamed the portable fMRI for this reason.

Considering the advantages and drawbacks of the fNIRS system, we calculated the features during each 1-min period throughout the dataset in this work. Each minute in the 30 min of data yielded a DCL value, which was used to discriminate between the well-rested and sleep-deprived conditions. In addition, oxygen consumption in the prefrontal cortex may represent cognitive workload or fatigue (Ayaz et al., 2012, 2013; Harrison et al., 2014; McKendrick et al., 2014). Therefore, it is likely that fNIRS may be a significant indicator of mental fatigue, and we are sure that employing multimodal data is quite useful in monitoring mental fatigue. Also, the prefrontal cortex is related closely to mental workload (Mandrick et al., 2013a)

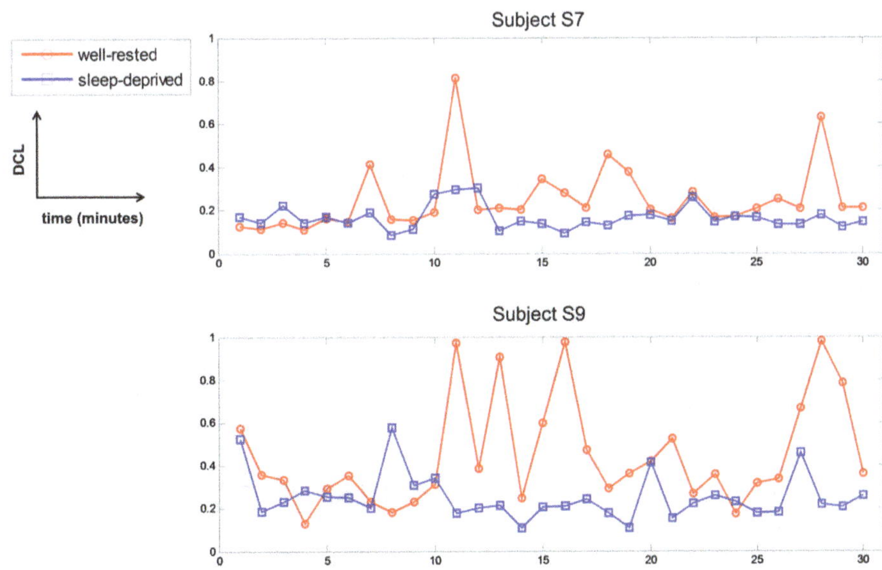

FIGURE 8 | Driving condition level of subject S7 and S9 in two conditions per 1 min over time. Red-circle and blue-square represent the driving condition level in well-rested and sleep-deprived conditions, respectively.

and the performance of cognitive tasks (Mandrick et al., 2013b). For these reasons, we introduced the prefrontal fNIRS in this work. However, whole head fNIRS would be beneficial and will be considered in our future work.

Limitations and Future Work

We proposed here an indicator of drivers' mental fatigue (Equation 4) that was able to discriminate the drivers' mental conditions well. To include equal contributions of EEG, ECG, and fNIRS features in the indicator, we normalized and summed all three. Further, all three were weighted equally to calculate the indicator, although this might not be an optimal method of quantification. Therefore, we calculated a new indicator using a weighting factor of $[DCL = a * norm\left(\frac{beta\ RPL}{alpha\ RPL}\right) + b * norm(HbO) + c * norm(HR)]$. Each weighting factor was defined between 0 and 1 with increments of 0.10; thus, we were able to search for the highest DCL difference in the two conditions (subtraction of sleep-deprived from well-rested). As a result, they had values comparable to those with equal weights and we observed no significant improvement. Even though we were able to apply elegant optimization methods, a somewhat better indicator may be achieved.

The primary reason to monitor drivers' mental fatigue is to prevent car accidents by providing drivers with a rapid and reliable alarm. To achieve this purpose, both making predictions before driving and monitoring a driver's condition in real-time are potential approaches. Our proposed rDCL (Equation 5) can predict a driver's fatigue prior to driving if training data can be obtained when the driver is in an alert state. Compared with DCL in the well-rested condition, the driver's condition prior to driving may be pre-checked by estimating the DCL. Although we used the entire dataset obtained during 30 min in the well-rested condition in this work, data of a shorter duration could be used for baseline. We are investigating the minimum duration needed to predict drivers' fatigue now. Another approach to accident prevention is to monitor drivers' fatigue in real-time.

We performed only an offline analysis in this work, and normalized DCL values were estimated each minute. For online monitoring, however, normalization of each modality's features is quite difficult to implement based on current methods available. One possible approach to solve the normalization issue is to record resting data before driving and use them as baseline data. Alternatively, an adaptive normalization method that updates feature values in real-time is a candidate. We are investigating the most appropriate normalization method for a subsequent online mental fatigue monitoring system.

In this work, we attempted to analyze multimodal data with simultaneous recordings of EEG/ECG/EOG and fNIRS. One of the advantages of multimodal signal integration is that each imaging method provides a physiologically and physically filtered view of one or more brain processes of interest. Thus far, the EEG-fMRI combination has been investigated widely, especially in epilepsy research, to help localize specific regions (Rosenkranz and Lemieux, 2010) by improving spatial and temporal resolution. Now, the EEG-fNIRS combination may be an alternative imaging method with merits that include low cost and simple implementation.

In this study, we custom-built an fNIRS that was already validated in previous study (Kim et al., 2015), and thus enabled us to design the experiment well. Although, a lengthy preparation time was required to attach the detectors and emitters, and test the quality of the light intensity for fNIRS measurement, this EEG-fNIRS integration may be quite beneficial in developing a monitoring system, as reported in the existing literature (Fazli et al., 2012; Wallois et al., 2012; Khan et al., 2014; Morioka et al., 2014; Putze et al., 2014; Koo et al., 2015; Yin et al., 2015). Another concern in analyzing multimodal data is how their differences (physical values, temporal resolution) are considered in an integrated frame. An in-depth investigation is needed to enhance the synergistic effect of multimodal data recording. Similarly, in this study, we were unable to guarantee that the EEG, ECG, and fNIRS, or their combined features, are related linearly to the fatigue level, although in the multimodal results, each modality influenced the fatigue level to some degree, as shown in **Figure 8**.

CONCLUSIONS

The purpose of this study was to use simultaneous EEG/ECG/EOG and fNIRS recordings to determine neuro-physiological correlates that can be used to discriminate sleep deprivation-induced mental fatigue in drivers by comparison to those who are well-rested. To achieve our purpose, we introduced two driving conditions (well-rested and sleep-deprived), and were able to extract significant features from their EEG, ECG, and fNIRS data. However, no significant feature was found in the EOG due to high variability in the subjects' data. The features observed allowed us to determine the mental condition of each driver, and also yielded good discriminative results between two driving conditions. Further, we investigated the synergistic effects of multimodal data to compare the various combinations at the classification level with a single modality. In conclusion, our proposed combined approach of simultaneous EEG/ECG and fNIRS data may be a promising tool with which to monitor drivers' mental fatigue.

AUTHOR CONTRIBUTIONS

SA, TN, HJ, JGK, and SCJ designed the experimental paradigm, and TN and JGK custom-built the fNIRS system. Data collection was conducted by SA, TN, and HJ, and analysis was performed by SA; the entire manuscript was written by SA and SCJ.

ACKNOWLEDGMENTS

This work was supported by Hyundai Next Generation Vehicle (NGV), the National Research Foundation of Korea (#2013R1A1A2009029), and the GIST Research Institute (GRI) in 2016.

REFERENCES

Ahn, M., Ahn, S., Hong, J. H., Cho, H., Kim, K., Kim, B. S., et al. (2013a). Gamma band activity associated with BCI performance: simultaneous MEG/EEG study. *Front. Hum. Neurosci.* 7:848. doi: 10.3389/fnhum.2013.00848

Ahn, M., Cho, H., Ahn, S., and Jun, S. C. (2013b). High theta and low alpha powers may be indicative of BCI-Illiteracy in motor imagery. *PLoS ONE* 8:e80886. doi: 10.1371/journal.pone.0080886

Ahn, M., and Jun, S. C. (2015). Performance variation in motor imagery brain–computer interface: a brief review. *J. Neurosci. Methods* 243, 103–110. doi: 10.1016/j.jneumeth.2015.01.033

Ahn, S., Ahn, M., Cho, H., and Jun, S. C. (2014). Achieving a hybrid brain-computer interface with tactile selective attention and motor imagery. *J. Neural Eng.* 11:066004. doi: 10.1088/1741-2560/11/6/066004

Alhola, P., and Polo-Kantola, P. (2007). Sleep deprivation: impact on cognitive performance. *Neuropsychiatr. Dis. Treat.* 3, 553–567.

Ayaz, H., Onaral, B., Izzetoglu, K., Shewokis, P. A., McKendrick, R., and Parasuraman, R. (2013). Continuous monitoring of brain dynamics with functional near infrared spectroscopy as a tool for neuroergonomic research: empirical examples and a technological development. *Front. Hum. Neurosci.* 7:871. doi: 10.3389/fnhum.2013.00871

Ayaz, H., Shewokis, P. A., Bunce, S., Izzetoglu, K., Willems, B., and Onaral, B. (2012). Optical brain monitoring for operator training and mental workload assessment. *Neuroimage* 59, 36–47. doi: 10.1016/j.neuroimage.2011.06.023

Bell, A. J., and Sejnowski, T. J. (1995). An information-maximization approach to blind separation and blind deconvolution. *Neural Comput.* 7, 1129–1159. doi: 10.1162/neco.1995.7.6.1129

Bergasa, L. M., Nuevo, J., Sotelo, M. A., Barea, R., and Lopez, M. E. (2006). Real-time system for monitoring driver vigilance. *IEEE Trans. Intell. Transp. Syst.* 7, 63–77. doi: 10.1109/TITS.2006.869598

Cho, H., Ahn, M., Kim, K., and Jun, S. C. (2015). Increasing session-to-session transfer in a brain–computer interface with on-site background noise acquisition. *J. Neural Eng.* 12:066009. doi: 10.1088/1741-2560/12/6/066009

Connor, J., Norton, R., Ameratunga, S., Robinson, E., Civil, I., Dunn, R., et al. (2002). Driver sleepiness and risk of serious injury to car occupants: population based case control study. *BMJ* 324:1125. doi: 10.1136/bmj.324.7346.1125

Cope, M., Delpy, D. T., Reynolds, E. O., Wray, S., Wyatt, J., and van der Zee, P. (1988). Methods of quantitating cerebral near infrared spectroscopy data. *Adv. Exp. Med. Biol.* 222, 183–189.

D'Orazio, T., Leo, M., Guaragnella, C., and Distante, A. (2007). A visual approach for driver inattention detection. *Pattern Recognit.* 40, 2341–2355. doi: 10.1016/j.patcog.2007.01.018

de Chazal, P., O'Dwyer, M., and Reilly, R. B. (2004). Automatic classification of heartbeats using ECG morphology and heartbeat interval features. *IEEE Trans. Biomed. Eng.* 51, 1196–1206. doi: 10.1109/TBME.2004.827359

Delorme, A., and Makeig, S. (2004). EEGLAB: an open source toolbox for analysis of single-trial EEG dynamics including independent component analysis. *J. Neurosci. Methods* 134, 9–21. doi: 10.1016/j.jneumeth.2003.10.009

Doi, H., Nishitani, S., and Shinohara, K. (2013). NIRS as a tool for assaying emotional function in the prefrontal cortex. *Front. Hum. Neurosci.* 7:770. doi: 10.3389/fnhum.2013.00770

Durmer, J. S., and Dinges, D. F. (2005). Neurocognitive consequences of sleep deprivation. *Semin. Neurol.* 25, 117–129. doi: 10.1055/s-2005-867080

Fazli, S., Mehnert, J., Steinbrink, J., Curio, G., Villringer, A., Müller, K.-R., et al. (2012). Enhanced performance by a hybrid NIRS-EEG brain computer interface. *Neuroimage* 59, 519–529. doi: 10.1016/j.neuroimage.2011.07.084

Gateau, T., Durantin, G., Lancelot, F., Scannella, S., and Dehais, F. (2015). Real-time state estimation in a flight simulator using fNIRS. *PLoS ONE* 10:e0121279. doi: 10.1371/journal.pone.0121279

Grandjean, E. (1979). Fatigue in industry. *Br. J. Ind. Med.* 36, 175–186.

Harrison, J., Izzetoglu, K., Ayaz, H., Willems, B., Hah, S., Ahlstrom, U., et al. (2014). Cognitive workload and learning assessment during the implementation of a next-generation air traffic control technology using functional near-infrared spectroscopy. *IEEE Trans. Hum. Mach. Syst.* 44, 429–440. doi: 10.1109/THMS.2014.2319822

Herman, J., Kafoa, B., Wainiqolo, I., Robinson, E., McCaig, E., Connor, J., et al. (2014). Driver sleepiness and risk of motor vehicle crash injuries: a population-based case control study in Fiji (TRIP 12). *Injury* 45, 586–591. doi: 10.1016/j.injury.2013.06.007

Homma, S., Fukunaga, T., and Kagaya, A. (1996). Influence of adipose tissue thickness on near infrared spectroscopic signal in the measurement of human muscle. *J. Biomed. Opt.* 1, 418–424. doi: 10.1117/12.252417

Horne, J., and Reyner, L. (1999). Vehicle accidents related to sleep: a review. *Occup. Environ. Med.* 56, 289–294.

Hu, S., and Zheng, G. (2009). Driver drowsiness detection with eyelid related parameters by support vector machine. *Expert Syst. Appl.* 36, 7651–7658. doi: 10.1016/j.eswa.2008.09.030

Ji, Q., Zhu, Z., and Lan, P. (2004). Real-time nonintrusive monitoring and prediction of driver fatigue. *IEEE Trans. Veh. Technol.* 53, 1052–1068. doi: 10.1109/TVT.2004.830974

Jouvet, M. (1969). Biogenic amines and the states of sleep. *Science* 163, 32–41. doi: 10.1126/science.163.3862.32

Kar, S., Bhagat, M., and Routray, A. (2010). EEG signal analysis for the assessment and quantification of driver's fatigue. *Transp. Res. Part F Traffic Psychol. Behav.* 13, 297–306. doi: 10.1016/j.trf.2010.06.006

Khan, M. J., Hong, M. J., and Hong, K.-S. (2014). Decoding of four movement directions using hybrid NIRS-EEG brain-computer interface. *Front. Hum. Neurosci.* 8:244. doi: 10.3389/fnhum.2014.00244

Khushaba, R. N., Kodagoda, S., Lal, S., and Dissanayake, G. (2011). Driver drowsiness classification using fuzzy wavelet-packet-based feature-extraction algorithm. *IEEE Trans. Biomed. Eng.* 58, 121–131. doi: 10.1109/TBME.2010.2077291

Kim, E., Lee, S., Phillips, Z., and Kim, J. G. (2015). A discrepancy of penile hemodynamics during visual sexual stimulation observed by near-infrared spectroscopy. *BMC Urol.* 15, 11. doi: 10.1186/s12894-015-0005-x

Kocsis, L., Herman, P., and Eke, A. (2006). The modified Beer-Lambert law revisited. *Phys. Med. Biol.* 51, N91–N98. doi: 10.1088/0031-9155/51/5/N02

Koo, B., Lee, H.-G., Nam, Y., Kang, H., Koh, C. S., Shin, H.-C., et al. (2015). A hybrid NIRS-EEG system for self-paced brain computer interface with online motor imagery. *J. Neurosci. Methods* 244, 26–32. doi: 10.1016/j.jneumeth.2014.04.016

Kripke, D. F., Garfinkel, L., Wingard, D. L., Klauber, M. R., and Marler, M. R. (2002). Mortality associated with sleep duration and insomnia. *Arch. Gen. Psychiatry* 59, 131–136. doi: 10.1001/archpsyc.59.2.131

Lal, S. K. L., and Craig, A. (2001). A critical review of the psychophysiology of driver fatigue. *Biol. Psychol.* 55, 173–194. doi: 10.1016/S0301-0511(00)00085-5

Lal, S. K. L., and Craig, A. (2002). Driver fatigue: electroencephalography and psychological assessment. *Psychophysiology* 39, 313–321. doi: 10.1017/S0048577201393095

Lal, S. K. L., Craig, A., Boord, P., Kirkup, L., and Nguyen, H. (2003). Development of an algorithm for an EEG-based driver fatigue countermeasure. *J. Safety Res.* 34, 321–328. doi: 10.1016/S0022-4375(03)00027-6

Li, G., and Chung, W.-Y. (2013). Detection of driver drowsiness using wavelet analysis of heart rate variability and a support vector machine classifier. *Sensors* 13, 16494–16511. doi: 10.3390/s131216494

Li, Z., Zhang, M., Zhang, X., Dai, S., Yu, X., and Wang, Y. (2009). Assessment of cerebral oxygenation during prolonged simulated driving using near infrared spectroscopy: its implications for fatigue development. *Eur. J. Appl. Physiol.* 107, 281–287. doi: 10.1007/s00421-009-1122-6

Lin, C.-T., Huang, K.-C., Chao, C.-F., Chen, J.-A., Chiu, T.-W., Ko, L.-W., et al. (2010). Tonic and phasic EEG and behavioral changes induced by arousing feedback. *Neuroimage* 52, 633–642. doi: 10.1016/j.neuroimage.2010.04.250

Lin, C.-T., Huang, K.-C., Chuang, C.-H., Ko, L.-W., and Jung, T.-P. (2013). Can arousing feedback rectify lapses in driving? Prediction from EEG power spectra. *J. Neural Eng.* 10:056024. doi: 10.1088/1741-2560/10/5/056024

Lin, C.-T., Wu, R.-C., Liang, S.-F., Chao, W.-H., Chen, Y.-J., and Jung, T.-P. (2005). EEG-based drowsiness estimation for safety driving using independent component analysis. *IEEE Trans. Circuits Syst. Regul. Pap.* 52, 2726–2738. doi: 10.1109/TCSI.2005.857555

Mandrick, K., Derosiere, G., Dray, G., Coulon, D., Micallef, J.-P., and Perrey, S. (2013a). Prefrontal cortex activity during motor tasks with additional mental load requiring attentional demand: a near-infrared spectroscopy study. *Neurosci. Res.* 76, 156–162. doi: 10.1016/j.neures.2013.04.006

Mandrick, K., Derosiere, G., Dray, G., Coulon, D., Micallef, J.-P., and Perrey, S. (2013b). Utilizing slope method as an alternative data analysis for functional near-infrared spectroscopy-derived cerebral hemodynamic responses. *Int. J. Ind. Ergon.* 43, 335–341. doi: 10.1016/j.ergon.2013.05.003

Maquet, P., Degueldre, C., Delfiore, G., Aerts, J., Péters, J.-M., Luxen, A., et al. (1997). Functional neuroanatomy of human slow wave sleep. *J. Neurosci.* 17, 2807–2812.

Matcher, S. J., Elwell, C. E., Cooper, C. E., Cope, M., and Delpy, D. T. (1995). Performance comparison of several published tissue near-infrared spectroscopy algorithms. *Anal. Biochem.* 227, 54–68. doi: 10.1006/abio.1995.1252

McKendrick, R., Ayaz, H., Olmstead, R., and Parasuraman, R. (2014). Enhancing dual-task performance with verbal and spatial working memory training: continuous monitoring of cerebral hemodynamics with NIRS. *Neuroimage* 85 (Pt 3), 1014–1026. doi: 10.1016/j.neuroimage.2013.05.103

Morioka, H., Kanemura, A., Morimoto, S., Yoshioka, T., Oba, S., Kawanabe, M., et al. (2014). Decoding spatial attention by using cortical currents estimated from electroencephalography with near-infrared spectroscopy prior information. *Neuroimage* 90, 128–139. doi: 10.1016/j.neuroimage.2013.12.035

Okogbaa, O. G., Shell, R. L., and Filipusic, D. (1994). On the investigation of the neurophysiological correlates of knowledge worker mental fatigue using the EEG signal. *Appl. Ergon.* 25, 355–365.

Parasuraman, R. (2003). Neuroergonomics: research and practice. *Theor. Issues Ergon. Sci.* 4, 5–20. doi: 10.1080/14639220210199753

Parasuraman, R., and Rizzo, M. (eds.). (2008). *Neuroergonomics: The Brain at Work.* New York, NY: Oxford University Press.

Parasuraman, R., and Wilson, G. F. (2008). Putting the brain to work: neuroergonomics past, present, and future. *Hum. Factors* 50, 468–474. doi: 10.1518/001872008X288349

Patel, M., Lal, S. K. L., Kavanagh, D., and Rossiter, P. (2011). Applying neural network analysis on heart rate variability data to assess driver fatigue. *Expert Syst. Appl.* 38, 7235–7242. doi: 10.1016/j.eswa.2010.12.028

Pettersson, K., Jagadeesan, S., Lukander, K., Henelius, A., Hæggström, E., and Müller, K. (2013). Algorithm for automatic analysis of electro-oculographic data. *Biomed. Eng. OnLine* 12:110. doi: 10.1186/1475-925X-12-110

Pfurtscheller, G., Allison, B. Z., Brunner, C., Bauernfeind, G., Solis-Escalante, T., Scherer, R., et al. (2010). The hybrid BCI. *Front. Neurosci.* 4:42. doi: 10.3389/fnpro.2010.00003

Putze, F., Hesslinger, S., Tse, C.-Y., Huang, Y., Herff, C., Guan, C., et al. (2014). Hybrid fNIRS-EEG based classification of auditory and visual perception processes. *Neuroprosthetics* 8:373. doi: 10.3389/fnins.2014.00373

Rihs, T. A., Michel, C. M., and Thut, G. (2007). Mechanisms of selective inhibition in visual spatial attention are indexed by α-band EEG synchronization. *Eur. J. Neurosci.* 25, 603–610. doi: 10.1111/j.1460-9568.2007.05278.x

Rosenkranz, K., and Lemieux, L. (2010). Present and future of simultaneous EEG-fMRI. *Magn. Reson. Mater. Phys. Biol. Med.* 23, 309–316. doi: 10.1007/s10334-009-0196-9

Sahayadhas, A., Sundaraj, K., and Murugappan, M. (2012). Detecting driver drowsiness based on sensors: a review. *Sensors* 12, 16937–16953. doi: 10.3390/s121216937

Sato, H., Yahata, N., Funane, T., Takizawa, R., Katura, T., Atsumori, H., et al. (2013). A NIRS-fMRI investigation of prefrontal cortex activity during a working memory task. *Neuroimage* 83, 158–173. doi: 10.1016/j.neuroimage.2013.06.043

Sauseng, P., Klimesch, W., Stadler, W., Schabus, M., Doppelmayr, M., Hanslmayr, S., et al. (2005). A shift of visual spatial attention is selectively associated with human EEG alpha activity. *Eur. J. Neurosci.* 22, 2917–2926. doi: 10.1111/j.1460-9568.2005.04482.x

Schalk, G., McFarland, D. J., Hinterberger, T., Birbaumer, N., and Wolpaw, J. R. (2004). BCI2000: a general-purpose brain-computer interface (BCI) system. *IEEE Trans. Biomed. Eng.* 51, 1034–1043. doi: 10.1109/TBME.2004.827072

Schleicher, R., Galley, N., Briest, S., and Galley, L. (2008). Blinks and saccades as indicators of fatigue in sleepiness warnings: looking tired? *Ergonomics* 51, 982–1010. doi: 10.1080/00140130701817062

Shen, K.-Q., Li, X.-P., Ong, C.-J., Shao, S.-Y., and Wilder-Smith, E. P. V. (2008). EEG-based mental fatigue measurement using multi-class support vector machines with confidence estimate. *Clin. Neurophysiol.* 119, 1524–1533. doi: 10.1016/j.clinph.2008.03.012

Simon, M., Schmidt, E. A., Kincses, W. E., Fritzsche, M., Bruns, A., Aufmuth, C., et al. (2011). EEG alpha spindle measures as indicators of driver fatigue under real traffic conditions. *Clin Neurophysiol* 122, 1168–1178. doi: 10.1016/j.clinph.2010.10.044

Tanaka, M., Shigihara, Y., Ishii, A., Funakura, M., Kanai, E., and Watanabe, Y. (2012). Effect of mental fatigue on the central nervous system: an electroencephalography study. *Behav. Brain Funct.* 8:48. doi: 10.1186/1744-9081-8-48

Åkerstedt, T., Knutsson, A., Westerholm, P., Theorell, T., Alfredsson, L., and Kecklund, G. (2004). Mental fatigue, work and sleep. *J. Psychosom. Res.* 57, 427–433. doi: 10.1016/j.jpsychores.2003.12.001

Uludağ, K., and Roebroeck, A. (2014). General overview on the merits of multimodal neuroimaging data fusion. *Neuroimage* 102, (Pt 1), 3–10. doi: 10.1016/j.neuroimage.2014.05.018

Wallois, F., Mahmoudzadeh, M., Patil, A., and Grebe, R. (2012). Usefulness of simultaneous EEG-NIRS recording in language studies. *Brain Lang.* 121, 110–123. doi: 10.1016/j.bandl.2011.03.010

Wang, Y.-T., Huang, K.-C., Wei, C.-S., Huang, T.-Y., Ko, L.-W., Lin, C.-T., et al. (2014). Developing an EEG-based on-line closed-loop lapse detection and mitigation system. *Neuroprosthetics* 8:321. doi: 10.3389/fnins.2014.00321

Worden, M. S., Foxe, J. J., Wang, N., and Simpson, G. V. (2000). Anticipatory biasing of visuospatial attention indexed by retinotopically specific α-bank electroencephalography increases over occipital cortex. *J. Neurosci.* 20:RC63.

Yang, G., Lin, Y., and Bhattacharya, P. (2010). A driver fatigue recognition model based on information fusion and dynamic Bayesian network. *Inf. Sci.* 180, 1942–1954. doi: 10.1016/j.ins.2010.01.011

Yeo, M. V. M., Li, X., Shen, K., and Wilder-Smith, E. P. V. (2009). Can SVM be used for automatic EEG detection of drowsiness during car driving? *Saf. Sci.* 47, 115–124. doi: 10.1016/j.ssci.2008.01.007

Yin, X., Xu, B., Jiang, C., Fu, Y., Wang, Z., Li, H., et al. (2015). A hybrid BCI based on EEG and fNIRS signals improves the performance of decoding motor imagery of both force and speed of hand clenching. *J. Neural Eng.* 12:036004. doi: 10.1088/1741-2560/12/3/036004

Yoshino, K., Oka, N., Yamamoto, K., Takahashi, H., and Kato, T. (2013). Functional brain imaging using near-infrared spectroscopy during actual driving on an expressway. *Front. Hum. Neurosci.* 7:882. doi: 10.3389/fnhum.2013.00882

Zhao, C., Zhao, M., Liu, J., and Zheng, C. (2012). Electroencephalogram and electrocardiograph assessment of mental fatigue in a driving simulator. *Accid. Anal. Prev.* 45, 83–90. doi: 10.1016/j.aap.2011.11.019

6

Efficient Workload Classification based on Ignored Auditory Probes: A Proof of Concept

Raphaëlle N. Roy[1,2]*, *Stéphane Bonnet*[1,3], *Sylvie Charbonnier*[1,2] *and Aurélie Campagne*[1,4]

[1] Université Grenoble Alpes, Grenoble, France, [2] Gipsa-Lab, Centre National de la Recherche Scientifique, Grenoble, France, [3] CEA LETI, Grenoble, France, [4] Laboratoire de Psychologie et NeuroCognition, Centre National de la Recherche Scientifique, Grenoble, France

***Correspondence:**
Raphaëlle N. Roy
roy.raphaelle@gmail.com

Mental workload is a mental state that is currently one of the main research focuses in neuroergonomics. It can notably be estimated using measurements in electroencephalography (EEG), a method that allows for direct mental state assessment. Auditory probes can be used to elicit event-related potentials (ERPs) that are modulated by workload. Although, some papers do report ERP modulations due to workload using attended or ignored probes, to our knowledge there is no literature regarding effective workload classification based on ignored auditory probes. In this paper, in order to efficiently estimate workload, we advocate for the use of such ignored auditory probes in a single-stimulus paradigm and a signal processing chain that includes a spatial filtering step. The effectiveness of this approach is demonstrated on data acquired from participants that performed the Multi-Attribute Task Battery – II. They carried out this task during two 10-min blocks. Each block corresponded to a workload condition that was pseudorandomly assigned. The easy condition consisted of two monitoring tasks performed in parallel, and the difficult one consisted of those two tasks with an additional plane driving task. Infrequent auditory probes were presented during the tasks and the participants were asked to ignore them. The EEG data were denoised and the probes' ERPs were extracted and spatially filtered using a canonical correlation analysis. Next, binary classification was performed using a Fisher LDA and a fivefold cross-validation procedure. Our method allowed for a very high estimation performance with a classification accuracy above 80% for every participant, and minimal intrusiveness thanks to the use of a single-stimulus paradigm. Therefore, this study paves the way to the efficient use of ERPs for mental state monitoring in close to real-life settings and contributes toward the development of adaptive user interfaces.

Keywords: workload, classification, auditory evoked potentials, spatial filtering

INTRODUCTION

Mental workload is frequently defined as task difficulty and the associated mental effort (Gevins and Smith, 2007). It is therefore of critical interest to better assess this state to the human factor community who aims at developing smart technologies that enhance operator's safety and performance. The impact of workload on behavior has been extensively documented. Participants' reaction time is known to increase linearly with the increase in the number of items to memorize

(Sternberg, 1969), as well as with the number of tasks to perform in parallel (Cain, 2007). However, behavioral responses are not always enough for mental state monitoring (MSM) systems, mainly due to their latency of occurrence, and to the fact that some mental states are not necessarily or systematically reflected by a specific response. Physiological data give more insight into the operator's state, especially electroencephalography (EEG), a method that allows for direct mental state assessment. The use of physiological markers derived from the cerebral activity for human factor purposes has given rise to a new field: neuroergonomics (Parasuraman et al., 2012).

Amongst the various markers derived from the EEG activity, event-related potentials (ERPs) are frequently used for MSM. ERPs correspond to the EEG activity that is temporally locked to the appearance of a given stimulation, or probe. Although, ERPs only allow for a discontinuous evaluation of the operator's mental state -unlike frequency measures, according to Roy et al. (2016) frequency measures are very sensitive to mental fatigue and vigilance states whereas ERPs are more robust to these states. Therefore, ERPs may be more suitable for ecological settings. Moreover, the literature describes numerous workload-related ERP modulations, such as early and late components' amplitude decreases. Hence, the P300 component's amplitude is reduced by an increase in workload (Kok, 2001; Schultheis and Jameson, 2004; Gomarus et al., 2006; Holm et al., 2009; Friedrich et al., 2011), and so is the N1, N2, and P2 components' amplitude (Kramer et al., 1995; Ullsperger et al., 2001; Gomarus et al., 2006; Allison and Polich, 2008; Miller et al., 2011; Boonstra et al., 2013). In the specific context of simulated flight, the P300 component's amplitude elicited by auditory probes has also been shown to decrease when the primary task's complexity increases (Natani and Gomer, 1981; Kramer et al., 1987; Sirevaag et al., 1993).

In order to determine an operator's mental state to modify the behavior of a system, one needs to compute an index or a class of workload to be fed as an input. This can be done using machine learning algorithms developed for brain–computer interfaces (BCIs). When those algorithms are used for applications that are not directed toward the voluntary control of an effector, those systems are often referred to as passive BCIs (Zander and Kothe, 2011; van Erp et al., 2012). Although, the number of publications regarding mental workload assessment has drastically increased this decade, only a few articles actually propose a classification based on ERPs. Brouwer et al. (2012) used seven electrodes and achieved 64% of correct binary classifications. Recently, it was proved that ERP spatial filtering could significantly enhance workload classification (Mühl et al., 2014; Roy et al., 2015). The authors achieved 72 and 98% of correct classifications using respectively a Fisher spatial filtering (FSF; Hoffmann et al., 2006) and a canonical correlation analysis filtering (CCA; Hotelling, 1936). However, these authors used task-dependent probes, i.e., items that were paramount for the task at hand, which is therefore quite unrealistic for real-life settings. Very recently, Roy et al. (2016) showed that ERPs elicited by visual task-independent probes could be used for mental workload estimation. They inserted a basic detection task in a Sternberg memory task and used the ERPs elicited by the targets to classify the workload level of the memory task. They reached 91% of correct binary classifications by filtering the ERPs using a CCA. This is very promising, however the probes, although task-independent, still required an overt answer from the participant. This kind of dual task setting can therefore lead to decreased attentional engagement to the primary task, which seems rather unwelcome for operators' monitoring in hazardous work situations (e.g., driving, plant monitoring, custom control). Hence, the best approach to use ERPs in ecological settings would be a stimulation paradigm with task-independent and ignored probes. And as the ultimate goal should be to develop systems based on minimally intrusive probes, these stimulations should be as scarce as possible. As reported by Mertens and Polich (1997), the ERPs elicited in a single-stimulus paradigm by visual or auditory probes are a viable alternative to the traditional oddball procedure, although late components' amplitude is reduced when the stimuli are ignored compared to when they are counted or await a motor response. The authors even report that auditory probes elicit ERPs that are more robust to response type. That is to say that ignored auditory stimuli generate early and late components which amplitude is quite similar to that of stimuli awaiting an active answer. This makes them very good candidates for the features to use in a mental workload estimation procedure.

This study intends to provide an evaluation of the efficiency of a workload estimation based on the ERPs elicited by infrequent, task-independent and ignored auditory probes. Workload was modulated by modulating the number of tasks to perform in parallel with the Multi-Attribute Task Battery – II (MATB; Comstock and Arnegard, 1992). A single-stimulus paradigm was used to elicit ERPs which were then spatially filtered with a CCA and classified. The performance of this processing chain was also compared to that of a simpler chain without spatial filtering. The contributions of this paper are threefold: (1) to assess the validity of the single-stimulus paradigm for effective mental workload estimation; (2) to assess the relevance of a processing chain that includes a spatial filtering step in order to classify accurately the auditory evoked potentials (AEPs) of those ignored, infrequent probes; (3) to assess the relevance of both the stimulation paradigm and the processing chain for an ecologically valid task, the MATB.

MATERIALS AND METHODS

This research was promoted by Grenoble's clinical research direction (France) and was approved by the French ethics committee (ID number: 2014-A00040-47) and the French health safety agency (B140052-31).

Experimental Setup

Eight healthy right-handed volunteers (three females; 29.9 years old ± 5.9) performed two 10-min experimental blocks of the Multi-Attribute Task Battery-II, the last version of task developed by NASA to study divided attention and multitasking (Comstock and Arnegard, 1992; **Figure 1**). In this experimental setup, each block corresponded to a different workload level (low/high), which was pseudo-randomly assigned. In the low

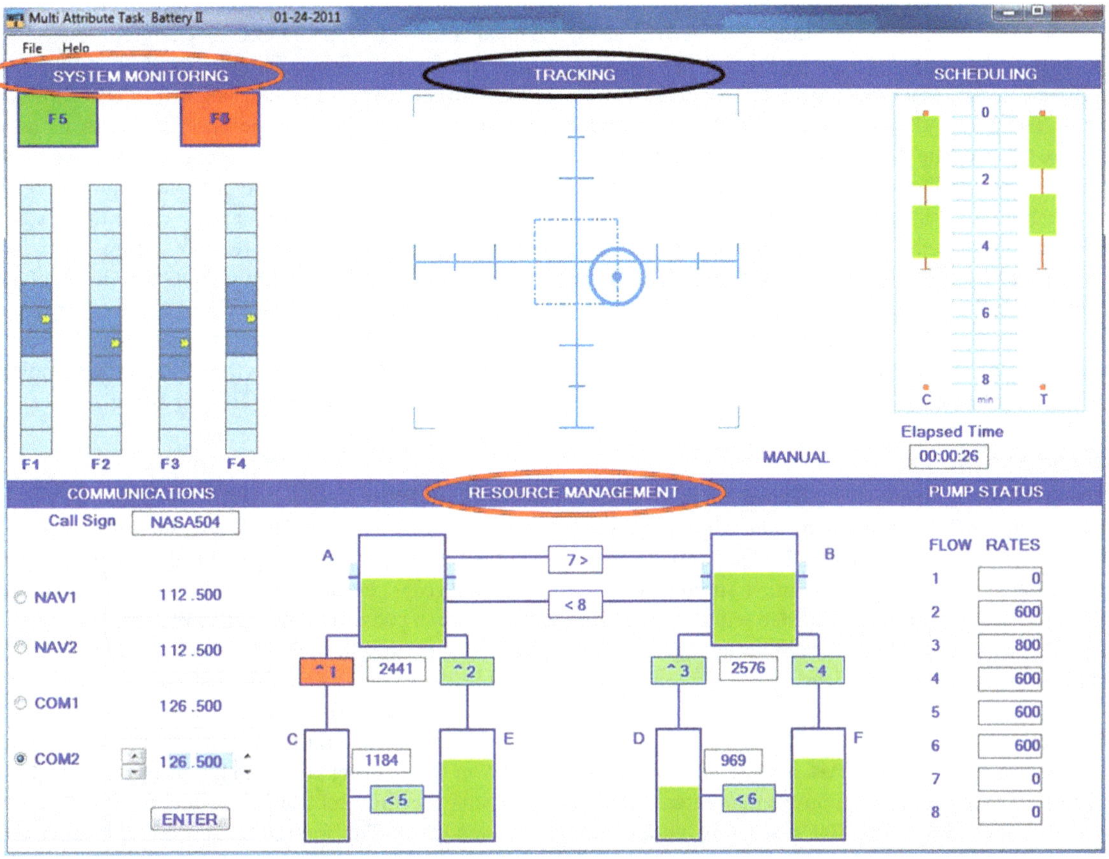

FIGURE 1 | Multi-Attribute Task Battery – II. The participants performed two out of three of the circled sub-tasks during the low workload condition (system monitoring and resource management tasks), and an additional third task during the high workload condition (tracking task).

workload condition, the participants performed two monitoring tasks using the keyboard, i.e., the system monitoring and the resource management tasks. The system monitoring task was presented in the upper left window of the display. As explained in the article of Comstock and Arnegard (1992), the demands of monitoring gages and warning lights were simulated here. The participants had to respond to the absence of the green light, the presence of the red light, and to monitor the four moving pointer dials deviation from midpoint. Regarding the resource management task, it simulated the demands of fuel management. The participants had to maintain tanks A and B at 2500 units each. This was done by turning on or off any of the eight pumps, which can sometimes fail.

In the high workload condition, they had an additional tracking task to manage in parallel. The tracking task was located in the upper middle window and simulated the demands of manual control. The participants had to keep the target at the center of the window using the joystick. Therefore, in both the low and high workload conditions perceptual, attentional, and decision making processes are recruited, along with motor preparation and performance. The difference between the low and the high workload conditions only stems in the additional workload imposed by the additional task.

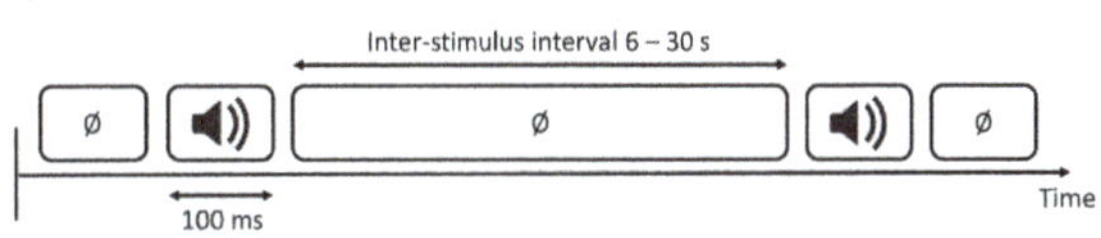

FIGURE 2 | Single-stimulus paradigm using ignored and infrequent auditory probes.

In addition to the visual stimulations induced by the MATB-II, the participants received auditory stimuli. They were instructed to ignore these auditory stimuli and to focus on the task at hand. These stimuli were sent by the Eprime software (E-prime Psychology Software Tools, Inc., Pittsburgh, PA, USA) into their Sennheiser audioset. In a similar fashion to the single-stimulus paradigm of Allison and Polich (2008), they consisted of 100 ms 1000 Hz pure tones (10 ms rise/fall, 65 dB SPL), with a random 6–30 s inter-tone interval (**Figure 2**). A minimum of 30 stimulations per block were presented.

Data Acquisition

Data acquisition was performed at the IRMaGe Neurophysiology facility (Grenoble, France). The participants' answers to the Rating Scale Mental Effort questionnaire (RSME; Zijlstra, 1993) and their resource management task root mean square (RMS) error scores were recorded, as well as their EEG activity using an Acticap® (Brain Products, Inc.) equipped with 32 Ag-AgCl unipolar active electrodes that were positioned according to the 10–20 system. The reference and ground electrodes used for acquisition were those of the Acticap, i.e., FCz for the reference, and AFz for the ground. The electro-oculographic activity was also recorded using two electrodes positioned at the eyes outer canthi, and two respectively above and below the left eye. Impedance was kept below 10 kΩ for all electrodes. The signal was amplified using a BrainAmp™ system (Brain Products, Inc.) and sampled at 500 Hz with a 0.1 Hz high-pass filter and a 0.1 μV resolution. Participants were instructed to limit eye and body movements during the task.

Signal Processing

The processing chain is detailed in **Figure 3**. In a general manner, the raw data was preprocessed, then spatially filtered, and lastly classified. Details are given in the following subsections regarding each step of this chain. It should be noted that the same processing chain was replicated without the spatial filtering step in order to evaluate if spatial filtering enhances the discriminability of the two workload levels.

Preprocessing

The digital EEG signal was band-pass filtered between 1 and 40 Hz, and re-referenced to a common average reference. The signal was then epoched starting 100 ms before and ending 600 ms after the auditory stimulation. Next, artifacts related to ocular movements (saccades and blinks) were corrected using the signal recorded from the electrooculographic electrodes (EOG) and the Second Order Blind Identification algorithm (SOBI; Belouchrani et al., 1997). This algorithm was chosen to perform the source decomposition because thanks to its assumption of non-correlation -and not mutual independence- it has been shown to be more suitable for electrophysiological data by Congedo et al. (2008). In order to get closer to a system that could be implemented on-line in a real-life setting, the two sources that were the most correlated to the EOG activity were canceled. All trials were kept for analysis. The AEPs were then extracted by subtracting a 100 ms baseline (i.e., mean signal amplitude) to the 600 ms segment that starts at the onset of the stimulation. Lastly, the data was decimated to 100 Hz using a five-point moving average.

Spatial Filtering

Then, the preprocessed data $\mathbf{X}$ (N_s – number of samples × N_e – number of channels) were spatially filtered, resulting in the signal $\mathbf{Z} = \mathbf{WX}$ (N_s – number of samples × N_f – number of spatial filters). Each column of the matrix $\mathbf{W}$ contains a spatial filter with its spatial pattern in the corresponding column of $\mathbf{A} = (\mathbf{W}^{-1})^{\mathrm{T}}$. In this paper, we use CCA as a spatial filtering method. As Spüler et al. (2014) detailed it , in a two-class scenario the CCA filters are computed in order to maximize the correlation between the EEG signal $\mathbf{X}$ and the matrix $\mathbf{Y} = \mathbf{D}_1\mathbf{P}_1+\mathbf{D}_2\mathbf{P}_2$ that contains the time replication of the average ERP responses $\mathbf{P}_i$ for each class. The matrix $\mathbf{D}_i$ is a Toeplitz binary matrix that indicates the stimulation onset for the ith class (Rivet et al., 2009).

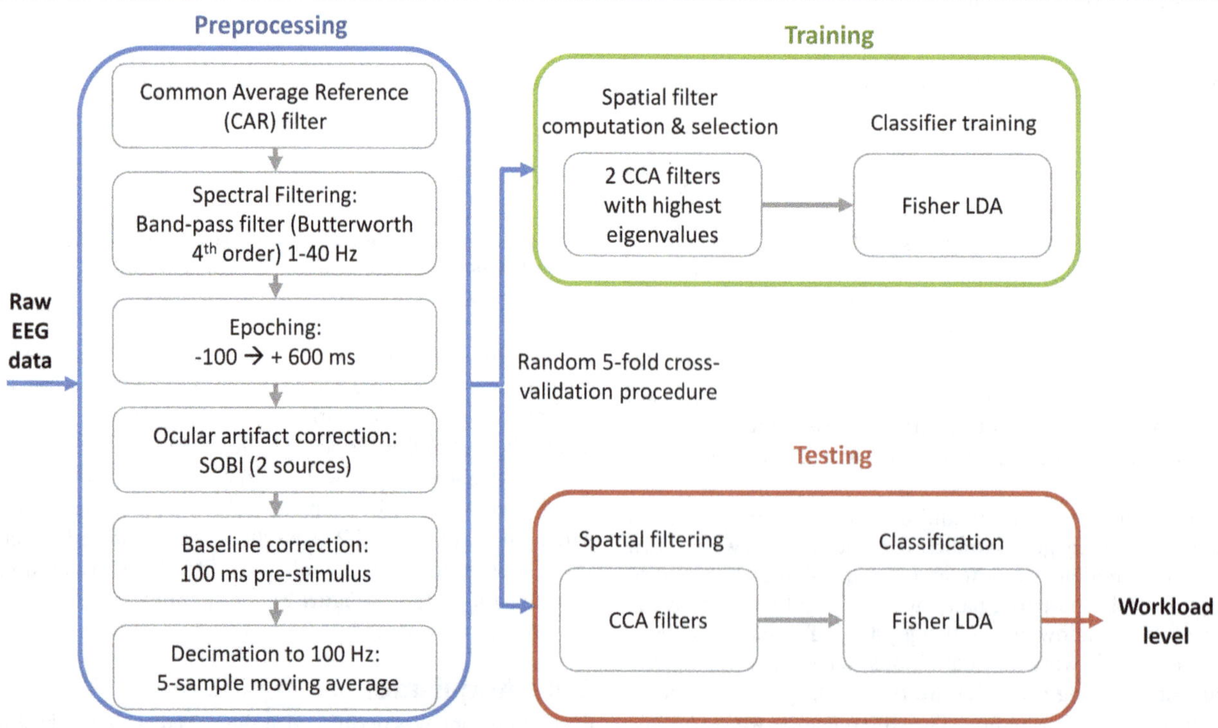

FIGURE 3 | Flow diagram of the signal processing chain applied on the EEG data in order to estimate mental workload.

Several methods have been proposed to solve CCA by computing orthonormal bases for the data matrices either by QR or singular value decomposition - SVD (Björck and Golub, 1973).

The CCA spatial filters were computed using the training data only. Then, the spatial filters with the two highest associated canonical correlations were selected. When these filters are applied on the testing data, the feature vector for the jth trial is given by the column concatenation $\mathbf{f}_j = \text{vec}(X_j[\mathbf{w}_1 \mathbf{w}_2])$ with dimension 120x1 (i.e., 60 samples × 2 virtual electrodes). In order to have the same number of features for both processing chains (with and without spatial filtering), for the chain without spatial filtering the feature vector was composed of the concatenated signals of the C3 and Pz electrodes (chosen visually using the average spatial patterns presented in Section "Spatial patterns").

Classification

A single-trial classification was performed on the feature vector **f** using a Fisher linear discriminant analysis (FLDA), with a shrinkage estimation of the covariance matrices (Schäfer and Strimmer, 2005). As explained by Blankertz et al. (2011), this estimation method allows the use of LDA with high dimensional features and gives good results that can generalize well (Blankertz et al., 2011). We used a random fivefold cross-validation procedure. The spatial filters were learned on the training set, and applied on the testing set. In the same way, the shrinkage estimation was learned on the training set. The performance of the processing chains was assessed based on their intra-subject binary classification accuracy.

Statistical Analyses

Statistical analyses were carried out on all results, i.e., subjective results from the RSME questionnaire, N1, P1, N2, P2, and P3 peak amplitude and latency from the AEP components, and classification results obtained using the processing chains with and without spatial filtering. All results were compared between themselves using repeated measures ANOVAs and Tukey *post hoc* tests. The significance level was set at 0.05.

RESULTS

Behavioral and Subjective Data

In a similar manner to Fournier et al. (1999), behavioral responses were standardized within each participant by dividing their response times to the resource management tasks by their proportion of correct responses. There was a significant effect of workload on this performance score ($t = 2.99$, $p < 0.05$), the participants' performance was significantly degraded in the high workload condition compared to the low workload condition ($m1\_perf = 0.33$; $sd1\_perf = 0.12$; $m2\_perf = 0.43$; $sd2\_perf = 0.12$). Moreover, the participants reported having furnished a significantly bigger effort in the high workload condition than in the low workload one [$F(1,7) = 38.04$, $p < 0.01$; $m1\_RSME = 45.5$; $sd1\_RSME = 18.2$; $m2\_RSME = 71.6$; $sd2\_RSME = 24.3$].

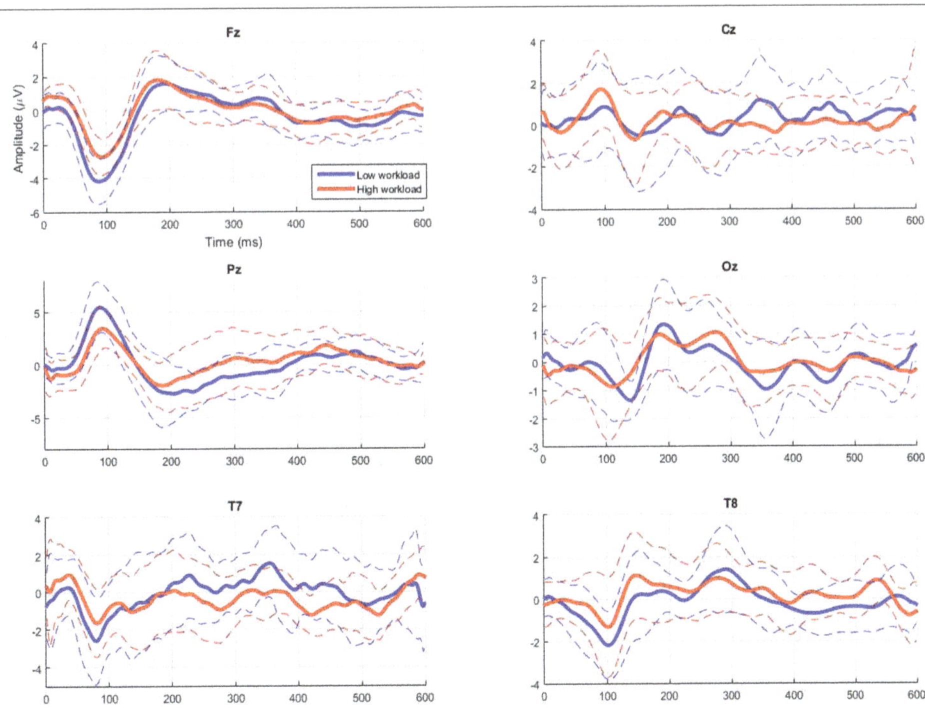

FIGURE 4 | Grand average (in bold) and standard deviation (dotted line) of the auditory evoked potentials (AEPs) elicited by the ignored infrequent auditory probes depending on workload condition at major midline electrode sites (Fz, Cz, Pz, and Oz), as well as at auditory processing relevant sites (T7 and T8).

Auditory Evoked Potentials

Figure 4 gives the grand-average AEPs across participants at major median electrode sites (Fz, Cz, Pz, and Oz), as well as at electrode sites located close to the auditory cortex (T7 and T8). **Figure 5** also gives the individual AEPs for the eight participants at the Pz electrode site (chosen to illustrate the results that follow regarding early components). The typical components reported to be modulated by workload can be noticed, i.e., N1, P1, P2, N2, and P3 (Kramer et al., 1995; Kok, 2001; Ullsperger et al., 2001; Schultheis and Jameson, 2004; Gomarus et al., 2006; Allison and Polich, 2008; Holm et al., 2009; Miller et al., 2011; Boonstra et al., 2013). However, the statistical analyses revealed only few significant results at the group level, which is understandable given the mostly overlapping variance of both signals (see standard deviations in **Figure 4**). Indeed, with increasing workload there were only trends at the Pz electrode for a decrease in amplitude of the P1 component ($p = 0.11$; **Figure 5**) and for a decrease in latency of the N1 component ($p = 0.07$). Moreover, when workload increased there was a significant decrease in latency of the P2 component at all electrode sites [$F(1,7) = 6.74, p < 0.05$].

Spatial Patterns

The topographical representation of each of the two CCA spatial patterns obtained for each participant using the processing chain proposed in this paper are presented respectively in **Figures 6** and 7 (average across training folds). The first spatial pattern reveals that in order to better discriminate workload levels, our first selected spatial filter enhances the activity from centro-parieto-occipital regions -consistent with attentional processing, while the second one enhances the activity from temporal regions -consistent with auditory processing- as well as prefrontal areas which could be related to ocular activity.

Filtered EEG Signal

The filtered EEG signals obtained from the testing sets for each participant using the first and second CCA filters are presented respectively in **Figures 8** and **9** (grand average across cross-validation folds). Both filters seem to mainly enhance the ERP activity of the low workload condition while decreasing it for the high workload condition from around 50 to 400 ms. This is particularly true for participants 3 and 4 for the early components. The signal's polarity fluctuates in a different manner depending on the participant and the filter, however, a general pattern emerges. Particularly, for both filters we can see an enhancement in the low workload condition of the amplitude of the early components that peak between 80 and 250 ms, be it in the negative or in the positive range. Therefore it seems that the filters act in a way so that they enhance the relevance of early auditory evoked components but not so much of later components.

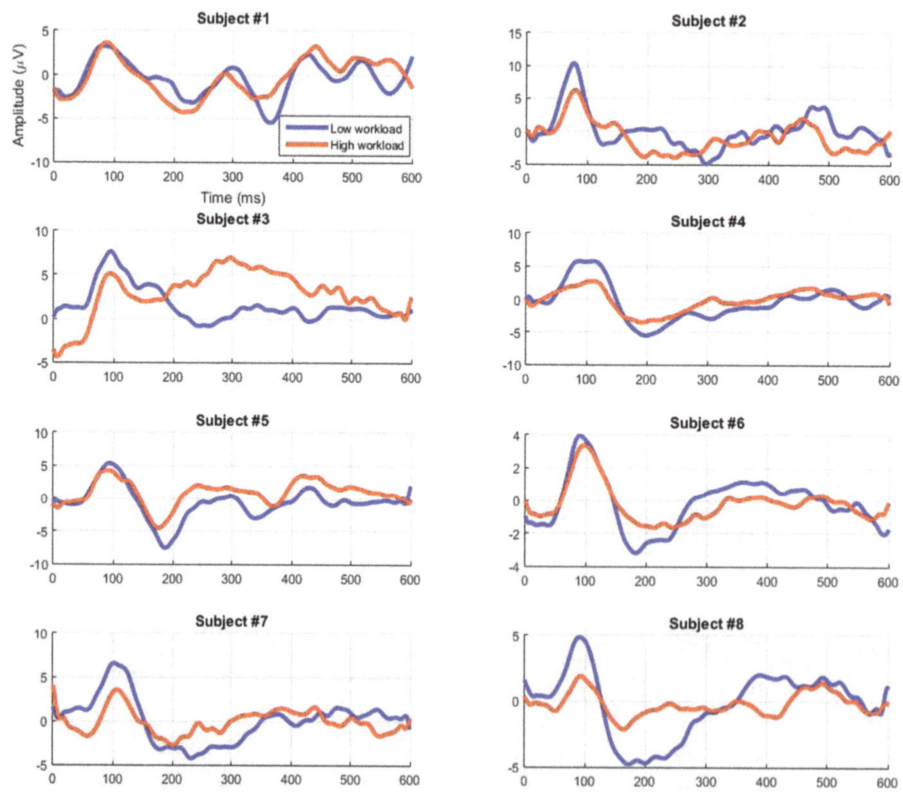

FIGURE 5 | Auditory evoked potentials elicited by the ignored infrequent auditory probes depending on workload condition at the Pz electrode site for all participants (grand average across trials).

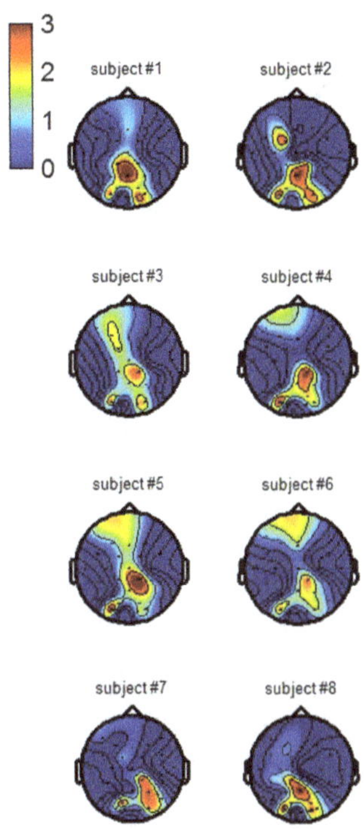

FIGURE 6 | Individual CCA spatial patterns of the first filter used to enhance the discrimination of the workload condition (grand average across training folds).

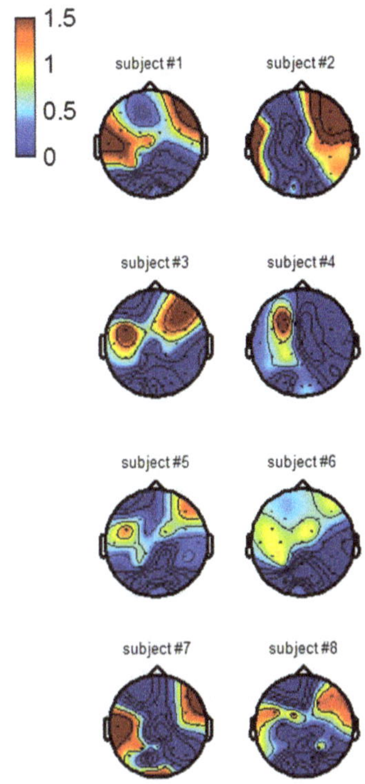

FIGURE 7 | Individual CCA spatial patterns of the second filter used to enhance the discrimination of the workload condition (grand average across training folds).

Classification Accuracy

The workload level classification results obtained using the single-stimulus paradigm and both the processing chain that includes a CCA spatial filtering step and the simpler processing chain without spatial filtering are given by **Figure 10** for each participant. There was a significant effect of the type of processing chain [$F(1,7) = 39.90, p < 0.001$]. Indeed, the chain that included the CCA spatial filtering step gave higher classification results than the one that didn't. The mean percentage of correct binary classification across the eight participants was 90.51% (± 10.7 SD) and 71.49% (± 15.9 SD) respectively for the processing chains with and without spatial filtering. Using the chain that included the CCA filtering, the performance was optimal for participant 4 with a classification accuracy of 100% and a null standard deviation, and the lowest performance was obtained for participant 7 with a classification accuracy of 80% and a very large standard deviation of 21.73.

DISCUSSION

Studies have demonstrated that workload modulates the ERPs elicited by attended or ignored auditory probes in a classical oddball paradigm involving deviant and standard tones (Kramer et al., 1995). Allison and Polich (2008) had also demonstrated this phenomenon using only infrequent standard tones (i.e., single-stimulus paradigm). However, to our knowledge, there was no literature regarding effective workload *classification* based on ignored auditory probes. Indeed, no signal processing chain had been applied to estimate workload in an automatic way from the ERPs of ignored auditory stimuli. Hence, this study was intended to bring new light on the potential use of ignored infrequent task-independent probes to efficiently and *automatically* assess mental workload in a minimally intrusive way. In order to do so, a single-stimulus paradigm similar to that of Allison and Polich (2008) was used, along with a processing chain that included a CCA spatial filtering step. The participants rated their effort as significantly higher for the high workload condition than for the low one and also exhibited a decrease in performance in the high workload condition compared to the low workload condition akin to that observed by Fournier et al. (1999). Their ERPs revealed only trends for a decrease in P1 amplitude and N1 latency, as well as a significant decrease in P2 latency. These results are in line with the literature regarding resource allocation processes. In a general manner, the amplitude of the ERP components that occur within the first 250 ms following stimulus onset has been demonstrated to be influenced by attentional capacity allocated to the eliciting stimulus and task operations (for a review see Kok, 1997). For instance, the P1 component amplitude is larger in active relative to passive viewing conditions (Fu et al., 2010). As for the N1 and the

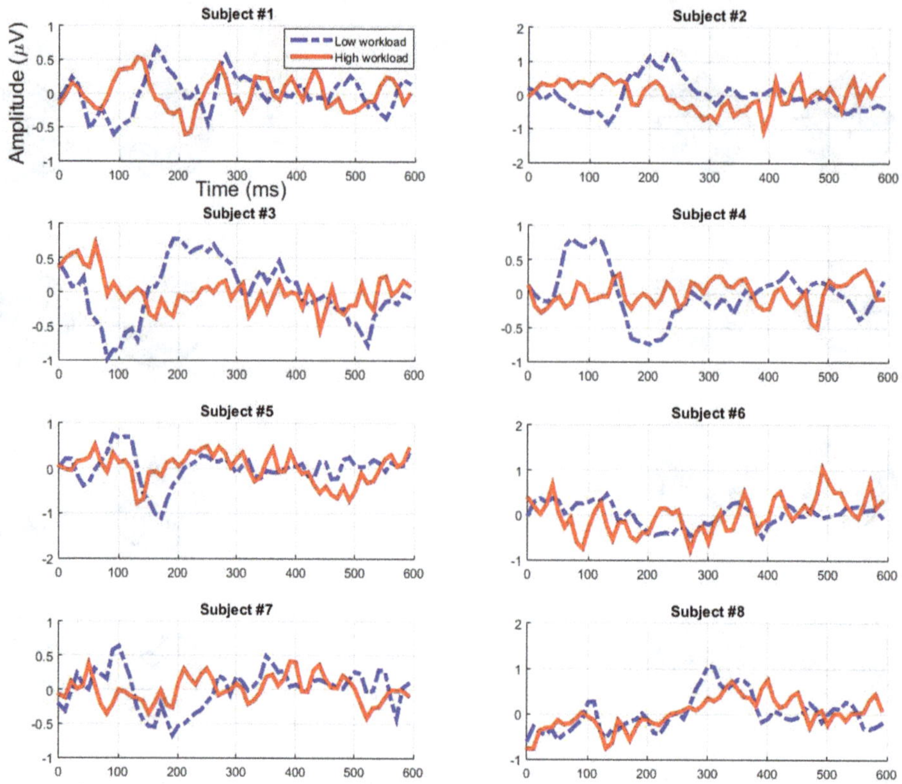

FIGURE 8 | Individual filtered test data – using the first CCA filter – depending on workload condition (grand average across cross-validation folds).

P2 latency, it has also been shown to decrease with a decrease in allocated attentional resources (Okita, 1979; Callaway and Halliday, 1982). However, more differences in amplitude were expected based on articles that describe workload modulations for ERPs elicited by task-dependent stimuli, specifically on late ERP components' amplitude (Kok, 2001; Ullsperger et al., 2001; Schultheis and Jameson, 2004; Gomarus et al., 2006; Holm et al., 2009; Miller et al., 2011; Boonstra et al., 2013). Yet, Kramer et al. (1995) had found that only the early components of the ERPs elicited by ignored task-irrelevant probes were relevant to perform a non-intrusive workload assessment, and that the late P300 component was not a good marker for such a goal. Our results confirm theirs as to which components are significantly modulated by workload using ignored auditory probes.

Despite the few significant results obtained at the group level regarding AEP components' amplitude, very accurate mental workload estimations were obtained using a signal processing chain that included a CCA spatial filtering step with at least 80% of correct binary classification accuracy for all participants, and an average of 90.51%. This result is in line with the literature that shows that classifiers can reveal statistical differences when standard statistical tests between ERPs do not (Noh and de Sa, 2014). Also, here the use of the CCA spatial filtering step significantly enhanced the estimation performance, as already demonstrated by Roy et al. (2015), and also reduced the variance in the results. Besides, this is only slightly lower than what Roy et al. (2016) obtained using task-independent visual probes -91%. This is very promising given that here, opposite to their protocol, the task-independent probes required no overt response and were ignored by the participants. Moreover, the probes used in this experiment are auditory while they were visual in their protocol. Lastly, those results are also higher than that obtained by previous studies that classified raw or spatially filtered ERPs elicited by task-dependent probes (Brouwer et al., 2012; Mühl et al., 2014). Therefore, the use of the single-stimulus paradigm coupled to a processing chain that includes a spatial filtering step allows a precise estimation of mental workload for a task that is very close to an actual work task. A limitation to this study is the number of trials, although in ecological settings it will be difficult to use more probes and to remain minimally intrusive. Nevertheless, according to Combrisson and Jerbi (2015), if we have more than 20 trials our performance should be over 70% in order to account for a significant detection with a $p < 0.05$ significance rate. Here, using the spatial filtering step we obtained at least 80% of correct detections, and an average of 90.51% with a minimum of 30 trials per condition. Therefore, we can say that our results were significantly above chance and that our method is quite efficient.

The spatial patterns of the selected CCA filters revealed that an enhancement of temporal and centro-parietal activity allowed reaching such high classification results. This is in accordance with the auditory nature of our probes. It is interesting to note that the activity that was enhanced by the spatial filters in the

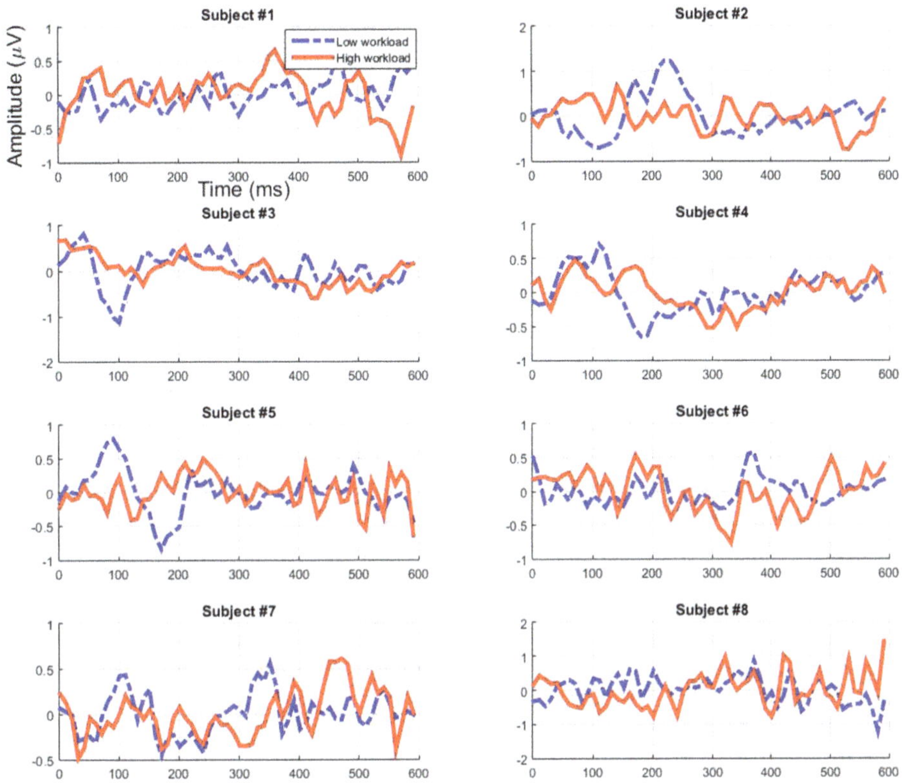

FIGURE 9 | Individual filtered test data – using the second CCA filter – depending on workload condition (grand average across cross-validation folds).

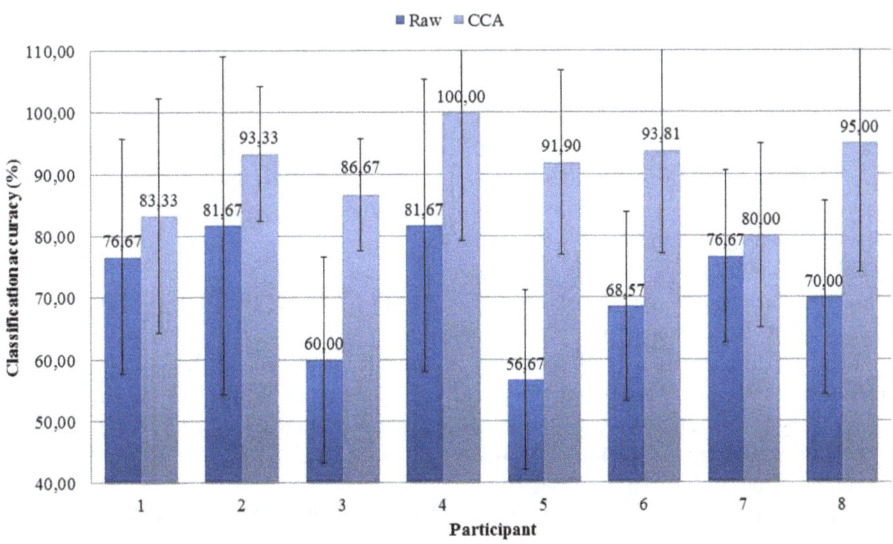

FIGURE 10 | Workload level classification accuracy reached for each participant using the raw data of two electrodes or a CCA spatial filtering step (mean and standard deviation of the percentage of correct binary classification across the random fivefold cross-validation procedure).

previously mentioned study of Roy et al. (2016) who used task-independent visual probes originated from the occipital sites, in accordance with the visual nature of their stimuli. In our study, given that the probes were auditory, we observed a specific enhancement of the activity from the temporal electrode sites. The signal from the centro-parietal sites was also enhanced in their study as in ours. These sites are known to be involved with attentional processing, and more generally with resource engagement (Kok, 1997). Additionally, the patterns also revealed an implication of prefrontal sites, which could stem from an under-efficient ocular artifact correction step in our processing chain. Indeed, in order to preserve the cerebral activity as much as possible, we only deleted the 2 out of 32 sources that were the most correlated to respectively the vertical and horizontal EOG channels. Also, given that the MATB-II is a task that is very close to a real work task, it elicits more ocular movements than classical laboratory tasks during which participants are asked to fixate the center of the screen and to limit eye movements and blinks. In any case, if it is indeed ocular activity that our second spatial filter enhanced, it means that this ocular activity allows efficient mental workload estimation. This is not surprising given that blink frequency has been reported to vary depending on task difficulty (Holland and Tarlow, 1972; Tanaka and Yamaoka, 1993). Moreover, it is known that the appearance of an unexpected stimulation leads to a startle eyeblink reflex. This reflex is attenuated during a multiple-task -high workload- compared to a single-task condition -low workload (Neumann, 2002). Therefore, the ocular activity produced in response to an infrequent auditory probe could be an efficient marker of task engagement and mental workload. As Roy et al. (2014) already argued , if ocular activity is helping to discriminate workload levels, why remove it? Hence, it might be interesting for future developments to use a processing chain that either does not include an ocular artifact correction step, or, that does but performs classification by fusing two feature vectors, a clean EEG one and an ocular activity one. Multimodality in terms of origin of the physiological markers (e.g., cerebral or ocular) could therefore be the key to enhance classification accuracy for real-life implementations.

Besides, this study evaluates the relevance of a stimulation paradigm and its dedicated processing chain for an ecological task which is the MATB. Although still in a laboratory setting, this task is very close to that performed by pilots and air traffic controllers. However, it modulates workload only by varying the number of tasks to perform in parallel, that is to say by varying the participants' degree of divided attention. In order to pursue the evaluation of the relevance of this stimulation paradigm, future work should focus on an evaluation of its relevance for several tasks that modulate workload based on different cognitive functions, e.g., working memory load, divided attention, executive functions. To our knowledge, only Berka et al. (2007) assessed the relevance of an EEG marker across several types of tasks. But, they focused on frequency power in the classical EEG bands. Thus, in order to progress toward an efficient estimation in real-life settings, the literature still lacks a thorough comparison of ERP modulations due to workload across several tasks. Also, although the participants of our study told us that they were not annoyed by the auditory infrequent stimulations and generally entirely forgot about it, a more thorough investigation of the real cost of such a paradigm in terms of operator fatigue and efficiency should be carried out. What's more, in order to increase the practicality of EEG measures, the number of electrodes should be diminished. However, this study, along with that of Roy et al. (2015) clearly establishes the relevance of a spatial filtering step in order to enhance the discriminability between the two workload levels. Therefore, future studies should evaluate how to reduce the number of electrodes while keeping enough channels to efficiently apply such a filtering step.

Consequently, this study contributes to the neuroergonomics research topic on mental workload estimation by uncovering three main points. First, the single-stimulus paradigm in which participants are probed by infrequent task-independent and ignored probes allows minimally intrusive workload estimation. Second, a spatial filtering step such as a CCA filtering enables a very accurate AEP-based workload classification. Lastly, the combination of this single-stimulus paradigm with infrequent ignored probes and its dedicated processing chain allows efficient workload estimation for an ecologically valid task such as the MATB.

CONCLUSION

This study has demonstrated as a proof-of-concept that a single-stimulus paradigm based on infrequent ignored auditory probes and its dedicated processing chain could allow a very accurate estimation of mental workload with a classification performance above 80% for every participant. This is also the first study to effectively classify workload based on ERPs elicited by ignored stimuli for a task that is very close to a real-life work situation. It paves the way toward the efficient use of ERPs for MSM and brings us closer to the implementation of user adaptive systems in ecological settings.

AUTHOR CONTRIBUTIONS

Study conception and design: RR, SB, SC, AC. Acquisition of data: RR. Analysis and interpretation of data: RR, SB. Drafting of manuscript: RR. Critical revision: SB, SC, AC.

ACKNOWLEDGMENTS

Grenoble Neurophysiology facility IRMaGe was partly funded by the French program "Investissement d'Avenir" run by the "Agence Nationale pour la Recherche": Grant "Infrastructure d'Avenir en Biologie Santé" (ANR-11-INBS-0006).

REFERENCES

Allison, B. Z., and Polich, J. (2008). Workload assessment of computer gaming using a single stimulus event-related potential paradigm. *Biol. Psychol.* 77, 277–283. doi: 10.1016/j.biopsycho.2007.10.014

Belouchrani, A., Abed-Meraim, K., Cardoso, J.-F., and Moulines, E. (1997). A blind source separation technique using second-order statistics. *IEEE Trans. Signal Process.* 45, 434–444. doi: 10.1109/78.554307

Berka, C., Levendowski, D. J., Lumicao, M. N., Yau, A., Davis, G., Zivkovic, V. T., et al. (2007). EEG correlates of task engagement and mental workload in vigilance, learning, and memory tasks. *Aviat. Space Environ. Med.* 78, 231–244.

Björck, A., and Golub, G. H. (1973). Numerical methods for computing angles between linear subspaces. *Math. Comput.* 27, 579–594. doi: 10.2307/2005662

Blankertz, B., Lemm, S., Treder, M., Haufe, S., and Müller, K.-R. (2011). Single-trial analysis and classification of ERP components: a tutorial. *Neuroimage* 56, 814–825. doi: 10.1016/j.neuroimage.2010.06.048

Boonstra, T. W., Powell, T. Y., Mehrkanoon, S., and Breakspear, M. (2013). Effects of mnemonic load on cortical activity during visual working memory: linking ongoing brain activity with evoked responses. *Int. J. Psychophysiol.* 89, 409–418. doi: 10.1016/j.ijpsycho.2013.04.001

Brouwer, A.-M., Hogervorst, M. A., van Erp, J. B. F., Heffelaar, T., Zimmerman, P. H., and Oostenveld, R. (2012). Estimating workload using EEG spectral power and ERPs in the n-back task. *J. Neur. Eng.* 9:045008. doi: 10.1088/1741-2560/9/4/045008

Cain, B. (2007). *A Review of the Mental Workload Literature 1.0.* Technical report, Defense Research and Development, Toronto, ON.

Callaway, E., and Halliday, R. (1982). The effect of attentional effort on visual evoked potential N1 latency. *Psychiatry Res.* 7, 299–308. doi: 10.1016/0165-1781(82)90066-X

Combrisson, E., and Jerbi, K. (2015). Exceeding chance level by chance: the caveat of theoretical chance levels in brain signal classification and statistical assessment of decoding accuracy. *J. Neurosci. Methods* 250, 126–136. doi: 10.1016/j.jneumeth.2015.01.010

Comstock, J. R. Jr., and Arnegard, R. J. (1992). *The Multi-Attribute Task Battery for Human Operator Workload and Strategic Behavior Research (NASA TM-104174).* Hampton, VA: NASA Langley Research Center.

Congedo, M., Gouy-Pailler, C., and Jutten, C. (2008). On the blind source separation of human electroencephalogram by approximate joint diagonalization of second order statistics. *Clin. Neurophysiol.* 119, 2677–2686. doi: 10.1016/j.clinph.2008.09.007

Fournier, L. R., Wilson, G. F., and Swain, C. R. (1999). Electrophysiological, behavioral, and subjective indexes of workload when performing multiple tasks: manipulations of task difficulty and training. *Int. J. Psychophysiol.* 31, 129–145. doi: 10.1016/S0167-8760(98)00049-X

Friedrich, E. V., Scherer, R., Sonnleitner, K., and Neuper, C. (2011). Impact of auditory distraction on user performance in a brain-computer interface driven by different mental tasks. *Clin. Neurophysiol.* 122, 2003–2009. doi: 10.1016/j.clinph.2011.03.019

Fu, S., Fedota, J. R., Greenwood, P. M., and Parasuraman, R. (2010). Dissociation of visual C1 and P1 components as a function of attentional load: an event-related potential study. *Biol. Psychol.* 85, 171–178. doi: 10.1016/j.biopsycho.2010.06.008

Gevins, A., and Smith, M. E. (2007). "Electroencephalography (EEG) in neuroergnomics," in *Neuroergonomics: The Brain at Work*, eds R. Parasuraman and M. Rizzo (New York, NY: Oxford University Press Inc), 15–31.

Gomarus, H. K., Althaus, M., Wijers, A. A., and Minderaa, R. B. (2006). The effects of memory load and stimulus relevance on the EEG during a visual selective memory search task: an ERP and ERD/ERS study. *Clin. Neurophysiol.* 117, 871–884. doi: 10.1016/j.clinph.2005.12.008

Hoffmann, U., Vesin, J., and Ebrahimi, T. (2006). "Spatial filters for the classification of event-related potentials," in *Proceeding of the European Symposium Artificial Neural Networks*, Bruges.

Holland, M. K., and Tarlow, G. (1972). Blinking and mental load. *Psychol. Rep.* 31, 119–127. doi: 10.2466/pr0.1972.31.1.119

Holm, A., Lukander, K., Korpela, J., Sallinen, M., and Müller, K. M. I. (2009). Estimating brain load from the EEG. *ScientificWorld J.* 9, 639–651. doi: 10.1100/tsw.2009.83

Hotelling, H. (1936). Relations between two sets of variates. *Biometrika* 28, 321–377. doi: 10.2307/2333955

Kok, A. (1997). Event-related-potential (ERP) reflections of mental resources: a review and synthesis. *Biol. Psychol.* 45, 19–56. doi: 10.1016/S0301-0511(96)05221-0

Kok, A. (2001). On the utility of P3 amplitude as a measure of processing capacity. *Psychophysiology* 38, 557–577. doi: 10.1017/S0048577201990559

Kramer, A. F., Sirevaag, E. J., and Braune, R. (1987). A psychophysiological assessment of operator workload during simulated flight missions. *Hum. Factors* 29, 145–160.

Kramer, A. F., Trejo, L. J., and Humphrey, D. (1995). Assessment of mental workload with task-irrelevant auditory probes. *Biol. Psychol.* 40, 83–100. doi: 10.1016/0301-0511(95)05108-2

Mertens, R., and Polich, J. (1997). P300 from a single-stimulus paradigm: passive versus active tasks and stimulus modality. *Electroencephalogr. Clin. Neurophysiol.* 104, 488–497. doi: 10.1016/S0168-5597(97)00041-5

Miller, M. W., Rietschel, J. C., McDonald, C. G., and Hatfield, B. D. (2011). A novel approach to the physiological measurement of mental workload. *Int. J. Psychophysiol.* 80, 75–78. doi: 10.1016/j.ijpsycho.2011.02.003

Mühl, C., Jeunet, C., and Lotte, F. (2014). EEG-based workload estimation across affective contexts. *Front. Neurosci.* 8:114. doi: 10.3389/fnins.2014.00114

Natani, K., and Gomer, F. E. (1981). *Electrocortical Activity and Operator Workload: A Comparison of Changes in the Electroencephalogram and in Event-Related Potentials.* McDonnell Douglas Technical Report E2427. Long Beach CA: McDonnell Douglas Corporation.

Neumann, D. L. (2002). Effect of varying levels of mental workload on startle eyeblink modulation. *Ergonomics* 45, 583–602. doi: 10.1080/00140130210148546

Noh, E., and de Sa, V. R. (2014). "Discriminative dimensionality reduction for analyzing EEG data," in *Proceedings of the 36th Annual Meeting of the Cognitive Science Society*, Austin, TX, 1090–1095.

Okita, T. (1979). Event-related potentials and selective attention to auditory stimuli varying in pitch and localization. *Biol. Psychol.* 9, 271–284. doi: 10.1016/0301-0511(79)90027-9

Parasuraman, R., Christensen, J., and Grafton, S. (2012). Neuroergonomics: The brain in action and at work. *Neuroimage* 59, 1–3. doi: 10.1016/j.neuroimage.2011.08.011

Rivet, B., Souloumiac, A., Attina, V., and Gibert, G. (2009). xDAWN algorithm to enhance evoked potentials: application to brain-computer interface. *IEEE Trans. Biomed. Eng.* 56, 2035–2043. doi: 10.1109/TBME.2009.2012869

Roy, R. N., Bonnet, S., Charbonnier, S., Jallon, P., and Campagne, A. (2015). A comparison of ERP spatial filtering methods for optimal mental workload estimation. *Conf. Proc. IEEE Eng. Med. Biol. Soc.* 2015, 7254–7257. doi: 10.1109/EMBC.2015.7320066

Roy, R. N., Charbonnier, S., and Bonnet, S. (2014). Eye blink characterization from frontal EEG electrodes using source separation and pattern recognition algorithms. *Biomed. Signal Process. Control* 14, 256–264. doi: 10.1016/j.bspc.2014.08.007

Roy, R. N., Charbonnier, S., Campagne, A., and Bonnet, S. (2016). Efficient mental workload estimation using task-independent EEG features. *J. Neural Eng.* 13:026019. doi: 10.1088/1741-2560/13/2/026019

Schäfer, J., and Strimmer, K. (2005). A shrinkage approach to large-scale covariance matrix estimation and implications for functional genomics. *Stat. Appl. Genet. Mol. Biol.* 4, 1175–1189.

Schultheis, H., and Jameson, A. (2004). Assessing cognitive load in adaptive hypermedia systems: physiological and behavioral methods. *Lect. Notes Comput. Sci.* 313, 225–234. doi: 10.1007/978-3-540-27780-4_26

Sirevaag, E., Kramer, A., Wickens, C. D., Reisweber, M., Strayer, D., and Grenell, J. (1993). Assessment of pilot performance and mental workload in rotary wing aircraft. *Ergonomics* 36, 1121–1140. doi: 10.1080/00140139308967983

Spüler, M., Walter, A., Rosenstiel, W., and Bogdan, M. (2014). Spatial filtering based on canonical correlation analysis for classification of evoked or event-related potentials in EEG data. *IEEE Trans. Neural Syst. Rehabil. Eng.* 22, 1097–1103. doi: 10.1109/TNSRE.2013.2290870

Sternberg, S. (1969). Memory-scanning: mental processes revealed by reaction-time experiments. *Am. Sci.* 57, 421–457.

Tanaka, Y., and Yamaoka, K. (1993). Blink activity and task difficulty. *Percept. Mot. Skills* 77, 55–66. doi: 10.2466/pms.1993.77.1.55

Ullsperger, P., Freude, G., and Erdmann, U. (2001). Auditory probe sensitivity to mental workload changes - an event-related potential study. *Int. J. Psychophysiol.* 40, 201–209. doi: 10.1016/S0167-8760(00)00188-4

van Erp, J., Lotte, F., and Tangermann, M. (2012). Brain-computer interfaces: beyond medical applications. *Computer* 45, 26–34. doi: 10.1109/MC.2012.107

Zander, T. O., and Kothe, C. (2011). Towards passive brain–computer interfaces: applying brain–computer interface technology to human–machine systems in general. *J. Neural Eng.* 8:025005. doi: 10.1088/1741-2560/8/2/025005

Zijlstra, F. R. H. (1993). *Efficiency in Work Behavior.* Doctoral dissertation, Technical University, Delft.

7

Toward a Wireless Open Source Instrument: Functional Near-Infrared Spectroscopy in Mobile Neuroergonomics and BCI Applications

Alexander von Lühmann [1,2], Christian Herff [3], Dominic Heger [3] and Tanja Schultz [3]*

[1] Machine Learning Department, Computer Science, Technische Universität Berlin, Berlin, Germany, [2] Institute of Biomedical Engineering, Karlsruhe Institute of Technology, Karlsruhe, Germany, [3] Cognitive Systems Lab, Karlsruhe Institute of Technology, Karlsruhe, Germany

***Correspondence:**
Alexander von Lühmann
a.vonluehmann@campus.tu-berlin.de

Brain-Computer Interfaces (BCIs) and neuroergonomics research have high requirements regarding robustness and mobility. Additionally, fast applicability and customization are desired. Functional Near-Infrared Spectroscopy (fNIRS) is an increasingly established technology with a potential to satisfy these conditions. EEG acquisition technology, currently one of the main modalities used for mobile brain activity assessment, is widely spread and open for access and thus easily customizable. fNIRS technology on the other hand has either to be bought as a predefined commercial solution or developed from scratch using published literature. To help reducing time and effort of future custom designs for research purposes, we present our approach toward an open source multichannel stand-alone fNIRS instrument for mobile NIRS-based neuroimaging, neuroergonomics and BCI/BMI applications. The instrument is low-cost, miniaturized, wireless and modular and openly documented on www.opennirs.org. It provides features such as scalable channel number, configurable regulated light intensities, programmable gain and lock-in amplification. In this paper, the system concept, hardware, software and mechanical implementation of the lightweight stand-alone instrument are presented and the evaluation and verification results of the instrument's hardware and physiological fNIRS functionality are described. Its capability to measure brain activity is demonstrated by qualitative signal assessments and a quantitative mental arithmetic based BCI study with 12 subjects.

Keywords: open source, functional near-infrared spectroscopy (fNIRS), brain computer interface (BCI), modularity, wearable devices, neuroergonomics

1. INTRODUCTION

Functional Near-Infrared Spectroscopy (fNIRS) is an increasingly established technology pioneered by Jöbsis (1977) that allows non-invasive, comparatively low-cost, compact and hazard-free continuous measurement of cerebral oxygenation levels using near-infrared light.

While first generation instruments were rather bulky and expensive, using Laser Diodes with Photo Multiplier Tubes (PMTs) (Cope and Delpy, 1988; Cope, 1991; Rolfe, 2000;

Schmidt et al., 2000) and later Avalanche Photo Diodes (APDs) (Boas et al., 2001; Coyle et al., 2004, 2007), today's devices often take advantage of Light Emitting Diodes (LED) and Photo Diodes (PDs) (Vaithianathan et al., 2004; Bunce et al., 2006; Chenier and Sawan, 2007; Ayaz et al., 2013; Safaie et al., 2013; Piper et al., 2014) which allow safe, more compact and mobile applications. After the initial development of laboratory and bedside-monitoring devices for monitoring of local oxygenation levels e.g., in newborn infants (Cope and Delpy, 1988; Cope, 1991), in the 2000s many research groups focused on the design of imaging instruments for brain activity mapping from topographic information [functional Near-Infrared Imaging (fNIRI)] (Schmidt et al., 2000; Boas et al., 2001; Vaithianathan et al., 2004). Recently, fNIRS and fNIRI have entered neuroscience as a reliable and trustworthy research tool for research based on investigating groups of subjects (Scholkmann et al., 2014), offering potentially complementary information to fMRI, PET and EEG (e.g., oxygenation information or cytochrome oxidase as marker of metabolic demands; Strangman et al., 2002). But also in adjacent fields such as Brain Computer Interfaces (BCI) and neuroergonomics, defined as the study of the human brain in relation to performance at work, (Parasuraman, 2003, 2011), fNIRS technology opens new possibilities (see e.g., Matthews et al., 2008, for an introduction in hemodynamics for Brain-Computer Interfaces). It is increasingly built for and used in single-trial fNIRS applications for BCIs for control (Naseer and Hong, 2013; Schudlo and Chau, 2015) and rehabilitation (Kanoh et al., 2009; Yanagisawa et al., 2010) and has successfully been used for cognitive workload assessment (Son and Yazici, 2006; Ayaz et al., 2012), brain dynamics monitoring during working memory training and expertise development (Ayaz et al., 2013), hybrid NIRS-EEG based signal processing tasks (Safaie et al., 2013; Putze et al., 2014) and recently also in combination with trans-cranial direct current stimulation (tDCS; McKendrick et al., 2015). Furthermore, fNIRS is found to be a promising multimodal expansion to EEG-based BCI (Pfurtscheller et al., 2010; Biessmann et al., 2011; Fazli et al., 2012). The major limitation of fNIRS is the relatively slow onset of hemodynamic processes. However, especially in the field of passive BCI (Zander and Kothe, 2011), reaction times do not necessarily have to be extremely fast.

An increasing number of approaches using fNIRS in the field of mobile brain imaging (e.g., Piper et al., 2014) and neuroergonomics (Fairclough, 2009) shows the demand for wireless, miniaturized and customizable fNIRS technology. So far, researchers either relied on costly and mainly static commercial devices, or designed their own fNIRS equipment from scratch. Trying to overcome the restrictions of commercial tabletop instruments, the latter was done by groups such as Ayaz et al. (2013), Safaie et al. (2013), Lareau et al. (2011) and Atsumori et al. (2007), using LEDs with Si PDs/APDs for new generation instruments that generally enable a mobile use. To the best of our knowledge however, only very few of even newer generation devices (Safaie et al., 2013) are truly miniaturized, stand-alone, unobtrusive and mobile and can be carried on the body without a backpack while still enabling free movement and data transmission/processing at the same time, as often external static instrumentation such as DAQ-equipment, lock-in amplifiers and power sources are required. Also, in many cases, signal extraction technologies like lock-in amplification seem to be sacrificed for the sake of miniaturization or complexity. Probe and attachment designs proposed in the last years, such as the use of flexible PCBs (Vaithianathan et al., 2004; Bozkurt et al., 2005; Bunce et al., 2006; Son and Yazici, 2006; Rajkumar et al., 2012), eeg-cap like optodes (Kiguchi et al., 2012; Piper et al., 2014) and mechanical mounting structures (Coyle et al., 2007) are usually limited to static applications and/or in case of flexible PCB to a fixation on the forehead due to obstruction by hair. An often reported issue in the field of mobile applications, that seems not to be resolved satisfactorily so far, is the optode attachment to the head for both stable optical contact, sufficient light levels and comfortable wearing.

While the recent trend of new system designs for portability and mobility can also increasingly be observed in commercial devices, researchers will always need custom solutions for innovative approaches. To help reducing the time and effort in these cases, we present the design and a first evaluation of a configurable, miniaturized, modular, fully mobile (wireless) multichannel fNIRS system that is provided open source on www.opennirs.org under a CC BY-NC 4.0 license with a detailed documentation. It is a customizable low-cost research tool that enables both stand-alone use and the combination with custom or external DAQ equipment. Also, the device makes use of a new detailed spring-loaded optode fixation concept to tackle the above mentioned optode attachment issue.

2. MATERIALS AND METHODS

2.1. Instrument Requirements

We identified aspects that are crucial to be fulfilled for a fNIRS device in the context of mobile BCI and neuroergonomics. Besides the criterion for the hardware to be comparatively low cost, these can be assigned to four groups:

- **Usability:** Miniaturization and mobility of the device, unobtrusiveness and robustness of the optode attachment.
- **Signal Quality:** Low inter channel crosstalk, low drifts of light sources and overall system signals, high signal sensitivity/amplifier precision, robustness to background light and high dynamic range.
- **Safety:** Low heat development, harmless light intensities and galvanic isolation to power lines.
- **Configuration/Customization:** Scalability of channel number, modularity, configuration of light intensities and receiver gain, interface to custom hard-/software.

The following subsections will provide detailed information on our approach to fulfill these requirements on a concept, hardware and software level.

2.2. Instrumentation Design

2.2.1. System Concept

The system concept of the modular open instrument is shown in **Figure 1**. It consists of one or more stand alone 4-channel

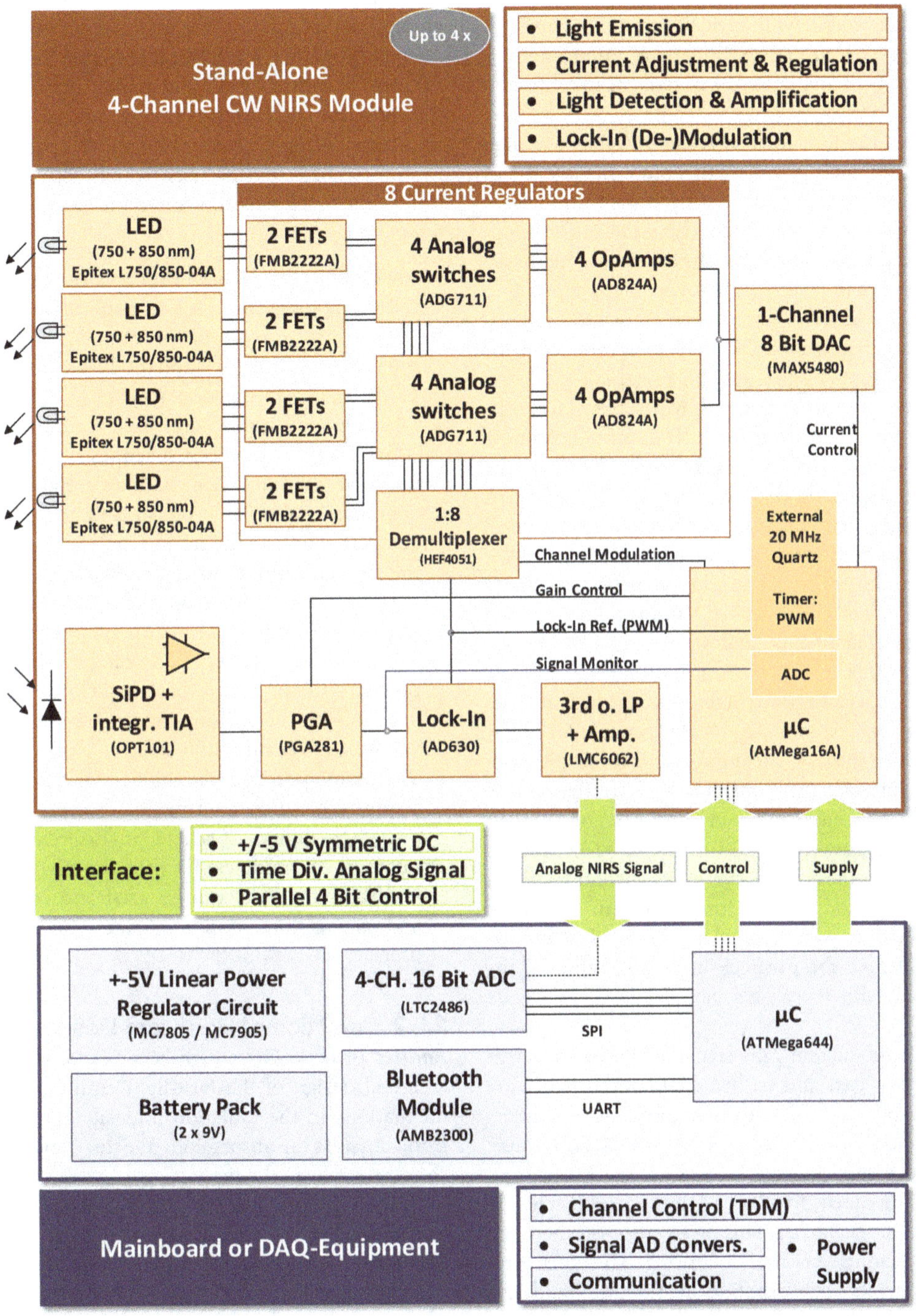

FIGURE 1 | System Concept.

Continuous Wave NIRS modules and a mainboard. Each module is controlled by the mainboard via a simple parallel 4 Bit control interface. The mainboard provides the power supply rails, AD-conversion of the NIRS signals and an UART communication interface and can be replaced by any custom data acquisition (DAQ-) equipment when the control interface and symmetric ±5 V power rail are supplied. This enables full customization of the instrument with respect to physical channel number, power consumption and conversion rate and depth, while spatially distributing the hardware components (and weight), and performing local hardware signal amplification and processing, thus minimizing noise and interferences.

The fNIRS modules were designed considering the current understanding of fNIRS instrumentation technology as reviewed by Scholkmann et al. (2014) and others (Obrig and Villringer, 2003; Son and Yazici, 2006) with special regard to hardware design and wavelength-selection for SNR maximization/crosstalk minimization and considering potential hazards as identified by Bozkurt and Onaral (2004).

Each module provides four dual wavelength fNIRS channels using 750 and 850 nm multi-wavelength *Epitex L750/850-04A* LEDs. While the LEDs have a broader emission spectrum ($\Delta\lambda =$ 30/35 nm) than sharp peaked laser diodes (typically $\Delta\lambda \approx 1$ nm), their incoherent and uncollimated light allows for a higher tissue interrogation intensity and direct contact with the scalp due to less heating and is safer with the human eyes.

The LED current is regulated by adjustable current regulator circuits based on high precision amplifiers (*Analog Devices AD824A*) and field effect transistors (FMB2222A). Channel activation and current modulation for lock-in amplification is performed by analog switches (*Analog Devices ADG711*) that are accessed via an analog 1:8 demultiplexer (*NXP HEF4051*). After tissue interrogation, NIR light is detected by a central Si photo detector with integrated trans-impedance amplifier for output noise minimization (*Texas Instruments OPT101*, 1 MΩ feedback resistor, bandwidth 14 kHz) and is then amplified and lock-in demodulated (using Analog Devices AD630). An 8 Bit *Atmel Corp. AtMega16A* microcontroller's PWM module creates the 3.125 kHz square wave reference for lock-in (de-)modulation using an external 20 MHz crystal for jitter minimization. It also processes incoming control signals from the 4 Bit control interface and operates and configures the on board hardware. For adjustment of the LED currents, an 8 Bit digital-to-analog converter (DAC; *Maxim MAX5480*) is implemented. It supplies the voltage level at the current regulator inputs that is the command variable for the current regulation level. A programmable gain amplifier (*Texas Instruments PGA281*) is implemented for pre lock-in amplification of the detected NIR signal with a variable gain from $G = 0.688$ to 88.

During lock-in demodulation, the signal is filtered by a 3rd-order Butterworth low-pass and is then again amplified ($G = 5.1$) and stabilized by a set of two high precision amplifiers (*Texas Instruments LMC6062*) before leaving the fNIRS module for external AD conversion.

The system is designed for Time-Division Multiplexing (TDM) of the fNIRS channels. This is a trade-off between minimizing inter-channel crosstalk, heating (Bozkurt and Onaral, 2004) and battery consumption on the one hand and sacrificing SNR, which is limited by the width of the applied time windows. For demultiplexing of the locked-in output branches, a variable (sample rate dependent) dwell time is inserted after each onset of a single channel activation before sampling the steady state photo detector signal on the mainboard or with custom DAQ equipment.

Configurable PGA gain ($G = 0.6875$–88) and LED-intensity (256 DAC levels) in combination with a feedback "signal monitor" line allow the signal dependent adaption for maximum amplification in the lock-in demodulation process without reaching the dynamic range limit of one of the components.

Modularity: The above described design of the fNIRS modules allows operation in many configurations—only requiring compatibility with the above mentioned interface consisting of 4 Bit control, power supply and analog output. For an extension of the total channel count, several modules can be used. Changes in set-up and module count only affect the control unit and its routines chosen by the user, which activate the time division multiplexed channels and convert the analog fNIRS signals from the modules:

- As the objective of this work was the design of miniaturized fNIRS modules for mobile applications, a microcontroller (*Atmel AtMega644*) based mainboard was developed for mobile data acquisition and module control. Using a 4 channel 16 Bit analog-to-digital converter (ADC; *Linear Technologies LTC2486*) and a Bluetooth wireless controller (*Amber Wireless AMB2300*), the mainboard acquires the fNIRS signal(s) from up to 4 modules (16 channels), transmits the data to a computer via serial protocol and processes incoming user controls. To scale the number of channels, the user connects the desired number of modules and configures the channel administrator routine on the mainboard's microcontroller (see also Section 2.2.3). The symmetric ±5 V power rail is created from battery DC voltage using a stabilized linear power regulator circuit (based on *ON Semiconductor MC7805 and MC7905* ICs). Running on batteries and using only low voltages also ensures user safety.
- The mainboard is a placeholder for any (custom) peripheral acquisition and control hardware. With DAQ-devices providing digital I/Os and an external power supply, any number of modules (limited by the desired dwell time and sampling rate) can be used and controlled by control- and acquisition routines written and customized by the user.

2.2.2. Selection of Hardware Design Aspects

Emitter Branch: For a high accuracy of the fNIRS instrument, a careful design of the NIR-light emitting circuit is crucial, as fluctuations in the radiation intensity cannot be discriminated from changes in absorption due to changes in chromophore concentrations in the tissue.

To keep the current through the LED semiconductor junctions constant and independent from variations in supply voltage and temperature, and at the same time allow intensity adjustment and current modulation for the lock-in amplification process, a customized current regulator circuit was designed (see **Figure 2**).

Similar to a solution proposed by Chenier and Sawan (2007), an analog switch is used in the OpAmp based regulation circuit for square-wave modulation of the current. However, instead of disrupting the regulation process at the transistor base, analog switches (ADG711) are used at the inputs of the regulator circuits to pull the regulator inputs low when deactivated. fNIRS channel activation and modulation is thus realized by simply feeding through the square wave reference to the corresponding current regulator switch selected by the multiplexer.

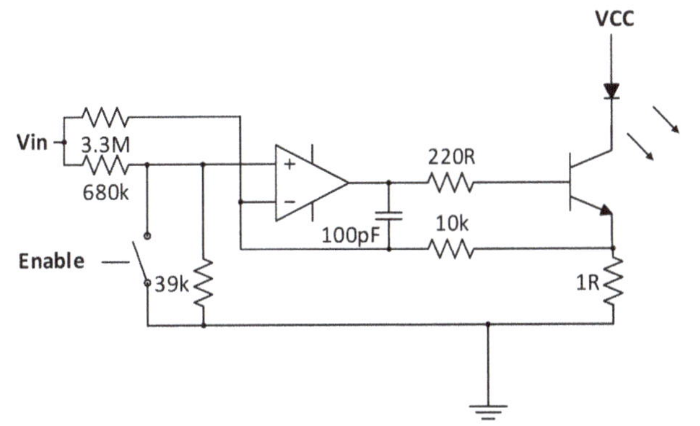

FIGURE 2 | Current regulator/modulator circuit.

As the regulator is modulated in the kHz-range, over- and undershoots influence the ideally square-wave shape of the current. To optimize the shape, a passive negative RC feedback was added and evaluated for best performance.

***Receiver Branch*:** The receiver branch was designed to maximize SNR by minimizing noise influences from shot, thermal and $1/f$ noise, dark currents and stray light from external light sources.

Shot noise is based on the quantum nature of the photons and therefore unavoidable and, for detectors without internal amplification, proportional to the square root of the average incident intensity (Scholkmann et al., 2014). To maximize SNR, the instrument is operated using the maximum NIR-light intensity level for the current regulators that is feasible in the experimental situation. Opaque cell rubber tubes are used to cover the sides of the NIR emitters and detector and the fNIRS module housing is covered with opaque paint to minimize shot noise influences from background radiation.

To reduce thermal noise influences, a Si photo diode with integrated trans-impedance amplifier circuitry (OPT101) was selected for detection. Lock-in extraction of the detected signal further reduces stray light, dark current and 1/f noise influences. Placing the PGA between the detection and lock-in extraction unit enables maximum pre-amplification of the signal while amplifier noise components added in the amplification process are reduced by the subsequent lock-in demodulation. Non-physiological high frequency components of the signal are attenuated by the 3rd order low pass filter of the lock-in demodulation unit.

2.2.3. Interfaces and Software Design

Figure 3 shows the software concept. The fNIRS module software sets up hardware components (PGA, DAC, MUX,...) and is controlled by an interrupt-based architecture that receives its control signals from the 4 Bit parallel interface. Therefore, interface operation and analog signal conversion can be done by the mainboard or any custom or standard DAQ-equipment with 4Bit programmable digital outputs (such as e.g., NI USB600x series). Using the mainboard, a channel administration routine both supervises data acquisition and acts as interface between the fNIRS modules and the PC by processing received user

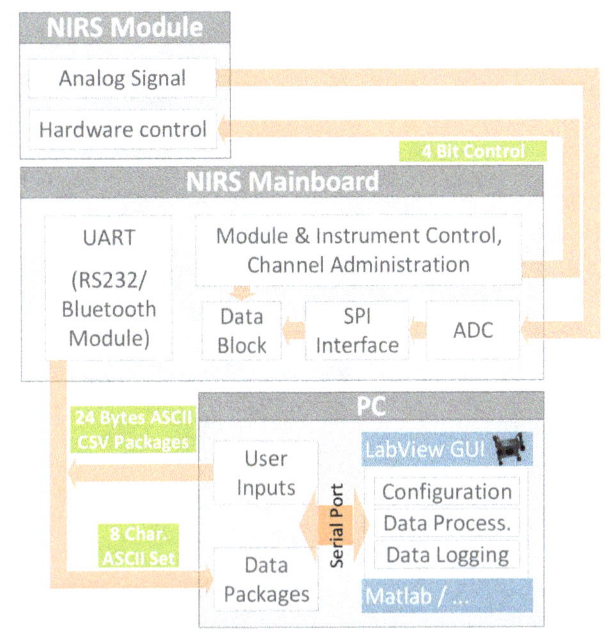

FIGURE 3 | Software and Interface Concept. Stand alone fNIRS module operated via parallel control interface by the mainboard or any custom control and data acquisition device. Function of the 4 Bit interface (3:RST, 2:TRIG, 1:CH1, 0:CH0): Bits CH1:CH0 select one of the four physical NIRS channels. A rising edge on the TRIG line activates the selected channel, always beginning with wavelength 750 nm of the corresponding LED. Each subsequent rising edge toggles the activation between 750 and 850 nm. When the RST line is pulled up, all channels are turned off. The next rising edge on the TRIG line starts the process again, beginning with 750 nm.

commands (configuration, start, stop...), translating them into signals for the 4 Bit fNIRS module interface(s) and sending acquired data packages via the UART interface. On the PC's operating system side, the user can control the instrument and directly read out the data packages in ASCII CSV format via a simple serial port command console or access the serial port with any software such as LabView or Matlab. A LabView graphical user interface was developed for easy configuration and control as well as display and logging of raw and modified Beer-Lambert Law data.

2.2.4. Mechanical and Probe Design

In the fNIRS instrument's mechanical design, the idea of modularity/scalability and robust fixation is continued by providing independent custom 3D printed solutions for the single fNIRS modules and the mainboard:

The Mainboard, Bluetooth module and batteries are worn on the upper arm of a subject in a chained multiple-unit housing (see also **Figure 5**, in the next section).

For the single fNIRS modules, a new mechanical spring-loaded design was approached to optimize signal quality, sensitivity and light penetration depth together with easy and robust, adaptive fixation of the optodes (see **Figure 4**). Based on a spherical approximation of the head with diameter $D = 20$ cm, the central NIR light detector and the four NIR LEDs are placed perpendicular to the scalp with a source-detector distance of $d =$

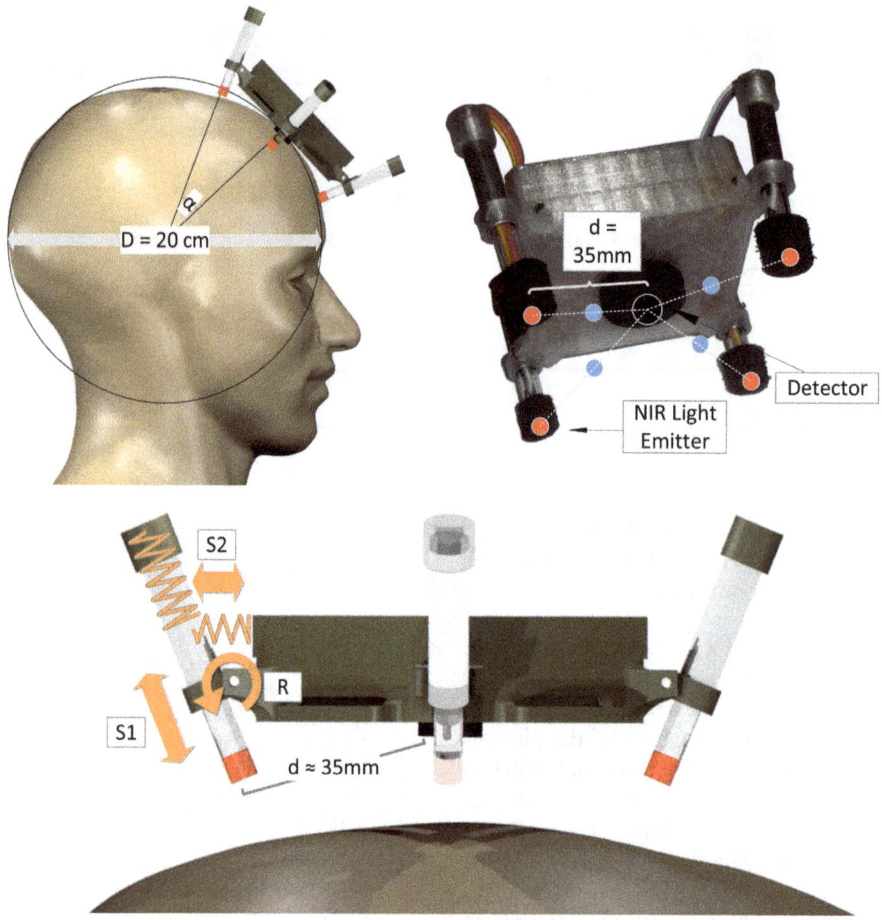

FIGURE 4 | Mechanical spring-loaded concept: Spherical head approximation (top left), geometric channel arrangement (red: NIR LEDs, black: photo detector, blue: measurement points of highest sensitivity; top right), spring-loaded mechanical design illustrated on one LED-holder (bottom). Spring S1 for alignment and buffering, spring S2 and rotatory joint R for perpendicular alignment.

35 mm. To enable perpendicular fixation of the emitters/detector and at the same time allow alignment to the natural unevenness of the head and its deviations from the spherical approximation, the NIR light LEDs are not stiffly connected to the module body housing but integrated in movable spring-loaded LED holders. These holders are based on two nested tubes that are spring-loaded against each other (S1) and against the module housing (S2) and are able to rotate around an axis (R): Spring S1 presses the LED toward the surface of the head, thus enabling alignment and preventing the loss of contact during movements. Spring S2 and the rotary joint R keep the LED perpendicular to the surface while enabling small deviations for comfort and alignment.

To minimize stray light influences and for cushioning purposes, the detector and emitters are encased by an opaque cell rubber tubing. To fixate a single module to the head, a flexible ribbon with hook-and-loop fastener can be used that is sewed to the module housing.

The mechanical concept was designed to allow the modules to be used on the forehead as well as over haired regions of the head: The single spring-loaded optodes are easily accessible due to their modular fixation without a cap or other concealing elements. This enables the user to manually brush aside obstructing hair from under the optodes for better optical contact. Even though we successfully conducted measurements over hairy regions of the head, it has to be pointed out that the usability of the modules on other regions than the forehead has not been proven under controlled conditions so far.

2.3. System Evaluation

2.3.1. Hardware Analysis

To enable a differentiated characterization of the instrument's hardware according to functional units, evaluation and analysis was split into emitter branch (current regulation and modulation), receiver branch (lock-in module), power supply stability and overall drift characteristics:

- *Current regulator/modulator speed and current shape/oscillation characteristics*: To evaluate and optimize the current regulator design characteristics for a stable and

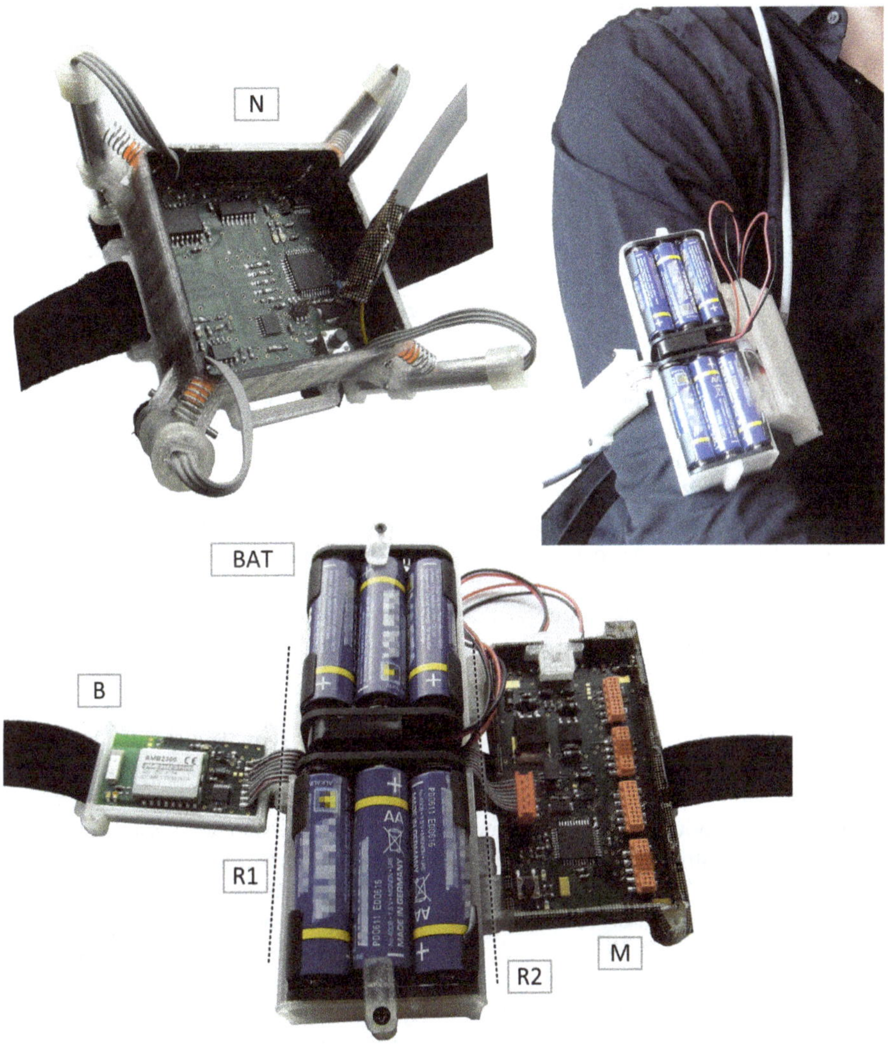

FIGURE 5 | Final System. (N): single 4 channel fNIRS module. Top right/bottom: Chained mainboard module. B, bluetooth module; BAT, batteries; R1/R2, Rotatory joints; M, mainboard.

minimally oscillating but steep square wave shape of the regulated current signal, both LTSpice simulations and measurements were conducted and the regulator design parameters iteratively improved using two high-precision operational amplifiers (Analog Devices AD824A and Linear Technologies LMC6064). To minimize transient oscillation and settling times, a negative feedback decoupling capacitor C was introduced to the regulator design. For the determination of its optimal value, the shape of the regulated square wave current signal was investigated in a range from $C = 0$ pF to $C = 330$ pF at different current levels.

- *Lock-in performance*: The sum of propagation delays that result from each hardware component in the emitter-detector-signal path leads to an overall phase shift between input and reference signal in the analog lock-in amplification process. Such a phase shift results in an attenuation of the signal during demodulation (Meade, 1982, 1983). To minimize this effect, all hardware elements in the signal path were selected with respect to high-speed/low delay times. The remaining overall phase shift $\Delta\Phi = \frac{\Delta t}{T} \cdot 2\pi$ between the reference signal (with period T) and the detected pre-amplified signal was measured before demodulation. Using the established straight forward mathematical model for square wave reference lock-in demodulation, as in Meade (1983), a phase shift dependent attenuation factor

$$A = cos(\Delta\Phi) \tag{1}$$

was used to estimate the resulting attenuation.

For an estimation of the receiver sensitivity using the noise equivalent power (NEP), dark voltage noise levels (no incident light to the photo detector) were measured at the output of the lock-in-module.

- *System drifts*: The following possible sources of system drift were considered: Changes in the 1 Ω LED current regulation resistance due to temperature changes, changes in the total radiated power of the LEDs due to semiconductor junction temperature and changes despite constant currents and supply voltage variations. Changes in stray light, amplifier and thermal resistor noise are strongly suppressed by the lock-in amplification process. To minimize signal drifts resulting from changes in the 1 Ω current regulator resistance, Panasonic current sensing resistors with a low temperature coefficient of resistance ($TCR = \pm 50 \cdot 10^{-6}/°C$) were chosen.

The overall system drift of a single fNIRS module was specified with 20 min continuous acquisition windows of a single active channel at maximum intensity (100 mA) with the PGA set to $G = 44$ and the module being placed at a fixed position in an opaque closed box.

- *Mainboard power supply stability*: DC supply voltage drifts during 20 min signal acquisition periods and current modulation impacts on the supply voltage were evaluated. As the 100 mA (max.) square wave 3.125 kHz modulation can influence the power supply voltage stability and noise it can degrade the performance of the signal detection and amplification elements. Their output signals during active modulation were acquired while zero optical input to the photo detector was ensured by encasing the active LED with an opaque metal box. For customization, the layout of the fNIRS module allows both separate and common supply of the LED currents and module hardware.

2.3.2. Physiological Verification

Simple qualitative experiments were conducted using a channel at 10–20 point Fp1 to verify significant strength of physiological information in the raw signal and its power spectrum. Amongst others, visibility and strength of pulse artifacts are indicators for the signal quality and have been widely documented in fNIRS literature with the pulse artifact's amplitude being in the order of metabolic variations due to brain activity (Boas et al., 2004; Lareau et al., 2011; Scholkmann et al., 2014). Thus, with the fNIRS module pressed firmly against the head to reduce the sensitivity to scalp signals (decreased blood flow under the optodes), a clearly visible pulse artifact is a first indicator for sufficient signal quality to measure brain activation. The pulse rate was verified with conventional reference pulse measurements.

For verification and quantification of the device's capability to measure metabolic brain activity, a mental arithmetic BCI experiment was conducted with 12 subjects. In this experiment, it is shown that the measured hemodynamic responses can be classified on a single-trial basis, i.e., each trial can be classified as containing mental arithmetic or relaxation, instead of measuring only the difference in the average hemodynamic response.

Mental arithmetic tasks are known to illicit strong hemodynamic reactions in frontal brain areas and have been investigated in a variate of studies with fNIRS (Ang et al., 2010; Herff et al., 2013; Bauernfeind et al., 2014). Here, 30 trials of mental arithmetic data were recorded for each participant. During each 10 s trial, participants were asked to repeatedly subtract a number between 7 and 19 (excluding 10) from a number between 501 and 999). Both numbers were presented on a screen at a distance of roughly 50 cm. After each mental arithmetic trial, participants were asked to relax for 25–30 s. These pause intervals were indicated by a fixation cross on the screen. A longer resting period of variable length was included after 15 trials to allow participants to rest and drink. No data of these extended resting periods were used in our analysis.

The open fNIRS device was placed on the forehead and fixated around the head with the flexible ribbon with hook-and-loop fastener sewed to its housing. It was placed such that both active emitters were placed on the locations Fp1 and Fp2 of the international 10–20-system. The light detector was placed on AFz resulting in an emitter-detector distance of approximately 3.5 cm.

All subjects were informed prior to the experiment and gave written consent.

The signal processing of the recorded data was performed in a straight-forward and simple manner, since we focus on the developed hardware in this paper. More advanced methods have been shown to improve accuracies for classification in neuroimaging (Calhoun et al., 2001; Blankertz et al., 2008; Lemm et al., 2011; Heger et al., 2014). The raw optical densities were transferred to concentration changes of oxygenated and deoxygenated hemoglobin (HbO and HbR, respectively) using the modified Beer-Lambert Law (Sassaroli and Fantini, 2004). HbO and HbR values were then linearly detrended in windows of 300 s. Low frequency noise was attenuated by subtracting a moving average of the mean of 30 s prior and after every sample. Finally the data was low-pass filtered using an elliptic IIR filter with filter order 6 and a cut-off frequency of 0.5 Hz to reduce high-frequency systemic noise like pulse artifacts.

After preprocessing, trials were extracted based on the experiment timings. For the pause blocks, we extracted the last 10 s of the 25–30 s pause intervals, to ensure that hemoglobin levels have returned to baseline. For each mental arithmetic trial, we extracted 10 s of data starting 5 s after stimulus presentation, to ensure that the hemodynamic response has already developed. Labels were assigned to the trials referring to either mental arithmetics or pause data. For each trial, we extracted the slope of a straight line fitted to the HbO and HbR data of each channel as a feature. The line was fitted using linear regression with a least-squares approach. Slope features have been shown to work well in previous studies (Herff et al., 2014).

Evaluation was performed using a 10-fold cross-validation and classification by Linear Discriminant Analysis. In addition to the single trial analysis, the average hemodynamic response is calculated by averaging over all mental arithmetics or all pause trials.

3. RESULTS

The developed open modular multichannel fNIRS system (see **Figure 5**) proved functionality, fast set up and easy application in all testing conditions. Wearing the mainboard module on the upper arm and the fNIRS module on the head using flexible ribbons and hook-and-loop fastener, the user can move freely and is bothered minimally by the instrument while signal quality and robustness to movement showed promising results. It should be noted however, that the physiological signals used for evaluation results in this paper were acquired from sitting subjects to reduce possible error sources and thus allow a more explicit first performance assessment of the new open source hardware.

The final instrument is characterized by:

- Modularity, customization and stand-alone functionality.
- Optimized adjustable current regulation and modulation with negative decoupling.
- A lock-in-based signal extraction module with programmable amplification.
- A 4-channel spring-loaded mechanical concept for fNIRS probe attachment to improve user comfort and robustness against movement artifacts.
- A microcontroller and Bluetooth based mainboard as interchangeable peripheral control, acquisition and transmission hardware with a Bluetooth range of max. 20 m (optimal open field conditions).

Low cost components were used for the design. The total cost of the instrument's hardware for one 4 channel fNIRS module and one mainboard mainly depends on PCB fabrication costs and is approximately 200 *EUR*/250 *USD*.

A full documentation including detailed descriptions, schematics, and evaluation can be found in the supplementary materials for this article/on the web: www.opennirs.org. In the following, we present the main evaluation results of the steps described in section 2.

3.1. Current Regulation/modulation Circuit

Mostly due to its higher slew rate, the AD824A showed a much faster current regulation and lower transient oscillations than the LMC6064. The experimental results for the minimization of oscillation and settling times with different decoupling capacitor values C (see **Figure 6**) showed higher settling oscillations for low C at low current levels, higher transient oscillation for high C at higher current levels and allowed the identification of the optimal C: $C = 100$ pF showed the best tradeoff between minimal oscillations and maximal edge steepness for all current levels.

3.2. System Drifts

The signal drift of a continuously active channel in Volts per second was calculated using linear least squares regression on the acquired 20 min. raw signals, yielding a negative drift coefficient of $C_D = -1 \cdot 10^{-6}$ V/s (measured fNIRS signals typically—dependent on the device configuration—being in the order of several hundred mV) and a respective long term stability coefficient of $< -0.42\%$ for both wavelengths. It was observed that independent from the fNIRS module, power supply heating on the peripheral hardware can add additional drifts of up to one order of magnitude by effecting the analog-to-digital converter. This points out the importance of careful selection/design of peripheral hardware for the acquisition of the fNIRS module's analog signal.

3.3. Lock-in Amplification, SNR and Dynamic Range

For an approximation of the total effective phase shift between reference and demodulator input signal in the lock-in unit, the delays between both signals were measured at the 50% levels of both respective rising (t_{dr}) and falling edges (t_{df}). It is the sum of times where the logical levels of both signals do not match and was measured as $\Delta t = t_{dr} + t_{df} = 18.5 + 7.2$ µs. To estimate the attenuation caused by non-phase-synchronous demodulation of the signal A, Equation (1) is used with the measured Δt and reference signal cycle duration $T = 320$ µs, and yields $A \approx 0.875$, which does not affect the overall accuracy significantly. Evaluation of the single component phase delays in the signal path revealed that further minimization approaches should first target the PGA ($\Delta t_{PGA} = 7.0 + 4.5$ µs).

For the evaluation of the detector's sensitivity and dynamic range, the mean dark voltage signal μ_d (no incident light on the

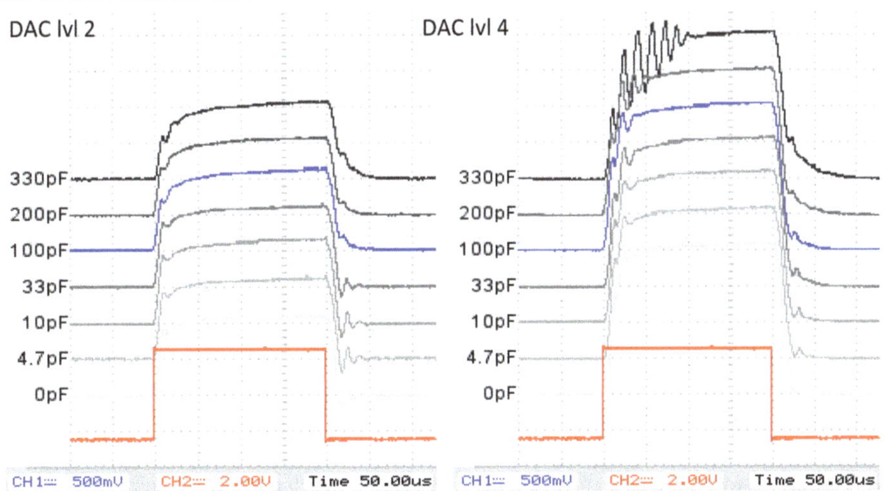

FIGURE 6 | Current regulator/moulator evaluation: 3.125 kHz PWM modulation reference (red) and regulated LED currents with different decoupling capacitor values and DAC levels (blue: selected value for design).

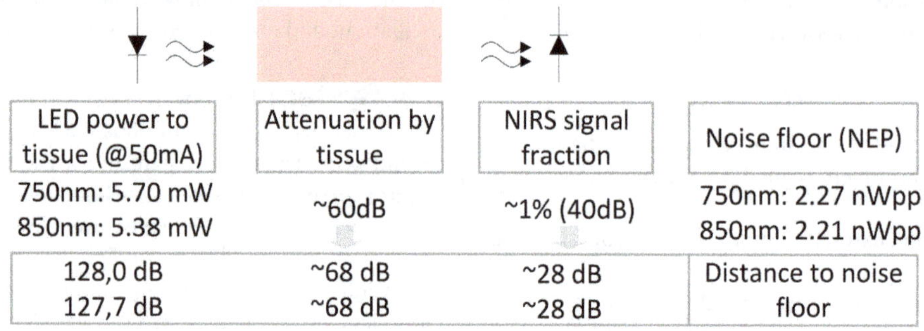

FIGURE 7 | Estimation of signal and noise in the instrument: With the NEPs identified to be 2.27/2.21 nWpp, the distance between these optical powers equivalent to the noise floor of the detection circuit and the measured powers incident to the tissue (5.70 mW/5.38 mW) at medium LED illumination can be determined to be approximately 128 dB/127.7 dB, respectively. The degree of optical loss of the incident light in the tissue is subject dependent. Here, we estimate it to be in the order of at least 40–60 dB. With the actual metabolic fNIRS signal being in the order of 1% of the measured optical signal, the distance of the fNIRS signals to the noise floor is approximately 28 dB.

photodetector) at the output of the lock-in amplifier and post amplification branch was measured to be $\mu_d = 0.101$ Vrms with a standard deviation of $\sigma_d = 3.99$ mVrms at a typical PGA gain of $G = 44$ and fixed lock-in filter gain of $G = 5.1$. Using the mean dark voltage plus standard deviation and the responsivities R_λ of the OPT101 photodiode ($R_{750} = 0.55$ V/μW and $R_{850} = 0.60$ V/μW), the Noise Equivalent Powers of the whole detector branch for a SNR of one

$$NEP_\lambda = \frac{\mu_d + \sigma_d}{R_\lambda \cdot G_{total}} \tag{2}$$

were estimated to be $NEP_{750} = 2.27$ nWpp $= 0.80$ nWrms and $NEP_{850} = 2.21$ nWpp $= 0.78$ nWrms.

The optical powers radiated by the LED at medium intensity ($I_F = 50$ mA) were measured to be 5.70 mW for 750 nm and 5.38 mW for 850 nm. Using these incident powers and the NEPs allows an estimation of the signal to noise distances (for an overview see **Figure 7**): The wavelength dependent ratio of incident light to light not longer detectable as its signal is drowning in noise, yields signal to noise distances of 128 dB_{750} and 127.7 dB_{850}. These distances are largely decreased by the optical loss due to tissue scattering and absorption that is subject dependent and assumed to be in the order of > 60 dB. With the physiological fNIRS signal usually being around 1% of the measured optical signal, the distance between the fNIRS signal components and the noise floor of the detection circuit is further decreased by ≈40 dB and estimated to be in the order of 28 dB.

Saturation of the detection branch occurs, when the upper input voltage limit of the ADC, here 2.5 Vpp, is reached for the lowest PGA gain setting of $G = 0.6875$, which is the case at 1.296/1.188 μWpp incident light (750 nm/850 nm). Using these results, the minimum system dynamic range, expressed as the ratio of signal saturation to the NEPs, is estimated to be in the order of 55.13/54.6 dB. It should be stated, that the configuration of the LED intensities (25–100 mA) on the emitter side can further increase the dynamic range of the instrument. **Table 1** summarizes the performance characteristics.

TABLE 1 | Performance characteristics of the fNIRS Module.

Parameter	Value
OPT101 Dark noise voltage	300 μVrms @0.1–20 kHz
OPT101 Responsivity	$R_{750} \approx 0.55$ V/μW
	$R_{850} \approx 0.60$ V/μW
Noise equivalent power	$NEP_{750} \approx 0.80$ nWrms
	$NEP_{850} \approx 0.78$ nWrms
Power to tissue (at peak wavelength)	
@$I_{LED} = 50$ mA	$P_{750} = 5.70$ mW
	$P_{850} = 5.38$ mW
@$I_{LED} = 100$ mA	$P_{750} = 11.10$ mW
	$P_{850} = 10.30$ mW
Est. signal to noise distance	
@$I_{LED} = 50$ mA	≈ 28 dB
Eff. dynamic range	> 55 dB
Signal drift	$< -1 \cdot 10^{-6}$ V/s/ < −0.5%
Sampling rate	Variable, dwell time dependent

3.4. Mainboard Power Supply

The ±5 V DC supply voltage drift measurements showed a stable supply voltage of +4.959 V and −4.960 V with less than 500 μV total drift in 20-min measurement periods. Evaluation of the maximum impact of the current modulation on the detecting components via the power supply revealed that current modulation flanks can create a ±2 mV high-frequency(kHz) noise around the photo detector output baseline signal that is further amplified by the PGA to strong ±100 mV peaks (at $G = 44$) when supplying the LED current either directly from the battery or from the regulated +5 V rail for the other fNIRS module hardware. However, as the supply variations are synchronous with the signals and as high-frequency noise is effectively suppressed by the 3rd-order lock-in low-pass of the fNIRS module, influences on the baseline of the lock-in demodulated signal were not observed.

3.5. Physiological Measurements

Qualitative physiological experiments showed very clear signals and proved the basic functionality of the instrument. **Figure 8** shows a representative raw signal (750 nm) during three mental arithmetics trials performed by a subject (a) and the power spectrum computed over the whole session for the same subject (b). The latter shows the typical power law appearance and peaks by systemic artifacts that have widely been reported for fNIRS signals in the literature (e.g., Fekete et al., 2011).

The average hemodynamic response (see **Figure 9A**) over all subjects of the mental arithmetics experiment shows the expected behavior, i.e., an increase in HbO peaking after approximately 10 s during mental arithmetics. During the average pause interval, HbO levels still slowly return to baseline after the preceding activation.

Discrimination between pause and mental arithmetics yielded an average of 65.14% accuracy. Of the 12 recorded participants, 9 yielded accuracies significantly higher than chance level (one-sided t-test, $p < 0.05$). Classification results for all participants can be seen in **Figure 9B**). In a similar study by Herff et al. (2013), mental arithmetics could be discriminated from pause with 71.17% using 8 channels and 67.26% when using only two channels at similar positions as in this study.

4. DISCUSSION AND CONCLUSION

4.1. Key Findings

In the beginning of this paper, we identified system requirements for mobile fNIRS based neuroergonomics/BCI applications. The results indicate, that the presented open source device satisfies the requirements.

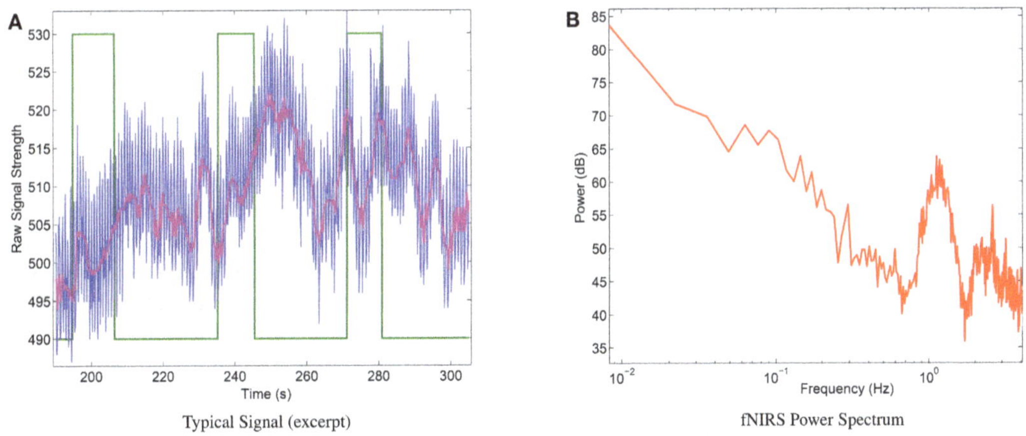

FIGURE 8 | (A) Excerpt of typical raw signal (blue) during mental arithmetics. Green line: binary label (high states: m. arithmetics. low states: relax), magenta line: median filtered signal). **(B)** Typical power spectrum of raw signal of the same subject and complete session, showing expected shape (power spectrum follows power law) and deviations caused by systemic artifacts.

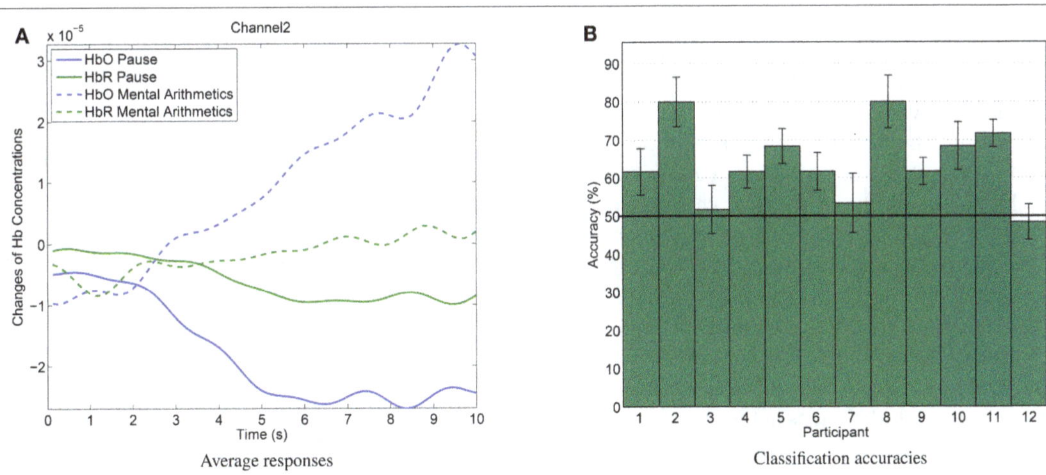

FIGURE 9 | (A) Average hemodynamic response over all subjects during mental arithmetics and pause. **(B)** Classification results for single-trial discrimination between pause and mental arithmetics. Whiskers indicate standard errors. Solid line shows chance level.

In the course of the experiments, both, experimentators and subjects, appraised the usability of the device to be high. Miniaturization of the modules and mobility through Bluetooth based wireless transmission allowed free movement, the use of commercial reference systems usually required longer preparation times for optode fixation and was often uncomfortable and static because of the weight of the optical fiber guides and the lack of cushioning of the optodes. In contrast, the new wearable system could be applied within several seconds and was generally perceived less cumbersome during the experiments.

The hardware evaluation results and physiological verification of the designed miniaturized fNIRS instrument indicated a sufficient signal quality and system performance for brain activity measurements with an approximated signal to noise distance of 28 dB. The lock-in amplifier, detector sensitivity, current modulation precision and drift evaluation of the device showed satisfying results comparable to other documented fNIRS devices. The physiological measurements showed the expected hemodynamic responses, classification accuracies in single-trial analysis exceeded chance level for 9 out of 12 participants and yielded results comparable to those measured with a commercial device in a similar study (Herff et al., 2013) using 2 of 8 channels at similar positions (65.14 vs. 67.26%). The open fNIRS device can thus be used for mobile fNIRS-based BCI and neuroergonomics applications.

Battery supply and wireless communication, low heating due to time multiplexing of the channels and the use of LEDs as light sources assured a safe usage of the device.

The scalable modular concept, configurable light intensities and detector amplification gains and the flexible parallel interface of the fNIRS modules allow easy customization and configuration of the hardware.

However, there are still several elements in the design that can be optimized to further improve instrument performance in the future.

4.2. Limitations and Next Steps

4.2.1. Mainboard/Data Acquisition and Control

An obvious but crucial component for the use of the fNIRS module is the data acquisition unit. When using custom hardware for data acquisition, the design and selection of the analog-to-digital converter (ADC) determine not only quantization depth but also the frequency resolution of the time division multiplexed fNIRS channels, as the ADC sampling rate has to be shared by the up to 4 active channels of one module. The ADC (LTC2486) first used on the mainboard offered 16 Bit conversion depth and exceptional DC accuracy but significantly limited time resolution due to a conversion time of type 80.3 ms. Additional experiments indicated that, using ADCs with significantly higher sample rate but lower resolution, down to 10 Bit quantization depth can suffice for reliable brain activation measurements. Future designs of the mainboard/DAQ hardware should therefore aim to use a better suited (faster) ADC to prevent the sampling frequency bottleneck. Here, the modular concept is advantageous, as the DAQ-unit can be customized and optimized independent from the hardware of the fNIRS modules.

Power supply and current modulation impact evaluation showed, that even though the implemented linear-voltage-regulator-based symmetric supply appeared to be sufficient, several improvements can be suggested for use with the fNIRS module:

To minimize crosstalk between the modulated NIR-LED current and the regulated ± 5 V supply voltage rail for the detection hardware, supplying the LEDs with a separate additional voltage regulator circuit is preferable over the use of a common regulator or direct battery connection in the design. Implementation of additional high-frequency filters and enhanced stabilization are also recommended in future approaches to reduce noise pickup from external sources and further minimize LED current modulation influences on the rest of the system. The use of voltage regulators with higher efficiency can further enhance battery life and decrease heating effects, which also can—dependent on the supplying and acquisition hardware's design and layout—influence system drifts.

4.2.2. fNIRS Module

The phase delay dependent attenuation of approximately 0.875 by the lock-in detector is acceptable as it does not significantly decrease overall system accuracy. However, it can be further minimized: To improve the lock-in performance, an analog adjustment of the PWM reference phase could be implemented for overall phase shift compensation. Alternatively, a potentially superior approach for a next-generation design would be digital lock-in demodulation based on a microcontroller/DSP. This bears several advantages: reduced cost of hardware components, reduced power consumption and an adjustable phase shift correction and thus higher precision.

The four channel set up per module using four LEDs and one photodiode was necessary for this first approach using a single-channel analog lock-in receiver branch for a simple interface in favor of modularity. However, to further reduce energy consumption and increase channel density, future approaches should utilize configurations with more PDs measuring simultaneously. Additionally, although the fNIRS module is already compact and provides stand-alone functionality, further miniaturization is possible. A next step will be the development of entirely stand-alone modules to redundantize peripheral hardware such as the mainboard. Integrating the above mentioned insights and data acquisition, digital lock in, power management and wireless transmission components onto a further miniaturized multichannel fNIRS module could enable even more applications in and out of the lab.

The instrument can be improved and evaluated in several more ways. However, providing this fNIRS device open source, we hope that aspects of this work will be helpful to further simplify and reduce time and effort in future custom fNIRS based mobile BCI and neuroergonomics approaches.

ACKNOWLEDGMENTS

We acknowledge support by Deutsche Forschungsgemeinschaft and Open Access Publishing Fund of Karlsruhe Institute of Technology.

REFERENCES

Ang, K., Guan, C., Lee, K., Lee, J., Nioka, S., and Chance, B. (2010). "A brain-computer interface for mental arithmetic task from single-trial near-infrared spectroscopy brain signals," in *International Conference on Pattern Recognition* (Istanbul), 3764–3767.

Atsumori, H., Kiguchi, M., Obata, A., Sato, H., Katura, T., Utsugi, K., et al. (2007). "Development of a multi-channel, portable optical topography system," in *Engineering in Medicine and Biology Society, 2007. EMBS 2007. 29th Annual International Conference of the IEEE* (Lyon), 3362–3364.

Ayaz, H., Onaral, B., Izzetoglu, K., Shewokis, P. A., McKendrick, R., and Parasuraman, R. (2013). Continuous monitoring of brain dynamics with functional near infrared spectroscopy as a tool for neuroergonomic research: empirical examples and a technological development. *Front. Hum. Neurosci.* 7:871. doi: 10.3389/fnhum.2013.00871

Ayaz, H., Shewokis, P. A., Bunce, S., Izzetoglu, K., Willems, B., and Onaral, B. (2012). Optical brain monitoring for operator training and mental workload assessment. *Neuroimage* 59, 36–47. doi: 10.1016/j.neuroimage.2011.06.023

Bauernfeind, G., Steyrl, D., Brunner, C., and Muller-Putz, G. R. (2014). "Single trial classification of fnirs-based brain-computer interface mental arithmetic data: a comparison between different classifiers," in *Engineering in Medicine and Biology Society (EMBC), 2014 36th Annual International Conference of the IEEE* (Chicago, IL: IEEE), 2004–2007.

Biessmann, F., Plis, S., Meinecke, F., Eichele, T., and Muller, K. (2011). Analysis of multimodal neuroimaging data. *Biomed. Eng. IEEE Rev.* 4, 26–58. doi: 10.1109/RBME.2011.2170675

Blankertz, B., Tomioka, R., Lemm, S., Kawanabe, M., and Muller, K.-R. (2008). Optimizing spatial filters for robust eeg single-trial analysis. *Signal Process. Mag. IEEE* 25, 41–56. doi: 10.1109/MSP.2008.4408441

Boas, D., Brooks, D., Miller, E., DiMarzio, C., Kilmer, M., Gaudette, R., et al. (2001). Imaging the body with diffuse optical tomography. *Signal Process. Mag. IEEE* 18, 57–75. doi: 10.1109/79.962278

Boas, D. A., Dale, A. M., and Franceschini, M. A. (2004). Diffuse optical imaging of brain activation: approaches to optimizing image sensitivity, resolution, and accuracy. *Neuroimage* 23(Suppl.1), S275–S288. doi: 10.1016/j.neuroimage.2004.07.011

Bozkurt, A., and Onaral, B. (2004). Safety assessment of near infrared light emitting diodes for diffuse optical measurements. *Biomed. Eng. Online* 3:9. doi: 10.1186/1475-925X-3-9

Bozkurt, A., Rosen, A., Rosen, H., and Onaral, B. (2005). A portable near infrared spectroscopy system for bedside monitoring of newborn brain. *Biomed. Eng. Online* 4:29. doi: 10.1186/1475-925X-4-29

Bunce, S., Izzetoglu, M., Izzetoglu, K., Onaral, B., and Pourrezaei, K. (2006). Functional near-infrared spectroscopy. *Eng. Med. Biol. Mag. IEEE* 25, 54–62. doi: 10.1109/MEMB.2006.1657788

Calhoun, V., Adali, T., Pearlson, G., and Pekar, J. (2001). Spatial and temporal independent component analysis of functional mri data containing a pair of task-related waveforms. *Hum. Brain Mapp.* 13, 43–53. doi: 10.1002/hbm.1024

Chenier, F., and Sawan, M. (2007). "A new brain imaging device based on fnirs," in *Biomedical Circuits and Systems Conference, 2007. BIOCAS 2007.* (Montreal, QC: IEEE), 1–4.

Cope, M. (1991). *The Application of Near Infrared Spectroscopy to Non Invasive Monitoring of Cerebral Oxygenation in the Newborn Infant.* Ph.D. thesis, Department of Medical Physics and Bioengineering, University College London.

Cope, M., and Delpy, D. (1988). System for long-term measurement of cerebral blood and tissue oxygenation on newborn infants by near infra-red transillumination. *Med. Biol. Eng. Comput.* 26, 289–294. doi: 10.1007/BF02447083

Coyle, S., Ward, T., and Markham, C. (2007). Brain-computer interface using a simplified functional near-infrared spectroscopy system. *J. Neural Eng.* 4, 219–226. doi: 10.1088/1741-2560/4/3/007

Coyle, S., Ward, T., Markham, C., and McDarby, G. (2004). On the suitability of near-infrared systems for next generation brain computer interfaces. *Physiol. Meas.* 25, 815–822. doi: 10.1088/0967-3334/25/4/003

Fairclough, S. H. (2009). Fundamentals of physiological computing. *Interact. Comput.* 21, 133–145. doi: 10.1016/j.intcom.2008.10.011

Fazli, S., Mehnert, J., Steinbrink, J., Curio, G., Villringer, A., Müller, K.-R., et al. (2012). Enhanced performance by a hybrid nirs-eeg brain computer interface. *Neuroimage* 59, 519–529. doi: 10.1016/j.neuroimage.2011.07.084

Fekete, T., Rubin, D., Carlson, J. M., and Mujica-Parodi, L. R. (2011). The nirs analysis package: noise reduction and statistical inference. *PLoS ONE* 6:e24322. doi: 10.1371/journal.pone.0024322

Heger, D., Herff, C., and Schultz, T. (2014). "Combining feature extraction and classification for fnirs bcis by regularized least squares optimization," in *Engineering in Medicine and Biology Society (EMBC), 2014 36th Annual International Conference of the IEEE* (IEEE), 2012–2015.

Herff, C., Heger, D., Fortmann, O., Hennrich, J., Putze, F., and Schultz, T. (2014). Mental workload during n-back task-quantified in the prefrontal cortex using fnirs. *Front. Hum. Neurosci.* 7:935. doi: 10.3389/fnhum.2013.00935

Herff, C., Heger, D., Putze, F., Hennrich, J., Fortmann, O., and Schultz, T. (2013). "Classification of mental tasks in the prefrontal cortex using fnirs," in *Engineering in Medicine and Biology Society (EMBC), 2013 35th Annual International Conference of the IEEE* (Osaka), 2160–2163.

Jöbsis, F. (1977). Noninvasive, infrared monitoring of cerebral and myocardial oxygen sufficiency and circulatory parameters. *Science* 198, 1264–1267. doi: 10.1126/science.929199

Kanoh, S., Murayama, Y.-M., Miyamoto, K.-I., Yoshinobu, T., and Kawashima, R. (2009). "A nirs-based brain-computer interface system during motor imagery: system development and online feedback training," in *Engineering in Medicine and Biology Society, 2009. EMBC 2009. Annual International Conference of the IEEE* (Minneapolis, MN), 594–597.

Kiguchi, M., Atsumori, H., Fukasaku, I., Kumagai, Y., Funane, T., Maki, A., et al. (2012). Note: wearable near-infrared spectroscopy imager for haired region. *Rev. Sci. Instrum.* 83, 056101. doi: 10.1063/1.4704456

Lareau, E., Simard, G., Lesage, F., Nguyen, D., and Sawan, M. (2011). "Near infrared spectrometer combined with multichannel eeg for functional brain imaging," in *Medical Information Communication Technology (ISMICT), 2011 5th International Symposium on* (Montreux), 122–126.

Lemm, S., Blankertz, B., Dickhaus, T., and Müller, K.-R. (2011). Introduction to machine learning for brain imaging. *Neuroimage* 56, 387–399. doi: 10.1016/j.neuroimage.2010.11.004

Matthews, F., Pearlmutter, B. A., Ward, T., Soraghan, C., and Markham, C. (2008). Hemodynamics for brain-computer interfaces. *Signal Process. Mag. IEEE* 25, 87–94. doi: 10.1109/MSP.2008.4408445

McKendrick, R., Parasuraman, R., and Ayaz, H. (2015). Wearable functional near infrared spectroscopy (fnirs) and transcranial direct current stimulation (tdcs): expanding vistas for neurocognitive augmentation. *Front. Syst. Neurosci.* 9:27. doi: 10.3389/fnsys.2015.00027

Meade, M. L. (1982). Advances in lock-in amplifiers. *J. Phys. E* 15, 395. doi: 10.1088/0022-3735/15/4/001

Meade, M. L. (1983). *Lock-in Amplifiers: Principles and Applications.* London, UK: Peter Peregrinus Ltd.

Naseer, N., and Hong, K.-S. (2013). Classification of functional near-infrared spectroscopy signals corresponding to the right-and left-wrist motor imagery for development of a brain–computer interface. *Neurosci. Lett.* 553, 84–89. doi: 10.1016/j.neulet.2013.08.021

Obrig, H., and Villringer, A. (2003). Beyond the visible - imaging the human brain with light. *J. Cereb. Blood Flow Metab.* 12, 1–18. doi: 10.1097/00004647-200301000-00001

Parasuraman, R. (2003). Neuroergonomics: research and practice. *Theor. Issues Ergon. Sci.* 4, 5–20. doi: 10.1080/14639220210199753

Parasuraman, R. (2011). Neuroergonomics: brain, cognition, and performance at work. *Curr. Dir. Psychol. Sci.* 20, 181–186. doi: 10.1177/0963721411409176

Pfurtscheller, G., Bauernfeind, G., Wriessnegger, S. C., and Neuper, C. (2010). Focal frontal (de)oxyhemoglobin responses during simple arithmetic. *Int. J. Psychophysiol.* 76, 186–192. doi: 10.1016/j.ijpsycho.2010.03.013

Piper, S. K., Krueger, A., Koch, S. P., Mehnert, J., Habermehl, C., Steinbrink, J., et al. (2014). A wearable multi-channel fNIRS system for brain imaging in freely moving subjects. *Neuroimage* 85, 64–71. doi: 10.1016/j.neuroimage.2013.06.062

Putze, F., Hesslinger, S., Tse, C.-Y., Huang, Y., Herff, C., Guan, C., et al. (2014). Hybrid fnirs-eeg based classification of auditory and visual perception processes. *Front. Neurosci.* 8:373. doi: 10.3389/fnins.2014.00373

Rajkumar, E. R., Safaie, J., Gupta, R., Pattnaik, D., Abrishamimoghaddam, H., Grebe, R., et al. (2012). "Development of an autonomic portable single-board computer based high resolution nirs device for microcirculation analysis," in *Engineering in Medicine and Biology Society (EMBC), 2012 Annual International Conference of the IEEE* (San Diego, CA), 3235–3238.

Rolfe, P. (2000). *In vivo* near infra-red spectrophotometry. *Annu. Rev. Biomed. Eng.* 2, 315–354. doi: 10.1146/annurev.bioeng.2.1.715

Safaie, J., Grebe, R., Moghaddam, H. A., and Wallois, F. (2013). Toward a fully integrated wireless wearable eeg-nirs bimodal acquisition system. *J. Neural Eng.* 10:056001. doi: 10.1088/1741-2560/10/5/056001

Sassaroli, A., and Fantini, S. (2004). Comment on the modified beer-lambert law for scattering media. *Phys. Med. Biol.* 49, N225–N257. doi: 10.1088/0031-9155/49/14/n07

Schmidt, F., Fry, M., Hillman, E., Hebden, J., and Delpy, D. (2000). A 32-channel time-resolved instrument for medical optical tomography. *Rev. Sci. Instrum.* 71, 256–265. doi: 10.1063/1.1150191

Scholkmann, F., Kleiser, S., Metz, A. J., Zimmermann, R., Pavia, J. M., Wolf, U., et al. (2014). A review on continuous wave functional near-infrared spectroscopy and imaging instrumentation and methodology. *Neuroimage* 85, 6–27. doi: 10.1016/j.neuroimage.2013.05.004

Schudlo, L. C., and Chau, T. (2015). Single-trial classification of near-infrared spectroscopy signals arising from multiple cortical regions. *Behav. Brain Res.* 290, 131–142. doi: 10.1016/j.bbr.2015.04.053

Son, I.-Y., and Yazici, B. (2006). "Near infrared imaging and spectroscopy for brain activity monitoring," in *Advances in Sensing with Security Applications*, ed J. Byrnes (NATO Security Through Science Series-A: Chemistry and Biology, Springer), 341–372. Available on line at: http://www.springer.com/de/book/9781402042843?wt_mc=ThirdParty.SpringerLink.3.EPR653.About_eBook

Strangman, G., Culver, G., Thompson, J., and Boas, D. (2002). A quantitative comparison of simultaneous bold fmri and nirs recordings during functional brain activation. *Neuroimage* 17, 719–731. doi: 10.1006/nimg.2002.1227

Vaithianathan, T., Tullis, I. D. C., Everdell, N., Leung, T., and Gibson, A. (2004). Design of a portable near infrared system for topographic imaging of the brain in babies. *Rev. Sci. Instrum.* 75, 3276–3283. doi: 10.1063/1.1775314

Yanagisawa, K., Asaka, K., Sawai, H., Tsunashima, H., Nagaoka, T., Tsujii, T., et al. (2010). "Brain-computer interface using near-infrared spectroscopy for rehabilitation," in *Control Automation and Systems (ICCAS), 2010 International Conference on* (Gyeonggi-do), 2248–2253.

Zander, T. O., and Kothe, C. (2011). Towards passive brain–computer interfaces: applying brain–computer interface technology to human–machine systems in general. *J. Neural Eng.* 8:025005. doi: 10.1088/1741-2560/8/2/025005

8

The Impact of Expert Visual Guidance on Trainee Visual Search Strategy, Visual Attention and Motor Skills

Daniel R. Leff[1†], David R. C. James[1†], Felipe Orihuela-Espina[1,2], Ka-Wai Kwok[1], Loi Wah Sun[1], George Mylonas[1], Thanos Athanasiou[1], Ara W. Darzi[1] and Guang-Zhong Yang[1]*

[1] Hamlyn Centre for Robotic Surgery, Imperial College London, London, UK, [2] National Institute for Astrophysics, Optics and Electronics (INAOE), Tonantzintla, Mexico

***Correspondence:** Guang-Zhong Yang, Hamlyn Centre for Robotic Surgery, Imperial College London, Level 4, Bessemer Building, South Kensington Campus, London, SW7 2AZ, UK g.z.yang@imperial.ac.uk*

Minimally invasive and robotic surgery changes the capacity for surgical mentors to guide their trainees with the control customary to open surgery. This neuroergonomic study aims to assess a "Collaborative Gaze Channel" (CGC); which detects trainer gaze-behavior and displays the point of regard to the trainee. A randomized crossover study was conducted in which twenty subjects performed a simulated robotic surgical task necessitating collaboration either with verbal (control condition) or visual guidance with CGC (study condition). Trainee occipito-parietal (O-P) cortical function was assessed with optical topography (OT) and gaze-behavior was evaluated using video-oculography. Performance during gaze-assistance was significantly superior [biopsy number: (mean $\pm$ SD): control = 5.6 $\pm$ 1.8 vs. CGC = 6.6 $\pm$ 2.0; $p < 0.05$] and was associated with significantly lower O-P cortical activity [ΔHbO_2 mMol $\times$ cm [median (IQR)] control = 2.5 (12.0) vs. CGC 0.63 (11.2), $p < 0.001$]. A random effect model (REM) confirmed the association between guidance mode and O-P excitation. Network cost and global efficiency were not significantly influenced by guidance mode. A gaze channel enhances performance, modulates visual search, and alleviates the burden in brain centers subserving visual attention and does not induce changes in the trainee's O-P functional network observable with the current OT technique. The results imply that through visual guidance, attentional resources may be liberated, potentially improving the capability of trainees to attend to other safety critical events during the procedure.

Keywords: functional near infrared spectroscopy, optical topography, neuroergonomics, graph theory, collaborative gaze, visual attention, skills assessment, mentoring

Highlights

1. A randomized crossover study assessing the impact of trainer visual guidance upon trainee visual cognition, occipito-parietal (O-P) brain function and technical performance.
2. Visual guidance is associated with enhanced gaze behavior, improved technical accuracy and attenuated activity across O-P cortices.
3. Parameters of network performance such as cost and global efficiency are not detrimentally effected by visual guidance.

Introduction

In high-risk industry, collaboration between operators is integral to performing goal-orientated tasks successfully (e.g., pilots, air-traffic controller, surgeons, etc). Regarding surgery, collaboration is necessary between surgeons and their assistant(s), theatre nurse(s) and occasionally members of allied specialties. Recent developments in technologies for robotic surgery such as dual console systems (e.g., da Vinci® Si) enable two surgeons to operate simultaneously, facilitating both high-level co-operation and mentorship as well as potentially streamlining the operators' cognitive resources towards improved safety. However, in this scenario, it is important that communication between both surgeons is effective to enable a seamless flow of information between the two operators and ensure an efficient workflow. Similarly, excellent communication facilitates technical skills training in surgery. During "open" surgery, expert trainers' employ a variety of methods for communication with trainees that include a combination of verbal instruction, physical pointing or actual demonstration(s). However, during robotic minimally invasive surgery (MIS), there may be circumstances in which the trainee or collaborating surgeon is using both instruments simultaneously within the operative field of view, constraining the trainer/master surgeon and rendering them reliant solely on verbal communication.

Within MIS and robotic surgery, techniques exist such as telestration that aid information transfer between surgeons and/or between trainer and trainee. Telestration allows information to be "*drawn*" onto a monitor at a remote site by the surgeon guiding the procedure. This information is then displayed on the operator's screen with the aim of guiding performance and may be undertaken either remotely or locally (Ferguson and Stack, 2010). Remote guidance or telementoring enables surgeons to be guided by a mentor at a location remote from the operation. This form of instruction has been applied to better enable regional experts to guide surgeons at local centers and to provide assistance and mentoring from surgical experts in other countries (Micali et al., 2000; Schlachta et al., 2010).

There has been interest in the role that gaze behavior may have in improving the flow of communication between collaborating subjects. For example, it has been demonstrated that shared gaze during visual collaboration enables a more efficient search strategy when compared to verbal collaboration alone (Brennan et al., 2008). Therefore, it is anticipated that observing a guiding surgeon's point of regard instead of, or in conjunction with their verbal instruction(s) will significantly improve the performance of the operating surgeon by providing supplementary cues critical to task success. Based on this concept, a new system referred to as "*collaborative gaze control*" (CGC) was developed to enable an operating surgeon to be directed by visual guidance as opposed to or in conjunction with verbal instruction(s) from an expert (Kwok et al., 2012). With CGC enabled, the trainer's gaze behavior is extracted in real-time. Their point of regard is subsequently relayed to the trainee's screen, which may be in a remote location. Therefore, the trainee's operative manoeuvres can be directed more precisely, potentially obviating the dependence on verbal instruction(s). Importantly, in manipulating target salience, visual search is modulated leading to enhanced behavioral performance (Avraham et al., 2008).

More recently, there is evidence that workload can be inferred from saccadic eye movements (Tokuda et al., 2011), pupillary responses (Zheng et al., 2015) and blink frequency (Zheng et al., 2012). Challenging, effortful visual search results in greater visual cortical (V1) excitation (Kojima and Suzuki, 2010). Evaluating the impact that technological manipulation of visual search has on an operator's cortical function helps to determine whether performance enhancement is offset by the need for greater attentional demands at brain level. This is encompassed by "*neuroergonomics*" which concerns the investigation of the brain behavior at work (Parasuraman, 2003), a paradigm that has been applied to surgery in order to investigate how recruited brain regions may be modulated by novel performance-enhancing tools (James et al., 2010b, 2013).

In order to examine this effect, functional Near Infrared Spectroscopy (fNIRS) a non-invasive neuroimaging modality is utilized to measure task-evoked fluctuations in oxygenated and deoxygenated hemoglobin (HbO_2 and HHb respectively) within cortical tissues that reflects the magnitude of cortical activation (Jöbsis, 1977). This is based upon the principle that neuronal activity and the associated increased metabolic demand within the brain leads to local hemodynamic changes, so termed "*neurovascular coupling*" (Roy and Sherrington, 1890). Unlike functional magnetic resonance imaging (fMRI), fNIRS is relatively resistant to motion artifact and can be used in conjunction with ferromagnetic instruments and has been successfully applied to monitor the cortical responses in surgeons (Leff et al., 2008a,b,c; Ohuchida et al., 2009; James et al., 2011, 2013). Broadly, these studies highlight the importance of the prefrontal cortex (PFC) in supporting "cognitive phases" of skill learning (Leff et al., 2008a), evolution in PFC excitation with technical skills training (Leff et al., 2008c), and relative PFC redundancy amongst expert surgeons (Ohuchida et al., 2009). More recently, investigators have demonstrated the impact of the type of learning (e.g., implicit vs. explicit) and the influence of technology to stabilize performance and enhance neuronal efficiency amongst surgeons (Zhu et al., 2011; James et al., 2013).

Functional brain connectivity captured in coherence or cross-correlation between different brain regions can be used to investigate efficiency in brain networks (Zhu et al., 2011; James et al., 2013). Graph Theory, a popular method for interrogating brain networks, can model the organization, development and function of complex networks (Sporns et al., 2004; Bullmore and Sporns, 2009; Sporns, 2011) and has been successfully employed to networks derived from fNIRS data (Niu et al., 2012; James et al., 2013). In this regard, studies investigating graph topology such as the number of connections, cost and efficiency have demonstrated associations between task performance and brain network efficiency or cost-efficiency (Bassett et al., 2009). Despite the above, there have been no studies investigating the influence of varying trainer/mentor guidance on brain function or network architectures amongst trainees.

The aim of this paper is to investigate the influence of a gaze channel on changes in visual search strategies, technical performance, and brain behavior in a group of task naïve subjects being instructed to perform simulated biopsy using robotic MIS. Therefore, it is anticipated that compared to verbal guidance technical procedural skills may be superior during gaze-assistance owing to the improved perceptual flow of information to the trainee. The primary hypothesis is that increased target saliency will lead to a *"bottom-up"* search strategy, reflected in a more focused pattern of V1 activation and a reduction in the need for recruitment of extra-striatal visual association areas. Conversely, verbal communication (gold standard) is anticipated to lead to a more effortful *"top down"* visual search strategy, necessitating recruitment of additional cortical regions outside V1, manifest as greater excitation in centers of visual attention. The secondary hypothesis is that collaborative gaze may facilitate the flow of information transfer in the visual-parietal network manifest as reduced network costs, improved efficiency and reduced network burden.

Materials and Methods

Subjects

The study was carried out in accordance with the recommendations of the Local Regional Research Ethics Committee (LREC 05/Q0403/142) with written informed consent from all subjects. All subjects gave written informed consent in accordance with the Declaration of Helsinki. Following ethical approval a randomized control trial was conducted in which 20 subjects (1 female) were recruited from Imperial College London (mean age, years ± SD = 28.9 ± 1.5). Left-handed subjects and those with a history of neuropsychiatric illness or previous exposure to the task were excluded (Orihuela-Espina et al., 2010). Subjects were included on the basis that they were task naïve. The task was performed under both guidance conditions (order randomized) such that subjects served as their own controls and bias associated with learning or ordering effects was minimized.

Task Paradigm

The robotic surgical task entailed the subject (*"trainee"*) and an expert (*"trainer"*) collaborating in taking virtual biopsies from a simulated gastric mucosa in a shared surgical environment as depicted in **Figure 1**. Haptic manipulators (Phantom, Omni, SensAble Technologies, USA) were used to control robotic graspers in the virtual scene. The task necessitated the trainee take a virtual biopsy and pass the specimen to the guiding trainer. Both the trainee's and the trainer's graspers were visible within the same field of view with the former located inferiorly and the latter superiorly as depicted in **Figure 1** (panels i–iv). Within the operative field, seven nodules were visible to the trainee. The choice of nodule for biopsy was randomly determined and this selection was available only to the trainer. Therefore, the appropriate biopsy site had to be conveyed to the trainee either visually or verbally by the trainer. Once the biopsy was taken by the trainee, the specimen was passed towards the trainer's graspers and when successfully transferred to the trainer, it disappeared from the field of view. This process was repeated as many times as possible during the allotted task periods.

Prior to commencing the study, all subjects received a standardized period of task familiarization. All subjects performed the simulated biopsy task under verbal (control) and visual instruction (CGC; Kwok et al., 2012). The order was randomized (random number generator) in order to control for learning effects. Regarding the control task, the location of the biopsy site was described by the trainer using verbal instructions. With CGC enabled, a portable eyetracker (×50 eyetracker Tobii Technologies, Sweden) situated beneath the trainer's monitor detected their fixation point and conveyed this to the trainee's screen as a cross. Therefore, with CGC enabled, the trainer's target selection would be conveyed to the trainee. For each condition (verbal and CGC) a block design experiment was employed comprising a baseline rest period (30 s) followed by five task blocks each of which comprised alternating episodes of simulated nodule biopsy (30 s) and inter-trial rest periods (30 s). During rest periods, subjects were asked to remain still with their eyes open regarding a black screen on the task monitor. Within functional neuroimaging experiments, block design paradigms have the advantage of allowing the hemodynamic response to return to baseline between each session, therefore providing reliable indices of task-evoked cortical activity. Furthermore, the block design allows task data to be averaged, increasing the signal to noise ratio.

Cortical Activity

Brain activation was assessed using a commercially available 24-channel Optical topography (OT) system (ETG-4000, Hitachi Medical Corp., Japan). Sixteen optodes (8 emitters and 8 detectors) were positioned in a 4 × 4 array over the O-P cortices as displayed in **Figure 1**. A "channel" represents a banana-shaped volume of cortex where changes in absorption of near infrared light from the optode emitters are interpreted as changes in HbO_2 and HHb. The array was centered on "Oz" of the International 10–20 system (Jurcak et al., 2007) with the intention of capturing activation within the visual cortex. Cortical data was subject to both manual and automated data integrity checks (Orihuela-Espina et al., 2010) to identify and eliminate data contaminated with noise, optode movement and saturation-related artifacts (i.e., apparent non-recordings and "mirroring"). Since both ambient light and near infra-red light from eye-tracking systems have the potential to influence OT data (Orihuela-Espina et al., 2010), laboratory lights were dimmed and the probes were shielded using a combination of external fixation tapes and shower cap.

Technical Performance

The number of nodules that the trainee was able to successfully biopsy and transfer to the trainer's graspers across the task period and the trainee's instrument pathlength (metres) were recorded and used as objective metrics of technical performance. This was preferred to restricting the overall number of moves towards calculating time/nodule biopsied, and helped to ensure that subjects were focusing on the task quality and not the procedural time, or perceiving the number of movements.

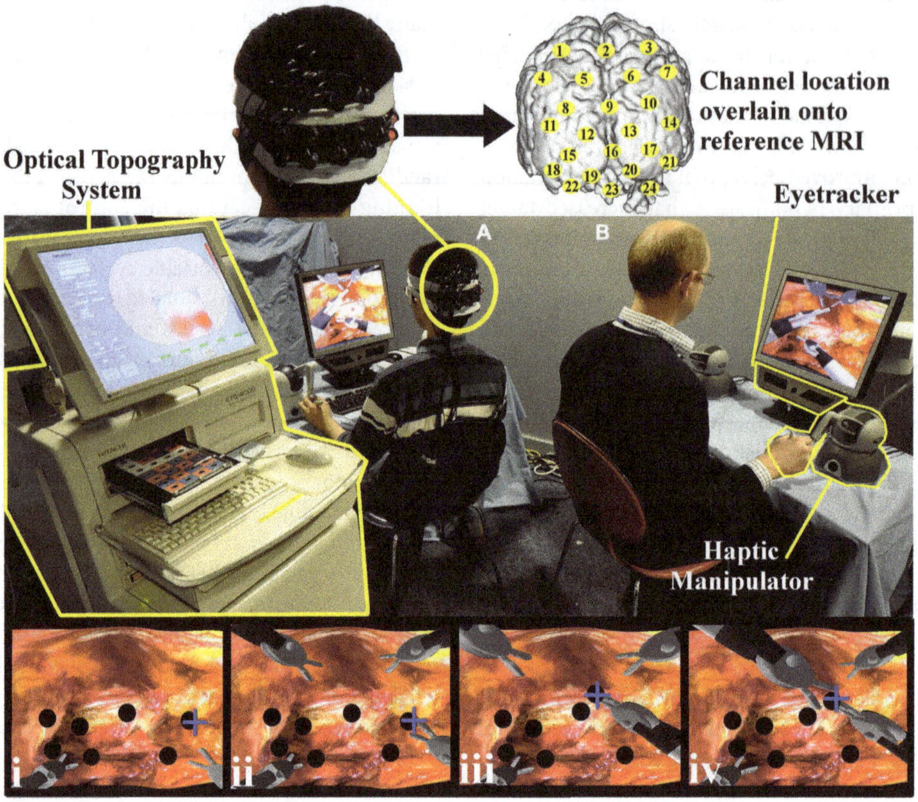

FIGURE 1 | Experimental task set up. Both the trainee **(A)** and trainer **(B)** control the virtual instruments, each with two haptic manipulators (Phantom Omni, SensAble Tech, USA). The trainer's right hand manipulator is highlighted (yellow). Gaze behavior is detected with portable eyetracker (X50 eyetracker, Tobii Technologies, Sweden) situated below both monitors (trainer eyetracker highlighted yellow). An Optical topography (OT) system (ETG-4000, Hitachi Medical Corp. Japan) positioned outside the trainee's field of view (left, highlighted) records cortical hemodynamic data from 24 cortical loci (channels). Appropriate channel locations (yellow circles) are understood by projecting 3D positional data onto a T1 weighted MRI image (upper subplot). The lowermost row of channels was centered on Oz of the International 10–10 system (Jurcak et al., 2007). Task images can be appreciated on trainer and trainee monitors and sample screen shots are represented in which the trainee's instruments are located inferiorly (i–iv). With the collaborative gaze channel (CGC) enabled, the trainee regards the blue cross indicating the intended biopsy target (i). The trainee then grasps the nodule (black circle) (ii) and passes it to the trainer's instrument (iii–iv). With the channel disabled, the trainee performs identical maneouvres but only with verbal instructions from the trainer.

Gaze Behavior

Subject and trainer gaze behavior was recorded throughout the study with portable eyetracking technology (×50 eyetracker, Tobii Technologies, Sweden) situated beneath the task monitor (as displayed in **Figure 1**). The gaze behavior of the trainer was interrogated to derive their fixation point in order to display this as a cross on the trainee's monitor thereby facilitating gaze-guidance in CGC (study condition). The trainer's fixation point was not visible to the trainee during episodes of verbal guidance (control condition). The trainee's fixation points were recorded to determine the time taken, termed "gaze latency" (GL, seconds), to fixate on the same area of the surgical scene as the expert.

Heart Rate Monitoring

A portable band electrocardiogram (Bioharness v2.3.0.5; Zephyr Technology Limited, USA) was used to acquire continuous heart rate data, from which heart rate variability (HRV) was derived and used to infer subject stress (Task Force of the European Society of Cardiology the North American Society of Pacing Electrophysiology, 1996).

Data Analysis

Cortical Hemodynamics

Cortical hemodynamic data and network graph econometrics were observed to be non-Gaussian and therefore analyzed using non-parametric tests of significance. Channel-wise cortical activation was determined as a task-evoked statistically significant increase in HbO_2 coupled to a significant decrease in HHb from baseline rest (Wilcoxon Rank Sign, $p < 0.05$). For each channel of data and hemoglobin species a variable ΔHb was computed (Hb task–Hb rest). To investigate the influence of the mode of guidance (CGC vs. control) and stress on cortical hemodynamics (i.e., ΔHbO_2 and ΔHHb) random effects models (REM) were generated (Intercooled Stata, v10.0 for windows, Stata Corporation, USA).

Cortical hemodynamic data was subsequently used to construct a task-evoked network of the 24 channels using graph theory (Bullmore and Sporns, 2009). A 24 × 24 bidimensional cross-correlation matrix was constructed by cross-correlating data between all channels, as previously described (James et al., 2013). This matrix represents the strength of functional associations within the network of 24 channels. Comparisons between graphs of different functional networks are potentially sensitive to the method used for thresholding, for which an optimal solution does not yet exist (van Wijk et al., 2010). Therefore, to evaluate the active network, the matrix was pruned to eliminate "inactive" graph nodes. This approach renders a network for each subject during each task condition.

Econometric data from these networks was then calculated to derive: (a) the number of network connections; (b) the maximum global efficiency (Achard and Bullmore, 2007); (c) the normalized cost (Achard and Bullmore, 2007); and (d) the task-induced *"network burden"* (James et al., 2010a). Network economy is defined as efficiency minus cost (Achard and Bullmore, 2007). The network burden is defined here as—economy which equates to "cost-efficiency". If a network is economical the cost-efficiency is high and accordingly the network burden is low. Network measures were also compared between the study and control groups using REM analysis to determine whether the mode of guidance (CGC vs. control) significantly influenced network econometrics. Statistical significance was set at p = 0.05.

Performance and Gaze Behavior

The number of nodules biopsied by each subject during the allotted task time and the instrument pathlength (metres) were determined. GL (seconds) was derived from the eye-tracking data stream. Behavioral performance and GL data was observed to be Gaussian and therefore analyzed using paired t-tests. These data were subsequently incorporated into the REM analysis in order to assess whether the guidance mode (control vs. CGC) was a predictor of performance accuracy and efficiency in visual search.

Heart Rate Analysis

HRV as calculated by the standard deviation of the R to R interval (SD_{RR}) was derived from the HR data stream (Task Force of the European Society of Cardiology the North American Society of Pacing Electrophysiology, 1996). The SD_{RR} decreases under stress and was incorporated into the REM analysis, to exclude any potential confounding effect that differences in HRV or changes in mean HR may exert on changes in cortical hemodynamics. Furthermore, HRV was utilized to determine which mode of guidance (verbal vs. CGC) trainee's found the most stressful by undertaking a univariate random effects analysis (p = 0.05).

Results

Technical Performance

Biopsy number and instrument pathlength was analyzed to determine whether CGC improved trainees' technical performance. As illustrated in **Figure 2A**, gaze-guidance

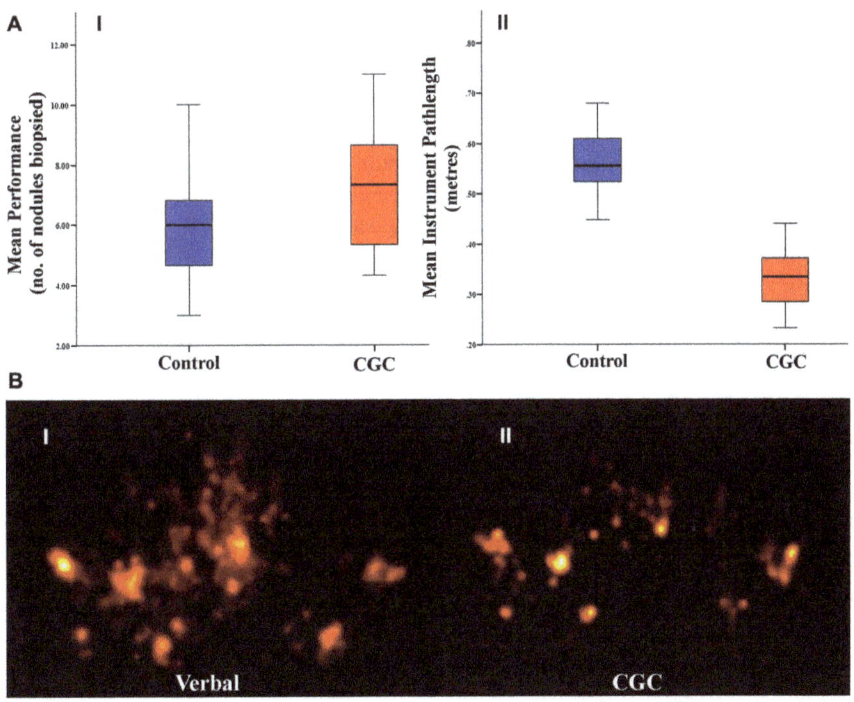

FIGURE 2 | (A) Technical performance as indexed by the number of biopsies retrieved (I) and instrument path length (II). Box plots indicate mean and error bars represent 95% confidence interval. **(B)** Gaze plots from a representative subject under control (I) and gaze guidance (II) demonstrate more focussed fixations during gaze-assistance.

TABLE 1 | The influence of guidance mode on technical performance, visual search behavior, changes in cortical hemodynamics, network topological properties and systemic effects.

Outcome variable	Control condition (Mean ± SD)	CGC condition (Mean ± SD)	*t*-value	*p*-value
Technical lerformance				
Biopsy number	5.6 ± 1.8	6.6 ± 2.0	−3.394	**0.003**
Instrument path length (m)	0.6 ± 0.1	0.3 ± 0.7	11.765	***0.000***
Visual search				
Gaze latency (s)	1.4 ± 0.3	0.8 ± 0.2	7.292	***0.000***
Outcome variable	**Control condition median (IQR)**	**CGC condition median (IQR)**	***z*-value**	***p*-value**
Cortical hemodynamics				
ΔHbO_2 (mMol × cm)	2.5 (12.0)	0.6 (11.2)	−4.049	***0.000***
ΔHHb (mMol × cm)	−1.4 (5.0)	−1.0 (4.5)	−1.098	0.272
ΔHbT (mMol × cm)	3.6 (13)	1.1 (11.6)	−6.064	***0.000***
Cortical network				
Normalized cost (a.u.)	0.10 (0.13)	0.19 (0.43)	−0.722	0.470
Global efficiency (a.u.)	0.03 (0.05)	0.02 (0.08)	−0.220	0.826
Network burden (a.u.)	0.09 (0.14)	0.18 (0.46)	−0.847	0.397
Network edges (a.u.)	56.0 (304.0)	81.0 (120.0)	−0.589	0.556
Systemic effect				
Heart rate (beatsmin^{-1})	71.2 (10.0)	73.4 (8.1)	−0.392	0.695
SD_{NN}	57.7 (42.0)	47.2 (36.9)	−0.784	0.433

$p < 0.05$ = bold, $p < 0.001$ = bold italic.

under the influence of CGC resulted in enhanced technical performance. **Table 1** highlights the differences in technical performance according to the mode of guidance. With gaze-assistance, trainees' biopsied a significantly greater number of nodules [biopsy number (mean ± SD): control = 5.6 ± 1.8 vs. CGC = 6.6 ± 2.0, $p < 0.05$] using significantly shorter instrument pathlength (metres) [mean ± SD: control = 0.6 ± 0.1 vs. CGC = 0.3 ± 0.7, $p < 0.001$]. This implies that trainees were faster, more productive and used virtual instruments more economically when operating from the CGC mode.

Gaze Behavior

GL which represents the temporal delay between trainer and trainee gaze fixation was analyzed to determine whether gaze guidance streamlined trainee visual search. **Figure 2B** depicts the visual search pattern acquired from a representative trainee under both guidance conditions. It is apparent that whilst operating under gaze guidance, trainee fixations appear to be more localized to the nodule to be biopsied. GL was significantly shorter in CGC mode [GL seconds (mean ± SD): control = 1.4 ± 0.3 vs. CGC = 0.8 ± 0.2, $p < 0.001$]. This suggests that gaze assistance manifests as more rapid fixation on the appropriate target nodule to be biopsied.

Cortical Activation

Cortical hemodynamic change was analyzed to compare trainee brain responses between verbal and gaze-assisted modes of operation, with the hypothesis that verbal guidance would induce higher amplitude and spatially broader O-P hemodynamic changes. Topograms of a representative subject depicting the

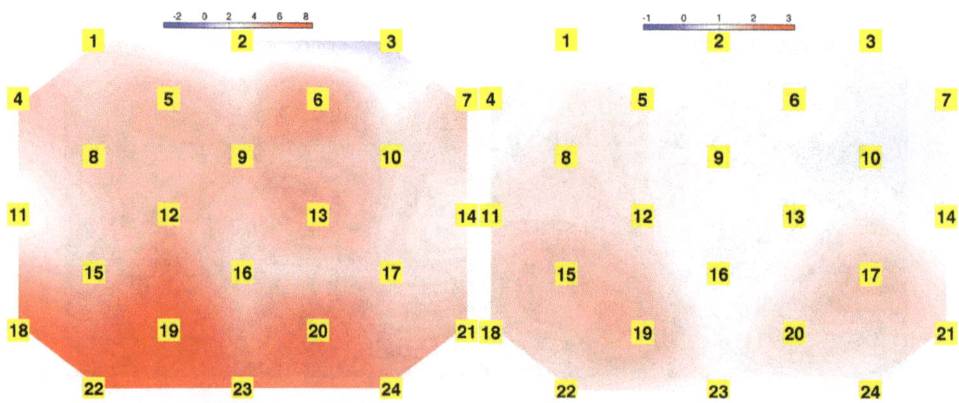

FIGURE 3 | Topograms derived from task averaged HbO_2 response of a representative subject for verbal (left) and gaze guidance (right) conditions, depicting spatially broader task-evoked oxygenated hemoglobin change during verbal guidance.

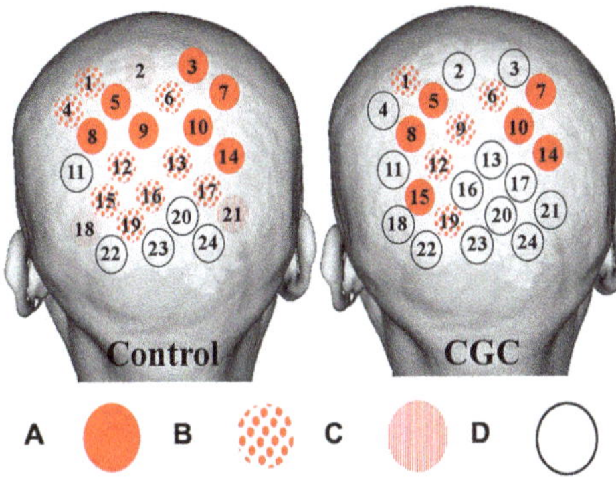

FIGURE 4 | Figure depicting group averaged (O-P) channel activation for verbal (left) and gaze guidance (right). Magnitude of statistical changes in cortical hemodynamics reflect intensity of brain activation as follows: **(A)** statistically significant ($p < 0.05$) increase in HbO_2 coupled to statistically significant ($p < 0.05$) decrease in HHb (red circles); **(B)** increase HbO_2 and decrease HHb with one species reaching statistical significance, $p < 0.05$ (spots); **(C)** increase HbO_2 and decrease HHb with neither species reaching statistical significance (stripes); and **(D)** no coupled increase HbO_2 and decrease HHb (clear circles). Verbal guidance resulted in a greater number of activating channels (control vs. CGC = 19/24 vs. 11/24).

average change in HbO_2 overlying the O-P cortices are displayed in **Figure 3**. **Table 1**, depicts cortical hemodynamic change as ΔHbO_2 (mMol × cm) averaged across the O-P cortices for both verbal and gaze-guidance. Cortical hemodynamic change evoked by verbal guidance was more diffuse as illustrated in **Figure 4** (CGC: 11/24 channels active vs. verbal: 19/24 channels active), more likely to involve bilateral parietal as well as bilateral visual cortices and was greater in magnitude than the response evoked by gaze guidance (ΔHbO_2 mMol × cm [median (IQR)]: control = 2.5 (12.0) vs. CGC = 0.63 (11.2), $p < 0.001$; ΔHbT mMol × cm [median (IQR)]: control = 3.6. (13.0) vs. CGC = 1.1 (11.6), $p < 0.001$). Overall, this data supports the primary hypothesis that training in CGC mode evokes an attenuated O-P brain response. The mode of guidance did not significantly influence the magnitude of ΔHHb [ΔHHb mMol × cm [median (IQR)]: control = −1.4 (5.0) vs. CGC = −1.0 (4.5), $p = 0.27$]. Similarly, as highlighted in **Table 2**, REM analysis revealed that guidance mode was a predictor of ΔHbO_2 ($p < 0.001$) but not of ΔHHb ($p = 0.19$).

Cortical Networks

Graph theoretical econometric data were computed and compared between guidance modes with the hypothesis that the performance of functional network in CGC mode would be associated with less cost and greater efficiency. **Figure 5** depicts the activated cortical network under control and CGC conditions for a representative subject. **Table 1** represent results of econometric analysis delineating the number of cortical connections, normalized cost, maximum global efficiency and cognitive burden. Differences in these network topological properties between modes guidance did not reach statistical threshold. Additionally, even when subject-level clustering was considered (**Table 2**) guidance mode was not found to predict network properties (e.g., cost, efficiency, etc). This suggests that CGC does not induce changes in the trainee's O-P functional network observable with the current OT technique.

Heart Rate Data

HR and SD_{RR} were monitored to determine the influence of guidance mode on stress-related change in systemic responses (**Table 1**). Between-condition differences in HR and SD_{RR} were not statistically significant [Median HR (IQR): control = 71.2 (10.0) vs. CGC = 73.4 (8.1) $p = 0.70$; Median SD_{RR} (IQR): control = 57.7 (42.0) vs. CGC = 47.2 (36.9), $p = 0.43$). Additionally, upon REM analysis, neither HR nor SD_{RR} were observed to be predictors for changes in cortical hemodynamics.

Harms

No harms occurred in the study.

Discussion

In this study, performance on a simulated surgical task has been improved by modulating the manner in which collaborating surgeons interact with one another. Communicating through collaborative gaze-driven control leads to a greater number of successful biopsies and a reduction in instrument path length, the latter being a measure of dexterity previously shown to reflect skill level in laparoscopic and open surgery (Bann et al., 2003; Xeroulis et al., 2009). The foundation for this improvement appears to be a change in visual search strategy manifest as a reduced GL indicating that with gaze-assistance, trainee fixation points more rapidly reach those of the expert. This was accompanied by an amelioration of cortical excitation across primary visual centers in the brain, but without an appreciable difference in O-P network costs or burden.

The current paper offers a potential mechanistic explanation for improvements observed in novices' performance when training under the influence of expert visual cues (Wilson et al., 2011; Chetwood et al., 2012). Experienced operators are known to utilize more effective gaze-strategies than novices, characterized by fixating on relevant target locations and adopting optimal psychomotor control (Wilson et al., 2011). Unlike novices who learn mapping rules by switching their point of regard between tool and target, experts utilize a target locking strategy and rarely need to check tool locations (Leong et al., 2008). As demonstrated by Wilson et al. (2011), novices trained to observe and then "mimic" the more focused gaze patterns of experts improve their laparoscopic performance and multi-tasking capabilities more than novices trained to observe expert performance without the benefit of expert gaze-cues. Similarly, Chetwood et al. (2012) observed improved completion times and reduced errors in novices guided by expert gaze vs. expert verbal instructions. However, unlike the current experiment, the aforementioned studies were not designed to explain the foundation for improved performance owing to gaze guidance, resulting instead in speculation regarding adaptation in visual

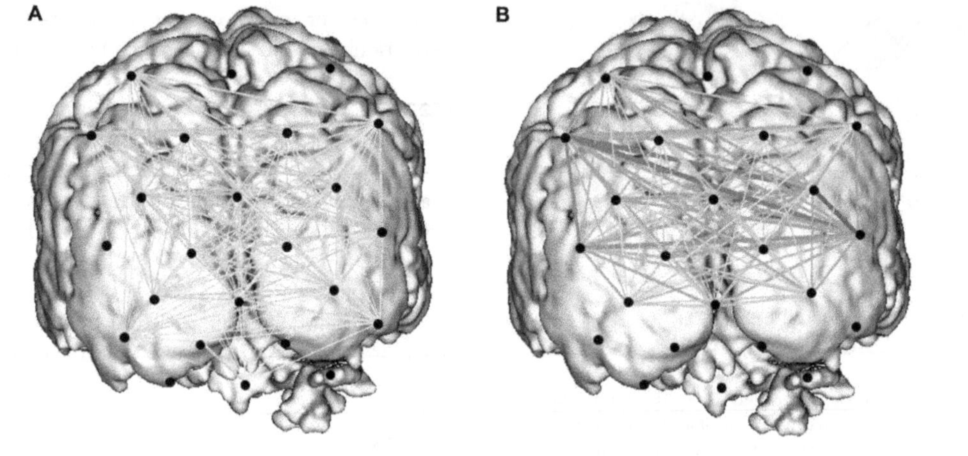

FIGURE 5 | Activity-guided cortical networks for a representative subject during the control condition (A) and study condition (B). Approximate channel locations (black circles) are overlain onto reference MRI atlas. The strength of functional associations between nodes in the network is represented by the boldness of network edges.

cognitive function. Here, improved performance as a result of expert gaze guidance is understood as a reduction in visual activation and hence attentional demand on the visual cortex. This is in line with studies demonstrating learning related plasticity in activation maps implying attenuation of attentional resources associated with training and expertise (Dayan and Cohen, 2011). By manipulating the visual behavior of novices in a way that they align more closely with those of experts it is conceivable that novices may bypass the early "cognitive" phases of visual-motor learning (Fitts and Posner, 1967). This notwithstanding confirming that the gaze behavior of trainees operating under gaze guidance was characterized by less random saccadic activity and was indeed more "expert" cannot be confirmed using GL alone and would necessitate a more elaborate analysis of eye-tracking data such as using exploit/explore ratio (Dehais et al., 2015) or visual entropy (Di Nocera et al., 2007).

There is evidence from functional neuroimaging studies that streamlined visual search strategies lead to reduced activation in the visual cortex (Kojima and Suzuki, 2010). For example, Kojima and Suzuki (2010) observed greater hemodynamic responses in fNIRS channels centred on the visual cortex during more effortful search strategies. However, it must be acknowledged that the introduction of a target feature into the surgical scene might be anticipated to increase visual attention owing to changes in visual saliency. This is relevant since the eye-tracking derived fixation point of the expert was projected to trainee as a visually salient target. Interestingly, shifts in visual attention secondary to manipulations in visual saliency as a result of gaze-guidance (i.e., the trainer's fixation point) did not manifest as greater activation in the visual cortex when compared to verbal instruction. Rather, the resultant visual search is potentially streamlined from a *"top-down"* to *"bottom-up"* strategy (van der Stigchel et al., 2009; Theeuwes, 2010). Specifically, if a target markedly differs from its background, it

TABLE 2 | Results of univariate random effect models (REM), evaluating the influence of the independent variable (mode of guidance) on dependent variables including performance, changes in cortical hemodynamics, cortical network metrics, heart rate (HR) and heart rate variability (HRV).

Dependent variable	Coefficient	*S.E.*	$p > z$	95% *C.I.*
Biopsy number	0.090	0.040	**0.025**	0.011 to −0.168
Instrument pathlength (m)	−3.20	0.312	***0.000***	−3.808 to −2.586
Gaze latency (s)	−0.761	0.118	***0.000***	−0.992 to −0.530
ΔHbO_2 (mMol × cm)	−1.294	0.326	***0.000***	−1.933 to −0.654
ΔHHb (mMol × cm)	−0.198	0.151	0.188	−0.494 to −0.097
ΔHbT (mMol × cm)	−1.094	0.303	***0.000***	−1.689 to −0.500
No. of connections	−0.000	0.000	0.754	−0.002 to −0.001
Normalized cost (a.u.)	−0.036	0.101	0.720	−0.234 to −0.161
Network burden (a.u.)	−0.333	0.097	0.732	−0.244 to −0.157
Global efficiency (a.u.)	−0.106	0.282	0.706	−0.659 to −0.446
Mean HR (beatsmin^{-1})	0.008	0.009	0.353	−0.009 to −0.025
SD_{NN}	−0.002	0.003	0.595	−0.008 to −0.004

($p < 0.05$ = bold, $p < 0.001$ = bold italic).

is visually salient and is more likely to be detected by a *"bottom-up"* search strategy guided by the saliency of the scene, whereas if a target requires greater cognitive input to be identified, a *"top down"* search ensues which is dependent on the PFC and parietal cortex (PC; van der Stigchel et al., 2009; Theeuwes, 2010). Bottom up saliency is not coded in the primary visual cortex (Betz et al., 2013), and this mode results in search simplification leading to a reduction in activity in visual association areas (Kojima and Suzuki, 2010). Enhanced saliency through visual guidance may parallel visual processing of natural stimuli (Einhäuser and König, 2010), whereby responses in V1 cells are optimally sparse (Vinje and Gallant, 2000). In the current study, this effect has been observed as a reduction in O-P cortical hemodynamic changes with comparatively fewer channels reaching statistical threshold for activation.

Parietal cortical activity is also associated with oculomotor intention and attention and may be important in planning eye movements (Kanwisher and Wojciulik, 2000). Verbal guidance may result in demanding visual search since it necessitates that auditory information be explicitly processed and translated into visual-spatial co-ordinates to understand the desired target's location, and parietal lobe activation has been shown to be important in spatial integration (Molholm et al., 2006). Conversely, gaze-guidance protocols may share many similarities with implicit learning protocols (Wilson et al., 2011). Implicit learning, a form of unconscious, incidental and procedural knowledge demands fewer attentional resources than explicit learning, a form of conscious, intentional or declarative knowledge. Implicit motor learning has been shown to reduce non-essential co-activation or connectivity between verbal-analytic and motor planning regions during laparoscopic performance (Zhu et al., 2011).

Here, as well as investigating connectivity (i.e., correlations), network topology has been explored with graph theory, which provides a powerful method for quantitatively describing the topology of brain connectivity (He and Evans, 2010). Graph theory has been utilized to interrogate cortical networks in both pathological and non-pathological brains (Achard and Bullmore, 2007; Bassett et al., 2009), and allows network parameters such as cost and efficiency to be determined (Bullmore and Bassett, 2011). Presently, graph theory was applied to experimental data in order to further appreciate the impact of a "gaze-channel" on functional brain networks. From the active network analysis (i.e., that which retains only activated nodes), it is evident that compared to verbal-guidance, gaze-assistance does not lead to significant differences in O-P network topologies, therefore disproving the secondary hypothesis. Therefore, our conclusion is that collaborative gaze exerts a positive effect on technical skills, alleviates burden on the visual cortices, and yet critically does not significantly alter performance of the functional O-P network.

Intuitively verbal instructions about target location are time consuming to deliver, more complex to interpret and harder to translate into the "visual" workspace, ultimately relying therefore on greater cognitive work as evidenced by enhanced task performance when visual guidance is employed (Chetwood et al., 2012). We suspect that gaze assistance makes the flow of information between the trainer and trainee more seamless by increasing the perceptual fidelity of the instruction given. Extrapolating this effect to the *in vivo* setting, a reduction in the attentional demands necessary to execute a procedure may manifest as a liberation of resources to devote to other safety critical aspects of clinical care (e.g., reacting to unexpected events, multitask decision making, planning operative steps, *etc.*). Future studies may capitalize on a framework that enables combined analysis of brain responses, visual behavior and HRV to improve the detection of changes in workload as has been demonstrated in pilots (Duratin et al., 2014). Furthermore, although not specifically investigated within the confines of this study, it is feasible that in using visual guidance the need to verbalize the intended target is bypassed and as such the trainer can focus on supplementary aspects of the procedure. For example, if the site of suture placement is already determined and displayed visually, a trainer can then focus verbal instruction on the technical aspects of suturing manoeuvres required to achieve accurate tissue apposition.

Conclusion

To summarize, this study demonstrates that capitalizing on visual behavior enhances communication between collaborating surgeons, and improves operator performance. This may be achieved through a *bottom up* allocation of resources within the visual cortex of the surgeon being instructed. It is plausible that trainees instructed in this fashion will be better able to devote neural resources to other safety critical aspects of the procedure. In investigating these hypotheses, fNIRS technology is well placed to make an impact, as it overcomes the limitations of traditional scanning environments (Cutini et al., 2012). However, future validation of graph theory measures for fNIRS connectivity analysis will necessitate comparison against models of anticipated responses and structural connectivity as have been observed using other neuroimaging technologies such as fMRI (van den Heuvel et al., 2009; Zhang et al., 2010). Critically, demonstration of correspondence between predicted and observed patterns of functional connectivity would support the feasibility and validity of fNIRS-derived connectivity measures.

Author Contributions

Study design and protocols were conceived by DRCJ, DRL, FO-E, LWS, K-WK, GM, G-ZY, and AWD. Data collection was performed by DRCJ, DRL, FO-E, LWS and K-WK. Data analysis was performed by DRCJ, FO-E, DRL, K-WK, LWS, GM and TA. The manuscript was written by DRCJ, DRL and FO-E and final critical editing was performed by DRL, LWS, GM, TA, G-ZY and AWD.

Funding

This work was funded in part by research grants from the Academy of Medical Sciences (Lecturer Starter Grant) and Cancer Research UK (Academic Lecturership).

References

Achard, S., and Bullmore, E. (2007). Efficiency and cost of economical brain functional networks. *PLoS Comput. Biol.* 3:e17. doi: 10.1371/journal.pcbi.0030017

Avraham, T., Yeshurun, Y., and Lindenbaum, M. (2008). Predicting visual search performance by quantifying stimulus similarities. *J. Vis.* 8:9. doi: 10.1167/8.4.9

Bann, S. D., Khan, M. S., and Darzi, A. W. (2003). Measurement of surgical dexterity using motion analysis of simple bench tasks. *World. J. Surg.* 27, 390–394. doi: 10.1007/s00268-002-6769-7

Bassett, D. S., Bullmore, E. T., Meyer-Lindenberg, A., Apud, J. A., Wienberger, D. R., and Coppola, R. (2009). Cogntive fitness of cost-efficient functional networks. *Proc. Natl. Acad. Sci. U S A* 106, 11747–11752. doi: 10.1073/pnas.0903641106

Betz, T., Wilming, N., Bogler, C., Haynes, J. D., and König, P. (2013). Dissociation between saliency signals and activity in the early visual cortex. *J. Vis.* 13:6. doi: 10.1167/13.14.6

Brennan, S. E., Chen, X., Dickinson, C. A., Neider, M. B., and Zelinsky, G. J. (2008). Coordinating cognition: the costs and benefits of shared gaze during collaborative search. *Cognition.* 106, 1465–1477. doi: 10.1016/j.cognition.2007.05.012

Bullmore, E., and Sporns, O. (2009). Complex brain networks: graph theoretical analysis of structural and functional systems. *Nat. Rev. Neurosci.* 10, 186–198. doi: 10.1038/nrn2575

Bullmore, E. T., and Bassett, D. S. (2011). Brain graphs: graphical models of the human brain connectome. *Ann. Rev. Clin. Psychol.* 7, 113–140. doi: 10.1146/annurev-clinpsy-040510-143934

Cutini, S., Basso Moro, S., and Bisconti, S. (2012). Functional near infrared optical imaging in cognitive neuroscience: an introductory review. *J. Near Infrared Spectrosc.* 20, 75–92. doi: 10.1255/jnirs.969

Chetwood, A. S., Kwok, K. W., Sun, L. W., Mylonas, G. P., Clark, J., Darzi, A., et al. (2012). Collaborative eye tracking: a potential training tool in laparoscopic surgery. *Surg. Endosc.* 26, 2003–2009. doi: 10.1007/s00464-011-2143-x

Dayan, E., and Cohen, L. G. (2011). Neuroplasticity subserving motor skill learning. *Neuron.* 72, 443–445. doi: 10.1016/j.neuron.2011.10.008

Dehais, F., Peysakhovich, V., Scanella, S., Fongue, J., and Gateau, T. (2015). ""Automation suprise" in aviation: real-time solutions," in *CHI'15 Proceedings of the 33rd Annual ACM Conference on Human Factors in Computing Systems* (Seoul: Republic of Korea), 2525–2534.

Di Nocera, F., Camilli, M., and Terenzi, M. (2007). A random glance at the Flight Deck: Pilots' scanning strategies and real-time assessment of mental workload. *J. Cogn. Eng. Decis. Mak.* 1, 271–285. doi: 10.1518/155534307X255627

Duratin, G., Gagnon, J. F., Tremblay, S., and Dehais, F. (2014). Using near infrared spectroscopy and heart rate variability to detect mental overload. *Behav. Brain Res* 259, 16–23. doi: 10.1016/j.bbr.2013.10.042

Einhäuser, W., and König, P. (2010). Getting real-sensory processing of natural stimuli. *Curr. Opin. Neurobiol.* 20, 389–395. doi: 10.1016/j.conb.2010.03.010

Ferguson, S., and Stack, B. C. (2010). Addition of a telestrator for teaching during video-based procedures. *Otolaryngol. Head Neck Surg.* 143, 159–160. doi: 10.1016/j.otohns.2009.12.043

Fitts, P. M., and Posner, M. I. (1967). *Learning and Skilled Performance in Human Performance.* Belmont, CA: Brooks/Cole.

He, Y., and Evans, A. (2010). Graph theoretical modeling of brain connectivity. *Curr. Opin. Neurol.* 23, 341–350. doi: 10.1097/wco.0b013e32833aa567

James, D. R., Leff, D. R., Orihuela-Espina, F., Kwok, K. W., Mylonas, G. P., Athanasiou, T., et al. (2013). Enhanced frontoparietal network architectures following "gaze-contingent" versus "free-hand" motor learning. *Neuroimage.* 64, 267–276. doi: 10.1016/j.neuroimage.2012.08.056

James, D. R. C., Orihuela-Espina, F., Leff, D. R., Sodergren, M. H., Athanasiou, T., Darzi, A. W., et al. (2011). The ergonomics of Natural Orifice Translumenal Endoscopic Surgery (NOTES) in terms of performance, stress and cognitive behaviour. *Surgery.* 149, 525–533. doi: 10.1016/j.surg.2010.11.019

James, D. R. C., Orihuela-Espina, F., Leff, D. R., Mylonas, G. P., Kwok, K. W., Darzi, A. W., et al. (2010a). Cognitive burden estimation for visuomotor learning with fNIRS. *Med. Image Comput. Comput. Assist. Interv.* 13, 319–326. doi: 10.1007/978-3-642-15711-0_40

James, D. R. C., Orihuela-Espina, F., Leff, D. R., Mylonas, G. P., Kwok, K. W., Darzi, A. W., et al. (2010b). Neuroergonomic assessment of the robotic enhancement of surgery. *Surg. Endosc.* 24, 192–269.

Jöbsis, F. F. (1977). Noninvasive, infrared monitoring of cerebral and myocardial oxygen sufficiency and circulatory parameters. *Science.* 198, 1264–1267. doi: 10.1126/science.929199

Jurcak, V., Tsuzuki, D., and Dan, I. (2007). 10/20, 10/10 and 10/5 systems revisited: their validity as relative head-surface-based positioning systems. *Neuroimage.* 34, 1600–1611. doi: 10.1016/j.neuroimage.2006.09.024

Kanwisher, N., and Wojciulik, E. (2000). Visual attention: insights from brain imaging. *Nat. Rev. Neurosci.* 1, 91–100. doi: 10.1038/35039043

Kojima, H., and Suzuki, T. (2010). Hemodynamic change in occipital lobe during visual search: visual attention allocation measured with NIRS. *Neuropsychologia.* 48, 349–352. doi: 10.1016/j.neuropsychologia.2009.09.028

Kwok, K. W., Sun, L. W., Mylonas, G. P., James, D. R., Orihuela-Espina, F., and Yang, G. Z. (2012). Collaborative gaze channelling for improved cooperation during robotic assisted surgery. *Ann. Biomed. Eng.* 40, 2156–2167. doi: 10.1007/s10439-012-0578-4

Leff, D. R., Elwell, C. E., Orihuela-Espina, F., Atallah, L., Delpy, D. T., Darzi, A. W., et al. (2008a). Changes in prefrontal cortical behaviour depend upon familiarity on a bimanual co-ordination task: an fNIRS study. *Neuroimage.* 39, 805–813. doi: 10.1016/j.neuroimage.2007.09.032

Leff, D. R., Leong, J. J., Aggarwal, R., Yang, G. Z., and Darzi, A. (2008b). Could variations in technical skills acquisition in surgery be explained by differences in cortical plasticity? *Ann. Surg.* 247, 540–543. doi: 10.1097/sla.0b013e31815fa42e

Leff, D. R., Orihuela-Espina, F., Atallah, L., Athanasiou, T., Leong, J. J., Darzi, A. W., et al. (2008c). Functional prefrontal reorganization accompanies learning-associated refinements in surgery: a manifold embedding approach. *Comput. Aided Surg.* 13, 325–339. doi: 10.3109/10929080802531482

Leong, J. H., Atallah, L., Mylonas, G. P., Leff, D. R., Emery, R. J., Darzi, A. W., et al. (2008). "Investigation of partial directed coherence for hand-eye coordination in laparoscopic training," in *Lecture Notes in Computer Science.* eds T. Dohi, I. Sakuma, and H. Liao (Berlin Heidelberg: Springer-Verlag), 270–278.

Micali, S., Virgili, G., Vannozzi, E., Grassi, N., Jarrett, T. W., Bauer, J. J., et al. (2000). Feasibility of telementoring between Baltimore (USA) and Rome (Italy): the first five cases. *J. Endourol.* 14, 493–496. doi: 10.1089/end.2000.14.493

Molholm, S., Sehatpour, P., Mehta, A. D., Shpaner, M., Gomez-Ramirez, M., Ortigue, S., et al. (2006). Audio-visual multisensory integration in superior parietal lobule revealed by human intracranial recordings. *J. Neurophysiol.* 96, 721–729. doi: 10.1152/jn.00285.2006

Niu, H., Wang, J., Zhao, T., Shu, N., and He, Y. (2012). Revealing topological organization of human brain functional networks with resting-state functional near infrared spectroscopy. *PLoS One* 7:e45771. doi: 10.1371/journal.pone.0045771

Ohuchida, K., Kenmotsu, H., Yamamoto, A., Sawada, K., Hayami, T., Morooka, K., et al. (2009). The frontal cortex is activated during learning of endoscopic procedures. *Surg. Endosc.* 2310, 2296–2301. doi: 10.1007/s00464-008-0316-z

Orihuela-Espina, F., Leff, D. R., James, D. R. C., Darzi, A. W., and Yang, G. Z. (2010). Quality control and assurance in functional near infrared spectroscopy (fNIRS) experimentation. *Phys. Med. Biol.* 55, 1–24. doi: 10.1088/0031-9155/55/13/009

Parasuraman, R. (2003). Neuroergonomics: research and practice. *Theor. Issues Erg.* 4, 5–20. doi: 10.1080/14639220210199753

Roy, C. S., and Sherrington, C. S. (1890). On the regulation of the blood-supply of the brain. *J. Physiol.* 11, 85–158. doi: 10.1113/jphysiol.1890.sp000321

Schlachta, C. M., Lefebvre, K. L., Sorsdahl, A. K., and Jayaraman, S. (2010). Mentoring and telementoring leads to effective incorporation of laparoscopic colon surgery. *Surg. Endosc.* 24, 841–844. doi: 10.1007/s00464-009-0674-1

Sporns, O., Chialvo, D. R., Kaiser, M., and Hilgetag, C. C. (2004). Organisation, development and function of complex brain networks. *Trends Cogn. Sci.* 8, 418–425. doi: 10.1016/j.tics.2004.07.008

Sporns, O. (2011). *Networks of the Brain.* Cambridge: MIT Press.

Task Force of the European Society of Cardiology the North American Society of Pacing Electrophysiology (1996). Heart rate variability. Standards of measurement, physiological interpretation and clinical use. Task Force of the European Society of Cardiology and the North American Society of Pacing and Electrophysiology. *Eur. Heart J.* 17, 354–381. doi: 10.1161/01.cir.93.5.1043

Theeuwes, J. (2010). Top-down and bottom-up control of visual selection. *Acta Psychologica.* 135, 77–99. doi: 10.1016/j.actpsy.2010.02.006

Tokuda, S., Obinata, G., Palmer, E., and Chaparro, A. (2011). Estimation of mental workload using saccadic eye movements in a free-viewing task. *Conf. Proc. IEEE Eng. Med. Biol. Soc.* 2011, 4523–4529. doi: 10.1109/iembs.2011.6091121

van den Heuvel, M. P., Mandl, R. C., Kahn, R. S. and Hulshoff Pol, H. E. (2009). Functionally linked resting-state networks reflect the underlying structural connectivity architecture of the human brain. *Hum. Brain Mapp.* 30, 3127–3141. doi: 10.1002/hbm.20737

van der Stigchel, S., Belopolsky, A. V., Peters, J. C., Wijnen, J. G., Meeter, M., and Theeuwes, J. (2009). The limits of top-down control of visual attention. *Acta. Psychologica.* 132, 201–212. doi: 10.1016/j.actpsy.2009.07.001

van Wijk, B. C., Stam, C. J., and Daffertshofer, A. (2010). Comparing brain networks of different size and connectivity density using graph theory. *PLoS One* 5:e13701. doi: 10.1371/journal.pone.0013701

Vinje, W. E., and Gallant, J. L. (2000). Sparse coding and decorrelation in primary visual cortex during natural vision. *Science.* 287, 1273–1276. doi: 10.1126/science.287.5456.1273

Wilson, M. R., Vine, S. J., Bright, E., Masters, R. S., Defriend, D., and McGrath, J. S. (2011). Gaze training enhances laparoscopic technical skill acquisition and multi-tasking performance: a randomized, controlled study. *Surgi. Endosc.* 25, 3731–3739. doi: 10.1007/s00464-011-1802-2

Xeroulis, G., Dubrowski, A., and Leslie, K. (2009). Simulation in laparoscopic surgery: a concurrent validity study for FLS. *Surg. Endosc.* 23, 161–165. doi: 10.1007/s00464-008-0120-9

Zhang, D., Snyder, A. Z., Shimony, J. S., Fox, M. D., and Raichle, M. E. (2010). Noninvasive functional and structural connectivity mapping of the human thalamocortical system. *Cereb. Cortex.* 20, 1187–1194. doi: 10.1093/cercor/bhp182

Zheng, B., Jiang, X., Tien, G., Mengeghetti, A., Panton, O. N., and Atkins, M. S. (2012). Workload assessment of surgeons: correlation between NASA TLX and blinks. *Surg. Endosc.* 26, 2746–2750. doi: 10.1007/s00464-012-p2268-6

Zheng, B., Jiang, X., and Atkins, M. S. (2015). Detection of changes in surgical difficulty: Evidence from pupil responses. *Surg. Innov.* doi: 10.1177/1553350615573582 [Epub ahead of print].

Zhu, F. F., Poolton, J. M., Wilson, M. R., Hu, Y., Maxwell, J. P., Masters, R. S., et al. (2011). Implicit motor learning promotes neural efficiency during laparoscopy. *Surg. Endosc.* 25, 2950–2955. doi: 10.1007/s00464-011-1647-8

9

The Role of Cognitive and Perceptual Loads in Inattentional Deafness

Mickaël Causse[1,2], Jean-Paul Imbert[3], Louise Giraudet[1], Christophe Jouffrais[4] and Sébastien Tremblay[2]*

[1] Département Conception et Conduite des Véhicules Aéronautiques et Spatiaux, Institut Supérieur de l'Aéronautique et de l'Espace (ISAE), Toulouse, France, [2] School of Psychology, Co-Dot Laboratory, Université Laval, Québec, QC, Canada, [3] Laboratoire d'Informatique Interactive (LII), École Nationale de l'Aviation Civile (ENAC), Toulouse, France, [4] Centre National de la Recherche Scientifique (CRNS) and Université de Toulouse, IRIT, Toulouse, France

***Correspondence:**
Mickaël Causse
mickael.causse@isae.fr

The current study examines the role of cognitive and perceptual loads in inattentional deafness (the failure to perceive an auditory stimulus) and the possibility to predict this phenomenon with ocular measurements. Twenty participants performed Air Traffic Control (ATC) scenarios—in the Laby ATC-like microworld—guiding one (low cognitive load) or two (high cognitive load) aircraft while responding to visual notifications related to 7 (low perceptual load) or 21 (high perceptual load) peripheral aircraft. At the same time, participants were played standard tones which they had to ignore (probability = 0.80), or deviant tones (probability = 0.20) which they had to report. Behavioral results showed that 28.76% of alarms were not reported in the low cognitive load condition and up to 46.21% in the high cognitive load condition. On the contrary, perceptual load had no impact on the inattentional deafness rate. Finally, the mean pupil diameter of the fixations that preceded the target tones was significantly lower in the trials in which the participants did not report the tones, likely showing a momentary lapse of sustained attention, which in turn was associated to the occurrence of inattentional deafness.

Keywords: inattentional deafness, cognitive load, perceptual load, pupil diameter, neuroergonomics

INTRODUCTION

The Air Traffic Control (ATC) environment involves supervisory control of emergency response, and security surveillance. Air traffic controllers must deal with dynamic and cognitively demanding tasks: guiding aircraft through a controlled airspace and optimizing trajectories whilst adhering to minimum distance and altitude separation minima requirement. This task must be completed in the face of temporal pressure, stress, and high-risk decision-making situations. Several research tried to identify the characteristics of the ATC environment that create cognitive demand (e.g., Manning et al., 2002; Loft et al., 2007). Manning et al. (2001) showed that these characteristics include, among others, the total number of aircraft controlled, the number of aircraft changing altitude, and the total conflict alert displayed. Other studies revealed that the dynamic density of the airspace at a given moment accounts for approximately half the variance in workload (Laudeman et al., 1998; Kopardekar and Magyarits, 2003). Although task demand has a strong relationship with workload, this relationship depends on the ATC operator capacity to select priorities and manage its cognitive resources (Loft et al., 2007).

The auditory channel is an essential means for air traffic controllers to exchange information with pilots and other controllers through radio and phone communications. They must also be vigilant and responsive to the occurrence of auditory alarms such as ground collision avoidance alerts or area infringement warnings that have been increasingly integrated into ATC workstations (Cabrera et al., 2005). Given that the auditory modality provides information without requiring head/gaze movements (Edworthy et al., 1991), it is particularly suitable for the transmission of alerts and warnings in emergency situations because perception is not dependent on the direction of gaze at a particular moment (Harris, 2011). However, research in the field of aviation has provided ample evidence that individuals can still remain unaware of unexpected task-relevant and often safety-critical auditory stimuli if deeply involved in demanding tasks (Dehais et al., 2012, 2014; Giraudet et al., 2015b).

Several studies support the notion of a central bottleneck of attention processing (Jolicoeur, 1999; Arnell and Larson, 2002; Lavie, 2005; Dux et al., 2006; Raveh and Lavie, 2015; Wahn and König, 2015) but other works propose modality-specific restrictions of attention (Duncan et al., 1997; Talsma et al., 2006; Martens et al., 2010; Keitel et al., 2013). In accordance with the first view, Tombu et al. (2011) proposed a central attentional bottleneck that includes the inferior frontal junction, superior medial frontal cortex, and bilateral insula that temporally limits cognitive processes such as perceptual encoding or decision-making. In contrast, other studies show support for modality specific limitations by demonstrating that attentional capacity between modalities is greater than attentional capacity within the same modality (Talsma et al., 2006). Furthermore, Martens et al. (2010) showed that an attentional blink is produced only when targets are both presented within the same modality (auditory or visual) but not cross-modally, thus favoring the idea of a modality-specific sensory system rather than a central amodal system. From a theoretical viewpoint, multiple resource theory (Wickens, 1980) posits that there are multiple, independent pools of resources and that tasks that share the same limited resource would interfere with each other but would not affect other tasks that require a different type of resource. For example, Kim et al. (2005), showed that Stroop interference increased when the type of working memory (WM) load overlapped with the type of information required for the target task. At the same time, Stroop interference decreased when the type of WM load overlapped with distractor processing. Beyond this debate between central vs. modality-specific attentional limitations, many studies show that WM load also affects the ability to process visual or auditory environmental stimuli. For example, Sörqvist et al. (2012) demonstrated that brain response to an irrelevant sound decreased as a function of central WM load, induced by a visual-verbal version of the n-back task. In the same way, it has been shown that manipulating the task load of the primary task reduced markedly the sensitivity to auditory distractors during a duration-discrimination task (Berti and Schröger, 2003).

Given the evidence for both sides of the amodal vs. modality-specific debate on attentional capacity, we might postulate the existence of both central limitations in the control of attention and executive control (Rossi et al., 2009), with a key role of the prefrontal cortex (Asplund et al., 2010) and higher-order multisensory cortices (Calvert and Thesen, 2004), and additional capacity limits in modality-specific sensory brain areas (Talsma and Kok, 2001). Such a hypothesis is supported by Vachon and Tremblay (2008) using an attentional blink paradigm. Their results tend to support the idea that attentional limitations are due to a mixture of both modality-specific and amodal resource constraints. Based on the results of Berti and Schröger (2003) and Sörqvist et al. (2012) showing the adverse effect of WM load, as well as similar fundamental works (Wood and Cowan, 1995; Spence and Read, 2003; Lavie et al., 2004; Hughes et al., 2013) and observations in flight and ATC simulators (Dehais et al., 2012, 2014; Giraudet et al., 2015a,b) indicating that a high cognitive load context can lead to the neglect of auditory alerts, we may reasonably postulate that the risk of missed alarms is quite important in complex activities such as ATC.

The high cognitive and perceptual loads typical of ATC operations may consume most of attentional resources, thus reducing the remaining attentional capacity for processing unexpected stimuli such as auditory alarms. This failure to perceive auditory stimuli has been called inattentional deafness (Macdonald and Lavie, 2011; Koreimann et al., 2014). Given the potential impact of inattentional deafness in safety-critical occupations, it is important to understand the factors that promote this phenomenon and to be able to detect its occurrence. When no visual feedback from the operator is available, or when the alarm is triggered by a system, it is almost impossible to interpret human reactions. However, recent studies have found electro-encephalographic indicators of the occurrence of inattentional deafness with diminution of the amplitude of the P300 evoked potential (Giraudet et al., 2015a,b). These results are promising since they allow an offline analysis to test alarm designs and to evaluate the conditions favoring inattentional deafness. However, the online detection of inattentional deafness with ERP is complex under ecological conditions given the low signal-to-noise ratio of the event-related EEG activity. A more robust way for detecting inattentional deafness online is still to be developed, but the ability to predict its occurrence using a physiological measure has excellent potential. With the visual modality monopolizing most of attentional resources, we suggest that recording eye movements while operators are exposed to alarms can inform about their auditory capacity in real time, particularly if they are displaying inattentional deafness. Eye-tracking has already proven very useful for interface design and for usability tests (Goldberg and Kotval, 1999). Several behavioral ocular metrics such as the number of fixations and their duration, the scanpath direction and length, or the switching rate between areas of interest can provide a non-invasive measure of cognitive activity (for a review see, Jacob and Karn, 2003). Evidence suggests that when the eye is free to move, fixation location is strongly correlated with where attention is focused (Findlay and Gilchrist, 2003). But while eye tracking is known to reflect visual cognition, it is uncertain whether ocular behavior could reflect further mental processes beyond basic visual encoding of task-relevant information. Also, the pupil diameter is a classic measure to index cognitive activity and is generally higher in context of high mental workload (Kahneman and Beatty, 1966; Palinko et al., 2010; Peysakhovich et al., 2015) or when the level of vigilance is high (Beatty, 1982). For example, Beatty (1982) showed that vigilance decrement was associated to decreased amplitude of the phasic task-evoked pupillary response during an auditory vigilance task, while tonic or baseline pupillary diameter exhibited no such relationship.

Inattentional deafness is generally studied by varying perceptual load (Koreimann et al., 2009, 2014; Macdonald and Lavie, 2011; Molloy et al., 2015; Raveh and Lavie, 2015), while the effects of variations in mental workload (central demand) are less well investigated (Giraudet et al., 2015b). Importantly, no studies have examined and compared the impact of these two loads on the ability to perceive auditory stimuli. The present study had two main objectives: to further understand how cognitive and perceptual loads impact auditory detection sensitivity, and to assess the possibility of eye-movements and pupil diameter to predict the occurrence of inattentional deafness. Twenty participants performed a realistic ATC simulation task called Laby (Imbert et al., 2014a) while an auditory oddball task was presented. Participants had to react to deviant tones (simulating auditory alarms) by button pressing, as an indicator of their detection of the sound. We separately examined the impact of cognitive and perceptual loads on auditory detection sensitivity with a 2 × 2 factorial design. The cognitive load varied with the number of central aircraft to control, and the perceptual load with the number of peripheral aircraft to monitor. In a previous study also using Laby, we demonstrated that the cerebral response (P300) to deviant auditory tones was diminished when the visual design of Laby was poor (Giraudet et al., 2015a). Also, this study showed that approximatively 6% of the deviant tones were missed in the high cognitive load condition with the poor visual design. To further understand the factors that promote the occurrence of inattentional deafness, in the present study we intended to increase the inattentional deafness rate by using a more engaging and complex version of the Laby. Inducing a high level of missed alarms would enable comparison between the ocular behavior of missed and reported alarms. We hypothesized that: (1) the high cognitive and perceptual load conditions should generate more missed alerts than the low cognitive and perceptual load conditions; (2) increased cognitive and perceptual load should impact ocular measurements; and (3) ocular measurements may predict the occurrence of inattentional deafness.

MATERIALS AND METHODS

Participants

Twenty participants, all students of Université Laval were recruited for this study (Mean age = 23.5 years, Standard Deviation (SD) = 4.2). None had a history of neurological disease, psychiatric disturbance, substance abuse, or took psychoactive medications. They all received full information on the experimental protocol, signed an informed consent and received compensation for their participation in the study.

Experimental Design

We used a 2 × 2 factorial design crossing two independent variables, cognitive and perceptual loads. The cognitive load was manipulated by the number of central aircraft in the corridor. The low cognitive load condition was the first half of the scenarios, with one aircraft to guide. The high cognitive load condition was the second half of the scenarios, with two aircraft to guide. The perceptual load was manipulated by the number of peripheral aircraft around the corridor (between 5 and 21). The perceptual load was unique for each scenario and the order in which low and high perceptual load scenarios was performed was counterbalanced across participants.

The Laby Microworld and The Auditory Oddball Task

The ATC Task

The Laby microworld is a functional simulation of ATC, developed to create and evaluate new designs for controller's visualization. It is built on the main task of guiding aircraft around a route shown on the center part of the screen (light green path). For the first half of the Laby scenario, there was only one aircraft to monitor. In order to increase the main task demand, at the beginning of the second half of the scenario, a second aircraft entered the corridor and participants had to guide both aircraft along the route (**Figure 1**).

In order to maintain the central aircraft within the corridor or to follow altitude instructions, participants had to regularly modify their heading and altitude, using drop-down menus (**Figures 2A,B**).

In addition to the central aircraft, participants had to monitor a set of static aircraft (5 in the low perceptual load condition, 21 in the high perceptual load condition) located around the main aircraft corridor (**Figure 1**). "Color-Blink" visual notifications were displayed in or around the radar label located in the vicinity of these peripheral aircraft (**Figure 3**). Color-Blink uses colored text with the word "ALRT" which switches from white to red (see **Figures 3A,B**). It is used in ATC operational radar visualization for high-priority short-term conflict alerts. The Laby interface design is similar to operational radar visualization, and has been used in a previous study comparing the performance of several visual notifications in peripheral vision (Imbert et al., 2014b). Compared to other enhanced designs, the Color-Blink notification was found to be less salient and had a lower detection rate among controllers (see, Imbert et al., 2014a). We thus selected the Color-Blink notification to increase the overall monitoring effort in the present study. In another study also with Laby (Giraudet et al., 2015a), we showed that a high cognitive load condition of the Laby was associated with 6% unreported ton. Also, as we intended to increase the inattentional deafness rate with a more engaging and complex versions of the Laby in the present study, two modifications were performed. In the present study, there was two aircraft to guide in the high cognitive load condition (one in the previous study). In addition, contrary to the previous studies in which the heading indications to give to the aircraft was already computed by the system and just had to be selected by the participants in a drop-down menus, in the present study, the participants had to mentally calculate the various heading that the aircraft should follow to turn and stay in the corridor. An orange heading indicator was displayed on the top left corner in order to help participants to transform direction into heading values in degree.

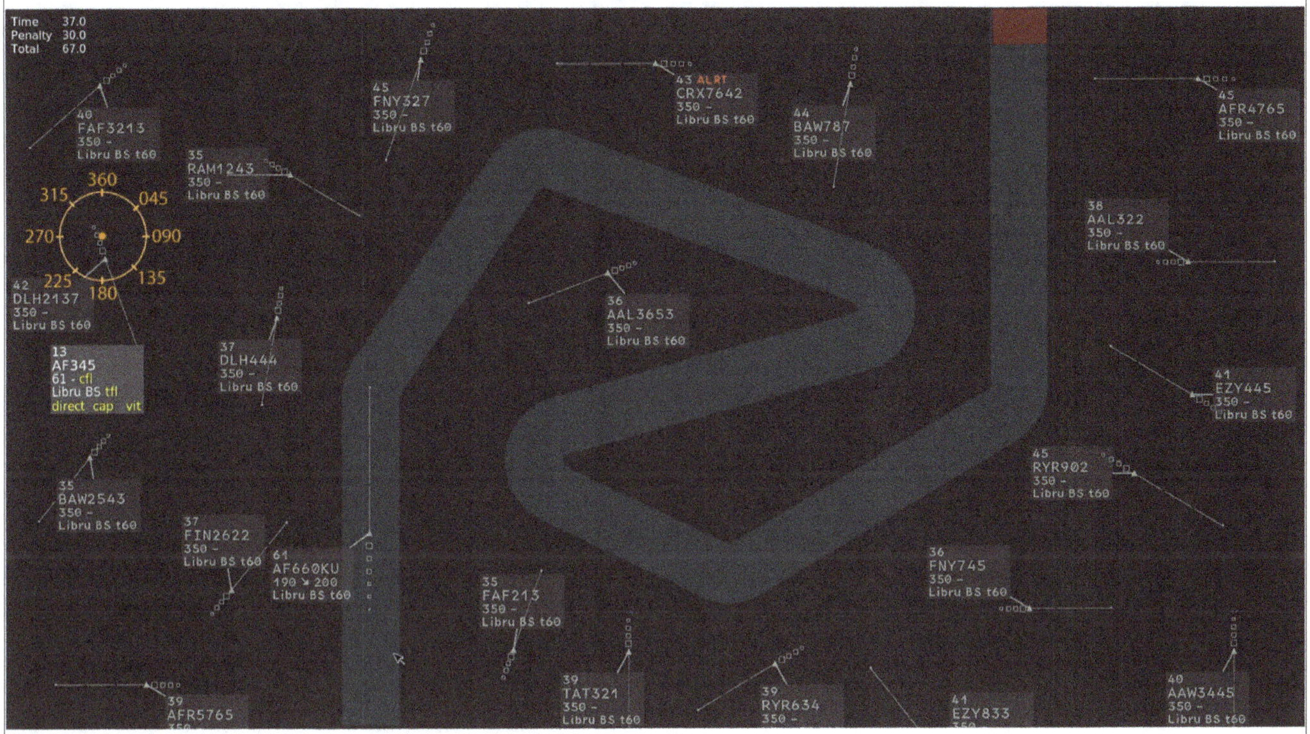

FIGURE 1 | Screenshot of the Laby microworld simulation. An example with 21 static peripheral aircraft positioned around the corridor. The central aircraft navigates through the corridor.

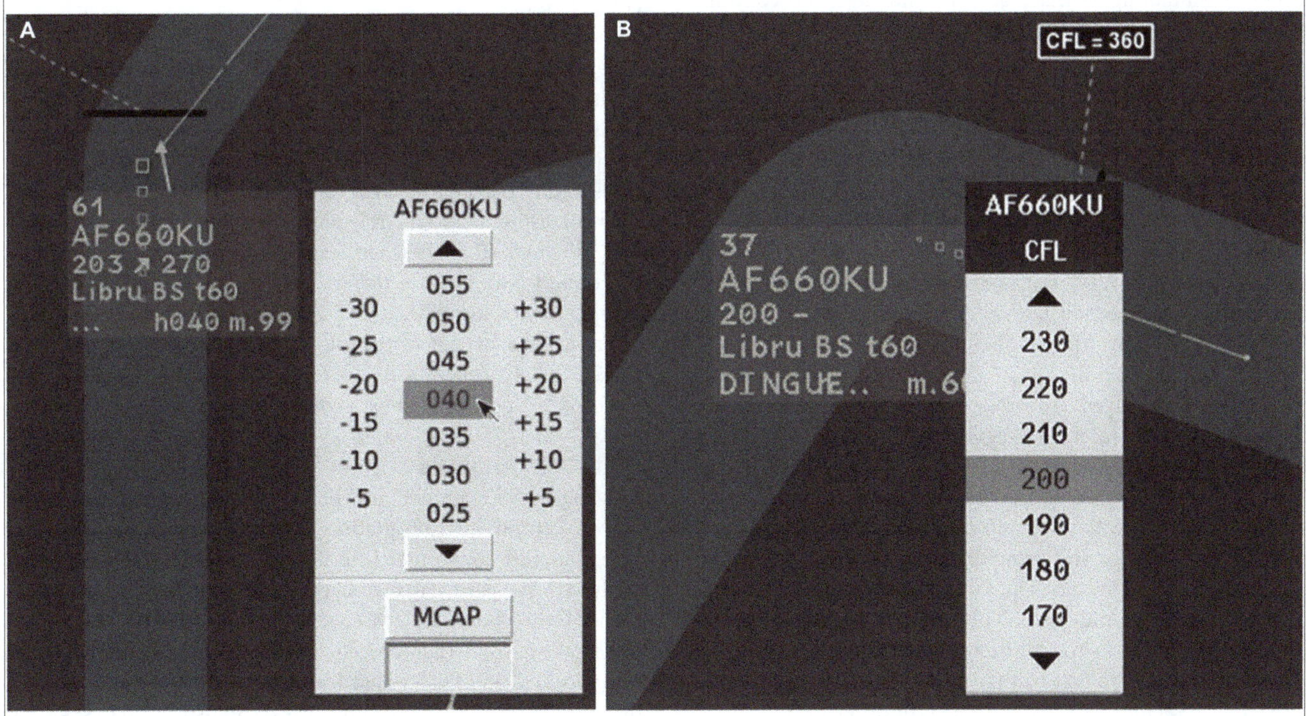

FIGURE 2 | Zoom on the Laby interface. (A) The menu used to select the heading of the central aircraft. **(B)** The menu used to select the altitude of the central aircraft. The menus appeared when clicking on the radar label.

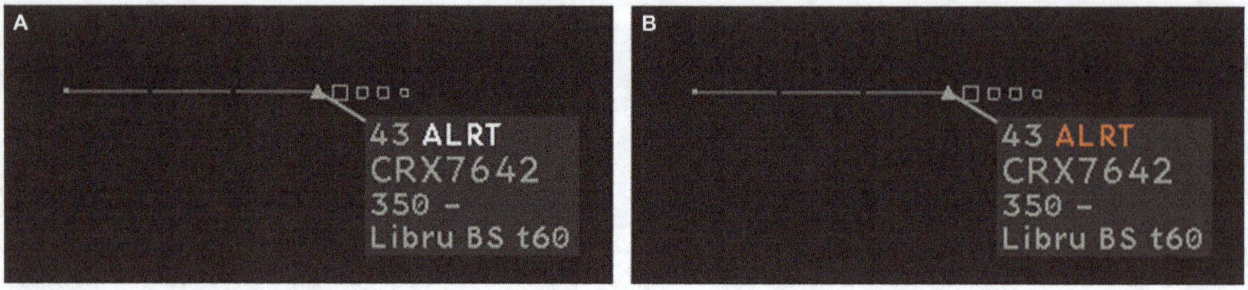

FIGURE 3 | The visual notification Color-Blink is inspired by operational warnings triggered in Air Traffic Control (ATC) radar screens when minimum separation between aircraft is lost. The text ALRT switches from white **(A)** to red **(B)** at a rate of 200 ms white/800 ms red.

Visual notifications were randomly displayed in the radar label located in the vicinity of these peripheral aircraft. Only one notification was issued at a time. The notification disappeared as soon as the participant clicked on the aircraft. If the participant did not react within a given time (5 s), the notification disappeared. Thirty-four visual notifications were displayed in each scenario.

A score was displayed on the top left of the screen. The score decreased for the following three reasons: first, when a participant led an aircraft outside the corridor; second, when he/she gave an incorrect altitude instruction; third, when he/she failed to click on a peripheral notification in the time limit. A deviation in the assigned route resulted in the aircraft crossing the border and initiating a visual alert in the center of the screen. An error in the altitude instructions resulted in the aircraft maintaining its trajectory, with no alert, and continued control. The score aimed to engage the participant in the ATC-like simulation in order to avoid them paying attention to the auditory alarm detection task only. The score was not considered in the analysis. The simulation ended as soon as the first aircraft reached the arrival area (colored red), at the end of the corridor.

Auditory Oddball to Simulate an Alarm Detection Task

In parallel to the ATC task, participants had to perform an auditory alarm detection task. Standard pure tones (1000 Hz, 52.5 dB SPL, 500 ms long, probability = 0.8) and deviant pure tones (2000 Hz, 52.5 dB SPL, 500 ms long, probability = 0.2) were randomly played. The tones were not representative of the auditory alerts recently integrated in ATC operations, their frequencies were chosen from previous works (Giraudet et al., 2014, 2015a,b). The mean time window between successive tones was 4.2 s. Participants were told to consider the deviant tones as auditory warnings and to report them as fast as possible by pressing a specific button. The auditory oddball detection task had no impact on the score. The number of auditory alarms (10) was the same in the four experimental conditions. There were ten tones in the first half (with one main aircraft) and ten tones in the second half (two aircraft). In order to increase the sound detection task difficulty, A 42 dB white noise was played continuously during each ATC scenario and the oddball control task. A control condition was also performed by the participant. They only had to react to the deviant auditory tones of the oddball while fixating a cross at the screen.

Procedure

The whole procedure lasted about 1 h. First, participants were seated comfortably at 60 cm from the 30″ screen in a sound-attenuated room with their right hand on the computer mouse and their left hand on the auditory alarm button. Second, they completed a training phase of 5 min to familiarize with the Laby microworld software, i.e., enter correctly path and altitude instructions by the drop-down menus, acknowledge visual notifications, and report deviant tones. After the training, the eye tracker was calibrated and participants completed the four ATC scenarios. Between scenarios, the eye tracker was recalibrated. Finally, participants performed the auditory oddball control task.

Eye Tracking Measurements and Data Processing

Continuous eye tracking was performed with a Tobii T1750 during the four ATC scenarios. The signal was recorded at a sampling rate of 300 Hz. For all eye movement analyses, the threshold to detect a fixation was set at 100 ms and the fixation field corresponded to a circle with a 30-pixel radius (equivalent to 1.15° of visual angle when seated at a distance of 50 cm). The position of both eyes on the screen was recorded. Data analysis was performed using MATLAB 7.1 (The Mathworks). Heatmaps visualizations of the distribution of fixations were generated using the open source software Open Gaze and Mouse Analyzer (OGAMA; Vosskühler et al., 2008).

Statistical Analysis

The impact of cognitive and perceptual loads on the accuracy to the central aircraft guiding task, peripheral notifications detection rate and missed auditory stimuli (rare tones) were analyzed. We also calculated the mean fixation duration on each of the four whole scenario and the mean duration of the fixation time that preceded the onset of a deviant tone (time-locked analysis) as well as the mean pupil diameter of this fixation (averaged on both eyes). Statistical analyses were performed using Statistica 10 (StatSoft©). Differences between the experimental conditions were investigated with the use of within-subjects analysis of variance (ANOVA) followed by *post hoc* testing (Tukey's honestly significant difference, Tukey HSD). We finally computed a multivariate logistic regression in order to further determine the variables that predicted inattentional deafness.

RESULTS

Effects of Cognitive and Perceptual Loads on Performance to The ATC Task

We examined if the performance in the ACT task depended on cognitive and perceptual loads, see **Figure 4**. The 2 × 2 (cognitive load × perceptual load) repeated measures ANOVA showed no significant effect of the cognitive and perceptual loads on the accuracy to the central aircraft guiding task (respectively, $F_{(1,19)} = 0.86$, $p > 0.05$, $\eta_p^2 = 0.04$; $F_{(1,19)} = 0.64$, $p > 0.05$, $\eta_p^2 = 0.03$). The interaction term was not significant ($F_{(1,19)} = 0.37$, $p > 0.05$, $\eta_p^2 = 0.01$). Regarding the peripheral notifications detection rate, the 2 × 2 (cognitive load × perceptual load) repeated measures ANOVA showed a significant effect of the cognitive load, with a lower performance in the high cognitive load condition ($F_{(1,19)} = 37.45$, $p < 0.001$, $\eta_p^2 = 0.66$). The perceptual load had a near significant impact ($F_{(1,19)} = 3.74$, $p = 0.06$, $\eta_p^2 = 0.16$). The interaction term was not significant ($F_{(1,19)} = 0.00$, $p > 0.05$, $\eta_p^2 = 0.00$).

Effects of Cognitive and Perceptual Loads on Ocular Behavior

The analysis of the dispersion of fixations across the Laby interface is shown in **Figure 5**. In the high cognitive load condition, there is an increase in the overall time spent fixating the central part of the Laby interface where the central aircraft are moving. Also, the time spent fixating peripheral aircraft is increased in the high perceptual load condition.

We analyzed the extent to which the overall fixation time, averaged across each whole condition duration, were affected by cognitive and perceptual loads (**Figure 6**). The 2 × 2 (cognitive load × perceptual load) showed a significant effect of cognitive load on fixation duration ($F_{(1,19)} = 7.69$, $p < 0.05$, $\eta_p^2 = 0.29$). The effect of the perceptual load was not significant ($F_{(1,19)} = 0.00$, $p > 0.05$, $\eta_p^2 = 0.00$) neither the interaction term ($F_{(1,19)} = 0.41$, $p > 0.05$, $\eta_p^2 = 0.02$). Overall average fixation durations were approximatively 420 ms (see **Figure 6**), which is consistent with a previous study using the same eye tracker during a simulated combat control system microworld. In this latter work, participants demonstrated average fixation durations above 300 ms in several experimental conditions (Hodgetts et al., 2015).

Fixation durations before a saccade have been shown to be modulated by the relative angle of the saccade (see, Wilming et al., 2013). The alternation between the two central planes in the high load condition could lead to systematic differences in the angle between subsequent saccades in comparison to the low load condition with only one central plane. This difference in angle by means of saccadic momentum can in turn lead to differences in fixation duration. Consequently, we compared the average angle between two saccades in the low vs. high cognitive load condition in order to examine a possible effect of momentum on fixation times. This analysis revealed that the mean angle slightly increased with increased cognitive load (low cognitive load = 84.64° (SD = 0.81); high cognitive load = 85.95° (SD = 1.08)) but the analysis did not reach the significance threshold ($F_{(1,19)} = 2.24$, $p > 0.05$, $\eta_p^2 = 0.10$). Saccadic momentum cannot explain by itself the variations of fixation times across the two cognitive load conditions.

Effects of Cognitive and Perceptual Loads on the Inattentional Deafness Rate

The control condition revealed that the inattentional deafness rate (missed alerts = 1-hit rate) was extremely low, with 2% (SD = 5.93) of missed alert. As a matter of fact, two participants omitted a few deviant tones whereas the 18 others reacted to 100% of the deviant tones. This result confirms that the

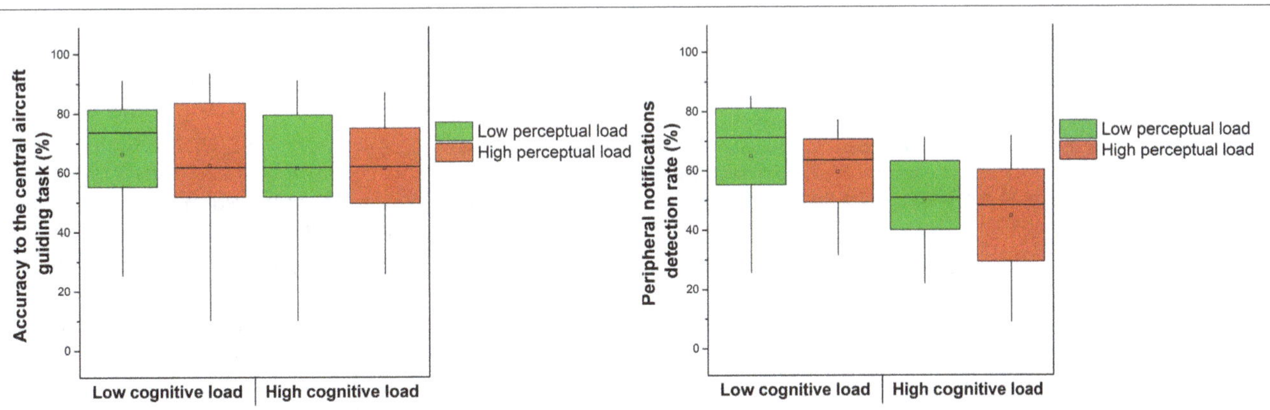

FIGURE 4 | Correct responses to the central aircraft guiding sub-task according to the levels of cognitive and perceptual loads. Validation of the peripheral aircraft sub-task according to the levels of cognitive and perceptual load. The square in the center of the boxes represent the mean, the horizontal line in the center of the boxes represent the 50th percentile (median), the end of the boxes represent the 25th and 75th percentiles, and the whiskers represent the 5th and 95th percentiles.

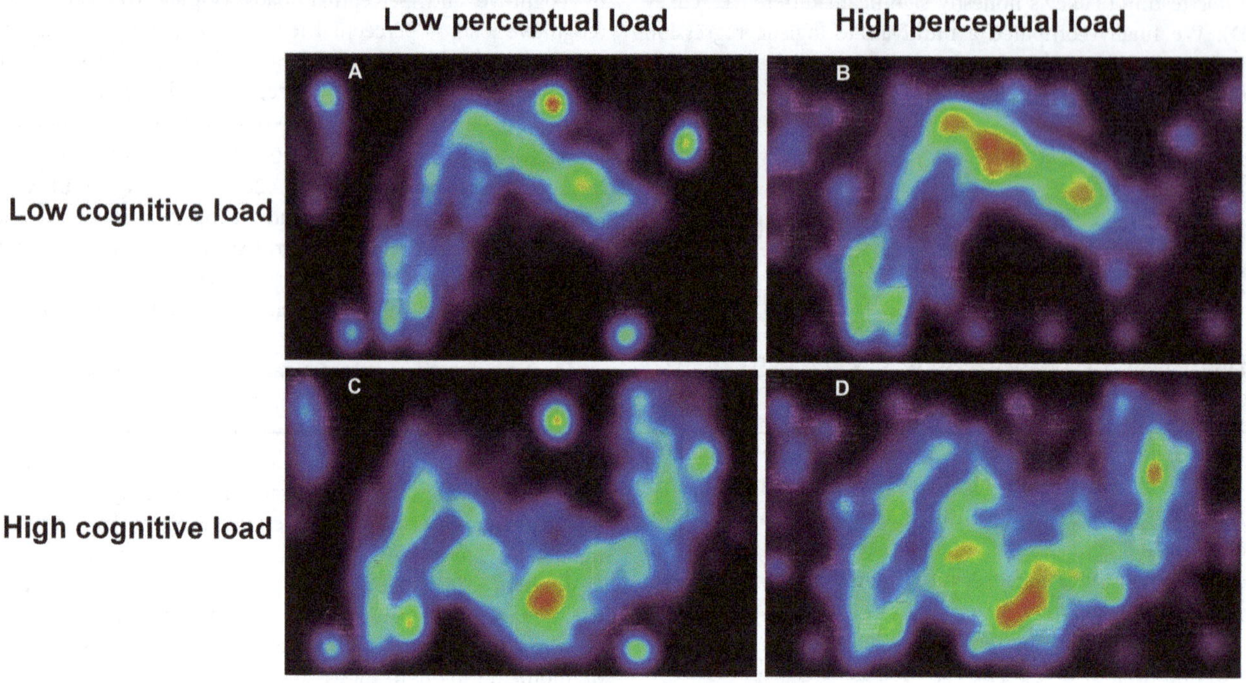

FIGURE 5 | Heatmap visualizations of the distribution of fixations on the Laby interface. (A) Low cognitive load/low perceptual load; **(B)** low cognitive load/high perceptual load; **(C)** high cognitive load/low perceptual load; **(D)** high cognitive load/high perceptual load.

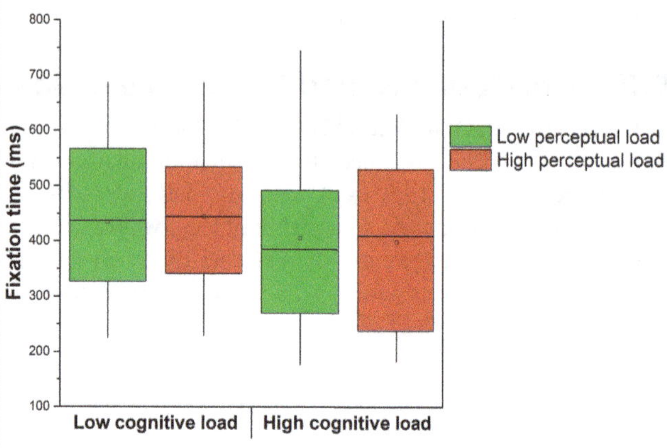

FIGURE 6 | Effect of the cognitive and perceptual loads on the fixation time averaged across the whole condition duration. The square in the center of the boxes represent the mean, the horizontal line in the center of the boxes represent the 50th percentile (median), the end of the boxes represent the 25th and 75th percentiles, and the whiskers represent the 5th and 95th percentiles.

tones were clearly perceptible despite the continuous white noise. We then examined if the inattentional deafness rate depended on cognitive and perceptual loads. The 2 × 2 (cognitive load × perceptual load) repeated measures ANOVA showed a significant effect of the cognitive load on the percentage of missed auditory alarms with an increased percentage of missed auditory stimuli in the high cognitive load condition ($F_{(1,19)} = 24.49$, $p < 0.001$, $\eta_p^2 = 0.56$), see **Figure 7**. The perceptual load had no significant impact ($F_{(1,19)} = 0.10$, $p > 0.05$, $\eta_p^2 = 0.00$). The interaction term was not significant ($F_{(1,19)} = 0.49$, $p > 0.05$, $\eta_p^2 = 0.02$). We finally examined if the specificity (true negative rate rate) and the discriminability index (d′ = Z(hit rate) − Z(false alarm rate); Stanislaw and Todorov, 1999) depended on cognitive and perceptual loads. A first 2 × 2 (cognitive load × perceptual load) repeated measures ANOVA revealed no significant main effect of cognitive load ($F_{(1,19)} = 1.23$, $p > 0.05$, $\eta_p^2 = 0.06$) and perceptual load ($F_{(1,19)} = 0.07$, $p > 0.05$, $\eta_p^2 = 0.00$) neither interaction effect ($F_{(1,19)} = 0.22$, $p > 0.05$, $\eta_p^2 = 0.01$) on the specificity. A second 2 × 2 (cognitive load × perceptual load) repeated measures ANOVA revealed significant main effect of cognitive load ($F_{(1,19)} = 18.88$, $p < 0.001$, $\eta_p^2 = 0.50$) but no effect of perceptual load ($F_{(1,19)} = 0.00$, $p > 0.05$, $\eta_p^2 = 0.00$) neither interaction ($F_{(1,19)} = 3.30$, $p > 0.05$, $\eta_p^2 = 0.14$) on the discriminability index. In summary, the cognitive load had a specific impact on the sensibility (hit rate), which increased the number of missed alerts. This is illustrated in **Figure 7**, the cognitive load had a specific impact on the true positive rate, not on the false positive rate. The d′ variations are only due to this effect of cognitive load on the true positive rate. We finally estimated if the variations in loads impacted the reaction time to alerts. In all four experimental conditions, mean reaction times were markedly below the mean time available to respond between two tones (i.e., 4.2 s), $M = 1.67$ s in low cognitive load condition; 1.53 s in high cognitive load condition; 1.65 s in low perceptual load condition; 1.55 s in the high perceptual load condition. The 2 × 2 repeated measures ANOVA showed no significant effect of

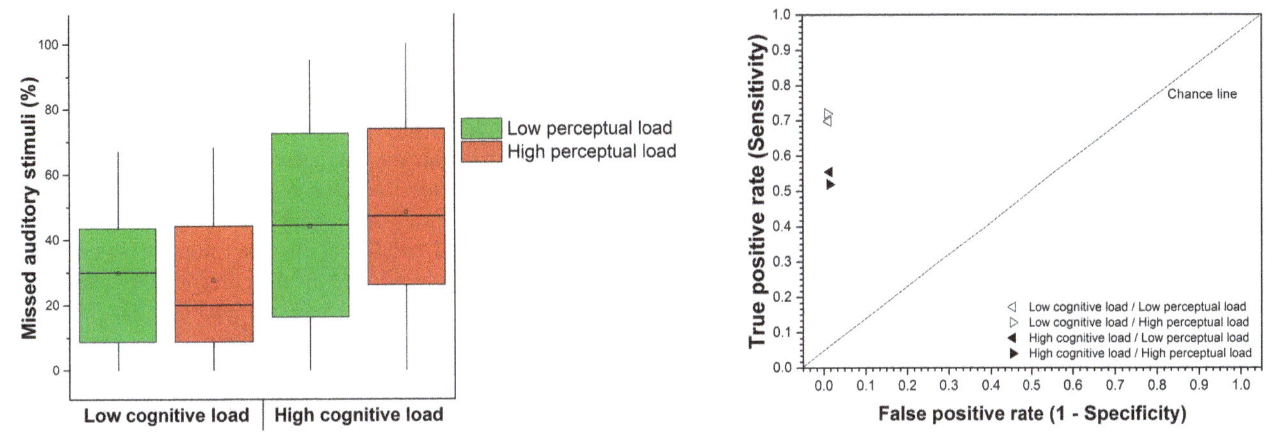

FIGURE 7 | Left: mean percentage of missed auditory stimuli according to the levels of cognitive and perceptual loads (referred to as inattentional deafness rate). The square in the center of the boxes represent the mean, the horizontal line in the center of the boxes represent the 50th percentile (median), the end of the boxes represent the 25th and 75th percentiles, and the whiskers represent the 5th and 95th percentiles. **Right:** true positive rate vs. false positive rate according to the levels of cognitive and perceptual loads.

cognitive ($F_{(1,19)} = 1.02, p > 0.05, \eta_p^2 = 0.05$) and perceptual load ($F_{(1,19)} = 1.03, p > 0.05, \eta_p^2 = 0.05$) neither significant interaction ($F_{(1,19)} = 0.06, p > 0.05, \eta_p^2 = 0.00$) on reaction times.

Multivariate Logistic Regression Analysis

In order to further investigate the factors that promote inattentional deafness, we performed a multivariate logistic regression analysis stratified by trial (trials with deviant tones only) with all participants grouped together (number of trials = 800). We used the occurrence of inattentional deafness (yes/no) as binary dependent variable and cognitive and perceptual load were introduced as categorical independent variables. Furthermore, the mean duration of the fixation that occurred just before the occurrence of the rare tone and the mean pupil diameter during this fixation were used as a continuous variable. The Wald chi-square p-values confirmed that the cognitive load was a significant predictor of the occurrence of inattentional deafness (Wald statistic = 14.38, $p < 0.001$) while perceptual load was not (Wald statistic = 0.77, $p > 0.05$). In addition, the regression also showed that pupil diameter of the fixation that preceded the rare sound was significantly lower in the trials in which the participants did not react to the target tones (Wald statistic = 18.66, $p < 0.001$) (see **Figure 8**). Finally, the duration of the previous fixation was not predictive (Wald statistic = 0.20, $p > 0.05$).

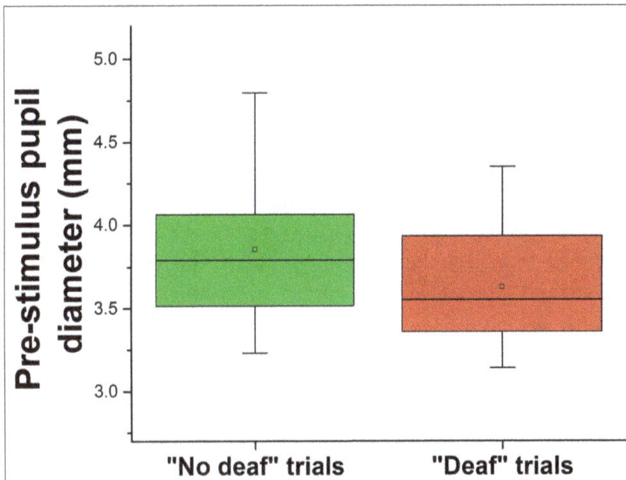

FIGURE 8 | Pre-stimulus pupil diameter (fixation $n-1$) for hit and missed auditory stimuli. The square in the center of the boxes represent the mean, the horizontal line in the center of the boxes represent the 50th percentile (median), the end of the boxes represent the 25th and 75th percentiles, and the whiskers represent the 5th and 95th percentiles.

DISCUSSION

Summary of Results

Our results showed that a high level of cognitive load, manipulated by the number of planes to guide, significantly increased the inattentional deafness rate whereas the perceptual load, manipulated by the number of peripheral aircraft to monitor, had no significant impact. The cognitive load also impacted ocular behavior with lower fixation time in the high load condition, while perceptual load had no significant effect. Finally, logistic regressions showed that the mean pupil diameter of the fixation that preceded the onset of the tones predicted inattentional deafness.

Effects of Cognitive and Perceptual Loads

Participants missed 28.76% of alarms in the low cognitive load condition (irrespective of the perceptual load) compared to 46.21% in the high cognitive load condition. This strikingly high rate of missed alerts cannot be attributed to sensorial difficulties as only 2% of alerts were missed in the control condition, in which the participant completed the tone detection task only (only 2 out of 20 participants missed any alerts). In the high cognitive load condition, participants engaged in greater mental effort by shifting their attention from one plane to the other, and also had a higher workload due to the need to calculate/modify heading and to change altitude parameters more often. These factors increased the chance of experiencing inattentional deafness.

Interestingly, perceptual load did not increase the missed alarm rate. In order to disentangle cognitive from perceptual load as much as possible, the high perceptual load did not generate a supplementary cognitive effort as the number of peripheral aircraft was increased while the number of associated peripheral alerts remained constant. Indeed, as demonstrated by Manning et al. (2001), the total conflict alert displayed contribute to increase cognitive effort. Inattentional deafness seems to be produced when an individual is engaged and monopolized in a task rather than when the individual is gazing more passively at visual information. One might argue that the additional number of peripheral aircraft was simply ignored by the participant which may explain this lack of effect of the high perceptual load condition. However, the heatmap illustrating the distribution of fixations clearly showed that fixations on the peripheral aircraft increased in the high perceptual load condition.

As demonstrated by the heatmaps and by a decline in the detection rate of peripheral notifications, the high load condition resulted in an important focus on the central aircraft, a behavior that can be compared to attentional tunneling (Wickens and Alexander, 2009; Régis et al., 2014). In general, fixation duration is known to reflect the attention (Findlay and Gilchrist, 2003) and mental effort (De Rivecourt et al., 2008) of an observer. In this last study on simulated flights, De Rivecourt et al. (2008) showed that momentary altitude changes can result in increased mean fixation duration. Variation of the fixation duration should be considered as task dependent: both shorter and longer fixations may indicate an increase in workload, and in particular shorter fixations indicated higher workload and increased temporal pressure in our study. This strong engagement of cognitive resources seemed to contribute to create a momentarily "deafness" to auditory stimuli.

One might also argue that this high inattentional deafness rate was due to an insufficient time window to report the alarm (i.e., mean time window = 4.2 s). Yet, in all four experimental conditions, mean reaction times were markedly below the mean time available to respond between two tones (around 1 s), and the reaction times did not significantly vary across the four experimental conditions. Even if we cannot completely eliminate the idea that a relatively small number of deviant tones were not reported because participants reacted too late, these two results tend to exclude this explanation as a major contributor of variation in the inattentional deafness rate with increased cognitive load. The analysis of d′ confirmed that the decline in the number of reported alerts in the high cognitive load condition is associated with a loss of sensitivity to deviant tones, and not due to an effect on the ability to discriminate the two tones. In this latter situation, the number of false alarms would have likely increased.

Importantly the inattentional deafness rate of the present study was considerably higher than in previous research using Laby (Giraudet et al., 2015a), whereby the percentage of unreported tones was 6% in the high cognitive load condition. To further understand the factors that promote the occurrence of inattentional deafness, the present study had employed two modifications to create a more engaging and complex version of the Laby task. First, there were two aircraft to guide in the high cognitive load condition whereas only one was displayed in the previous study. Second, in the current study participants had to mentally calculate the various headings that the aircraft should follow to turn and stay within the corridor, whereas previously these were pre-calculated by the system and just required selection from a drop-down menu. These modifications lead to a considerable rise in the incidence of inattentional deafness. It must be noted that in both studies, the importance of reporting the sounds was emphasized and that the time between the two tones was identical in both. The mental calculation of heading was undoubtedly a key factor in this increase of inattentional deafness as even in the low load condition, in which only one aircraft was displayed, the inattentional deafness rate was greater than three times that observed in the previous study in which the heading was given by the system.

Lower Pupil Diameter Predicts Inattentional Deafness

The multivariate logistic regression confirmed that cognitive load significantly predicted the occurrence of inattentional deafness. Most importantly, the regression also revealed that pupil diameter was lower during the fixation that preceded the onset of the target tones in the "deaf" trials. This result is counterintuitive as inattentional deafness was indubitably increased by the high cognitive load context, which is supposed in turn to increase the pupil diameter (Kahneman and Beatty, 1966; Palinko et al., 2010; Peysakhovich et al., 2015). Yet, as previously mentioned, Beatty (1982) showed that vigilance decrement was associated to decreased amplitude of the phasic task-evoked pupillary response during an auditory vigilance task, while tonic or baseline pupillary diameter exhibited no such relationship. In addition, a very recent study (Unsworth and Robison, 2016) indicated that pupillary diameter can index lapses of sustained attention. They showed that compared to focused states, inattentive and mind-wandering states are associated with lower pretrial baseline pupil responses and that distracted states are associated with larger pretrial baseline pupil diameter. These results support the notion that pupil diameter is sensitive to different types of lapses of attention, which is consistent with theories of locus coeruleus norepinephrine (LC-NE) functioning. In our study, despite a context of sustained high cognitive load, momentary lapses of sustained attention may have occurred, which could explain the relationship between lower phasic pupil diameter and inattentional deafness occurrence. This assumption can be also related to a past study that revealed that information overload resulted in a leveling of the dilation pattern, which suggested a momentary suspension of processing effort (Peavler, 1974).

Our results demonstrating an effect of cognitive load but not of perceptual load on inattentional deafness, are somewhat contradictory to a study by Macdonald and Lavie (2011) in which participants were engaged in a visual discrimination task of a cross shape. In the low visual load condition, this discrimination was made according to the line color and in the high visual-load condition, participants had to discriminate subtle line length. One brief pure tone was presented simultaneously at the final trial onset. Failures to notice the presence of this tone reached a rate of 79% in the high-visual-load condition, significantly greater than in the low-load condition. We could postulate that the type of perceptual load manipulated by the authors likely generated an indirect increase in mental effort and task engagement due to the comparison process of the line length. For example, Fierro et al. (2000) showed that the line-length comparison process engages the parietal cortex, indicating that spatial cognition is also taxed in such a task. Also, the paradigm used by Macdonald and Lavie (2011) was quite different as only one pure sound was presented in the study while 10 target tones per condition were presented in the current study. We believe that our paradigm is closer to a real life context or complex activity such as ATC in which the auditory environment is composed of a mixture of different sounds that can be repeated several times. As our paradigm can be related to "change deafness" studies, for example in which a subtle change between two voices is unnoticed (Vitevitch, 2003), a future study would look to reproduce the same paradigm but with only deviant tone.

Conclusion

The present study suggests that inattentional deafness is promoted by cognitive load rather than by a "passive" perceptual load that does not generate a supplementary amount of work. A strong engagement of cognitive resources in a given task can momentarily render one "deaf" to auditory stimuli. In our study, the key factor that promoted inattentional deafness was most likely the cognitive load generated by the mental calculation of heading and by the numerous tasks to conduct. This result confirmed previous studies showing that inattentional deafness drastically increases in the context of high cognitive load (Giraudet et al., 2015b), which can have serious consequences in safety-critical occupations like ATC. Finally, the mean pupil diameter of the period that just preceded the rare sound onset was significantly lower in the trials in which the participants did not react to the target tones, likely showing a momentary lapse of sustained attention, which in turn promoted the occurrence of inattentional deafness.

AUTHOR CONTRIBUTIONS

LG, J-PI and MC designed the experiment. LG conducted the experiments. LG, MC, J-PI analyzed and interpreted the data. MC, LG, ST and CJ wrote the article.

FUNDING

Financial support was provided by a Discovery grant from the National Sciences and Engineering Research Council of Canada (NSERC), awarded to Sébastien Tremblay [Grant number CG073877], by the Institut Supérieur de l'Aéronautique et de l'Espace to in the form of an operating grant to Mickaël Causse, and also by the Direction Générale de l'Armement in the form of a scholarship to Louise Giraudet.

ACKNOWLEDGMENTS

We would like to thank Danny Lebel for his technical support, and Marie-Kim Côté for her help running the experiment. We are also grateful to Zarrin Chua and Helen Hodgetts for proofreading earlier versions of the article.

REFERENCES

Arnell, K. M., and Larson, J. M. (2002). Cross-modality attentional blinks without preparatory task-set switching. *Psychon. Bull. Rev.* 9, 497–506. doi: 10.3758/bf03196305

Asplund, C. L., Todd, J. J., Snyder, A. P., and Marois, R. (2010). A central role for the lateral prefrontal cortex in goal-directed and stimulus-driven attention. *Nat. Neurosci.* 13, 507–512. doi: 10.1038/nn.2509

Beatty, J. (1982). Phasic not tonic pupillary responses vary with auditory vigilance performance. *Psychophysiology* 19, 167–172. doi: 10.1111/j.1469-8986.1982.tb02540.x

Berti, S., and Schröger, E. (2003). Working memory controls involuntary attention switching: evidence from an auditory distraction paradigm. *Eur. J. Neurosci.* 17, 1119–1122. doi: 10.1046/j.1460-9568.2003.02527.x

Cabrera, D., Ferguson, S., and Laing, G. (2005). "Development of auditory alerts for air traffic control consoles," in *Proceedings 119th Audio Engineering Society Convention* (New York, NY).

Calvert, G. A., and Thesen, T. (2004). Multisensory integration: methodological approaches and emerging principles in the human brain. *J. Physiol. Paris* 98, 191–205. doi: 10.1016/j.jphysparis.2004.03.018

De Rivecourt, M., Kuperus, M., Post, W., and Mulder, L. (2008). Cardiovascular and eye activity measures as indices for momentary changes in mental effort during simulated flight. *Ergonomics* 51, 1295–1319. doi: 10.1080/00140130802120267

Dehais, F., Causse, M., Régis, N., Menant, E., Labedan, P., Vachon, F., et al. (2012). "Missing critical auditory alarms in aeronautics: evidence for inattentional deafness?" in *Proceedings of the Human Factors and Ergonomics Society 56th Annual Meeting* (Boston), 1639–1643. doi: 10.1177/1071181312561328

Dehais, F., Causse, M., Vachon, F., Régis, N., Menant, E., and Tremblay, S. (2014). Failure to detect critical auditory alerts in the cockpit evidence for inattentional deafness. *Hum. Factors* 56, 631–644. doi: 10.1177/0018720813510735

Duncan, J., Martens, S., and Ward, R. (1997). Restricted attentional capacity within but not between sensory modalities. *Nature* 387, 808–810. doi: 10.1038/42947

Dux, P. E., Ivanoff, J., Asplund, C. L., and Marois, R. (2006). Isolation of a central bottleneck of information processing with time-resolved fMRI. *Neuron* 52, 1109–1120. doi: 10.1016/j.neuron.2006.11.009

Edworthy, J., Loxley, S., and Dennis, I. (1991). Improving auditory warning design: relationship between warning sound parameters and perceived urgency. *Hum. Factors* 33, 205–231.

Fierro, B., Brighina, F., Oliveri, M., Piazza, A., La Bua, V., Buffa, D., et al. (2000). Contralateral neglect induced by right posterior parietal rTMS in healthy subjects. *Neuroreport* 11, 1519–1521. doi: 10.1097/00001756-200005150-00030

Findlay, J. M., and Gilchrist, I. D. (2003). "Visual selection, covert attention and eye movements," in *Active Vision: The Psychology of Looking and Seeing Chapter 3*, (New York, NY: Oxford University Press), 35–54.

Giraudet, L., Berenger, M., Imbert, J.-P., Tremblay, S., and Causse, M. (2014). "Inattentional deafness in simulated air traffic control tasks: a behavioral and P300 analysis," in *AHFE 2014, 5th International Conference on Applied Human Factors and Ergonomics* (Kraków, Poland).

Giraudet, L., Imbert, J.-P., Bérenger, M., Tremblay, S., and Causse, M. (2015a). The neuroergonomic evaluation of human machine interface design in air traffic control using behavioral and EEG/ERP measures. *Behav. Brain Res.* 294, 246–253. doi: 10.1016/j.bbr.2015.07.041

Giraudet, L., St-Louis, M.-E., Scannella, S., and Causse, M. (2015b). P300 event-related potential as an indicator of inattentional deafness? *PLoS One* 10:e0118556. doi: 10.1371/journal.pone.0118556

Goldberg, J. H., and Kotval, X. P. (1999). Computer interface evaluation using eye movements: methods and constructs. *Int. J. Ind. Ergon.* 24, 631–645. doi: 10.1016/s0169-8141(98)00068-7

Harris, D. (2011). *Human Performance on the Flight Deck.* Farnham: Ashgate Publishing, Ltd.

Hodgetts, H. M., Tremblay, S., Vallières, B. R., and Vachon, F. (2015). Decision support and vulnerability to interruption in a dynamic multitasking environment *Int. J. Hum. Comput. Stud.* 79, 106–117. doi: 10.1016/j.ijhcs.2015.01.009

Hughes, R. W., Hurlstone, M. J., Marsh, J. E., Vachon, F., and Jones, D. M. (2013). Cognitive control of auditory distraction: impact of task difficulty, foreknowledge and working memory capacity supports duplex-mechanism account. *J. Exp. Psychol. Hum. Percept. Perform.* 39, 539–553. doi: 10.1037/a0029064

Imbert, J.-P., Hodgetts, H. M., Parise, R., Vachon, F., Dehais, F., and Tremblay, S. (2014a). Attentional costs and failures in air traffic control notifications. *Ergonomics* 57, 1817–1832. doi: 10.1080/00140139.2014.952680

Imbert, J.-P., Hodgetts, H. M., Parise, R., Vachon, F., and Tremblay, S. (2014b). "The LABY microworld a platform for research, training and system engineering," in *Proceedings of the Human Factors and Ergonomics Society Annual Meeting* (Chicago), 27–31.

Jacob, R., and Karn, K. S. (2003). "Eye tracking in human-computer interaction and usability research: ready to deliver the promises," in *The Mind's Eye: Cognitive and Applied Aspects of Eye Movement Research*, eds J. Hyona, R. Radach and H. Deubel (Oxford), 573–605.

Jolicoeur, P. (1999). Restricted attentional capacity between sensory modalities. *Psychon. Bull. Rev.* 6, 87–92. doi: 10.3758/bf03210813

Kahneman, D., and Beatty, J. (1966). Pupil diameter and load on memory. *Science* 154, 1583–1585. doi: 10.1126/science.154.3756.1583

Keitel, C., Maess, B., Schröger, E., and Müller, M. M. (2013). Early visual and auditory processing rely on modality-specific attentional resources. *Neuroimage* 70, 240–249. doi: 10.1016/j.neuroimage.2012.12.046

Kim, S.-Y., Kim, M.-S., and Chun, M. M. (2005). Concurrent working memory load can reduce distraction. *Proc. Natl. Acad. Sci. U S A* 102, 16524–16529. doi: 10.1073/pnas.0505454102

Kopardekar, P., and Magyarits, S. (2003). *Measurement and Prediction of Dynamic Density.* 5th Edn. Budapest, Hungary: Eurocontrol/FAA ATM R and D Seminar.

Koreimann, S., Gula, B., and Vitouch, O. (2009). Inattentional deafness under dynamic musical conditions. *Psychol. Res.* 78, 304–312. doi: 10.1007/s00426-014-0552-x

Koreimann, S., Gula, B., and Vitouch, O. (2014). Inattentional deafness in music. *Psychol. Res.* 78, 304–312. doi: 10.1007/s00426-014-0552-x

Laudeman, I. V., Shelden, S., Branstrom, R., and Brasil, C. L. (1998). Dynamic Density: An Air Traffic Management Metric. *Technical Report NASA/TM-1998-112226. Moffett Field, CA: National Aeronautics and Space Administration, Ames Research Center.*

Lavie, N. (2005). Distracted and confused? selective attention under load. *Trends Cogn. Sci.* 9, 75–82. doi: 10.1016/j.tics.2004.12.004

Lavie, N., Hirst, A., de Fockert, J. W., and Viding, E. (2004). Load theory of selective attention and cognitive control. *J. Exp. Psychol. Gen.* 133, 339–354. doi: 10.1037/0096-3445.133.3.339

Loft, S., Sanderson, P., Neal, A., and Mooij, M. (2007). Modeling and predicting mental workload in en route air traffic control: critical review and broader implications. *Hum. Factors* 49, 376–399. doi: 10.1518/001872007x197017

Macdonald, J. S., and Lavie, N. (2011). Visual perceptual load induces inattentional deafness. *Atten. Percept. Psychophys.* 73, 1780–1789. doi: 10.3758/s13414-011-0144-4

Manning, C. A., Mills, S. H., Fox, C., Pfleider, E., and Mogilka, H. J. (2001). *Investigating the Validity of Performance and Objective Workload Evaluation Research (POWER).* (Report No. DOT/FAA/AM-01/10). Washington, DC: FAA Office of Aerospace Medicine.

Manning, C., Mills, S., Fox, C., Pfleiderer, E., and Mogilka, H. (2002). The relationship between air traffic control communication events and measures of controller taskload and workload. *Air Traffic Control Qual.* 10, 69–83.

Martens, S., Kandula, M., and Duncan, J. (2010). Restricted attentional capacity within but not between sensory modalities: an individual differences approach. *PLoS One* 5:e15280. doi: 10.1371/journal.pone.0015280

Molloy, K., Griffiths, T. D., Chait, M., and Lavie, N. (2015). Inattentional deafness: visual load leads to time-specific suppression of auditory evoked responses. *J. Neurosci.* 35, 16046–16054. doi: 10.1523/JNEUROSCI.2931-15.2015

Palinko, O., Kun, A. L., Shyrokov, A., and Heeman, P. (2010). "Estimating cognitive load using remote eye tracking in a driving simulator," in *Proceedings of the 2010 symposium on eye-tracking research and applications* (Austin).

Peavler, W. S. (1974). Pupil size, information overload, and performance differences. *Psychophysiology* 11, 559–566. doi: 10.1111/j.1469-8986.1974.tb01114.x

Peysakhovich, V., Causse, M., Scannella, S., and Dehais, F. (2015). Frequency analysis of a task-evoked pupillary response: luminance-independent measure of mental effort. *Int. J. Psychophysiol.* 97, 30–37. doi: 10.1016/j.ijpsycho.2015.04.019

Raveh, D., and Lavie, N. (2015). Load-induced inattentional deafness. *Atten. Percept. Psychophys.* 77, 483–492. doi: 10.3758/s13414-014-0776-2

Régis, N., Dehais, F., Rachelson, E., Thooris, C., Pizziol, S., Causse, M., et al. (2014). Formal detection of attentional tunneling in human operator-automation interactions. *IEEE Trans. Hum. Mach. Syst.* 44, 326–336. doi: 10.1109/thms.2014.2307258

Rossi, A. F., Pessoa, L., Desimone, R., and Ungerleider, L. G. (2009). The prefrontal cortex and the executive control of attention. *Exp. Brain Res.* 192, 489–497. doi: 10.1007/s00221-008-1642-z

Sörqvist, P., Stenfelt, S., and Rönnberg, J. (2012). Working memory capacity and visual-verbal cognitive load modulate auditory-sensory gating in the brainstem: toward a unified view of attention. *J. Cogn. Neurosci.* 24, 2147–2154. doi: 10.1162/jocn_a_00275

Spence, C., and Read, L. (2003). Speech shadowing while driving on the difficulty of splitting attention between eye and ear. *Psychol. Sci.* 14, 251–256. doi: 10.1111/1467-9280.02439

Stanislaw, H., and Todorov, N. (1999). Calculation of signal detection theory measures. *Behav. Res. Methods Instrum. Comput.* 31, 137–149. doi: 10.3758/bf03207704

Talsma, D., Doty, T. J., Strowd, R., and Woldorff, M. G. (2006). Attentional capacity for processing concurrent stimuli is larger across sensory modalities than within a modality. *Psychophysiology* 43, 541–549. doi: 10.1111/j.1469-8986.2006.00452.x

Talsma, D., and Kok, A. (2001). Nonspatial intermodal selective attention is mediated by sensory brain areas: evidence from event-related potentials. *Psychophysiology* 38, 736–751. doi: 10.1111/1469-8986.3850736

Tombu, M. N., Asplund, C. L., Dux, P. E., Godwin, D., Martin, J. W., and Marois, R. (2011). A unified attentional bottleneck in the human brain. *Proc. Natl. Acad. Sci. U S A* 108, 13426–13431. doi: 10.1073/pnas.1103583108

Unsworth, N., and Robison, M. K. (2016). Pupillary correlates of lapses of sustained attention. *Cogn. Affect. Behav. Neurosci.* doi: 10.3758/s13415-016-0417-4 [Epub ahead of print].

Vachon, F., and Tremblay, S. (2008). Modality-specific and amodal sources of interference in the attentional blink. *Percept. Psychophys.* 70, 1000–1015. doi: 10.3758/pp.70.6.1000

Vitevitch, M. S. (2003). Change deafness: the inability to detect changes between two voices. *J. Exp. Psychol. Hum. Percept. Perform.* 29, 333–342. doi: 10.1037/0096-1523.29.2.333

Vosskühler, A., Nordmeier, V., Kuchinke, L., and Jacobs, A. M. (2008). OGAMA (Open Gaze and Mouse Analyzer): open-source software designed to analyze eye and mouse movements in slideshow study designs. *Behav. Res. Methods* 40, 1150–1162. doi: 10.3758/BRM.40.4.1150

Wahn, B., and König, P. (2015). Audition and vision share spatial attentional resources, yet attentional load does not disrupt audiovisual integration. *Front. Psychol.* 6:1084. doi: 10.3389/fpsyg.2015.01084

Wickens, C. D. (1980). "The structure of attentional resources," in *Attention and Performance VIII* (Vol. 8), ed. R. Nickerson (Hillsdale, NJ: Erlbaum), 239–257.

Wickens, C. D., and Alexander, A. L. (2009). Attentional tunneling and task management in synthetic vision displays. *Int. J. Aviat. Psychol.* 19, 182–199. doi: 10.1080/10508410902766549

Wilming, N., Harst, S., Schmidt, N., and König, P. (2013). Saccadic momentum and facilitation of return saccades contribute to an optimal foraging strategy. *PLoS Comput. Biol.* 9:e1002871. doi: 10.1371/journal.pcbi.1002871

Wood, N. L., and Cowan, N. (1995). The cocktail party phenomenon revisited: attention and memory in the classic selective listening procedure of Cherry (1953). *J. Exp. Psychol. Gen.* 124, 243–262. doi: 10.1037/0096-3445.124.3.243

10

Perception and Cognition of Cues Used in Synchronous Brain–Computer Interfaces Modify Electroencephalographic Patterns of Control Tasks

Luz María Alonso-Valerdi[1,2], Francisco Sepulveda[1] and Ricardo A. Ramírez-Mendoza[2]*

[1] Brain-Computer Interfaces (BCI) Group, School of Computing Science and Electronic Engineering, University of Essex, Colchester, UK, [2] Escuela de Ingeniería y Ciencias, Tecnológico de Monterrey – Campus Ciudad de México, Mexico City, Mexico

***Correspondence:**
Luz María Alonso-Valerdi
luzalonsoval@gmail.com

A motor imagery (MI)-based brain–computer interface (BCI) is a system that enables humans to interact with their environment by translating their brain signals into control commands for a target device. In particular, synchronous BCI systems make use of cues to trigger the motor activity of interest. So far, it has been shown that electroencephalographic (EEG) patterns before and after cue onset can reveal the user cognitive state and enhance the discrimination of MI-related control tasks. However, there has been no detailed investigation of the nature of those EEG patterns. We, therefore, propose to study the cue effects on MI-related control tasks by selecting EEG patterns that best discriminate such control tasks, and analyzing where those patterns are coming from. The study was carried out using two methods: standard and all-embracing. The standard method was based on sources (recording sites, frequency bands, and time windows), where the modulation of EEG signals due to motor activity is typically detected. The all-embracing method included a wider variety of sources, where not only motor activity is reflected. The findings of this study showed that the classification accuracy (CA) of MI-related control tasks did not depend on the type of cue in use. However, EEG patterns that best differentiated those control tasks emerged from sources well defined by the perception and cognition of the cue in use. An implication of this study is the possibility of obtaining different control commands that could be detected with the same accuracy. Since different cues trigger control tasks that yield similar CAs, and those control tasks produce EEG patterns differentiated by the cue nature, this leads to accelerate the brain–computer communication by having a wider variety of detectable control commands. This is an important issue for Neuroergonomics research because neural activity could not only be used to monitor the human mental state as is typically done, but this activity might be also employed to control the system of interest.

Keywords: brain–computer interface, motor imagery, classification accuracy, electroencephalographic patterns, human factors

INTRODUCTION

A brain–computer interface (BCI) is a system that enables humans to interact with their environment by translating their brain signals into control commands for a device of interest (Graimann et al., 2010). The mechanism of a BCI system fundamentally consists of two steps: (1) detecting and decoding the user intentions for controlling the system and (2) maintaining a continuous user-system communication. The *user intentions* of controlling a BCI system are changes in the user brain signals that are regulated through control tasks. A control task can be based on exogenous or endogenous paradigms (Jackson and Mappus, 2010). Particularly, the endogenous paradigm is based on the quantification of brain oscillations that are modulated via cognitive tasks such as motor imagery (MI). The *user-system communication* is established by a control interface. A control interface can be synchronous or asynchronous (Hassanien and Azar, 2015). In a synchronous interface, the user-system communication is allowed only in fixed time windows; whereas in an asynchronous interface, the user initiates the communication with the system at will. Both synchronous (Obermaier et al., 2003; Leeb et al., 2006; Maeder et al., 2012; Bamdadian et al., 2014) and asynchronous (Scherer et al., 2007; Galán et al., 2008; Lotte et al., 2008; Tseng et al., 2015) systems have been developed over the past few years. For real-world applications, the prototyping of asynchronous systems is preferred because these allow users to interact naturally with their environment. The relevance of synchronous systems cannot, however, be ignored, even in real applications. The cueing process facilitates the early and accurate detection of the user control tasks, despite the user ability for modulating his/her brain signals. This, in turn, raises confidence, persistency, and autonomy in the users toward the mastery of BCI skills. Furthermore, the identification of MI onset allows to analyze prior and post periods, which have been associated with the improvement of BCI performance and the recognition of the user cognitive state (Maeder et al., 2012; Bamdadian et al., 2014; Gutierrez et al., 2015).

As brain signals are modulated by neural networks that modify their degree of synchronization according to the sensory–cognitive input, it is not surprising that control tasks (particularly those based on MI) contain much more information than only that related to the user intention of controlling the system (Kropotov, 2010). MI-related control tasks are a source of information that has been exploited not only to generate control commands for a target device, but also to enhance BCI performance, to predict classification accuracy (CA), or to determine the user mental state. For example, Pfurtscheller and Neuper (2001), and then Obermaier et al. (2003), reported that left- and right-hand MIs were correctly discriminated as early as 250 ms after the onset of a specific visual cue. They attributed the early discrimination to the cue properties, concluding that the control tasks were the result of conscious (MI) and unconscious (visual stimulation) processes over the sensory–motor area of the brain. Furthermore, in a later and more detailed study, Pfurtscheller et al. (2008) found that distinct short-lasting brain patterns appeared within a time window of about 500–750 ms after cue onset. Those brain patterns produced different features for different imaginary movements (hands and feet), facilitating and accelerating the discrimination of MI-related control tasks in naïve subjects. Another example is the study carried out by Grosse-Wentrup and Scholkopf (2012) in which high gamma range (55–85 Hz) between two fronto-parietal networks were used to predict BCI performance on a trial-to-trial basis. Additional and important examples are two studies, respectively, undertaken by Maeder et al. (2012) and Bamdadian et al. (2014). Those researchers demonstrated that the user performance in classical synchronous BCIs can be predicted by quantifying the modulation of the brain signals on pre-cue stages because they reflected somehow the user cognitive state. Finally, and more recently, Scheel et al. (2015) found that visual and auditory cues provoked significant differences of the peak amplitude of movement-related cortical potentials in synchronous BCIs. They also found that potentials from the auditory-cue paradigm had a wider spatial distribution than those from the visual cue.

Overall, all aforementioned studies support the view that brain patterns extracted from MI-related control tasks can provide much more information than that used to control a target device. In particular, the cue effects on MI-related control tasks have been studied. Researchers in the field have shown that both perception (e.g., sensory–cognitive processing of the cue) and cognition (e.g., imaginary motor activity) are reflected on the brain signals wherefrom BCI control tasks are extracted. Studying the influence of human factors on BCI control tasks may help to design a more versatile human–machine interaction for this type of systems because of the active (e.g., extraction of control commands for manipulating a target device) and passive (e.g., monitoring of the level of attention of an individual) use of the brain signals. This work could have further applications in Neuroergonomics, where neural activity is registered in order to monitor human mental state. Making use of neural activity in an active and passive way may be much more fruitful.

So far, it has been shown that brain patterns before and after cue onset can reveal the user cognitive state and enhance the discrimination of MI-related control tasks. However, there has been no detailed investigation of the nature of those brain patterns. We, therefore, propose to study the cue effects on MI-related control tasks by selecting the brain patterns that best discriminate such control tasks, and analyzing where those patterns are coming from in order to answer two questions:

(1) If different cues provoke significant changes on MI-related control tasks, can different cues improve BCI performance as Scheel et al. (2015) suggested in their research? and
(2) If MI-related control tasks are defined by motor activity *per se* and the cue in use, do brain patterns proceed from sources (recording sites, frequency bands, and time intervals) not only associated with motor activity, but also related to the sensory–cognitive processing of the cue?

The present study was conducted as follows. First, brain activity was registered by means of electroencephalography (EEG). Second, the frequently used stimulation modalities (SMs) for cueing in training sessions were applied. These were auditory (Nijboer et al., 2008) and visual (Boostani et al., 2007) stimuli.

In addition, a bimodal cue (combination of auditory and visual stimuli) was included in the study because previous investigations in sensory encoding (Basar et al., 1999; Isoğlu-Alkaç et al., 2007) have shown that simultaneous presentation of auditory, visual, and somatosensory stimuli significantly enhances sensory responses. Third, as preparation and imagination of movements evoke similar neural desynchronization events over the sensory–motor areas (Neuper et al., 2006) and both of them are widely used as control task, the two motor activities were included in the study. Finally, given that brain oscillations occur in a wide range of EEG recording sites, frequency bands, and time intervals (Kropotov, 2010); brain patterns were analyzed using two methods: standard and all-embracing. The standard method was restricted to the well-established motor activity sources (Pfurtscheller et al., 2007), while the all-embracing method involved all the available EEG information.

MATERIALS AND METHODS

Experimental Procedure

Participant Recruitment and General Instructions

Nine participants (four females and five males) took part in this study, which was previously authorized by the Ethics Committee of the University of Essex. All of them were aged between 28 and 41 years. None of them reported auditory impairments, seven of them had normal vision, and two of them had corrected-to-normal vision. Eight of the nine reported to be right-handed and only one was left-handed.

The participants were informed about the experimental procedure and signed a consent form. Only two of the nine had previously engaged in cognitive tasks related to imagination of movements. At the beginning of the experiment, every participant was carefully instructed as follows:

- Get ready to imagine the movement of the hand that indicates a track playing "left" or "right" (audio), an arrow pointing to left or right (visual), or both of them (bimodal).
- Imagine yourself opening and closing your formerly pointed hand as soon as you listen to an increasing tone, see a green bulb, or perceive both of them.
- Stop the MI process and relax as soon as you listen to a decreasing tone, see a red bulb, or perceive both of them.

Organization of the Experiment

In order to collect sufficient EEG data, the participants attended two sessions. The sessions lasted 48 min each and followed an identical procedure. Every session consisted of six runs and one run had 50 trials. One trial took from 8500 to 9500 ms (**Figure 1**), resulting in runs of ~8 min. Within each trial, there were three phases: MP (0–2500 ms), MI (2500–6000 ms), and relaxing (6000–8500 ± 1000 ms). In the latter phase, a random variation of 1000 ms was included to reduce expectation effects.

As there were three SMs (audio, visual, and bimodal) and both hands (left and right) were involved, there were six categories of trials: audio-left, audio-right, visual-left, visual-right, bimodal-left, and bimodal-right. Each of these categories was randomly presented 50 times and distributed over the six runs. We thereby obtained 12 conditions (six categories of trials × two control tasks) and one condition had 100 trials (2 sessions × 50 trials).

Timing Protocol

The duration of the cues was standardized to 500 ms in accordance with sensory recognition and reaction time studies (Teichner, 1954; Shelton and Kumar, 2010). The movement preparation (MP) was adjusted to 2000 ms, which is the necessary period to achieve readiness in the neural networks over the sensory–motor area (Jeannerod, 2006; Neuper et al., 2006). The MI was limited to 3000 ms, as is commonly done in synchronous BCIs. The relaxation span varied from 2000 to 3000 ms, guaranteeing a proper recovery of the longest desynchronization process, i.e., the alpha one (Pfurtscheller et al., 1996). See **Figure 1**.

EEG Data Collection

The EEG signals were recorded by means of Biosemi equipment (Amsterdam, The Netherlands), the integration of ActiveTwo system and ActiView software (Honsbeek et al., 1998). The ActiveTwo system was configured to acquire the signals within a bandwidth between DC and 400 Hz, and at a sampling frequency of 2048 Hz. The ActiView software was programed to decimate the signals at 512 Hz. Such configuration limited the effective digital bandwidth to 104 Hz by default.

The EEG signals were sensed via 61 active electrodes, plus driven-right-leg and common-mode-sense electrodes. The 61 active electrodes were mounted on a head-cap labeled as stated in the 10/10 system. The other two electrodes were only used for referencing electrically the ActiveTwo system, but they were not recorded. In addition, three external electrodes were included for recording the eye movements (EOG). Two of them (EOG_L and EOG_R) were placed 1 cm below and above the lateral canthus of the left and right eyes, respectively. The third one was placed on the right mastoid (M_R) for referencing EEG and EOG signals (**Figure 2**). At the end of the experiments, we gathered 18 datasets (9 participants × 2 sessions).

Data Analysis

The datasets of one participant were excluded from the study. Those showed electrode-pop artifacts over the occipital area of the scalp. There were then 16 datasets for the study purposes.

Processing of Continuous EEG Data

To attenuate the interference in the EEG channels, these were processed by using the open-access toolbox for electrophysiological signal processing, EEGLAB (Delorme and Makeig, 2004). First, every channel from each of the 16 datasets was processed as follows: (1) referencing against M_R, (2) high-pass filtering at 0.1 Hz using a Butterworth filter of order 4, (3) low-pass filtering at 41 Hz using a Butterworth filter of order 7, and (4) down-sampling from 512 to 256 Hz. Second, every dataset was scanned to eliminate discontinuities and detect high-impedance electrodes. Up to three electrodes under this condition were detected per dataset. Third, independent component analysis was applied to each dataset for rejecting artifacts such as EOG and electrocardiography. Only EEG channels without high-impedance difficulties were involved

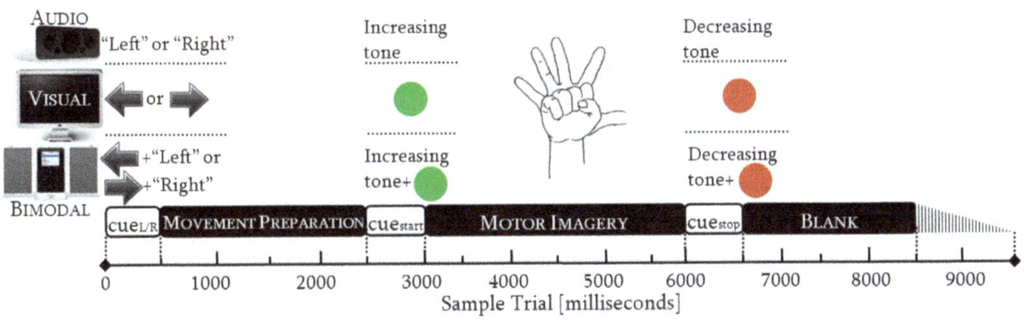

FIGURE 1 | Timing protocol: audio, visual, and bimodal stimuli for cueing MP and MI.

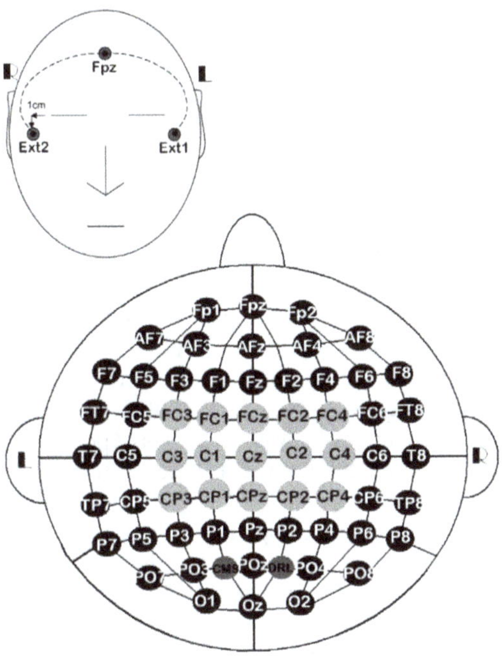

FIGURE 2 | 10/10 EEG layout of 61 channels, along with three external electrodes. All the EEG channels (■, ■) were used for the all-embracing method, 15 of them (■) were used for the standard method, EOG_L/EOG_R were used for recording eye movements, and M_R was used for referencing EEG and EOG signals.

in such analysis. EOG_L and EOG_R channels were used to identify all the independent components related to EOG activity. Finally, the EEG channels with high-impedance difficulties were replaced by interpolating their nearest neighboring channels as reported by Gargiulo et al. (2010). See **Figure 3**.

Processing of the Control Tasks (MP and MI)

The processing of the control tasks was carried out through the *miBCI* software[1], package published by Alonso-Valerdi and Sepulveda (2015). From every EEG channel of the 16 datasets, the control tasks were extracted in line with the cue onset (**Figure 1**). The MP and MI were thus 2500 and 3500 ms long, respectively. Having obtained the EEG signals of interest, they were spatially filtered via large Laplacian in order to obtain more localized electrical activity (Dornhege et al., 2007).

Feature Extraction

It is well-established that MP and MI provoke neural desynchronization with peak power around 10 and 20 Hz (Neuper et al., 2009). As band power (BP) estimation has been validated as a stable and consistent method for quantifying EEG power changes due to motor activity (Neuper et al., 2005), this was selected as feature extractor. BP estimation was applied in line with the methods described below.

Standard Method

Previous investigations have empirically established the following criteria to effectively discriminate hand imaginary movements. First, 18 central recording sites have been validated as the maximum number of EEG channels for satisfactory classification (Ramoser et al., 2000). Second, narrow frequency bands around the maxima 10 and 20 Hz have been widely used in synchronous BCI systems (Pfurtscheller et al., 2007; Neuper et al., 2009). Third, it has become common practice to discard 1 s post-cue, wherein evoked potentials are typically detected (Boostani et al., 2007). With these criteria in mind, we laid down the *standard method*. This method was based on 15 central recording sites (**Figure 2**), four frequency bands, and EEG segments taking place 1 s post-cue. The frequency bands were established as follows: lower alpha (α_L) from 8 to 10 Hz, upper alpha (α_U) from 10 to 12 Hz, lower beta (β_L) from 16 to 20 Hz, and upper beta (β_U) from 20 to 24 Hz.

All-Embracing Method

EEG signals are regulated by brain oscillators that adjust their state of synchrony according to sensory (e.g., cue decoding) and cognitive (e.g., MP and MI) events. These oscillators are neural networks that enter into synchrony in a wide range of resonant frequencies (from 0 up to about 80 Hz) and over specific periods of time (Krause, 2003). In view of this fact, we extended the scope of the standard method by establishing the

[1] Available at https://github.com/LuzAlondra/BrainComputerInterfaces/tree/master/MI-based_BCIsystem

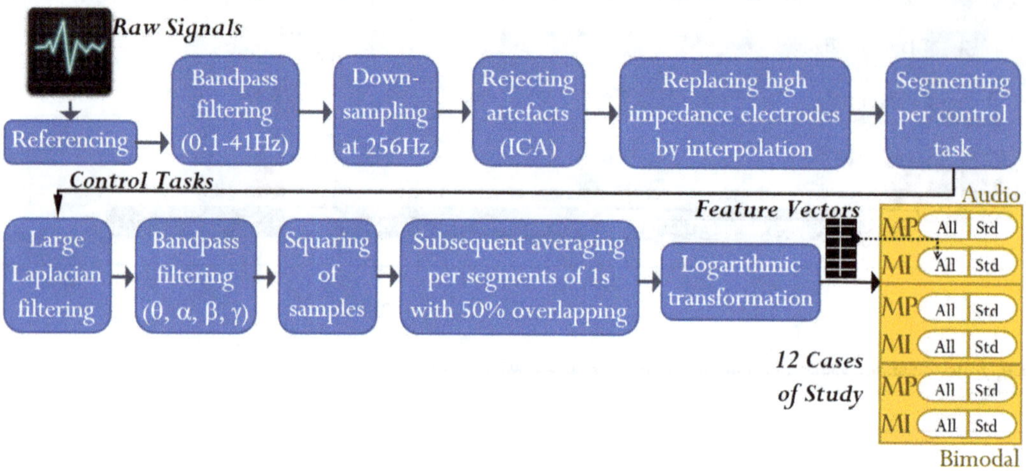

FIGURE 3 | EEG signal analysis: from raw signals to feature extraction. At the end of the analysis, feature vectors for 12 cases of study resulted. Note that the term "All" refers to all-embracing method, and the term "Std" refers to standard method.

all-embracing method. This method was based on 61 recording sites (**Figure 2**), seven frequency bands, and whole trace of MP and MI. In addition to the previously mentioned bands, the following ones were also considered: lower theta (θ_L) from 4 to 6 Hz, upper theta (θ_U) from 6 to 8 Hz, and gamma (γ) from 39 to 41 Hz. These bands were included in the analysis on the basis of the following evidence. Theta band rhythms resonate at the frequency band 4–8 Hz and emanate from the frontal midline due to audio–visual information encoding, attention demands, memory retrieval, and cognitive load. Moreover, these rhythms enhance after practice on the cognitive tasks at hand. They are more prevalent when the subject is focused and relaxed, and prolonged activity is related to selective attention (Basar et al., 1999; Krause, 2003; Kropotov, 2010). The upper theta band (6–8 Hz) generally reflects levels of alertness (Pineda, 2005). On the other side, gamma band rhythms oscillate near 40 Hz during sensory encoding, perceptual–cognitive functions, and motor behaviors. These rhythms are phase-locked to the stimulus and short-lasting, and appear 100 ms post-stimulus in sensory–motor tasks (Pfurtscheller and Lopes da Silva, 1999; Ward, 2003; Altermaller et al., 2005).

Bearing in mind the criteria of standard and all-embracing methods, we can now briefly describe the feature extraction based on BP. The MP/MI signals were first filtered through Butterworth band-pass filters of order 7, with cut-off frequencies defined by the afore-stated bands. Afterwards, the signals were squared per sample and segmented by using time windows of 500 ms length with 50% overlapping rate. Finally, the resulting time segments (herein denoted by δ_n) were averaged and logarithmically transformed (refer to **Figure 3**), obtaining nine features per MP signal and 13 features per MI signal.

By the standard method, there were 15 channels and 4 frequency bands under consideration. In addition, three time segments [δ_1 (0–500 ms), δ_2 (250–750 ms), and δ_3 (500–1000 ms)] were discarded. Hence, vectors of 300 features for MP and vectors of 540 features for MI were obtained. By the all-embracing method, vectors of 3843 features for MP and vectors of 5551 features for MI were similarly obtained.

Feature Selection and Classification

After the feature extraction, there were 24 types of feature vectors that proceeded from three SMs, two control tasks, two hands, and two methods. These feature vectors were grouped by merging left and right MIs. Having obtained 12 different cases of study (**Figure 3**), Davies–Bouldin indexes (DBIs) were determined in each case to increasingly sort the corresponding features (Sepulveda et al., 2004; Kovács et al., 2005). DBI is a method for measuring the linear separability among m classes (Equation 1). This metric is based on comparing the similarity (R) among classes. Such similarity is determined by the class dispersion (s) and the distance (d) between centroids (Eq. 2). The class dispersion is the average distance between every element (τ) in the class and the centroid of the class (v). See Eq. 3. Thereby, the features within each vector were ranked from the most to the least suitable feature in terms of linear separability between two classes: left and right (Kovács et al., 2005). Note that smaller DBIs correspond to major linear separability.

$$\mathrm{DBI} = \frac{1}{m}\sum_{i=1}^{m} R_i \tag{1}$$

where $R_i = \max\limits_{\substack{j=1,\ldots,m \\ i\neq j}} (R_{ij})$ and $i = 1,\ldots,m$

$$R_{ij} = \frac{s_i + s_j}{d_{ij}} = \frac{s_i + s_j}{d(v_i, v_j)} \tag{2}$$

$$s_i = \frac{1}{T_i}\sum d(\tau, v_i) \tag{3}$$

where T_i is the number of features in class i.

After ranking the features, a classification process took place in order to select the appropriate number of features that best

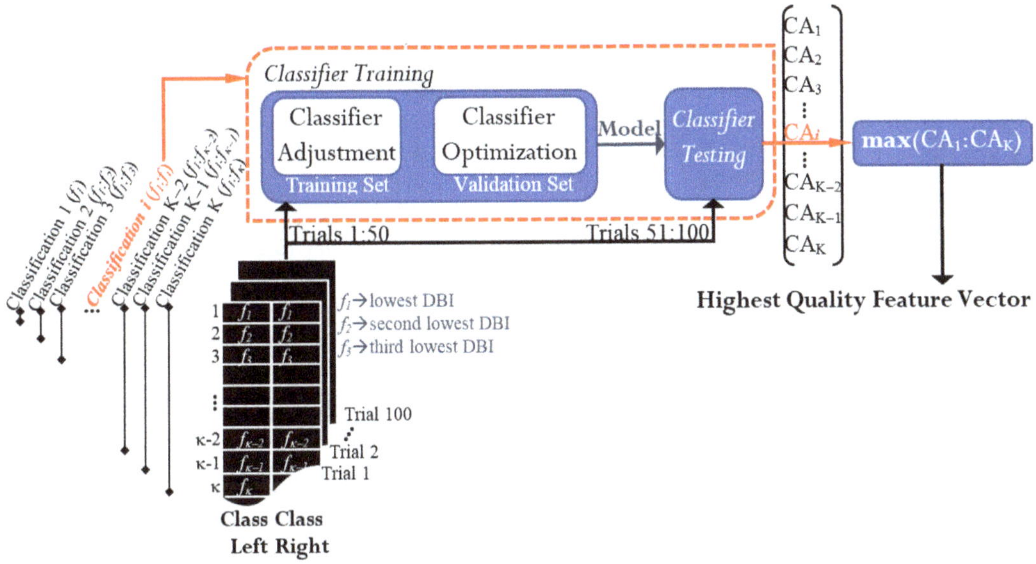

FIGURE 4 | Feature selection and classification: obtaining the highest quality feature vectors (HQFVs). For each case of study, a HQFV was obtained. A HQFV was the feature vector that reached the maximum CA and wherein each feature (*f*) was ranked according to DBI.

discriminated between left and right. If there were two classes and κ denoted the total number of features in each vector, K classifications were run for each case of study (**Figure 4**). From the K resulting CAs, the feature vector yielding the maximum performance was selected from each case of study. Thereby, we obtained 12 feature vectors for every participant. They were called the highest quality feature vectors (HQFVs). Note that the term "maximum performance" refers to 1.5 times the inter-quartile range plus the upper quartile of the general distribution of all the CAs obtained at the end of the process. As a result, any peak value that was beyond the 99% of the distribution was discarded.

Every classification process[2] was based on Fisher discriminant analysis (FDA) and consisted of two phases: training and testing. The 100 available trials per cluster were distributed half and half; that is, 50 trials (session 1) for training and 50 trials (session 2) for testing. The classifier was trained via 10-fold cross validation. That is, 50 training trials were split into a training set and a validation set. Through the validation set, the model was optimized by adjusting the regularization term that generally avoids overfitting problems due to the large number of features in use (Bishop, 2006). Once the classifier had been trained, this was tested by the rest of the trials and the percentage of the total number of correct predictions was estimated. The resulting CA in the testing phase was the parameter for acquiring the HQFVs. See **Figure 4**.

[2]Before undertaking the classification process, note that the features were normalized using normalization and standardization methods developed by *mlpy* (high-performance Python package for predictive modelling avaliable at http://mlpy.sourceforge.net/) developers, to avoid BP estimates in greater numeric ranges dominate those in smaller numeric ranges.

In this study, all statistical analyses were performed using the non-parametric method Kruskal–Wallis one-way ANOVA, and significance levels were set at 5%.

Statistical Evaluation of the HQFVs

The features of the HQFVs proceeded from specific recording sites (e.g., C3, Cz, or C4), frequency bands (e.g., α_L, α_U, β_L, or β_U) and time windows (δ_n). The origin of a feature in any of these three domains (location, frequency, and time) was referred as to *feature source*. On this basis, the HQFVs were statistically evaluated in accordance with those three domains and under two parameters: index of dispersion (ID) and *mode*.

The ID was calculated by using Eq. 4 and was an approach to quantify how spread a HQFV was over the feature sources in each domain. In Eq. 4, k is the number of feature sources in the domain of interest, f_i is the number of occurrences of each feature source, and N is the total number of features in the HQFV under analysis (Norman and Streiner, 2008). Note that ID is 0 when all the features fall into one feature source. By contrast, it is 1 when the features are equally divided among the k feature sources.

$$\mathrm{ID} = \frac{k\left(N^2 - \sum f_i^2\right)}{N^2\left(k-1\right)} \tag{4}$$

The *mode* was the central tendency of a HQFV, i.e., the most frequently occurring feature source in the domain at hand. Having gathered the *modes* of all the HQFVs, these were graphically represented via a 2D-histogram (*modal* distribution) for each domain. In every 2D-histogram, the number of occurrences of each *mode* (f_{mode}) was normalized by diving f_{mode} by N.

RESULTS

Classification Accuracy of the HQFVs

The CAs reached by the HQFVs are arranged in **Figure 5**. This figure indicates that there is no significant difference of CAs among SMs ($p = 0.935$). The figure also indicates that there is a significant increase of CAs ($p = 1.11 \times 10^{-16}$) between standard and all-embracing methods for both control tasks (MP and MI) and the three SMs (audio, visual, and bimodal). Finally, the figure shows that CAs ($p = 0.707$) between MP and MI are comparable for the three SMs and the two methods in use.

Index of Dispersion of the HQFVs in Location, Frequency, and Time

The IDs of the HQFVs, which were obtained from the standard method, are presented in **Figures 6A–C**. In location and time, the HQFVs are generally spread over all the feature sources showing IDs above 0.52 and 0.7, respectively. By contrast, IDs range between 0 and 1 in frequency. The IDs of the HQFVs, which resulted from the all-embracing method, are provided in **Figures 6D–F**. These IDs are above 0.85, 0.5, and 0.87 in location, frequency, and time, respectively. The statistical comparison of the IDs between both methods in location, frequency, and time resulted in the following *p*-values: 1.461×10^{-9}, 0.049, and 4.767×10^{-7}. Note that all the remarks mentioned in this section apply to MP and MI.

Modal Distribution of the HQFVs in Location, Frequency, and Time

Standard Method

Figure 7 presents the *modal* distribution of the HQFVs over the following feature sources: (a) 15 recording sites, (b) 4 frequency bands, and (c) 5/9 time windows for MP/MI. With regard to the location domain, **Figure 7A** shows that *modes* from audio cues mainly tend toward FC3 and C3, while those from visual cues mostly tend to FC2, FC4 (only applicable for MI), and C4. *Modes* from bimodal cues are essentially distributed among FC3, C3, FC4, and C4. In all the cases, MI displays greater tendencies than MP.

We can see from **Figure 7B** that the overriding band for the three SMs is α_U. In this case, the highest and the lowest tendencies are reached by *modes* from visual and bimodal cues, respectively. The MI control task shows a second dominant band. Such dominant band for *modes* from audio and visual cues is β_L, while that for *modes* from bimodal cues is β_U. The MP control task only shows a second dominant band for *modes* from bimodal cues, which is β_L. As in the location domain, MI reveals stronger tendencies in comparison with MP.

Lastly, **Figure 7C** provides the *modal* distribution in time. Keeping in mind that MP only involved five time windows (from δ_5 to δ_9), we can see that *modes* from the three SMs are evenly distributed along most of them. Although MI involved the nine time windows, the *modes* from the three SMs are mostly distributed across δ_5 and δ_9 as well. In both cases, the major *modal* tendencies for audio, visual, and bimodal cues are, respectively, the following: δ_7/δ_8 (1500–2000 ms), $\delta_6/\delta_8/\delta_9$ (1250–2500 ms), and δ_5/δ_9 (1000–1500 ms and 2000–2500 ms). There is additionally a relevant *modal* distribution over δ_{13} for the three SMs in MI, regardless of the decreasing trend of the foregoing time windows.

All-Embracing Method

Figure 8 provides the *modal* distribution of the HQFVs over the following feature sources: (a) 61 recording sites, (b) 7 frequency bands, and (c) 9/13 time windows for MP/MI. With respect to the location domain, **Figure 8A** indicates that *modes* from the three SMs are distributed over about 40% of the feature sources in both control tasks. Specifically, *modes* from audio cues are distributed among 24 of the 61 recording sites. From those, 62% are on central areas, 25% are on parieto-occipital areas, and 13% are on frontal areas. *Modes* from visual cues are also distributed among 24 of the 61 recording sites. However, those are differently spread. Over

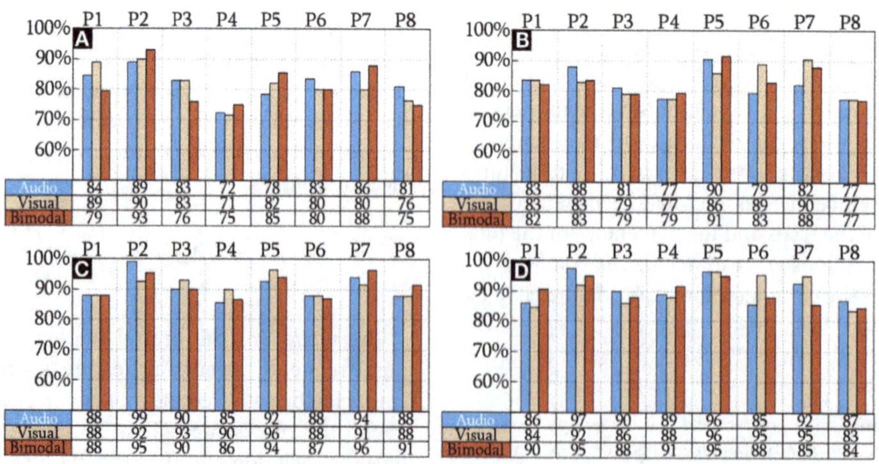

FIGURE 5 | CA of the HQFVs. MP and MI analyzed using the standard method are illustrated in **(A,B)**, respectively. MP and MI analyzed using the standard method are shown in **(C,D)**, respectively.

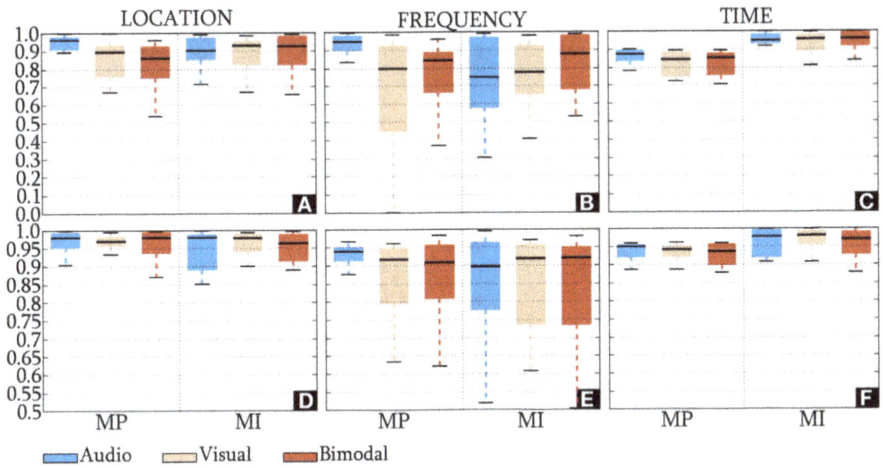

FIGURE 6 | IDs of the HQFVs. For the standard method, the indexes of the HQFVs over feature sources in location, frequency, and time are depicted in **(A–C)**, respectively. For the all-embracing method, the indexes of the HQFVs over feature sources in location, frequency, and time are presented in **(D–F)**, respectively.

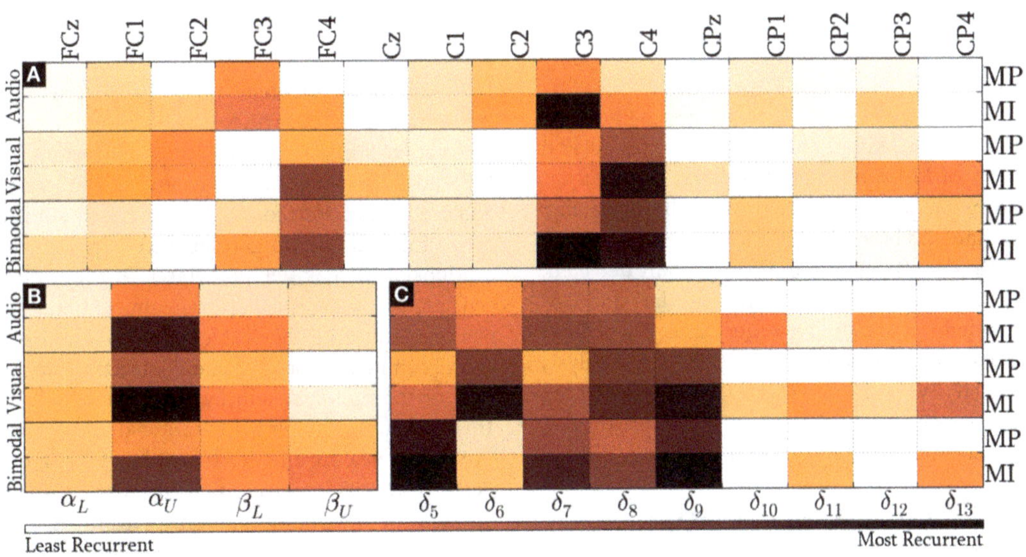

FIGURE 7 | *Modal* distribution of the HQFVs that resulted from the standard method. The *modal* distribution is illustrated in three domains: **(A)** 15 recoding sites, **(B)** 4 frequency bands, and **(C)** 5/9 time windows for MP/MI.

half of them are distributed between frontal and parieto-occipital areas (33% and 21%, respectively), while less than half of them are related to central areas (46%). *Modes* from bimodal cues are distributed among 27 of the 61 recording sites. From those, 56% are on central areas, 37% are on parieto-occipital areas, and 7% are on frontal areas.

Figure 8B illustrates the prevalence of α_U band in the *modes* from the three SMs in both MP and MI. The figure also reveals the secondary but not insignificant role of β_L band. The *modal* distribution between θ_L and α_L bands is moderate for the three SMs, whereas that between θ_U and β_U bands is negligible for the three SMs. Furthermore, the *modal* distribution over γ band is considerable for bimodal cues. In all these cases, MI shows much higher tendencies than MP.

Last but not least, **Figure 8C** depicts the *modal* distribution in time, considering that MP only involved 9 of the 13 time windows. It can be seen from this figure that the *modes* from audio cues are spread across δ_1 and δ_9 (0–2500 ms), while those from visual and bimodal cues are spread across δ_1 and δ_7 (0–2000 ms). Particularly for MI control tasks, the *modes* from audio, visual, and bimodal cues strongly tend toward δ_3 (500–1000 ms), δ_4 (750–1250 ms), and δ_2/δ_3 (250–1000 ms), respectively. In addition, there is an unexpected *modal* tendency to δ_{13} for the three SMs in MI.

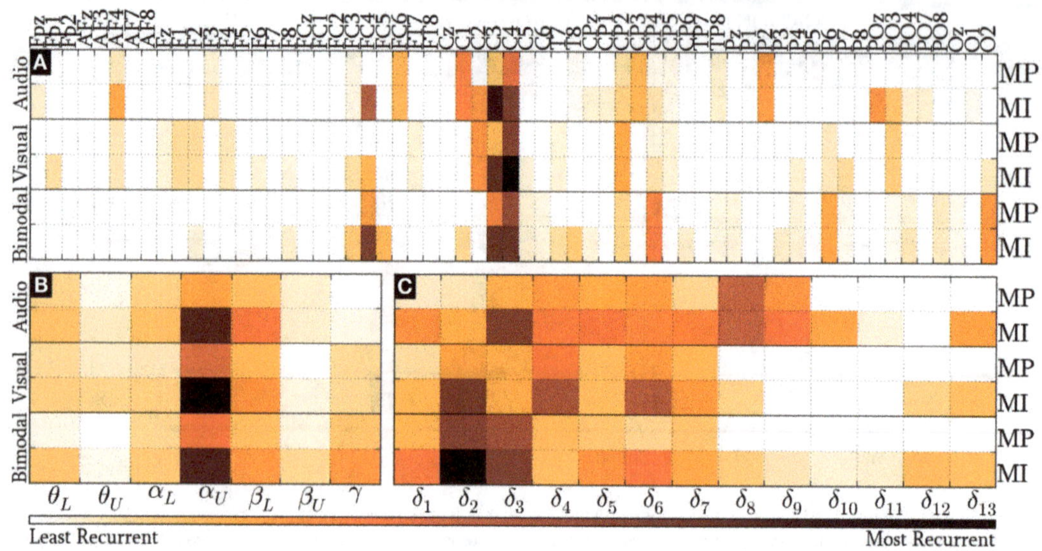

FIGURE 8 | *Modal* distribution of the HQFVs that resulted from the all-embracing method. The *modal* distribution is illustrated in three domains: **(A)** 61 recording sites, **(B)** 7 frequency bands, and **(C)** 9/13 time windows for MP/MI.

DISCUSSION

This paper set out with the aim of analyzing the cue effects on the discriminability of MP and MI control tasks. The analysis was carried out using two methods: standard and all-embracing. The standard method was based on feature sources, where the modulation of brain signals due to MP/MI is typically detected. For the all-embracing method, the scope of the standard method was extended by including a wider variety of feature sources, where not only motor activity is reflected. The analysis was limited to the HQFVs, i.e., the feature vectors that yielded the highest CAs during a DBI-FDA process. The following is a discussion of the most relevant results of the analysis.

Classification Accuracy of the HQFVs

On the question of improving CA by using different cues, we found that there was no significant difference in the discrimination of MI-related control tasks triggered by three SMs: audio, visual, and bimodal. However, there was a significant increase in the CA of control tasks analyzed under the all-embracing method over those analyzed using the standard method. These findings demonstrated that an unbiased approach in location, frequency, and time leads to a better performance, but different cues do not make a difference. Although Scheel et al. (2015) suggested that different stimuli might improve the CA of the control tasks at hand, this study has been unable to demonstrate that. Nevertheless, it is a fact that more distinguishable EEG patterns are extracted from no MI-related sources. Possibly, other type of stimuli could improve the differentiation of MI-related control tasks. In accordance with the findings of Pfurtscheller and Neuper (2001) and Obermaier et al. (2003), control tasks are result of conscious and unconscious processes. As different stimuli may evoke different unconscious processes, more differentiable EEG patterns could be found. However, this needs further investigation.

Another important result was the analogous performances of MP and MI for the three SMs and the two methods. It is well established that both control tasks generate similar event-related oscillations, but the "no-go" signal accompanying MI is frequently overlooked (Krepki et al., 2007). An imaginary movement activates motor areas of the brain almost to the same extent as a real one, except for the visible contractions. This means that the neural commands for muscular contractions are blocked at some level of the motor system by an active inhibitory mechanism. This questions whether MI in motor-disabled people takes place like that in healthy ones, or it is rather a real movement process (Jeannerod, 2006). In addition, the use of MI as control task involves the development of an electromyographic detector so as to eliminate undesirable muscular activity un- or consciously triggered by healthy BCI users. Based on these two factors and given that both control tasks achieved analogous performances, MP may be a better option for BCI systems.

Index of Dispersion of the HQFVs in Location, Frequency, and Time

For both methods, the distribution of the HQFVs over the available feature sources was much more even in location and time than in frequency. This indicates that the most gainful features for discriminating between left and right MIs mainly proceeded from the entire set of recording sites and the total duration of the control task, but only from a specific frequency band (α_U). The finding is in agreement with that of other studies (Pfurtscheller and Neuper, 2001; Neuper et al., 2009) which showed that the correct discrimination between left and right started 250–500 ms after cue onset and where the most discriminating frequency band was the α_U. With reference to the location domain, although this finding differs from some published studies (Ramoser et al., 2000; Leeb et al., 2006), it is consistent with those of Meckes et al. (2004) and Sepulveda et al. (2004). They suggested giving attention to non-motor locations, even when the mental task of interest was movement related.

The current study also found that the HQFVs tended to be more widely spread over the feature sources in the all-embracing method than in the standard method. It is worth mentioning that the inclusion of more feature sources increased the diversity of HQFVs. This result corroborate the ideas of Pfurtscheller and Neuper (2001) and Obermaier et al. (2003), who suggested that control tasks are result of the mental effort demanded by the control task (conscious process) and the sensory–cognitive processing of the cue (unconscious process).

Modal Distribution of the HQFVs in Location, Frequency, and Time

The *modes* of the HQFVs fundamentally tended toward the expected sources (Pineda, 2005). These were the C3/C4 recoding sites and the α_U/β_L frequency bands. The *modes* also revealed clear tendencies toward feature sources that reflected the nature of the cue in use. Before going on to discuss this further, it is necessary to mention that the *modal* tendencies were much greater in MI than in MP. The reason for this is not clear, but it may be due to the mental effort involved in each control task. MP is such an intention, whereas MI is a dynamic process that goes through many of the central phases of actual movements.

Standard Method

The *modes* from audio cues tended to the left hemisphere, where some language-related functions take place, whereas those from visual cues tended to the right hemisphere, where visual perception is processed (Kropotov, 2010). Being the bimodal cue, a composition of audio and visual cues, the corresponding *modal* tendency was to both hemispheres. This result suggests that the most discriminating features were defined not only by the MP/MI mechanisms but also by the sensory–cognitive processing of the cue in use. With respect to the frequency domain, the involvement of high frequency bands took importance successively in *modes* from audio, visual, and bimodal cues. This result may be related to previous work of Giannitrapani [whose work is cited in Kropotov (2010)], who found that high beta activity (21–33 Hz) increased when the stimulus structure complexity also increased. It is possible, therefore, that the cue complexity had played a significant role in the discrimination process of features as well. Regarding the time domain, the highest tendencies took more time (after the cue onset) to appear in *modes* from audio than from bimodal cues. Hence, it is also possible to hypothesize that more informative features were found earlier when a more direct cue was employed.

All-Embracing Method

The *modes* from audio cues mostly tended to central recording sites, where auditory evoked potentials are typically recorded (Proverbio and Zani, 2003), and to δ_3 (500–1000 ms) time window, where brain rhythms normally respond to the recognition and/or retrieval of acoustic stimuli (Krause, 2006). On the other hand, the visual stimulation is registered around 200 ms post-stimulus as a response to modulations of alpha band rhythms over parieto-occipital areas and beta band rhythms over fronto-parieto-occipital areas (Kropotov, 2010; Andreassi, 2013). This may be a reason why *modes* from visual cues tended to fronto-parieto-occipital recording sites, α_U band, and δ_2 (250–750 ms) time window. Finally, the *modes* from bimodal cues displayed a well-balanced distribution between central and fronto-parieto-occipital recording sites and between δ_2 (250–750 ms) and δ_3 (500–1000 ms). This finding confirms that bimodal stimuli require feature sources that are also required by audio and visual stimuli separately (Isoğlu-Alkaç et al., 2007). In the frequency domain, the remarkable tendency of these *modes* toward γ band accords with previous findings of Ward (2003), who found that the sensory decoding around 250 ms post-stimulus is reflected in modulation of γ band rhythms.

In the three SMs, one unanticipated finding was the minor role occupied by β_U band that is well-known as one of the major contributors in the discrimination process of MI activity. A possible explanation for the small contribution of this band is that neural desynchronization around 20 Hz has been considered as a harmonic response of desynchronization around 10 Hz, whereas the one around 16 Hz is an authentic response to motor activity (Pfurtscheller et al., 1996). Moreover, Pfurtscheller et al. (1999) found that the most discriminating frequency components throughout MI-related tasks were found within the α_U band in three of four subjects, while those were found within the β_U band only in one subject.

Lastly, it is worth noting the underlying tendency of *modes* from visual and bimodal cues toward the δ_9 (2000–2500 ms) time window in the standard method. There was also another clear tendency of *modes* from the three SMs toward the δ_{13} (3000–3500 ms) time window in both methods. For visual and bimodal stimulation, we believe that gaze fixation at the screen center provoked by cues "left"/"right" could have driven the participants to anticipate the upcoming cue "start." Similarly, the cue "start" appearance caused the cue "stop" expectation. For audio stimulation, once the participants had received the cue "start," and owing to the likeness between increasing and decreasing tones (cues "start" and "stop," respectively), the anticipation of the audio cue "stop" was likely to have arisen. This speculation is supported by the findings of Scherer et al. (2008), who found that the involuntary expectations for the approaching cues provoked false control commands during virtual navigation. Another interesting tendency of *modes* of the three SMs is toward δ_2 (250–750 ms) and δ_3 (500–1000 ms) time windows in the all-embracing method. These results are in agreement with the findings of Pfurtscheller et al. (2008), who showed that distinct short-lasting brain patterns appeared within a time window of about 500–750 ms after cue onset.

All these interpretations must be, however, taken with caution. More research on this topic need to be undertaken because these findings can only be conclusive in early training sessions. The effects observed in this study could diminish or vanish, either in further training sessions or in online applications. Another source of uncertainty is associated with the ambiguity of multivariate classifiers (such as FDA) to determine the brain regions, frequency, and time intervals where cognitive processes are reflected. Haufe et al. (2014) demonstrated that backward models (e.g., multivariate classifiers) combine information from different channels to separate the brain patterns of different classes. These models may, however, give significant weight to channels unrelated to brain processes of interest. By contrast, forward models (e.g., blind source separation) explain how the measure data are generated from the neural sources, providing a neurophysiological meaning of the outcomes. Furthermore, Haufe et al. showed that brain patterns were much smoother and covered more diverse cognitive-related areas, when those patterns were obtained via forward methods. These findings are of particular interest due the nature of our study. It seems that the present results are limited by the methods applied to select the features vectors. Possibly, by transforming the backward model in use (DBI-FDA process) into a forward model such as proposed Haufe et al. (selection of brain patterns according to the neurophysiological contribution of each EEG channel), a clearer feature distribution over unrelated MI sources could have been achieved.

Implications on Neuroergonomics Research

This is a key issue for Neuroergonomics research because neural activity could not only be used to monitor the human mental state, but this might be also employed to control a system of interest. In fact, Myrden and Chau (2015) have suggested to develop a BCI system on the basis of an overt adaptation to keep user mental within the optimal region, and a covert adaptation that automatically adjusts BCI parameters according to such mental state.

An important application may be on driver modeling and vehicle simulation environments (Xu et al., 2015). These two areas of research have been of interest to develop driver assistance systems for safer driving and intelligent transportation. For example, EEG signals of a driver can be used to model the driver neuromuscular dynamics (Bi et al., 2015) and, thus, improving the performance of a driver simulator. Such EEG signals can also be employed to detect the fatigue (Wang et al., 2014) and level of attention (Wang et al., 2015) of the driver to activate the driver simulator and, hence, preventing driving accidents. Furthermore, the performance of the driver simulator can be improved by analyzing the human reaction to traffic cues such as car horn, direction indicators, and traffic lights. All of these cues produce specific EEG patterns on the driver brain signals as has been shown in this study.

CONCLUSION

The findings of this study have provided a new understanding of how MI-related control tasks used to control a BCI system may become modified by their preceding cues. Although previous investigations have somehow studied the cue effects on MI-related control tasks; in this study, we have shown that the CA of those control tasks does not depend on the type of cue in use. Moreover, we found that the EEG patterns that best differentiate MI-related control tasks emerge from recording sites, frequency bands, and time windows well defined by the perception and cognition of the cue in use. An implication of this study is the possibility of obtaining different control commands that could be detected with the same accuracy. Since different cues trigger control tasks that yield similar CAs, and those control tasks produce EEG patterns differentiated by the cue nature, this leads to accelerate the brain–computer communication by having a wider variety of detectable control commands. This is an important issue for Neuroergonomics research because neural activity could not only be used to monitor the human mental state, but this might be also employed to control the system of interest.

ACKNOWLEDGMENTS

LA-V wishes to express her sincere gratitude to the National Council of Science and Technology of Mexico (CONACyT) for providing funding support to accomplish this research project (grant number: 306714). Authors also thank Alexander Bedborough (language advisor of the International Academy at the University of Essex) for his editorial help with the manuscript.

REFERENCES

Alonso-Valerdi, L. M., and Sepulveda, F. (2015). *Implementation of a Motor Imagery Based BCI System Using Python Programming Language*. Angers: SCITEPRESS Digital Library.

Altermaller, E. O., Munte, T. F., and Gerloff, C. (2005). "Neurocognitive functions and the EEG," in *Electroencephalography: Basic Principles, Clinical Applications and Related Fields*, 5th Edn, eds Niedermeyer E. and Lopes da Silva F. (Philadelphia, PA: Lippincott Williams and Wilkins), 661–683.

Andreassi, J. L. (2013). *Psychophysiology: Human Behaviour and Physiological Response*, 4th Edn. New York, NY: Psychology Press.

Bamdadian, A., Guan, C., Ang, K. K., and Xu, J. (2014). The predictive role of pre-cue EEG rhythms on MI-based BCI classification performance. *J. Neurosci. Methods* 235, 138–144. doi:10.1016/j.jneumeth.2014.06.011

Basar, E., Basar-Erouglu, C., Karakas, S., and Schumann, M. (1999). Are cognitive processes manifested in event-related gamma, alpha, theta and delta oscillations in the EEG? *Neurosci. Lett.* 259, 165–168. doi:10.1016/S0304-3940(98)00934-3

Bi, L., Wang, M., Wang, C., and Liu, Y. (2015). Development of a driver lateral control model by integrating neuromuscular dynamics into the queuing network-based driver model. *IEEE Trans. Intelligent Transportation Syst.* 16(5), 2479–2486.

Bishop, C. M. (2006). *Pattern Recognition and Machine Learning*. New York, NY: Springer.

Boostani, R., Graimann, B., Moradi, M. H., and Pfurtscheller, G. (2007). A comparison approach toward finding the best feature and classifier in cue-based BCI. *Med. Biol. Eng. Comput.* 45, 403–412. doi:10.1007/s11517-007-0169-y

Delorme, A., and Makeig, S. (2004). EEGLAB: an open source toolbox for analysis of single-trial EEG dynamics including independent component analysis. *J. Neurosci. Methods* 134, 9–21. doi:10.1016/j.jneumeth.2003.10.009

Dornhege, G., Krauledat, M., Müller, K.-R., and Blankertz, B. (2007). *Toward Brain-Computer Interfacing*. Cambridge, MA: MIT Press.

Galán, F., Nuttin, M., Lew, E., Ferrez, P. W., Vanacker, G., Philips, J., et al. (2008). A brain-actuated wheelchair: asynchronous and non-invasive brain-computer interfaces for continuous control of robots. *Neurophysiol. Clin.* 119, 2159–2169. doi:10.1016/j.clinph.2008.06.001

Gargiulo, G., Calvo, R. A., Bifulco, P., Cesarelli, M., Jin, C., Mohamed, A., et al. (2010). A new EEG recording system for passive dry electrodes. *Neurophysiol. Clin.* 121, 686–693. doi:10.1016/j.clinph.2009.12.025

Graimann, B., Allison, B., and Pfurtscheller, G. (2010). "Brain-computer interfaces: a gentle introduction," in *Brain-Computer Interfaces*, 1st Edn, ed. Graimann B. (Berlin: Springer), 1–27.

Grosse-Wentrup, M., and Scholkopf, B. (2012). High gamma-power predicts performance in sensorimotor-rhythm brain-computer interfaces. *J. Neural. Eng.* 9, 96–046001. doi:10.1088/1741-2560/9/4/046001

Gutierrez, D., Ramirez-Moreno, M. A., and Lazcano-Herrera, A. G. (2015). "Assessing the acquisition of a new skill with electroencephalography," in Proceedings of the 7th International IEEE EMBS Neural Engineering Conference, Montpellier.

Hassanien, A. E., and Azar, A. T. (2015). *Brain-Computer Interfaces: Current Trends and Applications*. 1st Edn. Berlin: Springer-Verlag.

Haufe, S., Meinecke, F., Görgen, K., Dähne, S., Haynes, J. D., Blankertz, B., et al. (2014). On the interpretation of weight vectors of linear models in multivariate neuroimaging. *Neuroimage* 87, 96–110. doi:10.1016/j.neuroimage.2013.10.067

Honsbeek, R., Kuiper, T., and van Rijn, C. M. (1998). *BIOSEMI*. Available at: http://www.biosemi.com/products.htm

Isoğlu-Alkaç, U., Kedzior, K., Keskindemirci, G., Ermutlu, N., and Karamursel, S. (2007). Event-related potentials to visual, auditory, and bimodal (combined auditory-visual) stimuli. *Int. J. Neurosci.* 117, 259–273. doi:10.1080/00207450500534118

Jackson, M. M., and Mappus, R. (2010). "Neural control interfaces," in *Brain-Computer Interfaces: Applying Our Minds to Human-Computer Interaction*, 1st Edn, eds Tan D. S. and Nijholt A. (London: Springer-Verlag), 21–35.

Jeannerod, M. (2006). *Motor Cognition: What Actions Tell the Self*. 5th Edn. Oxford: Oxford University Press.

Kovács, F., Legány, C., and Babos, A. (2005). "Cluster validity measurement techniques," in *6th International Symposium of Hungarian Researchers on Computational Intelligence*, Budapest.

Krause, C. M. (2003). "Brain electric oscillations and cognitive processes," in *Experimental Methods in Neuropsychology*, ed. Hugdahl K. (Amsterdam: Springer), 111–130.

Krause, C. M. (2006). Cognition- and memory-related ERD/ERS responses in the auditory stimulus modality. *Prog. Brain Res.* 159, 197–207. doi:10.1016/S0079-6123(06)59013-2

Krepki, R., Curio, G., Blankertz, B., and Müller, K.-R. (2007). Berlin brain-computer interface - the HCI communication channel for discovery. *Int. J. Hum. Comput. Stud.* 65, 460–477. doi:10.1016/j.ijhcs.2006.11.010

Kropotov, J. (2010). *Quantitative EEG, Event-Related Potentials and Neurotherapy*, 1st Edn. San Diego, CA: Academic Press - Elsevier.

Leeb, R., Keinrath, C., Friedman, D., Guger, C., Scherer, R., Neuper, C., et al. (2006). Walking by thinking: the brainwaves are crucial, not the muscles. *Presence* 15, 500–514. doi:10.1162/pres.15.5.500

Lotte, F., Renald, Y., and Lécuyer, A. (2008). "Self-paced brain-computer interaction with virtual worlds: a quantitative and qualitative study out of the lab," in *4th International Brain Computer Interface Workshop and Training Course*, Graz.

Maeder, C. L., Sannelli, C., Haufe, S., and Blankertz, B. (2012). Pre-stimulus sensorimotor rhythms influence brain-computer interface classification performance. *IEEE Trans. Neural Syst. Rehabil. Eng.* 20, 653–662. doi:10.1109/TNSRE.2012.2205707

Meckes, M. P., Sepulveda, F., and Conway, B. A., (2004). "1st order class separability using EEG-based features for classification of wrist movements with direction selectivity," in *Engineering in Medicine and Biology Society*, 2004. IEMBS '04. 26th Annual International Conference of the IEEE, San Francisco, CA, 4377–4379.

Myrden, A., and Chau, T. (2015). Effects of user mental state on EEG-BCI performance. *Front. Hum. Neurosci.* 9:308. doi:10.3389/fnhum.2015.00308

Neuper, C., Grabner, R. H., Fink, A., and Neubauer, A. C. (2005). Long-term stability and consistency of EEG Event-Related (de-) synchronization across different cognitive tasks. *Neurophysiol. Clin.* 116, 1681–1694. doi:10.1016/j.clinph.2005.03.013

Neuper, C., Scherer, R., Wriessnegger, S., and Pfurtscheller, G. (2009). Motor imagery and action observation: modulation of sensorimotor brain rhythms during mental control of a brain-computer interface. *Neurophysiol. Clin.* 120, 239–247. doi:10.1016/j.clinph.2008.11.015

Neuper, C., Wörtz, M., and Pfurtscheller, G. (2006). ERD/ERS patterns reflecting sensorimotor activation and deactivation. *Prog. Brain Res.* 159, 211–222. doi:10.1016/S0079-6123(06)59014-4

Nijboer, F., Furdea, A., Gunst, I., Mellinger, J., McFarland, D. J., Birbaumer, N., et al. (2008). An auditory brain-computer interface (BCI). *J. Neurosci. Methods* 167, 43–50. doi:10.1016/j.jneumeth.2007.02.009

Norman, G. R., and Streiner, D. L. (2008). *Biostatistics: The Bare Essentials*. 3rd Edn. Shelton: People's Medical Publishing House.

Obermaier, B., Müller, G., and Pfurtscheller, G. (2003). Virtual keyboard controlled by spontaneous EEG activity. *IEEE Trans. Neural. Syst. Rehabil. Eng.* 11, 422–426. doi:10.1109/TNSRE.2003.816866

Pfurtscheller, G., Müller-Putz, G. R., Alois Schlögl, Graimann, B., Scherer, R., Leeb, R. (2007). "Graz-brain-computer interface: state of research," in *Toward Brain-Computer Interfacing*, eds G. Dornhege, J. D. R. Millán, T. Hinterberger, D. J. McFarland, and K. R. Müller (Cambridge: The MIT Press), 65–84.

Pfurtscheller, G., and Lopes da Silva, F. H. (1999). "Functional meaning of event-related desynchronization (ERD) and synchronization (ERS)," in *Handbook of Electroencephalography and Clinical Neurophysiology*, eds Pfurtscheller G. and Lopes da Silva F. H. (Amsterdam: Elsevier), 51–65.

Pfurtscheller, G., and Neuper, C. (2001). Motor imagery and direct brain-computer communication. *Proc. IEEE* 89, 1123–1134. doi:10.1109/5.939829

Pfurtscheller, G., Neuper, C., Ramoser, H., and Müller-Gerking, J. (1999). Visually guided motor imagery activates sensorimotor areas in humans. *Neurosci. Lett.* 269, 153–156. doi:10.1016/S0304-3940(99)00452-8

Pfurtscheller, G., Scherer, R., Müller-Purtz, G. R., and Lopes de Silva, F. H. (2008). Short-lived brain state after cued motor imagery in naive subjects. *Eur. J. Neurosci.* 28, 1419–1426. doi:10.1111/j.1460-9568.2008.06441.x

Pfurtscheller, G., Stancák, A., and Neuper, C. (1996). Post-movement beta synchronization. A correlate of an idle motor area? *Electroencephalogr. Clin. Neurophysiol.* 98, 281–293. doi:10.1016/0013-4694(95)00258-8

Pineda, J. A. (2005). The functional significance of mu rhythms: translating "seeing" and "hearing" into "doing". *Brain Res. Rev.* 50, 57–68. doi:10.1016/j.brainresrev.2005.04.005

Proverbio, A. M., and Zani, A. (2003). "Electromagnetic manifestations of mind and brain," in *The Cognitive Electrophysiology of Mind and Brain*, eds Zani A. and Proverbio A. M. (San Diego, CA: Academic Press), 13–40.

Ramoser, H., Müller-Gerking, J., and Pfurtscheller, G. (2000). Optimal spatial filtering of single trial EEG during imagined hand movement. *IEEE Trans. Rehabil. Eng.* 8, 441–446. doi:10.1109/86.895946

Scheel, H., et al. (2015). "Influence of external cues on synchronized brain-computer interface based on movement related cortical potentials," in *2015 7th International IEEE/EMBS Conference on Neural Engineering (NER)*, Montpellier.

Scherer, R., Lee, F., Schlogl, A., Leeb, R., Bischof, H., and Pfurtscheller, G. (2007). "EEG-based interaction with virtual worlds: a self-paced three class brain-computer interface," in *BRAINPLAY 07 Brain-Computer Interfaces and Games Workshop at ACE (Advances in Computer Entertainment)* (Graz: Advances in Computer Entertainment).

Scherer, R., Lee, F., Schlogl, A., Leeb, R., Bischof, H., and Pfurtscheller, G. (2008). Toward self-paced brain-computer communication: navigation through virtual worlds. *IEEE Trans. Biomed. Eng.* 55, 675–682. doi:10.1109/TBME.2007.903709

Sepulveda, F., Meckes, M. P., and Conway, B. A. (2004). "Cluster separation index suggests usefulness of non-motor EEG channels in detecting wrist movement direction intention," in *IEEE Conference on Cybernetics and Intelligent Systems*, Singapore, 943–947.

Shelton, J., and Kumar, G. P. (2010). Comparison between auditory and visual simple reaction times. *Neurosci. Med.* 1, 30–32. doi:10.4236/nm.2010.11004

Teichner, W. H. (1954). Recent studies of simple reaction time. *Psychol. Bull.* 51, 128–149. doi:10.1037/h0060900

Tseng, K. C., Lin, B. S., Wang, A. M. K., and Lin, B. S. (2015). Design of a mobile brain computer interface based smart multimedia controller. *Sensors* 15, 5518–5530. doi:10.3390/s150305518

Wang, H., Zhang, C., Shi, T., Wang, F., and Ma, S. (2014). Real-time EEG-based detection of fatigue driving danger for accident prediction. *Int. J. Neural Syst.* 25, 1–14. doi:10.1080/00207721.2014.953798

Wang, Y. K., Jung, T. P., and Lin, C. T. (2015). EEG-based attention tracking during distracted driving. *IEEE Trans. Neural Syst. Rehabil. Eng.* 23(6), 1085–1094.

Ward, L. M. (2003). Synchronous neural oscillations and cognitive processes. *Trends Cogn. Sci.* 7, 553–559. doi:10.1016/j.tics.2003.10.012

Xu, L., Hu, J., Jiang, H., and Meng, W. (2015). Establishing style-oriented driver models by imitating human driving behaviors. *IEEE Trans. Intell. Transp. Syst.* 99, 1–9. doi:10.1109/TITS.2015.2459722

11

Prefrontal Cortex Activation Upon a Demanding Virtual Hand-Controlled Task: A New Frontier for Neuroergonomics

*Marika Carrieri[1], Andrea Petracca[1], Stefania Lancia[1], Sara Basso Moro[1], Sabrina Brigadoi[2], Matteo Spezialetti[1], Marco Ferrari[3], Giuseppe Placidi[1] and Valentina Quaresima[1]**

[1] Department of Life, Health and Environmental Sciences, University of L'Aquila, L'Aquila, Italy, [2] Department of Developmental Psychology, University of Padova, Padova, Italy, [3] Department of Physical and Chemical Sciences, University of L'Aquila, L'Aquila, Italy

***Correspondence:**
Valentina Quaresima
valentina.quaresima@univaq.it

Functional near-infrared spectroscopy (fNIRS) is a non-invasive vascular-based functional neuroimaging technology that can assess, simultaneously from multiple cortical areas, concentration changes in oxygenated-deoxygenated hemoglobin at the level of the cortical microcirculation blood vessels. fNIRS, with its high degree of ecological validity and its very limited requirement of physical constraints to subjects, could represent a valid tool for monitoring cortical responses in the research field of neuroergonomics. In virtual reality (VR) real situations can be replicated with greater control than those obtainable in the real world. Therefore, VR is the ideal setting where studies about neuroergonomics applications can be performed. The aim of the present study was to investigate, by a 20-channel fNIRS system, the dorsolateral/ventrolateral prefrontal cortex (DLPFC/VLPFC) in subjects while performing a demanding VR hand-controlled task (HCT). Considering the complexity of the HCT, its execution should require the attentional resources allocation and the integration of different executive functions. The HCT simulates the interaction with a real, remotely-driven, system operating in a critical environment. The hand movements were captured by a high spatial and temporal resolution 3-dimensional (3D) hand-sensing device, the LEAP motion controller, a gesture-based control interface that could be used in VR for tele-operated applications. Fifteen University students were asked to guide, with their right hand/forearm, a virtual ball (VB) over a virtual route (VROU) reproducing a 42 m narrow road including some critical points. The subjects tried to travel as long as possible without making VB fall. The distance traveled by the guided VB was 70.2 ± 37.2 m. The less skilled subjects failed several times in guiding the VB over the VROU. Nevertheless, a bilateral VLPFC activation, in response to the HCT execution, was observed in all the subjects. No correlation was found between the distance traveled by the guided VB and the corresponding cortical activation. These results confirm the suitability of fNIRS technology to objectively evaluate cortical hemodynamic changes occurring in VR environments. Future studies could give a contribution to a better understanding of the cognitive mechanisms underlying human performance either in expert or non-expert operators during the simulation of different demanding/fatiguing activities.

Keywords: functional near-infrared spectroscopy, neuroergonomics, hand-controlled task, LEAP motion controller, virtual reality, remote control, brain activation

INTRODUCTION

The term neuroergonomics was first introduced in 1997 for depicting an interdisciplinary area of research which involves the intersection of two disciplines: neuroscience and ergonomics (Parasuraman and Rizzo, 2007). The studies in this field, previously carried out using either mobile or immobile neuroimaging techniques, have been nicely reviewed by Mehta and Parasuraman (2013). Virtual reality (VR), a computer-based technology that allows the creation of multisensory simulated environments in which users can interact and receive real-time feedbacks on their performance, was claimed by Kearney et al. (2007) to be highly relevant for neuroergonomics. This because VR can replicate, with a greater control than that applicable in the real world, a wide range of conditions that are impractical or impossible to observe in the real situations; then allowing behavioral and neurophysiological observations of the mind and brain at work. Given its peculiarity, VR is also effectively used by human operators to accomplish their work in dangerous environments, thus avoiding any physical risk. For instance, applying gesture-based control interfaces, VR is usually employed for tele-operated applications such as driving robots, rovers and other devices remotely, with the operators at a certain distance from them (Chen et al., 2015; Liu and Zhang, 2015; Wei et al., 2015). The tele-operated systems are very expensive, unique neither replicable nor quickly replaceable, and from their proper use depends the success or failure of long-planned, critical, costly and challenging operations. Taking into account the high degree of responsibility inherent to operators' duties, their considerable physical/cognitive work should be evaluated objectively by neuroimaging techniques in the framework of neuroergonomics (for review, see Gramann et al., 2011, 2014; Mehta and Parasuraman, 2013).

Although the most widely used immobile functional neuroimaging modality has been undoubtedly represented by functional magnetic resonance imaging (fMRI), the development of portable and wearable neuroimaging devices, comprising electroencephalography (EEG) and functional near infrared spectroscopy (fNIRS; for review, see Mehta and Parasuraman, 2013; Gramann et al., 2014; Scholkmann et al., 2014) has considerably facilitated the approach of neuroergonomics. fNIRS, with its high degree of ecological validity and its very limited requirement of physical constraints to subjects, represents a valuable tool for monitoring cortical responses in the research fields of neuroergonomics (for reviews, see Ayaz et al., 2013; Derosière et al., 2013). Furthermore, compared to fMRI, fNIRS is silent, allowing to avoid any bias in the results due to difficulties in focusing on the task because of the high level of noise. Briefly, fNIRS is a non-invasive vascular-based functional neuroimaging technology which assesses, simultaneously from multiple measurement sites, concentration changes in oxygenated-deoxygenated hemoglobin (O_2Hb/HHb, respectively) at the level of the cortical microcirculation blood vessels (Scholkmann et al., 2014). O_2Hb/HHb, indeed, interact differently with near infrared light, so that both physiological indexes can be recovered from the measured signal. This is a further advantage of fNIRS over fMRI, the latter being able to recover only a single physiological index, namely the blood-oxygen level dependent (BOLD) signal. When a specific brain region is activated, cerebral blood flow increases in a temporally and spatially coordinated manner through a complex sequence of coordinated events, tightly linked to changes in neural activity (i.e., neurovascular coupling). The coupling between the neuronal activity and the cerebral blood flow is fundamental to brain function. fNIRS relies exactly on this coupling to reveal the activated cortical region by measuring the associated cortical blood oxygenation changes (i.e., the increase in O_2Hb and the decrease in HHb).

Since 1993, fNIRS has been employed for evaluating the spatiotemporal characteristics of the cortical activation during different motor tasks related to upper and/or lower limb exercise (for a review, see Leff et al., 2011). In most previous fNIRS studies, the activation of the sensory-motor cortex and the PFC has been widely investigated in different tasks of the lower limb like walking (Koenraadt et al., 2014; Mirelman et al., 2014), stepping (Huppert et al., 2013), precision stepping (Koenraadt et al., 2014), etc. Several fNIRS studies have also investigated the PFC activation during hand tasks such as: finger movement (Wriessnegger et al., 2012), passive finger movement (Chang et al., 2014), isometric grasping/grasping (Mandrick et al., 2013), handgrip exercise (Derosière et al., 2014), learning a hand motor skill (Hatakenaka et al., 2007), etc.

Since 2000, fNIRS has been also employed in real-world activities realized in VR environment for evaluating the PFC activation during the simulation of different hand-related demanding/fatiguing activities, like airplane piloting (Ayaz et al., 2012a; Durantin et al., 2014; Gateau et al., 2015), car driving (Tomioka et al., 2009), grasping (Holper et al., 2010, 2012), natural orifice transluminal endoscopic surgery (James et al., 2011), etc. Interestingly, the inferior frontal gyrus (Ayaz et al., 2012a) and the dorsolateral PFC (DLPFC;

Durantin et al., 2014; Gateau et al., 2015) were found activated during airplane piloting tasks. The bilateral ventrolateral PFC (VLPFC) was found activated during natural orifice transluminal endoscopic surgery when the simulation required a more difficult navigation path through an orifice (James et al., 2011).

It is well-known that the PFC, and in particular the VLPFC and DLPFC, are involved in the control of the motor actions. On one hand, it has been demonstrated that the VLPFC is involved in visuo-motor learning tasks (Yamagata et al., 2012; Hoshi, 2013). Moreover the reflexive orienting seems to be controlled by the right VLPFC (Corbetta et al., 2008), whereas the goal relevant information for the action control seems to be maintained and retrieved by the left VLPFC (Badre and Wagner, 2007; Souza et al., 2009). On the other hand, the DLPFC apparently plays a specific role in learning by trial and error (Halsband and Lange, 2006). Furthermore DLPFC, for its involvement in mediating and monitoring of actions, is considered to be the major anatomical correlate of the central executive (Baddeley, 2003; Gateau et al., 2015). Therefore, the VLPFC and the DLPFC are involved in associating visual information with motor responses (Halsband and Lange, 2006; Tanji and Hoshi, 2008).

The PFC plays not only a crucial role in single cognitive or motor tasks, but also in combined sensorimotor-cognitive task (i.e., dual-task; Gentili et al., 2013; Mandrick et al., 2013; Mirelman et al., 2014). Several fNIRS studies have reported that, in comparison to a single task, the attention-demanding dual-tasks (e.g., walking while talking, calculating while stepping, balancing a ball while walking, etc.) induced an increase of the PFC activation due to a greater cognitive load (Holtzer et al., 2011). For instance, Mandrick et al. (2013) investigated how an additional mental load (i.e., arithmetic task) during isometric grasping affects the PFC activation. The performance of the mental task was impaired when the motor task difficulty increased, suggesting that performing a dual-task requires more attentional resources than performing a single task.

In the last few years, the use of VR interfaces, driven by natural hand movements for remote control, is growing-up thanks to the development of innovative optical 3-dimensional (3D) systems for gesture recognition (Erden and Çetin, 2014). The key advantage of gesture recognition technology is that no physical contact is required between the human body and the gesture recognition device, so that the subjects can move freely. One of the most recent optical 3D sensors, based on stereo-vision, is the LEAP Motion Controller® (LEAP). The LEAP is a high-resolution 3D hand-sensing device, which allows the freehand natural interaction crucial for the implementation of real-time, realistic VR systems. This low cost non-bulky device has an extremely accurate reactivity (Bachmann et al., 2014). In addition, the 3D rendering technologies, including state of the art displays and visors specifically designed for VR (Dodgson, 2013; Desai et al., 2014; Nan et al., 2014), have permitted a large development of VR techniques. In particular, their high visual/rendering fidelity and an immersive wide field of view enables the sensation of presence and the feeling being actually inside the virtual scene with the possibility to have multi-sensorial feedbacks.

The aim of the present study was to investigate non-invasively by fNIRS the PFC responses in healthy subjects while performing a complex hand-controlled task (HCT) in a VR environment. This task emulated the interaction with a real, remotely-driven, system operating into a critical environment. The hand movements were captured by the LEAP, a high spatial and temporal resolution 3D hand-sensing device. The subjects were asked to move their right hand/forearm with the purpose of guiding a virtual ball (VB) over a virtual route (VROU). The VROU can be easily and purposely designed to replicate a real track that an operator should travel to carry on a given challenging operation. The HCT-related PFC response was monitored non-invasively by a 20-channel fNIRS system. The HCT involved the control of the hand/forearm movement, and the active interaction with the virtual environment through the hand/forearm motor actions. The attentional resources allocation and the integration of different executive functions (e.g., coordination, planning, decision making, etc.) are needed in performing the HCT. Taking into account the well-known role played by the VLPFC and the DLPFC in motor action preparation and in the allocation of the attentional resources to generate goals from current situations, it was hypothesized that either VLPFC or DLPFC or both of them would be activated bilaterally in subjects while performing the HCT.

MATERIALS AND METHODS

Participants

Fifteen University students (all males, age: 26.6 ± 2.9 years; level of education: 14.4 ± 2.1 years), without neurological or psychiatric illness and normal or corrected-to-normal vision were recruited in the study. In order to prevent any gender differences in emotional responses (Matud, 2004) and in visuo-motor abilities (Wang et al., 2015), only men were enrolled. To exclude left-handed subjects, all participants completed the Edinburgh Handedness Inventory assessing hand dominance. Following a full explanation of the protocol and its non-invasiveness, and prior to the starting of the experimental procedure, a written informed consent was obtained from each participant. All procedures were conducted in accordance with the Declaration of Helsinki and approved by the University Ethics Committee.

Experimental Setup

Hand-Controlled Task (HCT)

A VR HCT was implemented by integrating a LEAP Motion Controller® with a real-time 3D engine. The LEAP provides both a 3D hand model and real-time hand tracking information for enabling subjects to transpose their hand movements within the virtual 3D HCT (**Figure 1**). The LEAP is a small (1.3 cm × 3.2 cm × 8 cm) 3D sensor which uses two internal infra-red (IR) cameras and three IR

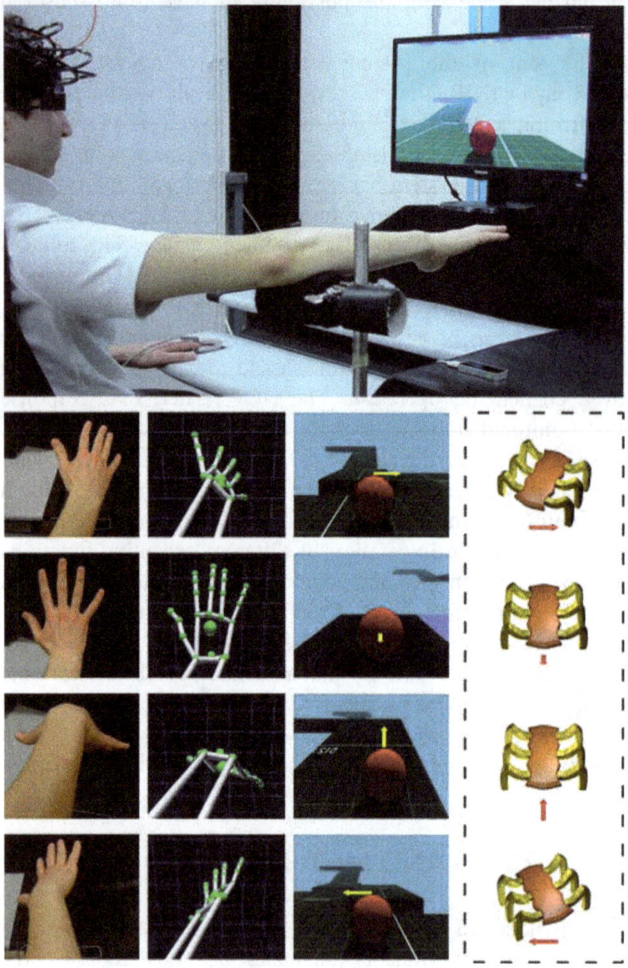

FIGURE 1 | Experimental setting for the execution of a virtual reality (VR) hand-controlled task (HCT). The upper large image shows the subject with the functional near-infrared spectroscopy (fNIRS) probe holder while sitting in front of a PC, and the positioning of the LEAP motion controller below the operator hand. The four columns of small images show (from left to right): the real position of the subject hand/forearm (first column); the corresponding hand/forearm virtual model (second column); the influence of the commands on the virtual ball (VB) during the HCT (third column); and the corresponding effects on a real, remote, spider-like rover (fourth column, in dashed line to indicate that the presence of the rover is just supposed). The yellow arrow indicates the direction of the guided VB and the red arrow indicates the corresponding effect on the rover. The length of the arrows indicates the force amplitude impressed by the operator. Note that, during the HCT, the hand/forearm virtual model (second column) was not shown to the operator and the visualization of the arrows (third column) was disabled.

light emitting diodes to detect objects within a dome of approximately 0.22 m^3 above it. Its spatial and temporal resolution is 1 mm and 15 ms, respectively. The LEAP, connected to a computer via a USB cable, is designed specifically to detect, in real-time, hand and finger motions and gestures, such as pinching fingers, closing hand, tapping, etc. This device, positioned under the palm center of the right hand at a distance of about 25 cm (**Figure 1**), was utilized to: (1) capture the movements of the hand; (2) associate hand movements to a virtual hand model; and (3) translate the movements of the virtual hand model to a set of commands in order to drive a VB within a virtual environment.

In the present study, the adopted virtual environment was aimed at simulating the driving action of a spider-like robot similar to the one developed by the National Aeronautics and Space Administration (NASA). Due to its high stability, equilibrium and ability to change quickly direction, this robot has been proven to be adapted for moving in very rough environments and in environments designed for humans (to go up and down stairs). The movements of the ball, in fact, simulated fairly those ones performed by the considered robot (lateral, ahead, behind, and stop). The aim of this adopted HCT was to move the VB over a VROU of a fixed length (42 m; **Figure 2**), trying to travel as long as possible the distance in a fixed time without falling (2 min). Either in the case of VB falling or in the case of accomplishment of a VROU in advance, subjects were requested to restart the VROU from the beginning. To calculate the whole distance traveled by each subject over the HCT, the completed VROU and the distance traveled until the task end were considered. The VROUs with failure were not considered. The VROU adopted in this study (**Figure 2**) was purposely designed to reproduce a narrow road including some critical points (i.e., stairs, turns, a slippery part, and climbs). The Torque 3D Engine[1], a cross-platform high performance real-time 3D engine, was used both for the editing and the rendering of the whole virtual 3D HCT. A controllable VB and a 3D VROU were created by using a customized version of Marble Motion, a well-known game[2]. In particular, the whole native source code was rewritten and enriched in order to fulfill the requirements of the task: (1) a time driven version of the task in which both the start and the end of the HCT were established by a fixed time interval; (2) the possibility of storing information related to the operator-task interaction process (including the number of times in which the VB was fallen out of the VROU, the position of the VB falls over the VROU, the distance traveled by the VB in the given time). The software allowed also the calculation of some dynamic parameters (followed trajectory, VB speed and acceleration). These last parameters have been considered to calculate the VB speed along the VROU, to get information about resting periods occurred during the HCT, and to evaluate the subject skills while executing the HCT. Moreover, to increase the subject's concentration and motivation during the HCT, the whole technical items, including elements of the VROU (textures and materials), were redefined utilizing some predefined items of the 3D engine editor (Torque 3D Editor[3].

The subject was asked to place his right forearm on a fixed and firm support in order to allow the hand capture (**Figure 1**). This support ensured the maintenance of the correct position of the forearm, and consequently of the hand, during the execution of the HCT. The task started with a stationary

[1] http://www.garagegames.com/products/torque-3d
[2] http://mit.garagegames.com/MarbleMotion-1-0b.zip
[3] http://www.garagegames.com/products/torque-3d/overview/editor

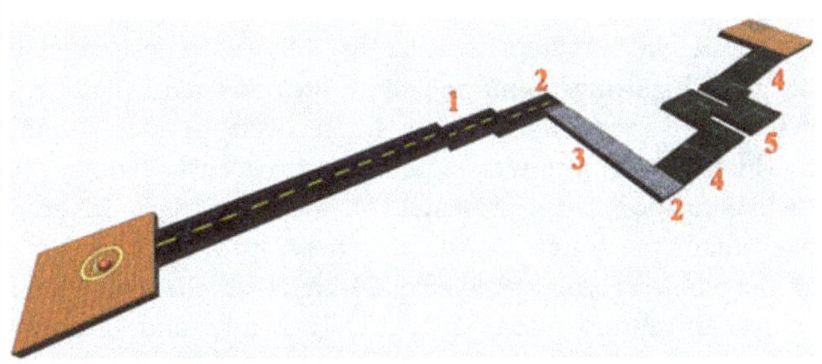

FIGURE 2 | A perspective view of the designed virtual route (VROU) which reproduces a narrow road including some critical points. 1: stairs; 2: turns; 3: slippery part; 4: climbs; and 5: sequential turns.

VB placed at the beginning of the VROU. The subject had to maintain his right hand opened over the LEAP device by keeping his forearm on the support with the center of the palm perpendicular to the center of the device and with all the five fingers extended (**Figure 1**). At the beginning of the HCT, the subject had to guide the VB over the VROU by using four commands (**Figure 1**). The first command (hand flexion) made the VB to proceed forward; the second command (hand extension) made the VB to decrease the speed (up to stop the VB) and to proceed backward; the third and the fourth commands (counter clockwise and clockwise rotations of the wrist) made the VB to move toward left or right, respectively (a combined use of the hand flexion/extension movements or the rotation of the wrist made the VB to stop). These hand movements had a real-time proportional impact on the VB. More specifically, the command chosen by the subject transmitted the direction and the "force" to the VB (e.g., a low hand downward flexion corresponded to a low "force" application to the VB in the forward direction), especially when the VB speed was depending on the inclination degree of the downward flexion and the time during which the hand was maintained at the same position. Thus, the HCT was purposely designed to combine the four main commands and when the subject assumed a pose of his hand halfway between two commands, the system merged both directions and "force" amplitude. In this way, the subject had the feeling to guide the VB without restrictions or constraints.

The effective range of the LEAP tracking system is limited to roughly 60 cm due to the low near infrared light intensity. In this study, the distance between the fNIRS head probe and the LEAP was always greater than 60 cm. Therefore, the LEAP should have not interfered with the fNIRS measurements. Interestingly, several fNIRS studies in combination with other near infrared based tracking systems such as Kinect or eye trackers have been published (Kita et al., 2010; Sukal-Moulton et al., 2014; Urakawa et al., 2015). Although those systems have utilized more powerful light emitters (than the LEAP), and the light emitters have been directly pointed toward the fNIRS head probe, the potential interference with the fNIRS data was not mentioned.

fNIRS Instrumentation and Data Processing

A two-wavelength continuous wave 20-channel fNIRS system (Oxymon Mk III, Artinis Medical Systems, Netherlands) was utilized to map non-invasively the changes in O_2Hb and HHb over the bilateral PFC. The details of this instrumentation have been previously reported (Basso Moro et al., 2013). The O_2Hb/HHb data from the 20 channels were acquired at 10 Hz. The O_2Hb/HHb concentration changes (expressed in $\Delta\mu M$), obtained by using the modified Beer-Lambert law and the age-dependent differential pathlenght factor ($4.99 + 0.067 \times Age^{0.814}$) were displayed in real-time on a PC monitor. Eight optical fiber bundles (length: 3.15 m; diameter: 4.5 mm) were utilized to transport the light to the left and the right PFC (four for each hemisphere), whereas ten optical fiber bundles of the same size (five for each hemisphere) were utilized to collect the light emerging from the PFC. The illuminating and collecting bundles were assembled into a flexible probe holder, consisting of two mirror-like units (9.7 cm × 8.9 cm each) held together by three flexible junctions. In 16 out of the 20 channels the illuminator-detector distance was set at 3.5 cm, while in the remaining four channels the illuminator-detector distance was set at 1 cm (short-separation channels or SS channels). In the 16 channels, the measurement points were defined as the midpoint of the corresponding illuminator-detector pairs. The probe holder was placed over the subject head by a Velcro brand fastener in order to get a stable optical contact with the scalp (**Figure 1**). In particular, the two frontopolar fibers bundles, collecting the light at the bottom of the holder, were centered (according to the International 10–20 system for the EEG electrode placement) on the Fp1 and Fp2 locations for the left and right hemisphere, respectively. The pressure created by the fastener was sufficient to induce a partial transient blockage of the skin circulation during the fNIRS study. The adopted procedure would suggest that a consistent reduction of forehead skin blood flow was occurring as a result of this approach. The Montreal Neurological Institute coordinates of the optodes and the relative 16 measurement points were calculated using a probe placement method. For the details of this procedure see Basso Moro et al. (2013). The measurement points 1, 2, 3, 9, 10, 11 corresponded to the DLPFC, which includes part of the Brodmann's Area (BA) 46; the measurement points 5, 6, 13, 14 corresponded to the frontopolar cortex, which includes part of the BA 10; and measurement points 4, 7, 8, 12, 15, 16 corresponded to the VLPFC, which includes part of the BA 45.

During the data collection procedure, the fNIRS signal quality as well as the absence of movement artifacts were verified on the PC monitor. The subject's heart rate (HR) was monitored by a pulse oximeter (N-600, Nellcor, Puritan Bennett, St. Louis, MO, USA) with the sensor clipped to the index finger of the left hand. The Homer2 NIRS processing package[4] was employed to analyze the data. Raw intensity data in each channel were converted into optical density changes (OD). Channels showing low intensity values were

[4]http://www.nmr.mgh.harvard.edu/PMI/resources/homer2/home.htm

excluded from further analyses. The Wavelet motion correction method was employed to correct motion artifacts. Based on the method developed by Molavi and Dumont (2012), it sets to zero all wavelet detail coefficients exceeding a predefined threshold (iqr = 0.1). The modified Beer-Lambert law was then applied to convert the corrected OD data into concentration changes. A General Linear Model (GLM) approach (hmrDeconvHRF_DriftSS) was utilized to recover the mean hemodynamic response function (HRF) for each subject and channel. The approach, consisting in adding the SS channel signal with the highest correlation with the analyzed standard channel signal in the design matrix, was able to reduce the contribution of the mean arterial blood pressure changes in task-evoked fNIRS signal. The less restrictive set of Gaussian functions with standard deviation (SD) of 3 s and with their means separated by 2 s was chosen as temporal basis functions (ranging between −20 before and 210 s after the starting of the HCT; Gagnon et al., 2011).

Experimental Design

A familiarization/training phase was carried out 3 days before the study. The subjects were informed about the procedures and familiarized with both the experimental setting and the HCT. During this phase, the fNIRS probe holder was placed over the head of the subjects who were trained to stay as firm as possible to avoid movement artifacts in fNIRS measurement during the HCT execution. After evaluating the joint mobility of their hand and wrist, the subjects were requested to pay attention to the presented four commands to be used for guiding properly the VB (hand flexion, hand extension, counter clockwise and clockwise rotations of the wrist). Later, the subjects were asked to place their right hand opened over the LEAP in order to verify the correctness of the estimated hand virtual model. Once this phase was completed, the subjects were asked to guide a VB over a VROU. In order to avoid a potential learning effect, a different VROU was used in this training phase. For each subject, the training phase was considered completed when he demonstrated his ability to guide properly the VB. After 3 days, at the same time of the training phase, the subjects participated in the study. A monetary reward was not given.

This study was carried out in a quiet and dimly lit room. The subject was asked to sit on a comfortable high-backed chair in front of a 17″ PC monitor, and to keep his forearm on the firm support with the right hand opened over the LEAP (see "The Hand-Controlled Task" Section; **Figure 1**). The HCT protocol lasted 6 min. Specifically, the protocol started with a 3 min baseline, during which subjects were asked to relax (observing a white fixation cross presented on a black screen) in order to get stable fNIRS signals. Then, a stationary VB came into view on the PC monitor, and a visual instruction informed the subjects that the 2 min HCT was starting. During the HCT, the subject had to guide the VB over the VROU through the four hand movements (see "The Hand-Controlled Task" Section). When the subject failed in guiding the VB over the VROU or the subject completed the VROU in less than 2 min, the VB was repositioned at the VROU starting point, and the route restarted. At the end of the HCT execution, there was a recovery period (1 min), in which the subject was requested to relax while observing a white fixation cross presented on a black screen. In order to evaluate the potential "state anxiety" provoked by HCT, all the subjects completed the 20-items of the State Trait Anxiety Inventory Form Y-1 (STAI) before and after the protocol.

Data Analysis and Statistics

The integral values of the O_2Hb/HHb ($_{INT}O_2Hb$/HHb) changes of the HRFs were calculated from the beginning (at 0 s) until the end of the HCT (at 120 s), for each measurement point and subject, and were used as metric for the following statistical analysis. The mean values of the HR changes (analyzed as percentage of control) were calculated from the beginning (at 0 s) until the end of the HCT (at 120 s). Both the $_{INT}O_2Hb$/HHb changes and the HR mean values were corrected for the baseline periods, calculated over the last 20 s before the starting of the HCT. The median of the values of the distance traveled by the guided VB was calculated to subdivide the subjects in two groups: best performers (above the median) and worst performers (below the median). The subject of the median value was not included in any group. Student's t-test was conducted in order to evaluate the presence of any difference, in terms of the distance traveled by the guided VB between the worst and best performers.

All data were examined for normality and sphericity using Shapiro–Wilk and Mauchly's Sphericity tests, respectively. Each level of the independent variables followed a normal or approximately normal distribution in all the dependent variables (O_2Hb, HHb and HR), permitting the use of parametric statistical analyses. When the sphericity was not assumed, the Greenhouse-Geisser correction was utilized.

In order to investigate the PFC activation in response to HCT, the two-way analysis of variance (ANOVA) was applied to $_{INT}O_2Hb$/HHb changes. The ANOVA included two factors: measurement point (16 levels) and cortical hemodynamic response (CHR; i.e., corrected task period vs. zero; 2 levels). To control for multiple significance tests, the Fisher's least significant difference adjustment was applied. A series of one-way ANOVAs was performed for the HCT in order to evaluate the influence of the CHR (2 levels) on the $_{INT}O_2Hb$/HHb changes. In particular, the one-way series of ANOVAs were performed only for the $_{INT}O_2Hb$/HHb changes related to the measurement points 7, 8, 15 and 16, chosen as descriptive measurement points of the hemodynamic response. For the HCT, the Pearson's correlation coefficient was calculated in order to evaluate the relation between the distance traveled by the guided VB and the $_{INT}O_2Hb$/HHb changes in the 7, 8, 15 and 16 measurement points. A one-way ANOVA was performed for the HCT in order to evaluate the influence of the CHR (2 levels) on the HR changes. The Pearson's correlation coefficient was also calculated for evaluating the relation between the distance traveled by the guided VB and the

HR. Student's *t*-tests were conducted in order to evaluate the presence of any difference in: (1) the anxiety state before and after the protocol; (2) $_{INT}O_2Hb/HHb$ changes in the 7, 8, 15 and 16 measurement points between the worst performers and best performers; and (3) the distance traveled by the guided VB of worst and best performers.

All statistical analyses were conducted with SPSS 20.0 (SPSS Inc., Chicago, IL, USA). Data were expressed as mean $\pm$ *SD*. The criterion for significance was $p < 0.05$.

RESULTS

The behavioral data analysis revealed the following main results. There was no significant difference ($t = 0.64$, $p = 0.53$) in the anxiety state before (28.8 $\pm$ 6.4) and after the protocol (28.9 $\pm$ 5.8). The distance traveled by the guided VB in the 15 subjects was: 21, 26, 36, 43, 51, 53, 56, 58, 61, 83, 88, 96, 101, 132, and 148 m, respectively. The median value was 58 m. The mean distance was 70.2 $\pm$ 37.2 m. The less skilled subjects failed several times in guiding the VB over the VROU. Therefore, the distance traveled by their guided VB was shorter. Indeed, the distance traveled by the guided VB was significantly different ($t = -4.89$, $p < 0.001$) between the worst performers (40.9 $\pm$ 13.7 m) and best performers (101.3 $\pm$ 29.7 m). The fNIRS data evidenced a heterogeneous O_2Hb/HHb response over the mapped cortical area in the subjects while performing the HCT (**Figure 3**). In particular, since the beginning of the HCT, a progressive O_2Hb increase and a concomitant progressive HHb decrease were observed in the measurement points 7, 8, 15 and 16, corresponding to the VLPFC, which includes part of the BA 45. About 15 s after the end of the HCT, a gradual return of O_2Hb/HHb to the corresponding baseline values, was observed. This delay is reasonable considering that the cerebral blood flow increase lasts over the period of the HCT. The statistical analysis revealed the following main results. The two-way ANOVA analysis, carried out on the $_{INT}O_2Hb$ changes, revealed a significant main effect of: (1) the measurement point ($F_{(2.67,37.47)} = 9.52$, $p < 0.001$), and (2) the measurement point * CHR interaction ($F_{(2.67,37.47)} = 9.52$, $p < 0.001$). The two-way ANOVA analysis, carried out on the $_{INT}HHb$ changes, revealed a significant main effect of the: (1) measurement point ($F_{(2.83,39.67)} = 15.70$, $p < 0.001$); (2) CHR ($F_{(1.00,14.00)} = 13.83$, $p = 0.002$); and (3) measurement point * CHR interaction ($F_{(2.83,39.67)} = 15.70$, $p < 0.001$). The two-way ANOVAs, carried out on the $_{INT}O_2Hb/HHb$ changes, revealed the main significant differences between the measurement points 7, 8, 15, 16 and all the others (*ps* < 0.05). The series of one-way ANOVAs, carried out on the $_{INT}O_2Hb$ changes of the measurement points 7, 8, 15, and 16, revealed a significant activation in all the measurement points ($F_{(1,14)} = 5.32$, $p = 0.037$; $F_{(1,14)} = 23.79$, $p < 0.001$; $F_{(1,4)} = 7.33$, $p = 0.017$; $F_{(1,14)} = 16.89$, $p = 0.001$).The series of one-way ANOVAs carried out on the $_{INT}HHb$ changes of the measurement points 7, 8, 15, and 16 revealed a significant cortical activation in all the measurement points ($F_{(1,14)} = 41.61$, $p < 0.001$; $F_{(1,14)} = 58.57$, $p < 0.001$; $F_{(1,14)} = 19.12$, $p = 0.001$; $F_{(1,14)} = 26.23$, $p < 0.001$). In the HCT, no correlation was found between the distance traveled by the guided VB and the corresponding $_{INT}O_2Hb/HHb$ changes (*ps* > 0.05). During the HCT, no differences (*ps* > 0.05) were found in the $_{INT}O_2Hb/HHb$ changes in the 7, 8, 15 and 16 measurement points between the worst performers and best performers. The one-way ANOVA analysis for the HR mean values revealed a significant main effect of the CHR ($F_{(2.88,40.40)} = 8.06$, $p < 0.001$). However, the mean values of the HR changes during the execution of the HCT increased only of about 15% with respect to the mean value of the baseline. No correlation was found between the HR and the distance traveled by the guided VB.

DISCUSSION

In this feasibility study, the bilateral PFC was investigated by a multi-channel fNIRS system while subjects performed a demanding VR HCT, a remotely-driven operation simulated by a high-resolution and low-cost 3D hand-sensing device. The observed involvement of the bilateral VLPFC supports the formulated hypothesis.

The results of the present study have indicated a consistent bilateral VLPFC activation (measured as O_2Hb increase and a concomitant HHb decrease) in response to the execution of the VR HCT (**Figure 3**). It has been reported that VLPFC is involved in associating visual information with motor responses (Tanji and Hoshi, 2008). In fact, the execution of the adopted HCT requires the combination of the contextual visual information in order to coordinate the hand/forearm movements for guiding the VB over the VROU. Although the tested subjects had the same age and level of education (University students), their skills in performing the HCT were different. Indeed, the distance traveled by the VB was heterogeneous: the distance traveled by the VB guided by the best performer was about seven times longer than the distance traveled by the VB guided by the worst performer. These results clearly confirm that the designed VROU (**Figure 2**) was really demanding. The diverse skills of the subjects could not be attributable to emotional factors, because no difference between anxiety state before and after the HCT, and no correlation between the distance traveled by the guided VB and the HR of the subjects were found. However, a bilateral VLPFC activation was observed indiscriminately in all the tested subjects, including the ones who never completed at least one VROU. Therefore, the present fNIRS data did not provide the possibility to discriminate the subjects according to their performance. This could be partly explained by the fact that other cortical areas were not investigated in this study and that subcortical areas and/or cortical-subcortical network are supposed to be responsible of the differences between the best and the worst performers. As well known, PFC is involved in the executive functions (e.g., attention, coordination, planning, decision making, etc.), the same required to perform the HCT regardless of the performer's skills. The combined use of a fNIRS-EEG system has evidenced a greater involvement of the deeper structures (e.g., hippocampus) in the "good performers group" compared with the "bad performers group" while executing a spatial navigation

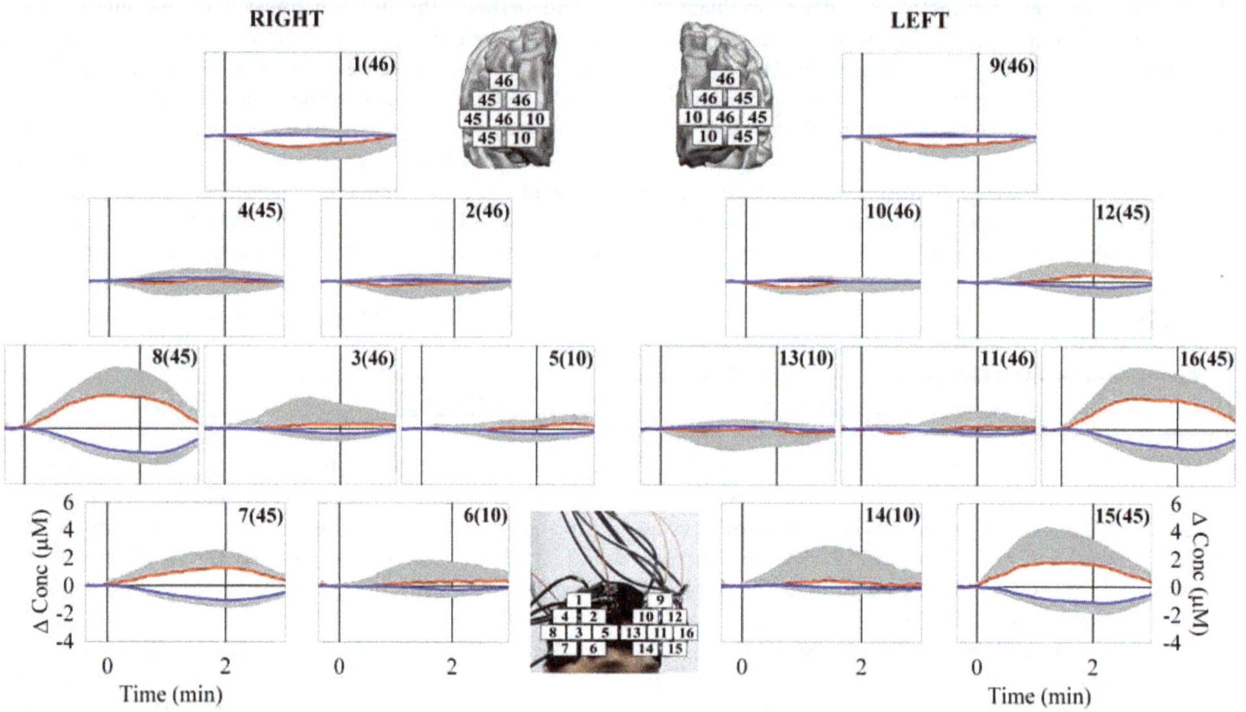

FIGURE 3 | Grand average of O_2Hb (red line) and HHb (blue line) changes observed over the bilateral PFC [16 measurement points of the right (from 1–8) and left (from 9–16) hemisphere] in response to the VR HCT. The corresponding numbers in the brackets refer to the associated Brodmann's Area (BA). The vertical solid lines limit the duration of the task execution. The major cortical activation was observed in the bilateral VLPFC (measurement points 7, 8, 15, and 16). *N* = 15; means ± *SD*.

task (Kober et al., 2013). Moreover, it has been reported that a complex sensorimotor-cognitive task, such as the adopted HCT, would require the involvement of different cortical-subcortical networks including: PFC, spinal cord, brainstem, cerebellum, basal ganglia, and motor cortex (Takakusaki, 2008). This suggests that the degree of the cognitive demand (measured by fNIRS), required for executing the HCT, is not associated with the subjects performance (measured as the distance traveled by the guided VB). This in part confirms the results of other VR fNIRS studies in which a dissociation between the mental work demanded to execute a complex task and the performance output was observed (Ayaz et al., 2012a; Boyer et al., 2015). In the present study, this dissociation could be also explained by the fact that tested subjects had only a short familiarization/training phase. A higher activation of the PFC was usually observed in non-expert subjects while executing a novel VR task compared to expert (Ayaz et al., 2012b). The non-expertise requires the employment of more attentional resources to perform a novel task. On the contrary, the expertise implies an increase of automaticity and does not require the same high level of attention and control (Ayaz et al., 2012b). The VLPFC activation, observed in the present study in non-expert subjects while performing the novel VR HCT, suggests that some of the well-known executive functions (e.g., attention, coordination, planning, decision making, etc.) are required in the learning phase. Then, it could be supposed that the amplitude of the observed VLPFC activation would become lower or even disappear in subjects very familiar with the VR HCT.

Several studies evidenced the advantages of using fNIRS technology for investigating non-invasively cortical responses in subjects while performing different VR tasks; the most representative studies are listed in **Table 1**. The common relevant finding is represented by the activation of different regions of the frontal cortex and the PFC. For example, the involvement of the medial PFC (mPFC) and the frontopolar cortex (Ayaz et al., 2012b) and the inferior frontal gyrus (Harrison et al., 2014) was observed in subjects while executing air traffic control tasks; an activation of the overall frontal cortex was observed in subjects while performing a train piloting task (Kojima et al., 2005). Very recently, the usefulness of fNIRS as a tool to conduct driving research has been nicely reviewed (Liu et al., 2015). For example, an activation of the right PFC (Tomioka et al., 2009) and an activation of the overall PFC (Tsunashima and Yanagisawa, 2009) were found in subjects while executing different simulated car driving tasks. However, in all of the above reported studies, no activation of the VLPFC, and in particular of the BA 45, was found.

The combined use of fNIRS-EEG would be an ideal tool for carrying out studies in the field of neuroergonomics. The pros of lightweight, high-density EEG and fNIRS recording

TABLE 1 | Selected fNIRS studies about the effects of VR tasks on different cortical areas.

VR Tasks	Subjects (patients)	Age (years)	D	Ch	Cortical areas	Main findings	Reference
Air traffic control	24	24–55	D1	16	FP, PFC	Medial FP/PFC activated	Ayaz et al. (2012b)
Air traffic control	12	NA	D1	16	PFC	PFC activated	Harrison et al. (2014)
Airplane piloting	9	36 ± 4	D7	1	FC	FC differently activated by task difficulty	Takeuchi (2000)
Airplane piloting	13	21–28	D1	16	FP, PFC	IFG differently activated by practice	Ayaz et al. (2012a)
Airplane piloting	12	25 ± 5	D1	16	PFC	Correlation DLPFC activation/ performance	Durantin et al. (2014)
Airplane piloting	19	27 ± 6	D1	16	FP, PFC	DLPFC activated bilaterally	Gateau et al. (2015)
Balancing (*swing*)	16	29 ± 5	D2	8	PFC	PFC activated bilaterally	Basso Moro et al. (2014)
Balancing (*tilt board*)	22	26 ± 4	D2	8	PFC	PFC activated bilaterally	Ferrari et al. (2014)
Balancing (*video game*)	9	18–42	D3	32	FC, MC, SC, TC	STG activated	Karim et al. (2012)
Boxing (*video game*)	20	18–40	D4	46	ATC, SMA	ATC and SMA differently activated	Kim et al. (2015)
Car driving	9	NA	D5	42	FC	FC less activated during ACC	Tsunashima and Yanagisawa (2009)
Car driving	14 (12 AD)	NA	D4	52	PFC	PFC less activated in AD	Tomioka et al. (2009)
Dancing	14	22 ± 1	D5	22	(L)PFC, (L)TC	Training-dependent PFC activation	Ono et al. (2015)
Dancing	26	NA	D6	22	(L)PFC, (L)TC	MTG activated	Noah et al. (2015)*
Grasping	23	NA	D8	4	M1, PC PMC, SMA	M1, PMC, SMA, PC activated	Holper et al. (2010)
Grasping	17	26 ± 4	D8	4	PMC, SMA	PMC/SMA differently activated by trials	Holper et al. (2012)
Lathe operation	7	24–26	D6	45	FC, MC	FC and MC activated	Hou and Watanuki (2012)
Line bisection	8	28	D9	20	OC, PC	OC and PC activated	Seraglia et al. (2011)
Line-tracking	2	NA	D8	4	PMC	PMC activated	Brand et al. (2011)
Maze	2	NA	D1	16	PFC	PFC more activated during BLK	Ayaz et al. (2011)
Maze	15 GP 12 BP	24 ± 1 28 ± 1	D4	24	(R)FC, (R)PC	PC activated	Kober et al. (2013)**
Missile defense	30	18–31	D9	2	PFC	PFC activated	Boyer et al. (2015)
Shopping	6 (10 BD)	61 ± 16 23 ± 1	D10	16	PFC	PFC more activated in BD	Okahashi et al. (2014)
Surgery	29	32 ± 6	D4	24	PFC	Lateral PFC more activated in experts	James et al. (2011)
Surgery	20	29 ± 2	D4	24	OC, PC	OC less activated by improved performance	Leff et al. (2015)
Surgery	7	23–26	D4	24	PC	IS activated	Miura et al. (2015)
Train driving	2	NA	D5	44	FC, OC	FC widely activated in manual condition	Kojima et al. (2005)
Walking (*haptic touch on treadmill*)	7 (1 CS)	25 ± 9	D4	44	PFC, PMC, SC, SMA	PFC and SMA widely/locally activated	Sangani et al. (2015)

*ACC, adaptive cruise control; AD, Alzheimer's disease; ATC, anterior temporal cortex; BD, brain damage patients; BLK, blocked order; BP, bad performers; Ch, number of channels; CS, chronic stroke patient; D, Device; D1, Imager 1000 (fNIR Devices, USA); D2, NIRO-200 (Hamamatsu Photonics, Japan); D3, CW6 (TechEn, USA); D4: ETG-4000 (Hitachi, Japan); D5, OMM-3000 (Shimadzu, Japan); D6, FOIRE-3000 (Shimadzu, Japan); D7, NIRO-500 (Hamamatsu Photonics, Japan); D8, Wireless prototype (Zurich University, Switzerland); D9, Imagent (ISS, USA); D10, OEG-16 (Spectratech Inc., Japan); DLPFC, dorsolateral prefrontal cortex; FC, frontal cortex; FP, frontopolar; GP, good performers; IFG, inferior frontal gyrus; IS, intraparietal sulcus; (L), left; M1, primary motor cortex; MC, motor cortex; MTG, middle temporal gyrus; NA, not available; OC, occipital cortex; PC, parietal cortex; PFC, prefrontal cortex; PMC, premotor cortex; (R), right; SC, somatosensory cortex; SMA, supplemental motor area; STG, superior temporal gyrus; TC, temporal cortex; VR, virtual reality; *fNIRS-fMRI study; **combined fNIRS-EEG study.*

to study natural human cognition have been previously reviewed (Gramann et al., 2011, 2014). Simultaneous fNIRS-EEG measurements offer complementary functional information about neuronal activity and hemodynamic changes in order to provide a wider perspective on different aspects of the cortical processes. To the best of our knowledge, Kober et al. (2013) have first compared neuronal responses of good and bad navigators during a VR spatial navigation task by a combined fNIRS-EEG system. The commercial fNIRS systems, utilized either by Kober et al. (2013) or in the present study, are equipped with fiber optic bundles. The disadvantage of using fiber optic bundles is that the fibers are often heavy and with a limited flexibility. Therefore, this kind of fNIRS instrumentation is not the best choice for studies in the neuroergonomics field. Since 2009, different battery operated multi-channel wearable/wireless fNIRS systems have been commercialized (Scholkmann et al., 2014). A 64-measurement point wireless fNIRS system was developed and integrated with simultaneous EEG and electrocardiography (ECG) monitoring in order to record data up to several days (Zhang et al., 2014). These most advanced versions of integrated fNIRS-EEG systems represent a suitable tool for evaluating brain activation in response to cognitive tasks executed in normal daily activities. To make fNIRS technology more suitable for neuroergonomics studies, in terms of robustness, mobility, user-friendliness and customization, a very recent and successful effort has been made to realize a dedicated fNIRS device (von Lühmann et al., 2015). Further future hardware developments will increase the production of miniaturized wireless integrated fNIRS-EEG devices and their use in neuroergonomics. It is noteworthy to mention that a 16-measurement point wireless fNIRS system has been recently coupled with transcranial direct current stimulation (tDCS) in order to investigate the effects of tDCS on spatial working memory (McKendrick et al., 2015). These authors have suggested the utility of using the combination of simultaneous tDCS and fNIRS techniques for future applications in the field of neuroergonomics: from enhanced/accelerated learning and training of complex human-machine systems to optimization of task load for improved safety and productivity. The neuroergonomics approaches can also provide sensitive and reliable assessment of mental workload in complex tasks and naturalistic work settings (Parasuraman, 2011). The mental workload has been defined as the degree of the effort to be made by the brain to meet the task demands (Young et al., 2015). Recently, Peck et al. (2014) have reviewed the use of fNIRS to measure mental workload in the real world tasks, and the different approaches for automatic detection of the workload.

The strengths and the limitations of the fNIRS technique have been previously discussed in detail (for review, see Scholkmann et al., 2014). The fNIRS equipment is transportable, completely safe and non-invasive. These advantages allow for the investigation of brain activity in natural conditions (e.g., while sitting on a chair) and during daily life activities (e.g., standing and/or walking). Therefore, with respect to other functional neuroimaging methods such as fMRI, fNIRS represents an useful tool for neuroergonomics research (for review, see Ayaz et al., 2013; Derosière et al., 2013), for studies in other fields of neuroscience such as brain-computer interface (for review, see Naseer and Hong, 2015), human-robot interaction (for review, see Canning and Scheutz, 2013), and cognitive states measurements (for review, see Strait and Scheutz, 2014). In addition, very recently the integration of fNIRS with a wearable technology, such as Google Glass, has been demonstrated (Afergan et al., 2015). For an adequate understanding of the current findings, some limitations should be pointed out: (1) this study has been conducted in a small sample of healthy young male adults subjects and the subjective cognitive load was not tested by NASA Task Load Index; (2) the duration of the adopted task and the length of the route were relatively short, hence, the effect of a longer duration of the VR HCT on the PFC hemodynamic response remains unknown; (3) this study did not imply a control session for example including/not including motor task with/without VR; (4) this study did not contemplate repeated trials on separate days in order to verify the reproducibility and the potential learning effect of the HCT; (5) the limited number of measurement points (16) made possible by the utilized fNIRS system did not allow the investigation of the supposed connectivity between the PFC and other cortical areas (e.g., premotor and motor cortices) likely involved in performing HCT; and (6) this study did not take into account the impact of the variability of the skull thickness amongst the 16 measurement points within subject and amongst subjects. This anatomical variability could be examined by acquiring structural T1-weighted MRI scans from each subject.

CONCLUSION

The results of the present study confirm the promising application of fNIRS technology to objectively evaluate cortical hemodynamic changes occurring in VR environments. The ongoing development of fNIRS technology, finalized to deliver more dedicated, sophisticated and wireless devices, together with the most advanced VR solutions, could provide the best combined approach for monitoring operators training and assessing mental work. Future studies could give a contribution to a better understanding of the cognitive mechanisms underlying human performance either in expert or non-expert operators.

AUTHOR CONTRIBUTIONS

Study design and protocols were conceived by MC, AP, SL, SBM, MS, MF, GP and VQ. Data collection was performed by MC, AP, SL, SBM, MS, MF, GP and VQ. Data analysis was performed by MC, AP, SL, SBM, SB, MS, MF, GP and VQ. The manuscript was written by MC, AP, SL, SBM, SB, MS, MF, GP and VQ.

ACKNOWLEDGMENTS

The study has been performed in the framework of the "Interdepartmental Research Centre for Molecular Diagnostics and Advanced Therapies". This work was supported in part by: (1) the 2014 grant from the "Fondazione Cassa di Risparmio della Provincia dell'Aquila", and (2) the "Abruzzo Earthquake Relief Fund" (Toronto, ON; purchase of the Artinis system). The authors wish to thank Dr. Simone Cutini, "Department of Developmental Psychology and Socialization", University of Padua, Italy for helping in the identification of the relative Brodmann's Areas, and Dr. Danilo Avola, "Department of Mathematics and Informatics", University of Udine, Italy for HCT implementation.

REFERENCES

Afergan, D., Hincks, S. W., Shibata, T., and Jacob, R. J. K. (2015). Phylter: a system for modulating notifications in wearables using physiological sensing. *Lect. Notes Comput. Sc.* 9183, 167–177. doi: 10.1007/978-3-319-20816-9_17

Ayaz, H., Cakir, M. P., Izzetoglu, K., Curtin, A., Shewokis, P. A., Bunce, S., et al. (2012a). "Monitoring expertise development during simulated UAV piloting tasks using optical brain imaging," in *Proceedings of the IEEE Aerospace Conference* (Big Sky, MN), 1–11.

Ayaz, H., Shewokis, P. A., Bunce, S., Izzetoglu, K., Willems, B., and Onaral, B. (2012b). Optical brain monitoring for operator training and mental workload assessment. *Neuroimage* 59, 36–47. doi: 10.1016/j.neuroimage.2011.06.023

Ayaz, H., Onaral, B., Izzetoglu, K., Shewokis, P. A., McKendrick, R., and Parasuraman, R. (2013). Continuous monitoring of brain dynamics with functional near infrared spectroscopy as a tool for neuroergonomic research: empirical examples and a technological development. *Front. Hum. Neurosci.* 7:871. doi: 10.3389/fnhum.2013.00871

Ayaz, H., Shewokis, P. A., Curtin, A., Izzetoglu, M., Izzetoglu, K., and Onaral, B. (2011). Using MazeSuite and functional near infrared spectroscopy to study learning in spatial navigation. *J. Vis. Exp.* 56:e3443. doi: 10.3791/3443

Bachmann, D., Weichert, F., and Rinkenauer, G. (2014). Evaluation of the leap motion controller as a new contact-free pointing device. *Sensors (Basel)* 15, 214–233. doi: 10.3390/s150100214

Baddeley, A. (2003). Working memory: looking back and looking forward. *Nat. Rev. Neurosci.* 4, 829–839. doi: 10.1038/nrn1201

Badre, D., and Wagner, A. D. (2007). Left ventrolateral prefrontal cortex and the cognitive control of memory. *Neuropsychologia* 45, 2883–2901. doi: 10.1016/j.neuropsychologia.2007.06.015

Basso Moro, S., Bisconti, S., Muthalib, M., Spezialetti, M., Cutini, S., Ferrari, M., et al. (2014). A semi-immersive virtual reality incremental swing balance task activates prefrontal cortex: a functional near-infrared spectroscopy study. *Neuroimage* 85, 451–460. doi: 10.1016/j.neuroimage.2013.05.031

Basso Moro, S., Cutini, S., Ursini, M. L., Ferrari, M., and Quaresima, V. (2013). Prefrontal cortex activation during story encoding/retrieval: a multi-channel functional near-infrared spectroscopy study. *Front. Hum. Neurosci.* 7:925. doi: 10.3389/fnhum.2013.00925

Boyer, M., Cummings, M. L., Spence, L. B., and Solovey, E. T. (2015). Investigating mental workload changes in a long duration supervisory control task. *Interact. Comput.* 27, 512–520. doi: 10.1093/iwc/iwv012

Brand, J., Geisseler, O., Holper, L., Hepp-Reimond, M. C., Morari, M., Kiper, D., et al. (2011). "The effects of manipulation of visual feedback in virtual reality on cortical activity: a pilot study," in *Proceedings of the IEEE International Conference on Virtual Rehab.*, Zurich, 1–2.

Canning, C., and Scheutz, M. (2013). Functional near-infrared spectroscopy in human-robot interaction. *J. Hum. Robot Interact.* 2, 62–84. doi: 10.5898/jhri.2.3.canning

Chang, P. H., Lee, S. H., Gu, G. M., Lee, S. H., Jin, S. H., Yeo, S. S., et al. (2014). The cortical activation pattern by a rehabilitation robotic hand: a functional NIRS study. *Front. Hum. Neurosci.* 8:49. doi: 10.3389/fnhum.2014.00049

Chen, S., Ma, H., Yang, C., and Fu, M. (2015). "Hand gesture based robot control system using leap motion," in *Intelligent Robotics and Applications*, eds H. Liu, N. Kubota, X. Zhu, R. Dillmann, and D. Zhou (Cham: Springer International Publishing), 581–591.

Corbetta, M., Patel, G., and Shulman, G. L. (2008). The reorienting system of the human brain: from environment to theory of mind. *Neuron* 58, 306–324. doi: 10.1016/j.neuron.2008.04.017

Derosière, G., Alexandre, F., Bourdillon, N., Mandrick, K., Ward, T. E., and Perrey, S. (2014). Similar scaling of contralateral and ipsilateral cortical responses during graded unimanual force generation. *Neuroimage* 85, 471–477. doi: 10.1016/j.neuroimage.2013.02.006

Derosière, G., Mandrick, K., Dray, G., Ward, T. E., and Perrey, S. (2013). NIRS-measured prefrontal cortex activity in neuroergonomics: strengths and weaknesses. *Front. Hum. Neurosci.* 7:583. doi: 10.3389/fnhum.2013.00583

Desai, R. P., Desai, N. P., Ajmera, D. K., and Mehta, K. (2014). A review paper on oculus rift-a virtual reality headset. *Int. J. Eng. Trends Tech.* 13, 175–179. doi: 10.14445/22315381/IJETT-V13P237

Dodgson, N. (2013). Optical devices: 3D without the glasses. *Nature* 495, 316–317. doi: 10.1038/495316a

Durantin, G., Gagnon, J. F., Tremblay, S., and Dehais, F. (2014). Using near infrared spectroscopy and heart rate variability to detect mental overload. *Behav. Brain Res.* 259, 16–23. doi: 10.1016/j.bbr.2013.10.042

Erden, F., and Çetin, A. (2014). Hand gesture based remote control system using infrared sensors and a camera. *IEEE Trans. Consum. Electron.* 60, 675–680. doi: 10.1109/tce.2014.7027342

Ferrari, M., Bisconti, S., Spezialetti, M., Basso Moro, S., Di Palo, C., Placidi, G., et al. (2014). Prefrontal cortex activated bilaterally by a tilt board balance task: a functional near-infrared spectroscopy study in a semi-immersive virtual reality environment. *Brain Topogr.* 27, 353–365. doi: 10.1007/s10548-013-0320-z

Gagnon, L., Perdue, K., Greve, D. N., Goldenholz, D., Kaskhedikar, G., and Boas, D. A. (2011). Improved recovery of the hemodynamic response in diffuse optical imaging using short optode separations and state-space modeling. *Neuroimage* 56, 1362–1371. doi: 10.1016/j.neuroimage.2011.03.001

Gateau, T., Durantin, G., Lancelot, F., Scannella, S., and Dehais, F. (2015). Real-time state estimation in a flight simulator using fNIRS. *PLoS One* 10:e0121279. doi: 10.1371/journal.pone.0121279

Gentili, R. J., Shewokis, P. A., Ayaz, H., and Contreras-Vidal, J. L. (2013). Functional near-infrared spectroscopy-based correlates of prefrontal cortical dynamics during a cognitive-motor executive adaptation task. *Front. Hum. Neurosci.* 7:277. doi: 10.3389/fnhum.2013.00277

Gramann, K., Ferris, D. P., Gwin, J., and Makeig, S. (2014). Imaging natural cognition in action. *Int. J. Psychophysiol.* 91, 22–29. doi: 10.1016/j.ijpsycho.2013.09.003

Gramann, K., Gwin, J. T., Ferris, D. P., Oie, K., Jung, T. P., Lin, C. T., et al. (2011). Cognition in action: imaging brain/body dynamics in mobile humans. *Rev. Neurosci.* 22, 593–608. doi: 10.1515/RNS.2011.047

Halsband, U., and Lange, R. K. (2006). Motor learning in man: a review of functional and clinical studies. *J. Physiol. Paris* 99, 414–424. doi: 10.1016/j.jphysparis.2006.03.007

Harrison, J., Izzetoglu, K., Ayaz, H., Willems, B., Hah, S., Ahlstrom, U., et al. (2014). Cognitive workload and learning assessment during the implementation of a next-generation air traffic control technology using functional near-infrared spectroscopy. *Proc. IEEE Trans. Hum. Mach. Sys.* 44, 429–440. doi: 10.1109/thms.2014.2319822

Hatakenaka, M., Miyai, I., Mihara, M., Sakoda, S., and Kubota, K. (2007). Frontal regions involved in learning of motor skill- A functional NIRS study. *Neuroimage* 34, 109–116. doi: 10.1016/j.neuroimage.2006.08.014

Holper, L., Kobashi, N., Kiper, D., Scholkmann, F., Wolf, M., and Eng, K. (2012). Trial-to-trial variability differentiates motor imagery during observation between low versus high responders: a functional near-infrared spectroscopy study. *Behav. Brain Res.* 229, 29–40. doi: 10.1016/j.bbr.2011.12.038

Holper, L., Muehlemann, T., Scholkmann, F., Eng, K., Kiper, D., and Wolf, M. (2010). Testing the potential of a virtual reality neurorehabilitation system during performance of observation, imagery and imitation of motor actions recorded by wireless functional near-infrared spectroscopy (fNIRS). *J. Neuroeng. Rehabil.* 7:57. doi: 10.1186/1743-0003-7-57

Holtzer, R., Mahoney, J. R., Izzetoglu, M., Izzetoglu, K., Onaral, B., and Verghese, J. (2011). fNIRS study of walking and walking while talking in young and old individuals. *J. Gerontol. A Biol. Sci. Med. Sci.* 66, 879–887. doi: 10.1093/gerona/glr068

Hoshi, E. (2013). Cortico-basal ganglia networks subserving goal-directed behavior mediated by conditional visuo-goal association. *Front. Neural Circuits* 7:158. doi: 10.3389/fncir.2013.00158

Hou, L., and Watanuki, K. (2012). Measurement of brain activity under virtual reality skills training using near-infrared spectroscopy. *J. Adv. Mech. Des. Syst.* 6, 168–178. doi: 10.1299/jamdsm.6.168

Huppert, T., Schmidt, B., Beluk, N., Furman, J., and Sparto, P. (2013). Measurement of brain activation during an upright stepping reaction task using functional near-infrared spectroscopy. *Hum. Brain Mapp.* 34, 2817–2828. doi: 10.1002/hbm.22106

James, D. R. C., Orihuela-Espina, F., Leff, D. R., Sodergren, M. H., Athanasiou, T., Darzi, A. W., et al. (2011). The ergonomics of natural orifice transluminal endoscopic surgery (NOTES) navigation in terms of performance, stress and cognitive behavior. *Surgery* 149, 525–533. doi: 10.1016/j.surg.2010.11.019

Karim, H., Schmidt, B., Dart, D., Beluk, N., and Huppert, T. (2012). Functional near-infrared spectroscopy (fNIRS) of brain function during active balancing using a video game system. *Gait Posture* 35, 367–372. doi: 10.1016/j.gaitpost.2011.10.007

Kearney, J. K., Rizzo, M., and Severson, J. (2007). "Virtual reality and neuroergonomics," in *Neuroergonomics: the Brain at Work*, eds R. Parasuraman and M. Rizzo (New York, NY: Oxford University Press), 253–274.

Kim, S., Biocca, F., Lee, K. M., Lee, S. W., and Chung, J. Y. (2015). "Neural correlates of embodied experiences through avatar self-identification," in *Proceeding of the 21st Annual Meeting of the Organization for Human Brain Mapping*, Hawaii, HI.

Kita, Y., Gunji, A., Sakihara, K., Inagaki, M., Kaga, M., Nakagawa, E., et al. (2010). Scanning strategies do not modulate face identification: eye-tracking and near-infrared spectroscopy study. *PLoS One* 5:e11050. doi: 10.1371/journal.pone.0011050

Kober, S. E., Wood, G., and Neuper, C. (2013). "Measuring brain activation during spatial navigation in virtual reality: a combined EEG-NIRS study," in *Virtual Environments: Developments, Applications and Challenges*, eds S. Trautman and F. Julien (New York, NY: NOVA Publisher), 1–24.

Koenraadt, K. L., Roelofsen, E. G., Duysens, J., Keijsers, N. L., Kojima, T., and Tsunashima, H. (2014). Cortical control of normal gait and precision stepping: an fNIRS study. *Neuroimage* 85, 415–422. doi: 10.1016/j.neuroimage.2013.04.070

Kojima, T., Tsunashima, H., Shizawa, T., Takada, H., and Sakai, T. (2005). Measurement of train driver's brain activity by functional near-infrared spectroscopy (fNIRS). *Opt. Quant. Electron* 37, 1319–1338. doi: 10.1007/s11082-005-4202-9

Leff, D. R., James, D. R. C., Orihuela-Espina, F., Kwok, K., Sun, L. W., Mylonas, G., et al. (2015). The impact of expert visual guidance on trainee visual search strategy, visual attention and motor skills. *Front. Hum. Neurosci.* 9:526. doi: 10.3389/fnhum.2015.00526

Leff, D. R., Orihuela-Espina, F., Elwell, C. E., Athanasiou, T., Delpy, D. T., Darzi, A. W., et al. (2011). Assessment of the cerebral cortex during motor task behaviours in adults: a systematic review of functional near infrared spectroscopy (fNIRS) studies. *Neuroimage* 54, 2922–2936. doi: 10.1016/j.neuroimage.2010.10.058

Liu, T., Pelowski, M., Pang, C., Zhou, Y., and Cai, J. (2015). Near-infrared spectroscopy as a tool for driving research. *Ergonomics* doi: 10.1080/00140139.2015.1076057 [Epub ahead of print].

Liu, Y., and Zhang, Y. (2015). "Toward welding robot with human knowledge: a remotely-controlled approach," in Vol. 12, *Proceedings of the IEEE Transaction on Automation Science and Engineering* (Gothenburg: IEEE), 769–774.

Mandrick, K., Derosière, G., Dray, G., Coulon, D., Micallef, J. P., and Perrey, S. (2013). Prefrontal cortex activity during motor tasks with additional mental load requiring attentional demand: a near-infrared spectroscopy study. *Neurosci. Res.* 76, 156–162. doi: 10.1016/j.neures.2013.04.006

Matud, M. P. (2004). Gender differences in stress and coping styles. *Pers. Individ. Dif.* 37, 1401–1415. doi: 10.1016/j.paid.2004.01.010

McKendrick, R., Parasuraman, R., and Ayaz, H. (2015). Wearable functional near infrared spectroscopy (fNIRS) and transcranial direct current stimulation (tDCS): expanding vistas for neurocognitive augmentation. *Front. Syst. Neurosci.* 9:27. doi: 10.3389/fnsys.2015.00027

Mehta, R. K., and Parasuraman, R. (2013). Neuroergonomics: a review of applications to physical and cognitive work. *Front. Hum. Neurosci.* 7:889. doi: 10.3389/fnhum.2013.00889

Mirelman, A., Maidan, I., Bernad-Elazari, H., Nieuwhof, F., Reelick, M., Giladi, N., et al. (2014). Increased frontal brain activation during walking while dual tasking: an fNIRS study in healthy young adults. *J. Neuroeng. Rehabil.* 11:85. doi: 10.1186/1743-0003-11-85

Miura, S., Kobayashi, Y., Kawamura, K., Nakashima, Y., and Fujie, M. G. (2015). Brain activation in parietal area during manipulation with a surgical robot simulator. *Int. J. Comput. Assist. Radiol. Surg.* 10, 783–790. doi: 10.1007/s11548-015-1178-1

Molavi, B., and Dumont, G. A. (2012). Wavelet-based motion artifact removal for functional near-infrared spectroscopy. *Physiol. Meas.* 33, 259–270. doi: 10.1088/0967-3334/33/2/259

Nan, X., Zhang, Z., Zhang, N., Guo, F., He, Y., and Guan, L. (2014). vDesign: a CAVE-based virtual design environment using hand interactions. *J. Multimodal User Interfaces* 8, 367–379. doi: 10.1007/s12193-014-0168-x

Naseer, N., and Hong, K. S. (2015). fNIRS-based brain-computer interfaces: a review. *Front. Hum. Neurosci.* 9:3. doi: 10.3389/fnhum.2015.00003

Noah, J. A., Ono, Y., Nomoto, Y., Shimada, S., Tachibana, A., Zhang, X., et al. (2015). fMRI validation of fNIRS measurements during a naturalistic task. *J. Vis. Exp.* 100:e52116. doi: 10.3791/52116

Okahashi, S., Mizumoto, H., Komae, A., Ueno, K., Yokoyama, M., Nagano, A., et al. (2014). An fNIRS-based study on prefrontal cortex activity during a virtual shopping test with different task difficulties in brain-damaged patients. *J. Behav. Brain Sci.* 4, 247–255. doi: 10.4236/jbbs.2014.46026

Ono, Y., Noah, J. A., Zhang, X., Nomoto, Y., Suzuki, T., Shimada, S., et al. (2015). Motor learning and modulation of prefrontal cortex: an fNIRS assessment. *J. Neural Eng.* 12:066004. doi: 10.1088/1741-2560/12/6/066004 [Epub ahead of print].

Parasuraman, R. (2011). Neuroergonomics: brain, cognition and performance at work. *Curr. Dir. Psychol. Sci.* 20, 181–186. doi: 10.1177/0963721411409176

Parasuraman, R., and Rizzo, M. (2007). *Neuroergonomics: The Brain at Work.* New York, NY: Oxford University Press.

Peck, E. M., Afergan, D., Yuksel, B. F., Lalooses, F., and Jacob, R. J. K. (2014). "Using fNIRS to measure mental workload in the real world," in *Advances in Physiological Computing*, eds S. H. Fairclough and K. Gilleade (London: Springer-Verlag), 117–139.

Sangani, S., Lamontagne, A., and Fung, J. (2015). Cortical mechanisms underlying sensorimotor enhancement promoted by walking with haptic inputs in a virtual environment. *Progr. Brain Res.* 218, 313–330. doi: 10.1016/bs.pbr.2014.12.003

Scholkmann, F., Kleiser, S., Metz, A., Zimmermann, R., Mata Pavia, J., Wolf, U., et al. (2014). A review on continuous wave functional near-infrared spectroscopy and imaging instrumentation and methodology. *Neuroimage* 85, 6–27. doi: 10.1016/j.neuroimage.2013.05.004

Seraglia, B., Gamberini, L., Priftis, K., Scatturin, P., Martinelli, M., and Cutini, S. (2011). An exploratory fNIRS study with immersive virtual reality: a new method for technical implementation. *Front. Hum. Neurosci.* 5:176. doi: 10.3389/fnhum.2011.00176

Souza, M. J., Donohue, S. E., and Bunge, S. A. (2009). Controlled retrieval and selection of action-relevant knowledge mediated by partially overlapping regions in left ventrolateral prefrontal cortex. *Neuroimage* 46, 299–307. doi: 10.1016/j.neuroimage.2009.01.046

Strait, M., and Scheutz, M. (2014). What we can and cannot (yet) do with functional near infrared spectroscopy. *Front. Neurosci.* 8:117. doi: 10.3389/fnins.2014.00117

Sukal-Moulton, T., de Campos, A. C., Stanley, C. J., and Damiano, D. L. (2014). Functional near infrared spectroscopy of the sensory and motor brain regions with simultaneous kinematic and EMG monitoring during motor tasks. *J. Vis. Exp.* 94:e52391. doi: 10.3791/52391

Takakusaki, K. (2008). Forebrain control of locomotor behaviors. *Brain Res. Rev.* 57, 192–198. doi: 10.1016/j.brainresrev.2007.06.024

Takeuchi, Y. (2000). Change in blood volume in the brain during a simulated aircraft landing task. *J. Occup. Health* 42, 60–65. doi: 10.1539/joh.42.60

Tanji, J., and Hoshi, E. (2008). Role of the lateral prefrontal cortex in executive behavioral control. *Physiol. Rev.* 88, 37–57. doi: 10.1152/physrev.00014.2007

Tomioka, H., Yamagata, B., Takahashi, T., Yano, M., Isomura, A. J., Kobayashi, H., et al. (2009). Detection of hypofrontality in drivers with Alzheimer's disease by near-infrared spectroscopy. *Neurosci. Lett.* 451, 252–256. doi: 10.1016/j.neulet.2008.12.059

Tsunashima, H., and Yanagisawa, K. (2009). Measurement of brain function of car driver using functional near-infrared spectroscopy (fNIRS). *Comput. Intell. Neurosci.* 2009:164958. doi: 10.1155/2009/164958

Urakawa, S., Takamoto, K., Ishikawa, A., Ono, T., and Nishijo, H. (2015). Selective medial prefrontal cortex responses during live mutual gaze interactions in human infants: an fNIRS study. *Brain Topogr.* 28, 691–701. doi: 10.1007/s10548-014-0414-2

von Lühmann, A., Herff, C., Heger, D., and Schultz, T. (2015). Towards a wireless open source instrument: functional near-infrared spectroscopy in mobile neuroergonomics and BCI applications. *Front. Hum. Neurosci.* 9:617. doi: 10.3389/fnhum.2015.00617

Wang, L., Krasich, K., Bel-Bahar, T., Hughes, L., Mitroff, S. R., and Appelbaum, L. G. (2015). Mapping the structure of perceptual and visual-motor abilities in healthy young adults. *Acta Psychol. (Amst)* 157, 74–84. doi: 10.1016/j.actpsy.2015.02.005

Wei, J. L., Sen, W. L., and Sani, Z. (2015). Leap motion underwater robotic arm control. *J. Teknologi* 74, 153–159. doi: 10.11113/jt.v74.4819

Wriessnegger, S. C., Bauernfeind, G., Schweitzer, K., Kober, S., Neuper, C., and Müller-Putz, G. R. (2012). The interplay of prefrontal and sensorimotor cortices during inhibitory control of learned motor behavior. *Front. Neuroeng.* 5:17. doi: 10.3389/fneng.2012.00017

Yamagata, T., Nakayama, Y., Tanji, J., and Hoshi, E. (2012). Distinct information representation and processing for goal-directed behavior in the dorsolateral and ventrolateral prefrontal cortex and the dorsal premotor cortex. *J. Neurosci.* 32, 12934–12949. doi: 10.1523/JNEUROSCI.2398-12.2012

Young, M. S., Brookhuis, K. A., Wickens, C. D., and Hancock, P. A. (2015). State of science: mental workload in ergonomics. *Ergonomics* 58, 1–17. doi: 10.1080/00140139.2014.956151

Zhang, Q., Ivkovic, V., Hu, G., and Strangman, G. E. (2014). Twenty-four-hour ambulatory recording of cerebral hemodynamics, systemic hemodynamics, electrocardiography and actigraphy during people's daily activities. *J. Biomed. Opt.* 19:047003. doi: 10.1117/1.JBO.19.4.047003

12

Pre-Trial EEG-Based Single-Trial Motor Performance Prediction to Enhance Neuroergonomics for a Hand Force Task

*Andreas Meinel[1], Sebastián Castaño-Candamil[1], Janine Reis[2] and Michael Tangermann[1]**

[1] Brain State Decoding Lab, Cluster of Excellence BrainLinks-BrainTools, Department of Computer Science, Albert-Ludwigs-University, Freiburg, Germany, [2] Department of Neurology, Albert-Ludwigs-University, Freiburg, Germany

Correspondence:
Michael Tangermann
michael.tangermann@blbt.uni-freiburg.de

We propose a framework for building electrophysiological predictors of single-trial motor performance variations, exemplified for SVIPT, a sequential isometric force control task suitable for hand motor rehabilitation after stroke. Electroencephalogram (EEG) data of 20 subjects with mean age of 53 years was recorded prior to and during 400 trials of SVIPT. They were executed within a single session with the non-dominant left hand, while receiving continuous visual feedback of the produced force trajectories. The behavioral data showed strong trial-by-trial performance variations for five clinically relevant metrics, which accounted for reaction time as well as for the smoothness and precision of the produced force trajectory. 18 out of 20 tested subjects remained after preprocessing and entered offline analysis. Source Power Comodulation (SPoC) was applied on EEG data of a short time interval prior to the start of each SVIPT trial. For 11 subjects, SPoC revealed robust oscillatory EEG subspace components, whose bandpower activity are predictive for the performance of the upcoming trial. Since SPoC may overfit to non-informative subspaces, we propose to apply three selection criteria accounting for the meaningfulness of the features. Across all subjects, the obtained components were spread along the frequency spectrum and showed a variety of spatial activity patterns. Those containing the highest level of predictive information resided in and close to the alpha band. Their spatial patterns resemble topologies reported for visual attention processes as well as those of imagined or executed hand motor tasks. In summary, we identified subject-specific single predictors that explain up to 36% of the performance fluctuations and may serve for enhancing neuroergonomics of motor rehabilitation scenarios.

Keywords: single-trial performance prediction, trial-by-trial variability, isometric force modulation, hand motor rehabilitation, visuomotor integration, EEG, oscillatory subspace, spatial filtering

1. INTRODUCTION

Motor training is utilized in rehabilitation scenarios to accelerate the re-gain of lost motor function after brain injury. State-of-the-art rehabilitation concepts are based on repetitive training tasks with the aim to reach a functional gain (Dobkin, 2004; Timmermans et al., 2009; Langhorne et al., 2011). Most prominent training paradigms comprise mirror training (French et al., 2007), constraint-induced movement therapy (Wolf et al., 2002), simultaneous bilateral training (Coupar et al., 2010), BCI-supported training (Ang and Guan, 2013) and robot-assisted techniques (Kwakkel et al., 2008). Recent rehabilitation approaches include the training of novel, unfamiliar motor skills instead of training well-known habitual motor tasks, attempting to optimize functional cortical reorganization.

Repetitive paradigms allow for the assessment of motor performance on a very fine-granular time scale. The performance of each single trial can be monitored by metrics such as the length, speed or smoothness of the produced movement trajectory. The distributions and temporal characteristics of trial-wise motor performance variations have been studied by different groups (Abe and Sternad, 2013; van Beers et al., 2013; Wu et al., 2014; Hadjiosif and Smith, 2015). While practicing a motor task over several sessions enables a user for skill acquisition (Lage et al., 2015), trial-by-trial variability of motor performance is a prominent feature which does not fully vanish with training (Cohen and Sternad, 2009; Osu et al., 2015). The underlying neural mechanisms of motor performance fluctuations on short time scales is subject of controversial discussion in literature and is not fully resolved yet (Faisal et al., 2008; Hadjiosif and Smith, 2015; Osu et al., 2015).

In the present work, we aim toward closing this gap. Therefore, trial-wise performance fluctuations of a sequential visuo-motor task (SVIPT; Camus et al., 2009; Reis et al., 2009; Fritsch et al., 2010 are investigated while registering a user's brain activity by EEG. In SVIPT trials, the quality of a movement changes within seconds and from repetition to repetition.

Our *hypothesis* is that subject-specific pre-trial brain signals can partially explain and temporally predict the trial-by-trial fluctuations of the upcoming motor performance. Given that such informative neural markers exist, then the SVIPT paradigm could be altered in order to meet the cognitive ergonomic requirements of each single user. Practically, the starting time point of the upcoming trial can be determined based on the information contained in this pre-trial neural marker. Ideally, such a neuroergonomic closed-loop gating strategy could provide control over the level of difficulty. This should allow to causally influence user performance and ultimately support SVIPT motor learning on the long run.

Paradigms which include *brain-state-dependent experimenting* (see Jensen et al., 2011; Horschig et al., 2014c) require that an informative neural marker can be extracted robustly from brain signals. Given the high dimensionality and noisy characteristic of most types of brain signals, the extraction and decoding of such individual neural markers is a challenging task.

Screening literature on relevant neural markers of visual and motor performance, it is important to make a distinction between the use of single-trial decoding in contrast to the extraction of statistical differences, which may even be reported as group averages. Neural features which correlate with the task performance on the grand average (GA) of a set of subjects have limited usefulness for closed-loop experimenting with a given individual. As inter-subject differences get lost during the averaging, GA features may have low predictive power when tested with data of a novel subject. Research in the field of brain-computer interfaces (BCI) has pushed forward methods for single-trial decoding of individual brain activity (mostly EEG signals) (Millán et al., 2010; Makeig et al., 2012). Results from this field affirm that brain signals and informative features vary strongly between individuals (Müller et al., 2008). To obtain optimal decoding results, BCI data processing pipelines thrive to identify subject-specific informative features. Technically, these are gained either from a calibration recording prior to the online use of the BCI (Blankertz et al., 2007), or by transfer learning methods (Kindermans et al., 2014) which exploit features from pre-trained machine learning models of earlier sessions or previous users. Furthermore, attention needs to be paid to temporal dependencies: brain features may correlate with previous behavior, with simultaneous behavior or may even be predictive for future behavior. Only the latter brain features can serve as a tool for brain-state-dependent experimenting.

Statistical correlates of visual perception performance are reported by several groups. For stimuli near the perception threshold, the pre-stimulus occipital alpha bandpower correlates with the detection performance (van Dijk et al., 2008), even on a single-trial basis using predictive features (Hanslmayr et al., 2007). In addition to bandpower, the pre-stimulus alpha phase was reported to correlate with the detection performance (Busch et al., 2009). Single-trial decoding methods were not applied in those auditory studies, but the reported correlates precede the perception, which may open the possibility for closed-loop experimenting. Based on the findings of Hanslmayr et al. (2007) and van Dijk et al. (2008), there are two examples that set up an online experiment based on occipital alpha bandpower features. Tonin et al. (2013) using EEG data and Horschig et al. (2014b), who employed MEG signals, both decoded covert visual attention in a closed-loop experiment by utilizing single-trial feedback on the detected attention shift. However, both groups did not fully close the loop e.g., by manipulating the perception performance, which may have been possible by selecting suitable brain states for stimulation. Gonzalez Andino et al. (2005) studied a cued reaction time task and identified that gamma band oscillatory activity observed in fronto-parietal regions prior to the stimulus onset correlates with reaction time. Similarly, Hoogenboom et al. (2010) stated that the strength of visually induced gamma band activity is predictive for the detection of stimulus motion. Somatosensory stimuli of low-intensity, but above threshold were delivered and combined with a distracting masker stimulus by Schubert et al. (2009). Investigating perceived vs. missed stimuli in an offline analysis, pre-stimulus beta bandpower over the left frontal cortex was found predictive for the perception performance on the grand average, as well as mu and beta bandpower over the pericentral sensorimotor areas.

In the motor domain, several groups have successfully decoded hand kinematics, using the center-out task as the dominating experimental approach. In their own work, Jerbi et al. (2011) provide a review over the decoding of hand movement parameters such as direction, position and velocity based on brain signals. ECoG signals were used by Pistohl et al. (2008) to decode two-dimensional hand movement trajectories using an autoregressive filtering approach. Considering non-invasive techniques, Waldert et al. (2008) have decoded (but not temporally predicted) the hand movement direction based on MEG and EEG. Neural correlates which encode the velocity of a movement have been investigated by Bradberry et al. (2009). The decoding of produced grip force based on a phase feature extracted from the beta range has been reported on data of three subjects by Logar et al. (2008). Zaepffel et al. (2013) reported an increased centro-parietal beta power during the planning period of grasping movements, but it was not investigated, if decoding may work on the basis of single trials. Focusing on single-trial methods, Lew et al. (2014) used slow cortical potentials of the EEG from fronto-parietal areas to predict self-paced movement directions a few hundred milliseconds prior to movement onset. Similarly, Hammon et al. (2008) inspected predictive EEG features for planning target directions using a cue-based paradigm.

In the field of BCI research, Maeder et al. (2012) studied a motor imagery paradigm. The single-trial decoding performance of left vs. right hand movement imagery tasks could be correlated to the level of pre-trial alpha bandpower over the sensorimotor cortices. Despite used offline, this neural marker would allow for a predictive intervention in a closed loop. In their statistical analysis, Yang et al. (2014) identified frontal alpha and beta bandpower features which correlate with performance metrics of a reaching task. Proceeding to single-trial methods, Meyer et al. (2014) reported on data of six subjects, who performed a hand positioning task. Their offline analysis revealed that the normalized time-to-target could be predicted based on pre-cue alpha-band activity of the EEG.

The state-of-the-art can be summed up as follows: In the perception domain, several studies have established single-trial performance prediction, partially even in closed-loop applications. The situation is different for the motor domain since only very few studies have investigated subject-specific motor performance prediction in single-trial upon a sufficiently large subject group. Closest to all of these requirements is the study by Meyer et al. (2014). Our research hypothesis builds exactly upon this point. In the context of a hand force task, we propose a generalized *workflow* which identifies subject-specific *predictive* oscillatory EEG features evaluated on a single trial basis.

First, by means of a simulated online analysis, an approach to extract robust and meaningful EEG components is developed. We evaluate, if the information contained in selected components is able to partially explain the trial-by-trial variation of SVIPT performance in a predictive fashion, i.e., the pre-trial component is required to predict the outcome of the upcoming trial. Second, the characteristics of the best performance predictors are investigated by a group-level analysis.

2. MATERIALS AND METHODS

2.1. Hand Motor Paradigm

In the context of hand motor skill learning, Reis et al. (2009) investigated the *Sequential Visual Isometric Pinch Task* (SVIPT), which demands an isometric force control of thumb and index finger. Interestingly, training-induced improvement of the SVIPT generalizes well to other hand motor control tasks, even though pinch grasp activities are rarely displayed during natural behavior patterns. Compared to the original SVIPT setup, brain activity is recorded using electroencephalogram (EEG) during a training session for *post-hoc* offline analysis. The resulting SVIPT setup follows the proposal in Meinel et al. (2015) and is sketched in **Figure 1**.

Each SVIPT trial consists of three phases: a light blue (inactive) cursor appears on the leftmost edge of the T0 field (corresponding to zero force), while the user is touching the sensor only slightly with his non-dominant left hand. The appearance of the cursor indicates the start of the *get-ready* phase, which corresponds to a waiting period with enhanced attention level. Its duration is varied randomly between 2 and 3 s. The transduction of force into cursor movements is deactivated during the get-ready phase. Fixating the cursor, the user will observe a distinct color change of the cursor from light to dark blue. This *go-cue* indicates the beginning of the *running* phase, in which the cursor position can be controlled by applying force to the sensor. As force is transduced into horizontal cursor position, increasing force will move the dark blue cursor to the rightmost position, which is pre-calibrated at session start to represent 30% of the user's maximum force. The user has been instructed to navigate the cursor as quickly and accurately as possible, in order to visit a sequence of target fields (T0, T1, and T2). Overshoots of the cursor are to be avoided. The current target field is visually indicated to the subject by a green shading (see **Figure 1**). Reaching a target field, a dwell time of 200 ms must be fulfilled in order to achieve a successful hit of this target field. Hit events are indicated visually by a switch of the target field (another field is shaded in green), or by the end of the trial. Trials were chosen randomly from two conditions, each with a specific required target field sequence (T1-T0-T2-T0 or T2-T0-T1-T0). A trial was finished by fulfilling the complete sequence – skipping a target was not allowed. Trial duration is presented visually as an immediate performance feedback during the *pause* phase between trials.

2.2. Subjects and Ethics

Overall, 20 right-handed *normally aged* subjects (8 female, average age: 53 years, std: 6 years) were recruited. The subject group resembles the target group of first-stroke patients with respect to age and gender (Ovbiagele and Nguyen-Huynh, 2011). The term *normally aged* was chosen to indicate our selection criteria: the participants did not have any known neurological or psychological history and were probably healthy—even though we can not exclude the possibility that some participants had a history of unrecognized micro stroke events.

The offline study was approved by the Ethics Committee of the University Medical Center Freiburg. Following the principles of the Declaration of Helsinki, written informed consent was given by subjects prior to participation. In one session of about 3–4 h (including EEG setup and washing the hair), every participant controlled the cursor with their left hand for 20 blocks of 20 trials each.

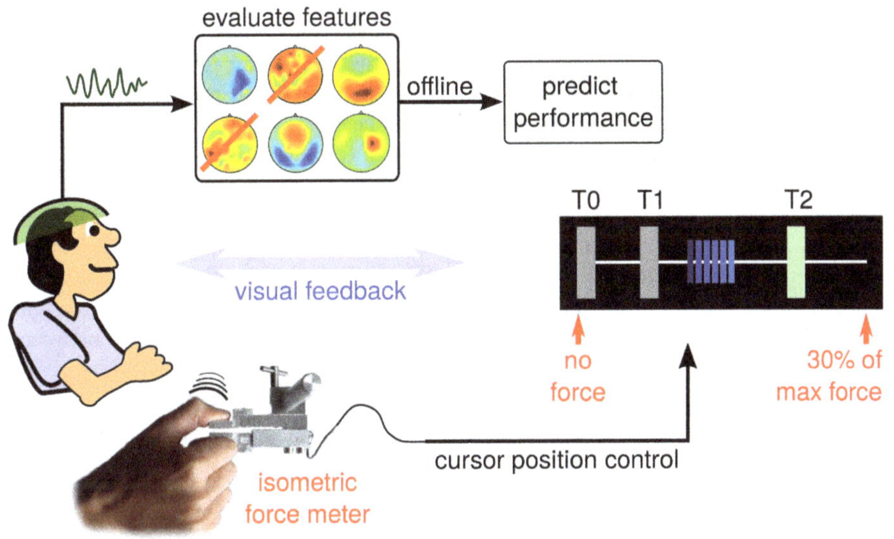

FIGURE 1 | Schematic setup of the EEG-tracked SVIPT. The subject applies force to a sensor using a pinch grasp. Force is transduced into positions of a horizontally moving cursor. EEG activity is recorded before, during and after repeated trials.

2.3. SVIPT Performance Scores

SVIPT enables to capture single trial motor performance. Given a high order motor control, the force profile $F(t)$ of a single-trial is characterized by a quick force ramp up upon the presentation of the go-cue and the avoidance of overshoots. The requested speed-accuracy trade-off can be translated into various performance scores of the SVIPT task. In Tangermann et al. (2015), the authors selected a set of scores, which describe the single-trial performance:

- **Reaction Time/RT**: A quick response upon the *go-cue* is a good start for a successful trial. The time interval between the *go-cue* at time t_{go} and the time point $t_{T0,exit}$, which indicates the cursor leaving the starting field T0, is defined as reaction time.
- **Duration/DUR**: Comparable to RT, a short time duration from the *go-cue* at time t_{go} until the hit of the first target field at time point t_{hit} characterizes a successful trial.
- **Cursor Path Length/CPL**: The total path length the cursor is moved from the *go-cue* to the hit of the first target field is described by the integral over the first temporal derivative of the force profile $F(t)$:

$$CPL \equiv \int_{t_{go}}^{t_{hit}} |\dot{F}(t)| \, dt'$$

- **Integrated Squared Jerk/ISJ**: The level of fine-granular motor control is reflected in variations of the trajectory smoothness. Therefore, jerk—defined as the third derivative of the force profile—is expressed by the ISJ metric, which is defined as:

$$ISJ \equiv \int_{t_{go}}^{t_{hit}} |\frac{d^3F(t)}{dt^3}|^2 \, dt'$$

- **Normalized Jerk/NJ**: A unit-free variant of ISJ captures smoothness variations. It is given by the *normalized* jerk:

$$NJ \equiv \sqrt{\frac{ISJ \cdot DUR^5}{2 \cdot CPL^2}}$$

Since there are two conditions of target field sequences, a standardization of the performance scores (except for RT) is the prerequisite for pooling trials of both conditions. Therefore, the extracted metrics of each condition were standardized (zero mean and standard deviation one) prior to pooling. Except RT, the metrics are defined with respect to some end point (e.g., t_{hit}). Choosing this boundary represents a trade-off between (a) harvesting a metric which is temporally close and thus related to the get-ready interval (the interval before the *go-cue*), and (b) including thorough information about the force trajectory of the current trial. To balance the two conflicting goals, we chose the hit of the first target field.

2.4. Data Acquisition and Preprocessing

During a single session, subjects were placed in a chair at 80 cm distance from a 24-inch flat screen. EEG signals from 63 passive Ag/AgCl electrodes (EasyCap) were recorded, which were placed according to the extended 10–20 system. Impedances were kept below 20 $k\Omega$. All channels were referenced against the nose. The signals were registered by multichannel EEG amplifiers (BrainAmp DC, Brain Products) at a sampling rate of 1 kHz. An analog lowpass filter of 250 Hz was applied before digitization. The signal of the force sensor was recorded by an additional amplifier system (BrainAmp ExG, Brain Products).

For outlier identification, the offline preprocessing consisted of high-pass filtering the raw EEG signals at 0.2 Hz, low-pass filtering at 48 Hz and sub-sampling to 500 Hz sample frequency. Therefore, linear butterworth filters of 5th order were applied.

For each trial and all 63 channels, an epoch of 2000 ms duration prior to the *go-cue* was extracted. In order to identify outlier epochs, three rejection methods were applied. First, EEG epochs violating a min-max threshold of 60 μV on frontal channels were excluded from further analysis. Second, a variance threshold on single epochs and channels was applied to remove high-frequent muscular artifacts. Therefore, the variance of single epochs needs to be within $P_{up} = $ 90th percentile and is not allowed to exceed $2 \cdot (P_{up} - P_{low})$ with $P_{low} = $ 10th percentile. Third, epochs belonging to extreme trials, represented by outliers of the motor performance metric, were removed. For this purpose, the following min-max thresholds were defined based on earlier pilot recordings (Meinel et al., 2015). The thresholds were [150, 900] ms for RT, [−1.5, 1.5] for ISJ, [−0.6, 0.6] for CPL, [−1.5, 2] for DUR, and [0, 1300] for NJ. They were applied prior to further data analysis. The total number of trials N_e entering the following offline analysis procedures varied across subjects and performance metrics. Only for 2 out of 20 subjects less than 150 out of the original 400 epochs were remaining after the EEG preprocessing. We discarded data of these subjects from the following analysis. The frequency filtering for our main analysis will subsequently be described in Section 2.6.

2.5. Single-Trial Performance Prediction

In the following, the multivariate variable $\mathbf{x}(t) \in \mathbb{R}^{N_c}$ characterizes the EEG signal recorded from N_c sensors. In addition, $\mathbf{s}(t)$ defines the time course of a neural source. The physics of volume conduction assumes a linear mapping of the source space to the sensor space. The forward (or generative) model thus reads :

$$\mathbf{x}(t) = \mathbf{A}\,\mathbf{s}(t) \tag{1}$$

where the matrix $\mathbf{A} \in \mathbb{R}^{N_c \times M}$ describes the projection of the M sources to the EEG sensor space.

The main goal is to approximate the true neural source $\mathbf{s}(t)$ by $\hat{\mathbf{s}}(t)$, whose power achieves the highest correlation with a predefined external variable $z(t)$, called *target variable* from this point onwards. Several methods can be used to estimate such a source, among them Blind Source Separation (BSS) and source reconstruction techniques. BSS techniques rely solely on an unsupervised framework, which may be a suboptimal approach given the availability of labels in the form of the target variable z. Source reconstruction techniques may provide a high level of interpretability for the results directly in the source space, and may describe non-stationarities in the data and other complex dynamics (Castaño-Candamil et al., 2015b). However, there are three potential drawbacks of source reconstruction approaches (Grech et al., 2008): First, the estimation of $\hat{\mathbf{s}}(t)$ usually creates a rather high computational burden. Second, the methods require a forward model $\mathbf{A}$ for each individual subject, which may not be available in most situations since it corresponds to the exact anatomical description of a subject's brain. Third, as source reconstruction problems are intrinsically ill-posed, the quality of an estimated source depends on additional assumptions, such as the density of sources or their location within the brain.

An alternative to both, BSS and source localization approaches is the family of the so-called supervised spatial-filtering methods. One widely known approach is the Common Spatial Patterns algorithm (CSP; Ramoser et al., 2000), which searches for spatial filters that enhance the contrast between two classes. Consequently, it is well suited for supervised classification problems. A more recent approach, the Source Power Comodulation algorithm (SPoC; Dähne et al., 2014) is adequate for regression problems. As the five SVIPT metrics are continuous variables, we preferred to include the SPoC algorithm into our data analysis framework.

SPoC learns an optimal spatial filter $\mathbf{w_{opt}} \in \mathbb{R}^{N_c \times 1}$ that allows to estimate the source as $\hat{\mathbf{s}}(t)$ by projecting $\mathbf{x}(t)$ into a subspace, which maximizes the correlation between the band power of $\hat{\mathbf{s}}(t)$ and the target variable $z(t)$:

$$\hat{\mathbf{s}}(t) = \mathbf{w_{opt}}^{\top}\mathbf{x}(t) \tag{2}$$

Without loss of generality, the objective function for SPoC may be defined in terms of the epoched data $\mathbf{x}(e)$, where e refers to the e-th epoch. Assuming that the EEG sensor signal has been bandpass-filtered to a narrow frequency band and that the norm of the spatial filter is constrained, e.g., $\mathrm{Var}[\mathbf{w}^{\top}\mathbf{x}(t)] \stackrel{!}{=} 1$, the optimization problem can be solved by maximizing the covariance:

$$\begin{aligned} \mathbf{w}_{opt} &= \underset{\mathbf{w}}{\mathrm{argmax}}\{\mathrm{Cov}[\Phi_x(e), z(e)]\}\ \forall\ e \\ &\text{s.t. } \mathrm{Var}[\mathbf{w}^{\top}\mathbf{x}(t)] \stackrel{!}{=} 1 \end{aligned} \tag{3}$$

where $\Phi_x(e) = \mathrm{Var}[\hat{\mathbf{s}}](e)$. This formulation of the algorithm – called SPoC$_\lambda$ – can be transformed into a generalized eigenvalue problem and thus delivers a set of N_c spatial filters $\mathbf{W} \in \mathbb{R}^{N_c \times N_c}$. In this paper, the SPoC$_\lambda$ algorithm is utilized which subsequently will be abbreviated by the term SPoC.

Applying a SPoC filter $\mathbf{w_{tr}}$ learned from training data $\mathbf{x_{tr}}(t)$, the method allows to estimate the target variable z_{est} on novel, unseen test data $\mathbf{x_{te}}(t)$ on a single-trial basis by calculating the bandpower of the narrowband subspace signal:

$$z_{est} = \mathrm{Var}[\mathbf{w_{tr}}^{\top}\mathbf{x_{te}}(t)](e) \tag{4}$$

Using this relation, we will focus on the prediction of single-trial SVIPT performance using EEG activity within the *get-ready* phase of the trial.

As Haufe et al. (2014) have been pointing out, there is an existing forward model of the form of Equation (1) for every backward model as in Equation (2). Thus, the corresponding spatial activation patterns can be obtained from the spatial filters $\mathbf{W}$ via the covariance matrix $\mathbf{C_x}$ of the data $\mathbf{x}(t)$ via:

$$\mathbf{A} = \mathbf{C_x}\mathbf{W} \tag{5}$$

Note, that any subspace components resulting from the SPoC analysis depend mainly on four hyperparameters. In the temporal domain, two of them define the epoching interval $[t_0, t_0 + \Delta t]$ where t_0 is the starting time relative to the *go-cue* and a duration Δt. In the frequency domain, the lower frequency f_0 and the band width Δf are the hyperparameters describing the band $[f_0, f_0 + \Delta f]$ in which $\mathbf{x}(t)$ is bandpass-filtered.

Even though simple regression of bandpower features on the channel level does not fulfill the requirements of the assumed forward model, we added this simple method for comparison with SPoC. Therefore, channel-wise bandpower features of the training and test set were calculated.

2.6. Selection Criteria for Informative Oscillatory Components

Performing a grid search across subjects and SPoC parameters, we restrict the evaluation to a fixed predictive time interval given by $t_0 = -800$ ms prior to the *go-cue* and a window size of $\Delta t = 750$ ms.

As sketched in **Figure 2**, logarithmically increasing and overlapping frequency bands ranging from $\approx$ 1–100 Hz (55 configurations in total) were evaluated from the original non-filtered signals. For bandpass filtering, linear butterworth filters of 5th order were utilized. As a trial-wise target variable z, the five different performance metrics introduced in Section 2.3 were considered. Evaluating SPoC across the complete study group of 18 subjects, using five different motor performance metrics, sweeping through 55 discrete frequency bands and selecting the highest-ranked components (see details below) per configuration, results in more than 12,000 oscillatory components. In this section, we will describe an offline selection strategy in order to identify a subset of the most robust and informative oscillatory components which qualify to predict single-trial motor performance.

Upon each parameter configuration, a K = 5-fold chronological cross-validation procedure was employed upon the calculation of SPoC (Lemm et al., 2011). Only trials were considered, which survived the data preprocessing (see Section 2.4). From these, N_e EEG pre-trial epochs and their corresponding target variable values z were extracted in chronological order and split into 5 equally-sized folds. Thus, 4-folds served as training data while the remaining one was used for validating the SPoC filter as described in Equation (4). Since each fold served as test fold once, the estimated target variable $z_{est,j}$ of fold j can be concatenated for all N_e epochs, resulting in $z_{est} = [z_{est,j}]_{j \in [1,K]}$. According to Equation (5), on each fold j the corresponding test pattern is given as

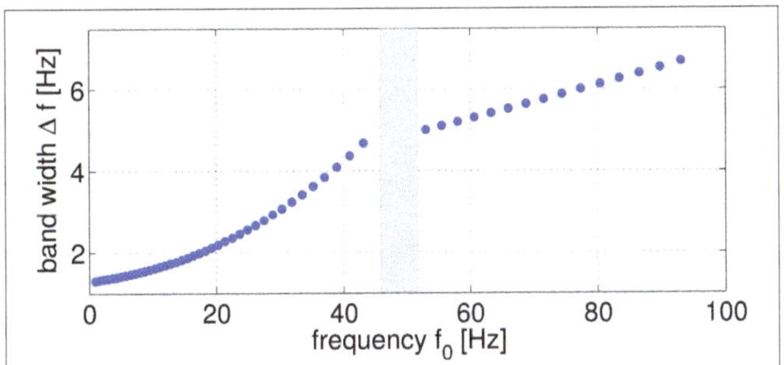

FIGURE 2 | Frequency parameter configurations characterized by the frequency f_0 and the corresponding band width Δf. In total, 55 configurations were used for computing SPoC filters. The omitted points (gray area) correspond to the power line frequency range.

$\mathbf{a_j} = \mathbf{C_{te,j}}\mathbf{w_{tr}}$ utilizing the covariance matrix $\mathbf{C_{te}}$ of the test data $\mathbf{x_{te}}(t)$.

The same cross-validation scheme was applied upon the linear regression model. The whole parameter space of 3600 configurations was screened. Note, that this number is smaller than the number of components delivered by SPoC analysis, since the latter may deliver more than one component per parameter configuration. The regression, which delivers a single component per configuration only, was trained on the training data and finally applied on test data such that an estimate z_{est} was gained on all $N(e)$ trials which had survived the data preprocessing step.

For a given parameter set, SPoC$_\lambda$ returns a set of N_c filters. As described in Tangermann et al. (2015), it is sufficient to take only the first-ranked components into consideration[1]. For this purpose, we applied a rank-based criterion. First, removed the linear trend from the ordered set of N_c eigenvalues. A threshold of $1.5 \cdot \sigma(r)$ relative to the standard deviation σ of the resulting N_c residuals r was defined. We restricted the investigation to positive eigenvalues.

Given a single component $\mathbf{w}$, the following set of scores enable to characterize its predictive strength and stability:

- **Correlation characteristics:** As a measure to verify the quality of the predictive strength of a SPoC configuration, the overall correlation of the N_e-many measured performance labels z_{true} with the corresponding predictions z_{est} can be considered:

$$R_{all} = \text{Corr}[z_{true}, z_{est}] \tag{6}$$

Similarly, the predictive strength in terms of single-trial performance can also be verified by checking the mean of the fold-wise correlations $R_j = \text{Corr}[z_{true,j}, z_{est,j}]$, which rewards temporally stable components:

$$R_{folds} = \frac{1}{K}\sum_{j=1}^{K} \text{Corr}[z_{true,j}, z_{est,j}] \tag{7}$$

The correlation based metrics R_{all} and R_{folds} come closest to the original optimization objective of the SPoC algorithm. If the trained spatial filters model trial-to-trial fluctuations well, R_{all} and R_{folds} will report a large value, but only R_{folds} allows to discriminate between single-trial predictors and session-trend models. Furthermore, a stable component requires that the correlation of each fold j shares the same sign with R_{all}. Thus, it is reasonable to require a high homogeneity H_{folds}:

$$H_{folds} = \sum_{j=1}^{K} \Theta(\text{sign}(R_{all}) \cdot \text{sign}(R_j)), \tag{8}$$

with $\Theta(x) = 1$ for $x \geq 0$ and $\Theta(x) = 0$ for $x < 0$ representing the unit-step function.

- **Separability of estimated performance:** Simulating the trial-wise online application, the continuous prediction is transferred into a two-class problem. Therefore, we split

[1] The components are sorted according to their eigenvalues. In case of SPoC$_\lambda$, they equal to the covariance between the bandpower features and the target variable.

the N_e prediction values z_{est} into two distributions ($z_{est,h}$ and $z_{est,l}$) based on the 50th percentiles of the true target variable distribution from z_{true}, thus representing high and low performance. The separability of $z_{est,h}$ and $z_{est,l}$ can be quantified by a statistical test. Here, the area under the receiver-operating-characteristic curve (Fawcett, 2006) is reported. It is denoted as z-AUC and has a chance level of 0.5.

- **Stressing the stability:** SPoC is a supervised method, which uses label information to guide the spatial filter calculation. Thus, the robustness of a resulting component can be stressed by introducing label noise. The concept of a step-wise reduction of the SNR of the labels has been introduced by Castaño-Candamil et al. (2015a). Here, SNR levels were varied from −20 dB to 10 dB by adding white noise. Applying SPoC, we estimated the target variable z_{est} for all N_e epochs using 5-fold cross-validation. At each SNR level, three sets of noisy labels z were calculated. For each SNR level, the separability of the resulting z_{est} distribution is verified by the z-AUC value. Regarding the z-AUC values as a function of the SNR, the area under this curve—referred to as AAUC_{SNR}—describes the stability of the component.

To finally identify and select robust and predictive components, we propose to apply three out of these five criteria in parallel. As a prerequisite, the data set needs to consist of at least $N_e = 150$ trials in order to ensure the convergence of the SPoC algorithm (see Dähne et al., 2014; Castaño-Candamil et al., 2015a):

1. The separability of the predicted performance z_{est} can be verified by the resulting z-AUC value. A corresponding threshold $\text{z-AUC}_{min} = 0.59$ was determined according to the 85th percentile across all configurations.
2. The stability of the component is assessed by the AAUC_{SNR}. Here, a threshold $\text{AAUC}_{min} = 0.18$ was determined from the 85th percentile.
3. As an additional stability criterion, we require all fold-wise correlations R_j to share equal sign as R_{all} such that $H_{folds,min} = 5$.

3. RESULTS

3.1. SVIPT Performance Metrics

Single-trial based SVIPT performance can be assessed by different metrics, as described in Section 2.3. In **Figure 3** examples of the trial-to-trial fluctuations of different metrics are visualized for two subjects. The visualization covers the full sessions, but omits trials removed during the preprocessing. **Figures 3A,D** show the metric reaction time (RT) for two subjects. It is not affected by a session trend. Its distribution is slight asymmetric, which is caused by a physiological limit for the minimal RT. The normalized jerk (NJ) in **Figures 3C,F** behaves in a similar manner. It is affected only slightly by a global trend, but shows a more skewed distribution compared to RT. In contrast, integrated squared jerk (ISJ) depicted in **Figure 3B**, and cursor path length (CPL) in **Figure 3E** both show a strong session trend, which can be explained by the user learning (data not shown here). A comparably strong session trend is present also in the duration metric DUR (data not shown).

The cross-correlations between all five metrics and the shape of their distributions were reported in Tangermann et al. (2015). Metrics ISJ, CPL and DUR showed strong correlations to each other, while RT as well as NJ both are rather independent from the four other metrics.

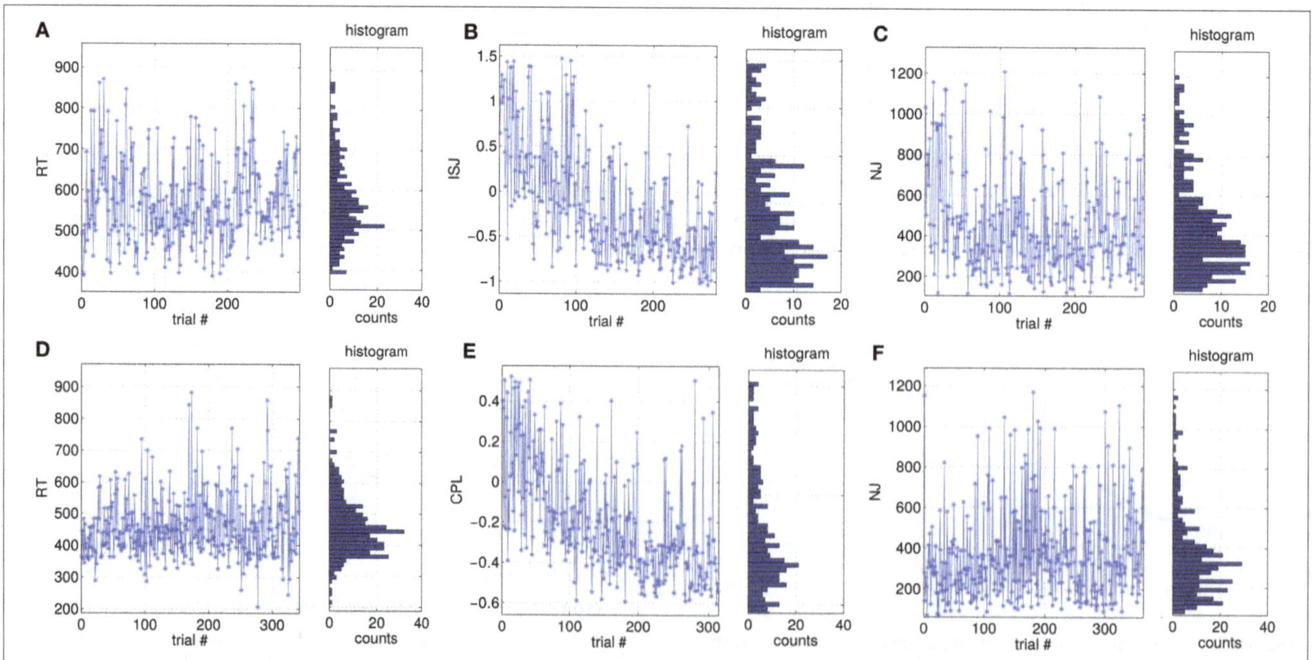

FIGURE 3 | Examples of trial-wise variations of different performance metrics over a full session, and their distributions. (A–C) are taken from data of subject S9, while **(D–F)** are from S13.

3.2. Contrasting SPoC with Linear Regression on Sensor Level

As a baseline comparison for the predictive power of SPoC components, a linear regression model employing channel-wise bandpower features was evaluated as described in Section 2.6. The resulting distributions of the overall correlation R_{all} and the performance separability z-AUC are reported in **Figure 4**. Across all configurations, SPoC delivers a median correlation $R_{all,med} = 0.07$ and a separability of z-$AUC_{med} = 0.54$, while on average the regression performs on chance level. While both methods come up with components revealing z-AUC values above chance level, those with the strongest predictive information are generated by the SPoC method.

3.3. Single-Trial Motor Performance Predictors

In **Figure 5**, five exemplary predictive and robust SPoC components, gained from five different subjects are characterized. Although SPoC components are computed from band-pass filtered data, the resulting filter **w** (gained on all available N_e trials) of a component can be re-applied to non-frequency-filtered epoched data. This spectral content of a SPoC component is shown in **Figure 5A**. The frequency band in which the component was extracted from is indicated by the dashed gray area. Using all available epochs, **Figure 5B** shows the spatial activity pattern gained via Equation (5). In **Figure 5C**, the SPoC filter weights on the 2D-scalp projection are shown. The scatter plot in **Figure 5D** reports on the measured performance metric z_{true} as a function of the predicted performance z_{est} according to the CV scheme described in Equation (4). The data points are colored by the fold index (1–5), which corresponds to the temporal order of the session. Fold 1 represents the beginning of the session, fold 5 its end. In addition, the overall correlation R_{all} reports on the predictive strength of the component. The distributions shown in **Figure 5E** illustrate the separability of the single-trial performance values z_{est}. For this purpose, the estimated labels z_{est} have been reduced to the lower and upper quartile. The corresponding true labels z_{true} were used to compute the quartiles $Q_{low,est}$ and $Q_{high,est}$ and were fitted by a kernel distribution (solid lines). In an ideal case, those quartiles would converge toward the extreme quartiles (Q_{low} and Q_{high}) of z_{true}, which are indicated by dashed lines. As a score of their separability, the score z-AUC as described in Section 2.6 is reported based on the 50th percentile.

The exemplary components in **Figure 5** are selected across the investigated frequency range depicted in **Figure 2**. The predictor of S7 can be assigned to the theta band, those of S9 and S13 correspond to the alpha range, the component for S5 originates from the beta range and the one of S8 was found in the gamma range. Regarding the scatter plots, there are two different types of patterns recognizable: single-trial predictors showing a confined point cloud without a clear trend over time (all examples except for S13), whereas the scatter plot of subject S13 shows a clear trend over the course of the session. The separability plots indicate that the predictive power of a single component nicely matches with the z-AUC value.

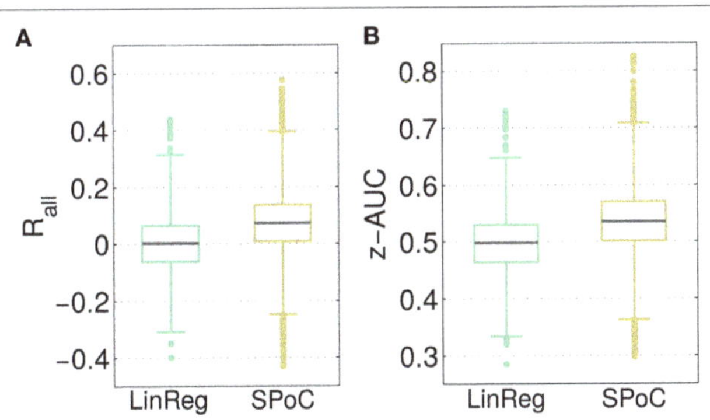

FIGURE 4 | Contrasting the predictive outcome of all 3600 tested parameter configurations for linear regression (LinReg) and over 12,000 configurations for SPoC. In **(A)**, the overall correlation R_{all} between predicted and estimated target variable values is depicted. **(B)** Shows the performance separability z-AUC. Gray lines indicate the median, boxes enclose the 25th to 75th percentile. The whisker length is set to two inter-quartile ranges.

3.4. Testing the Stability of SPoC Components

The stability of an oscillatory component can be challenged by varying the signal-to-noise ratio (SNR) of the target variable z. In **Figure 6**, the z-AUC score is investigated as a function of the SNR for two parameter configurations. **Figure 6A** shows a stable component, where z-AUC is expected to decrease, while for a non-informative component in **Figure 6B** the z-AUC can be expected around the noise floor. Thus, the resulting *area under the* z-AUC *curve* can be assessed as a tool for mapping the stability of the subspace component under challenging noise conditions. In **Figure 6C**, the distribution of this so-called $AAUC_{SNR}$ is reported for all evaluated SPoC components across all 18 subjects. The distribution of $AAUC_{SNR}$ values has its median at 0.07 and is slightly skewed.

3.5. Identification of Robust and Predictive Components

As described in Section 2.6, the first highest ranked components of each parameter configuration have been evaluated, resulting in about 12,000 different subspace components. In **Figure 7**, the configurations are characterized by their stability under noise ($AAUC_{SNR}$), which is plotted in **Figure 7A** as a function of the separability measure z-AUC, in **Figure 7B** as a function homogeneity of the fold-wise sign of the correlation H_{folds} and in **Figure 7C** as a function of the overall correlation R_{all}. A few observations can be made: First, the metrics are not centered at zero. Second, based on all initial configurations (blue data points), $AAUC_{SNR}$ correlates with the z-AUC as well as with R_{all}. The largest $AAUC_{SNR}$ values are evoked by the most homogeneous fold-wise correlation signs with $H_{folds} \geq 3$.

The threshold criteria applied to select the best of the 12,000 subspace components are indicated by red dashed lines, and red dots indicate the components finally selected. As shown in

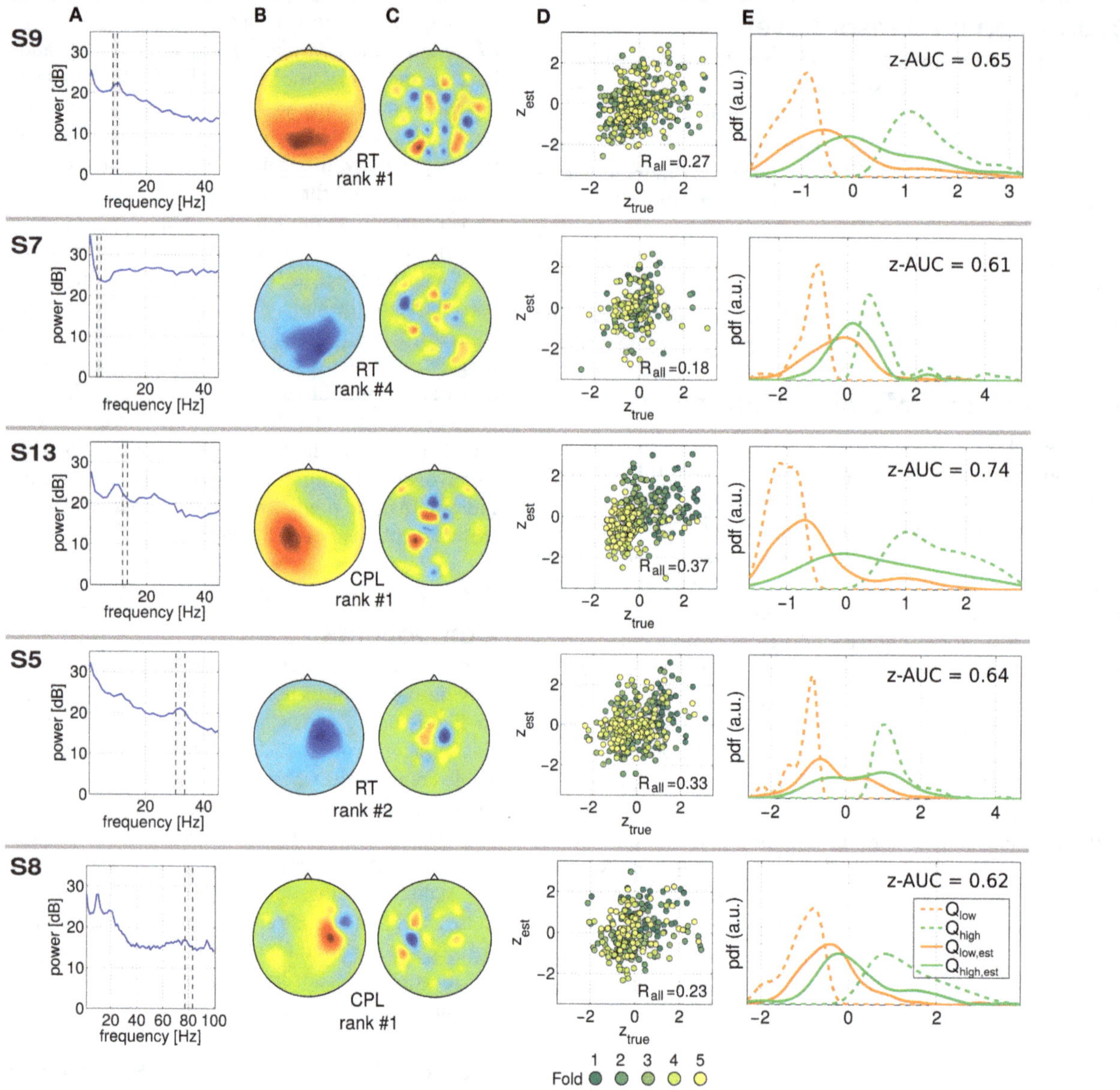

FIGURE 5 | Characterization of *exemplary* predictive SPoC features. Each component is characterized line-wise labeled by the used performance metric and the rank according to the full-session filters. **(A)** Power spectrum of the component applied on non-bandpass filtered full data. The frequency band where the component has been trained is marked by the dashed lines. Note that for the component of S8 a broader frequency range is visualized compared to the other examples. **(B)** Spatial activity pattern. **(C)** Filter weights visualized. **(D)** Scatter plot between true labels z_{true} and the predicted ones z_{est}, color coded by the fold of the chronological cross-validation. **(E)** To illustrate the separability of the prediction, the distribution of z_{true} values has been split using the corresponding trials of the upper and lower quartiles of z_{est}, which resulted in $Q_{low,est}$ and $Q_{high,est}$. As a reference, the extreme quartiles Q_{low} and Q_{high} of z_{true} are also given (dashed curves). In addition, the z-AUC value based on the 50th percentile split is reported.

Figure 8, the overall correlation R_{all} is strongly correlated with the z-AUC metric, such that an additional threshold criterion on R_{all} was not necessary. The most predictive components achieve a correlation value of up to 0.6, corresponding to $R_{all}^2 = 0.36$. Assuming a linear relationship between z_{true} and z_{est} as well as normally distributed data, this means that z_{est} can explain up to 36% of the performance variance contained in z_{true}.

In **Figure 9**, all 361 selected components are characterized by histograms in terms of their input parameters. **Figure 9A** displays the subject-wise grouping. In total, 11 out of 18 subjects contribute at least one component, for three subjects more than 50 configurations survive the selection procedure. **Figure 9B** shows the histogram over the number of trials available for the offline analysis. Note, that this histogram is dominated by the best three subjects reported in **Figure 9A**, who contributed a large number of the selected 361 configurations. **Figure 9C** characterizes the selected components assigned to their underlying frequency band $[f_0, f_0+\Delta f]$ (see **Figure 2**). Most components are gained from the alpha- and beta-band range. Interestingly, robust features detected in the gamma band were

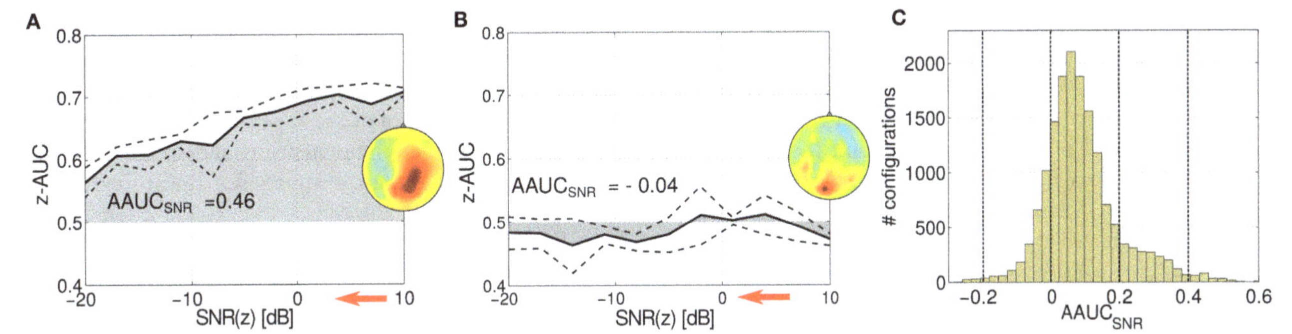

FIGURE 6 | Stressing the stability of two exemplary SPoC components for two different parameter configurations (A,B). While stepwise decreasing the SNR ratio (indicated by the red arrow), z-AUC-values (solid lines) describing the separability of the prediction are plotted together with standard deviations (dashed lines). The area under the z-AUC curve—further on called $AAUC_{SNR}$—describes the stability of the component under the challenge of added noise. **(C)** Shows the histogram of all $AAUC_{SNR}$ scores evaluated for the considered parameter configurations.

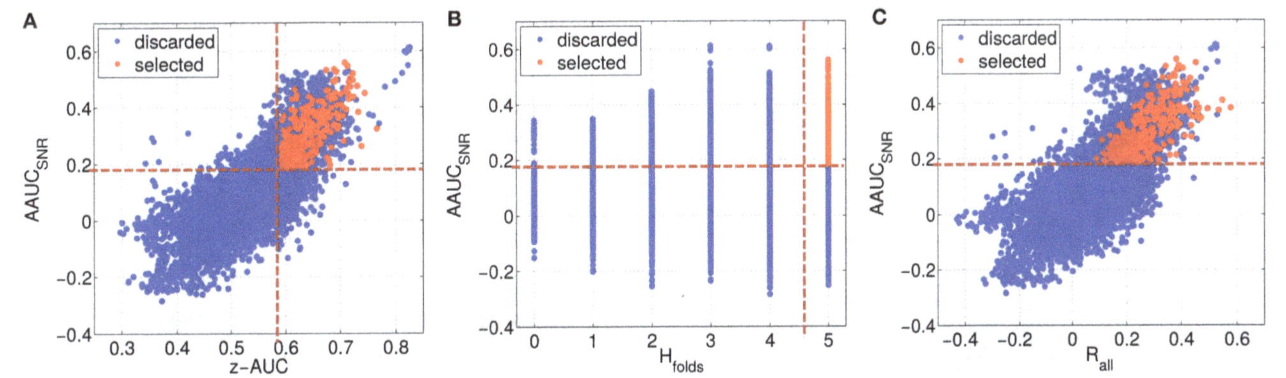

FIGURE 7 | Characterizing the space of SPoC components by several metrics, which describe their stability and predictive information. The SNR-challenged $AAUC_{SNR}$ is given as a function of the performance separability z-AUC **(A)**, in relation to the homogeneity of the correlation sign H_{folds} **(B)**, and dependent on the overall correlation R_{all} **(C)**. Red data points describe the selected SPoC components after applying thresholds (dashed red lines).

dominantly selected for their ability to predict CPL. The slow frequency (<4 Hz) components are dominated by artifactual subspaces. **Figure 9D** reports on the occurrences of the different performance metrics among the selected components. Most components could be extracted for RT (61%), followed by CPL (16%) while all other metrics contribute almost equally well with 6–8% of the selected components. **Figure 9E** provides an overview over the SPoC ranks of the surviving components. The rank ordering corresponds to the eigenvalue ordering of the complete data set. As the number of selected components drop with increased rank, the ranking is associated with the information content of the subspace component.

SPoC as a linear filtering method allows for a limited neurophysiological interpretation of spatial activity patterns. A representative subset of typical scalp topographies from the selected stable and informative subspaces are plotted in **Figure 10**. The components were assigned to three groups. About 70% of components fall into group G1, which comprises patterns ranging from activations in occipital, to central or frontal areas. The maximum activity of those components often is found over one of the hemispheres. About 10% of the components fall in group G2. They show patterns of probable non-neural sources and may represent e.g., eye artifacts, muscular activity or single noisy channels. Group G3 comprises noisy topographies. As indicated by patterns in the intersection area of the three groups, mixed components were observed as well. The detailed parameter configurations of each of the plotted components is listed in **Table 1**.

4. DISCUSSION

We hypothesized that subject-specific pre-trial brain signals contain information which allows to partially explain and temporally predict the trial-by-trial variability of the upcoming motor performance in SVIPT. To test the hypothesis, we developed a workflow which is capable to extract informative oscillatory EEG subspace components and to identify the most robust ones. Simulating an online application, our analysis revealed strong evidence that the band power of the selected components is predictive for the single-trial SVIPT performance. Major findings were that these components indeed exist, but need to be optimized for individual users. With 11 out of 18, not all, but a majority of the subjects revealed the desired informative features.

In the following we will first discuss the decision to utilize SPoC instead of other alternative analysis methods. In this context, the proposed selection procedure and the stability of SPoC components over time is discussed, with a special focus onto the role of SNR, frequency and the illiteracy phenomenon. In addition, the detected components will be related to existing literature and characterized on a group-level with respect to the covered frequency bands, sub-processes reflected by the components and the time courses revealed. Before concluding, we will describe a neuroergonomically enhanced rehabilitation paradigm as a possible use case of our contribution.

4.1. SPoC and its Alternatives

Designing the data analysis workflow, we built upon our background in BCI. Accordingly, we carefully selected algorithmic building blocks only, if they can be applied in single-trial analysis [e.g., the application of the spatial SPoC filter according to Equation (4)]. This decision should simplify the translation of the presented workflow to closed-loop experiments in the future. The choice of the supervised SPoC algorithm for extracting informative components is supported by its good performance compared to a supervised linear regression of bandpower features on the sensor level (see Section 3.2). This is in accordance with findings of Dähne et al. (2014). On data from an auditory steady-state evoked potential paradigm, these authors reported better results for SPoC compared to both, linear regression and an unsupervised subspace decomposition using independent component analysis (ICA). SPoC does not reconstruct sources of the brain, but instead performs a supervised subspace decomposition. Thus, a SPoC subspace component can not be expected to correspond to a single physical source or even a dipole source (even though such SPoC components are possible). Theoretically even several spread-out brain areas may contribute to a single SPoC component, if they share oscillatory activity which co-varies over time with the labels. The choice between SPoC and source reconstruction approaches (Gonzalez Andino et al., 2005) represents a trade-off—while the latter may facilitate the interpretation of results, SPoC components avoid several of the drawbacks mentioned in Section 2.5. As our workflow was aligned in terms of applicability for single-trial online paradigms, our decision was biased toward SPoC.

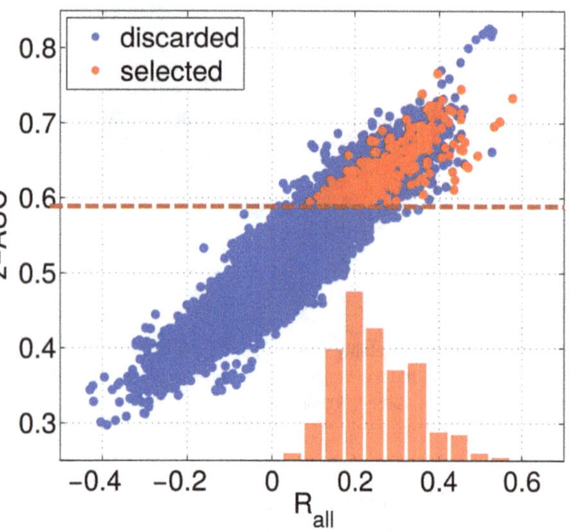

FIGURE 8 | Relation between separability metric z-AUC and the overall correlation R_{all} for all SPoC configurations (blue dots) and the selected ones (red dots). The dashed red line indicates the threshold z-AUC$_{min}$ applied to select most informative components. The red bars indicate the distribution of R_{all} values for the selected components.

4.2. Selection Criteria for Robust and Predictive Components

Over-fitting is a general issue for supervised methods and for SPoC in particular, as no form of regularization was applied. This requires some form of *post-hoc* selection of SPoC components. The situation is aggravated, as SPoC returns full rank filter matrices, which result in a very large numbers of subspaces. However, only a fraction of these can be expected to be informative about the labels. As robustness over time as well as with respect to label noise are important criteria for the potential closed-loop applicability of a component, a single selection criterion (e.g., a threshold on the correlation value) is not sufficient. By that, we selected three criteria (see Section 2.6), which suited best these requirements. Out of the initial five selection criteria, the two scores R_{all} and R_{folds} turned out to

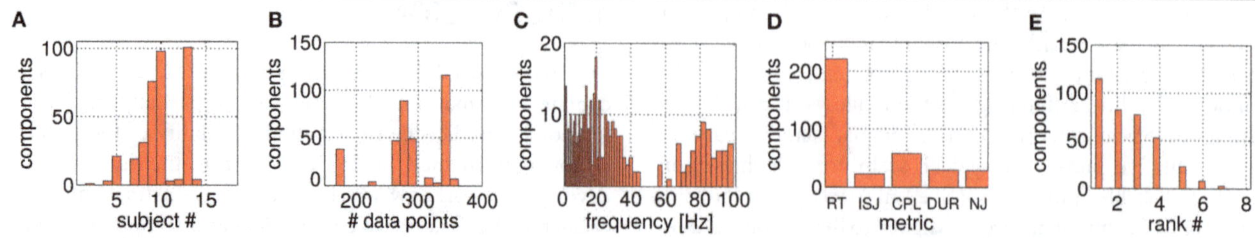

FIGURE 9 | Histograms of different parameters solely for the selected SPoC components. (A) Shows the assignment over the 18 subjects. **(B)** Gives the allocation over data set sizes N_e (with a lower limit of 150 trials). **(C)** Visualizes the distribution across frequency bands. **(D)** Depicts the spread of components over the five utilized motor performance metrics, while **(E)** shows the split according to their SPoC rank positions.

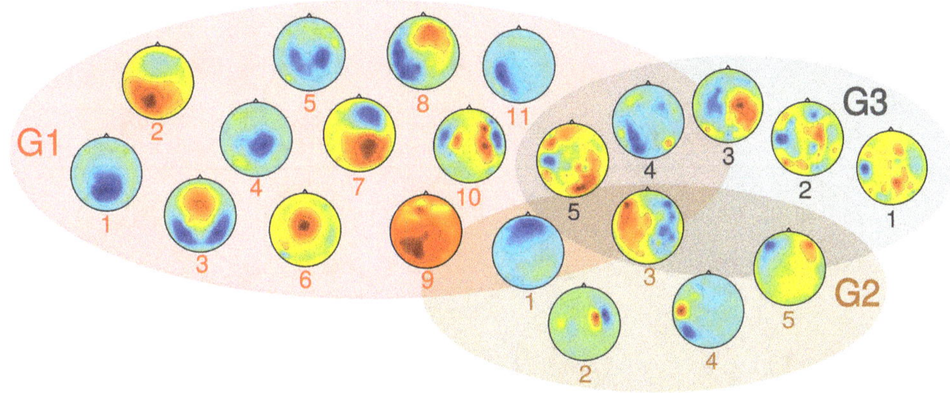

FIGURE 10 | Overview over typical activity patterns resulting from the selected components, grouped in three categories: G1 consists of components with neural origin, G2 comprises artifact-related subspaces and G3 captures non-informative components. Details on their parameter configurations are given in **Table 1**.

TABLE 1 | Parameter configurations for components of groups G1, G2 and G3 as visualized in Figure 10.

	G1				G2				G3			
Comp. no.	Subject	f_0 [Hz]	Metric	Rank	Subject	f_0 [Hz]	Metric	Rank	Subject	f_0 [Hz]	Metric	Rank
1	S13	7.9	NJ	2	S14	1.0	RT	2	S12	27.5	ISJ	1
2	S9	8.7	ISJ	3	S11	27.5	ISJ	1	S10	20.3	RT	1
3	S13	7.9	RT	3	S10	5.0	DUR	1	S9	8.7	ISJ	1
4	S13	8.7	NJ	2	S9	39.0	DUR	2	S15	19.2	CPL	1
5	S10	15.3	RT	6	S10	3.7	RT	3	S10	74.4	NJ	2
6	S5	30.4	RT	3								
7	S9	14.4	RT	5								
8	S9	10.2	ISJ	4								
9	S9	18.2	DUR	1								
10	S8	77.4	CPL	4								
11	S13	74.4	CPL	1								

be beneficial for characterizing the extracted components. Thus, they were omitted for the selection process, since a strong correlation between z-AUC and R_{all} was observed (see **Figure 8**). The same holds for the correlation between z-AUC and R_{folds} (not shown).

An alternative to the current selection procedure would be to relax the thresholds and combine it with additional methods to judge the plausibility of the remaining components *post-hoc*. For ICA components, workflows have been proposed, such as MARA, an automatic classification of artifactual components by Winkler et al. (2014). MARA uses features based on topology, time-frequency analysis and source reconstruction. Similar approaches have been proposed by Daly et al. (2015) and Grosse-Wentrup et al. (2013).

4.3. Influence of SNR on SPoC Components

By applying rather strict selection criteria, weaker but still informative components may have been removed. As a result, the data of some subjects did not reveal informative pre-go oscillatory components. Reasons may be a lower SNR of their data, which hides potential informative content from the SPoC analysis, especially in combination with the limited number of trials used. The work of Castaño-Candamil et al. (2015a) on robustness testing of SPoC components backs this interpretation. In this case, future improvements may be expected by regularization techniques introduced to SPoC, a reduction of the dimensionality prior to applying SPoC, using more data or from transfer learning approaches. However, we can not exclude that informative oscillatory components may not be visible to the EEG or may be absent in some subjects. This problem has been described as BCI "illiteracy." It has predominantly been studied in the context of motor imagery paradigms for the control of BCI applications (Hammer et al., 2012), where decoding the imagery class usually is not possible for a subset of subjects. The BCI illiteracy problem was tackled by novel experimental setups like hybrid BCI paradigms (Allison et al., 2012; Müller-Putz et al., 2015), but could also be alleviated by more advanced decoding methods (Sannelli et al., 2010).

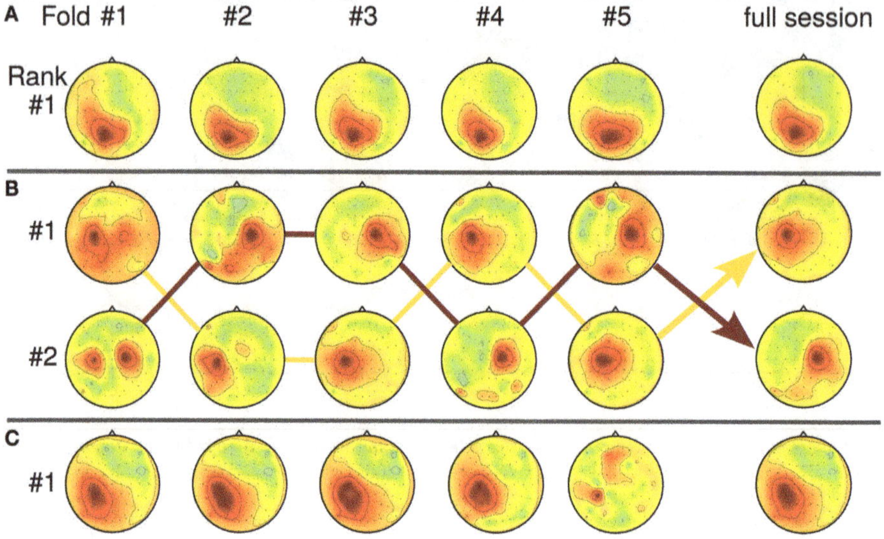

FIGURE 11 | Relation between SPoC rank stability and pattern homogeneity over five cross-validation folds (chronological order). (A) Stationary case: component is first-ranked across all five folds (data of subject S9, $f = [9.4, 11]$ Hz, RT). **(B)** Rank switching: Two almost stable components switch rank positions between folds (S5, $f = [27.5, 30.3]$ Hz, RT). Lines connect the corresponding topologies. **(C)** Intensity variation: intensity of first-ranked component decreases over time folds (S13, $f = [13.6, 15.3]$ Hz, CPL).

4.4. Rank Stability of SPoC Components over Time

In Section 4.3, the relation between SPoC solutions and the SNR of the data has been touched. As SPoC ranks the detected components according to their covariance values, solutions may seem unstable when only the first-ranked component is considered. In real-life data sets, variation of the SNR over time can induce rank switches or mixed components. Tracking a component over multiple runs of the subspace decomposition method is a challenging task, especially as mixtures theoretically can not be distinguished from a single source. However, as similar problems arise for online learning of blind source separation methods like ICA, practical solutions are available (Hsu et al., 2015). **Figure 11** gives examples of stable, stationary components (**Figure 11A**) and of unstable SPoC components (**Figures 11B,C**), both observed over the five chronological cross-validation folds. Instable components may be evoked if the stationarity assumption of SPoC is violated e.g., by slow temporal intensity variations due to user learning. For **Figure 11B**, arrows indicate a possible path through rank positions across folds by connecting corresponding components. Please observe, that SPoC generates cases with even severe variation between folds as those depicted in **Figures 11B,C**. However, such components typically have been removed during the selection process. While mixed, yet stable components may be hard to interpret, they can still be useful for predicting the task performance.

We have observed a high sensitivity of SPoC for small differences in the frequency parameters. Seemingly unstable components which display rank switching behavior (see **Figure 12** at 8.7 Hz) can sometimes be stabilized by slightly changing the frequency, e.g., to 9.4 Hz in this example. Further increase of the frequency to 10.2 Hz again induces instability in this example.

4.5. Characterization of Informative SPoC Components and Sub-Processes

The proposed SPoC workflow delivers a diverse set of oscillatory components, which vary in their topological patterns as well as in their underlying frequency band. This is not surprising, since SVIPT requires the interaction of several cognitive sub-processes in order to reach a good overall performance. For each sub-process, one or more specific neural features may exist, with all of them being informative about the overall outcome of the complex task.

The best components differ between subjects and predominantly occur in the alpha band, followed by beta and gamma band. Our findings are supported by informative features in the alpha and beta-range observed during pre-movement intervals of a hand grasping task (Zaepffel et al., 2013; Meyer et al., 2014; Yang et al., 2014). Furthermore, the informative frequency ranges for SVIPT are comparable to those reported for attention related tasks (Gonzalez Andino et al., 2005; Hoogenboom et al., 2010; van Ede et al., 2012). We obtained best results when using RT as a performance metric, which supports our earlier findings on disjunct data from younger subjects (Castaño-Candamil et al., 2015c; Meinel et al., 2015). RT of course does not automatically lead to a successful trial, but it can be seen as an indicator for a quick ramp-up phase and alertness. For fewer users, presumably those with highest SNR characteristics, informative oscillatory features could be identified for other performance metrics of the force task, too.

Comparing the topological plots of group G1 in **Figure 10** with those reported in literature, it can be observed that many

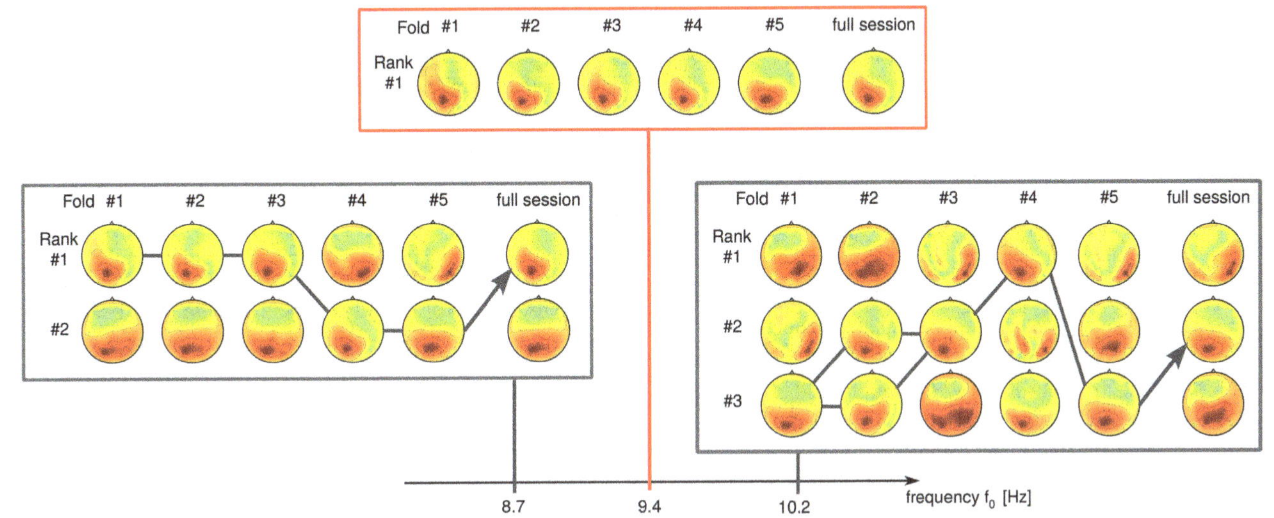

FIGURE 12 | Influence of the frequency band upon the rank stability. While stable at $f_0 = 9.4$ Hz, a component develops rank instability with slight increase/decrease of its frequency band (data of subject S9).

of them resemble patterns emerging for motor imagery tasks in BCI (Krauledat et al., 2008). These often display a clear maximum of activity in channels located over one of the sensorimotor areas (cp. pattern 5 of G1 in **Figure 10** and the pattern of S5 in **Figure 5**) or are located centrally over both hemispheres. While similarity of patterns are by no way a proof for an origin of these oscillatory components in the sensorimotor cortices, the hand force action required to succeed in the SVIPT task would allow for such components.

Other components show a maximum intensity over parietal and occipital areas and may reflect the involvement of the visual system in the SVIPT task. Pattern 2 of **Figure 10** and patterns in **Figure 11A** display a lateralization similar to patterns reported for *directed* and covert visual attention processes (Hanslmayr et al., 2007; Horschig et al., 2014a). Components with a centrally located maximum (cp. pattern 1 of **Figure 10** or the pattern of S9 in **Figure 5**), or with double wing shapes (e.g., pattern 3 of **Figure 10**) resemble components reported for generalized visual attention processes (van Dijk et al., 2008; Meyer et al., 2014). Again, most of these rather clear patterns originate from the alpha frequency band.

While the relevance of several of the selected components cannot be fully interpreted, we do consider these features as added value for neurologists, e.g., by tracking the power time course over sessions for a subject-specific component. Further insight into underlying sub-processes and participating brain areas may be obtained from a *post-hoc* source reconstruction applied upon single SPoC subspaces.

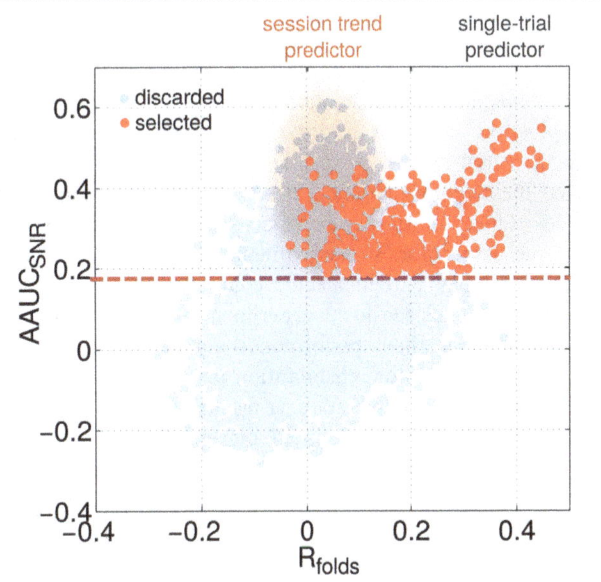

FIGURE 13 | The identification of session trends vs. single-trial variations of performance is possible by localizing a predictor's characteristic with respect to two selection criteria. The scatter plot visualizes $AAUC_{SNR}$ as a function of the mean correlation value across folds R_{folds} for all configurations (light blue) and the selected ones only (red). Two classes of predictors can be identified: single-trial predictors showing a high R_{folds} value while session-trend predictors show a very low R_{folds} value.

4.6. Behavioral Variability on Different Time Scales

Independent of the choice of the exact motor task, subjects generally display two types of performance variations (Chaisanguanthum et al., 2014). First, a large trial-to-trial performance variability is observed from behavioral data. Second, slow performance drifts can occur over the course of a session. Accordingly, SPoC can deliver components, which reflect either one of the two types of performance variations. To tell them apart, a comparison between R_{all} and R_{folds} is helpful. High values for R_{all}, but low for R_{folds} indicate a session trend. If both are high, then the component is informative for trial-by-trial variation (see *single-trial predictors* and *session trend predictors* in **Figure 13** as well as the examples given in **Figure 5**).

For the purpose of brain-state-informed closed-loop experimenting, single-trial predictors may be more suitable. Session trend predictors, however, may still be useful for pre-cleaning the performance labels. While session trend predictors may reflect an increasing fatigue or a learning effect, it is much harder to determine underlying mechanisms, which cause the rapidly changing trial-to-trial performance of the single-trial predictors (Wu et al., 2014; Hadjiosif and Smith, 2015; Osu et al., 2015). However, our identified components reveal strong evidence that the pre-trial brain activity is partially informative about trail-by-trial variability of motor performance. This in accordance with Churchland et al. (2006) who reported on monkey experiments that at least 30% of behavioral variability could be explained by the fluctuations of preparatory neural activity in the dorsal premotor cortex. However, Chaisanguanthum et al. (2014) stated only a weak relationship between motor cortex activity (PMd/M1) in monkeys and trial-wise fluctuations of behavior.

4.7. Closed-Loop Experimenting as Neuroergonomical Application

The predictive EEG features are extracted from a pre-go interval of each trial. Our pipeline carefully simulated an online scenario, but this approximation of course can not replace the evaluation within a future online study. However, the informative trial-by-trial performance predictors may serve to enhance the neureorgonomical needs of motor rehabilitation scenarios. Since motor performance variability was reported to become larger for stroke patients (Lodha et al., 2010), applying identified patient-specific components within brain-state dependent closed-loop experimenting may enable to causally influence their performance e.g., by manipulating difficulty levels in motor rehabilitation paradigms. So far, BCI methods in stroke rehabilitation (Ang and Guan, 2013) have been used to detect the attempted movement of the affected hand by analyzing informative ERD/ERS features of the EEG and subsequently close the feedback loop for the patient either by triggering a simulated hand movement on a screen (Pichiorri et al., 2015) or by triggering a passive movement of the affected hand, e.g., via an external robotic device or an active orthesis (Ramos-Murguialday et al., 2013).

When implemented in future closed-loop applications, it may be worth to combine SPoC features across multiple frequency bands e.g., by a regression approach. This might allow for enhancing the trial-wise performance prediction, in case the information contained in different frequency bands is independent. Similarly, the combination of predictors based on different performance metrics might serve to gain an enhanced performance estimate.

5. CONCLUSION

In summary, we have shown that the proposed workflow is a suitable basis to identify subject-specific single-trial based neural markers which are predictive for the performance of an upcoming motor task. Those predictors may be valuable building blocks for neuroergonomic applications since they are informative about the status of the visual subsystem as well as the sub-processes involved in hand motor control. Moreover, exploiting those features in future closed-loop experimenting, e.g., by temporal gating of upcoming trials, they will allow for brain-state-informed rehabilitation paradigms. Furthermore, the group-level analysis motivated to utilize our workflow to gain a better understanding of trial-to-trial variations of cognitive sub-processes, which are relevant for a successful rehabilitation outcome.

AUTHOR CONTRIBUTIONS

Conceived and designed the experiments: AM, SC, JR, and MT. Performed the experiments: AM, SC, and MT. Analyzed the data: AM and MT. Contributed reagents/materials/analysis tools: AM, SC, JR, and MT. Wrote the paper: AM and MT.

ACKNOWLEDGMENTS

This work was fully supported by BrainLinks-BrainTools Cluster of Excellence funded by the German Research Foundation (DFG), grant number EXC 1086. The analysis was partly performed on the computational resource bwUniCluster funded by the Ministry of Science, Research and the Arts Baden-Württemberg and the Universities of the State of Baden-Württemberg, Germany, within the framework program bwHPC. The article processing charge was funded by the German Research Foundation (DFG) and the Albert-Ludwigs-University Freiburg in the funding programme Open Access Publishing. The authors would like to thank to Eva-Maria Schlichtmann for her support with the data collection.

REFERENCES

Abe, M. O., and Sternad, D. (2013). Directionality in distribution and temporal structure of variability in skill acquisition. *Front. Hum. Neurosci.* 7:225. doi: 10.3389/fnhum.2013.00225

Allison, B. Z., Brunner, C., Altstätter, C., Wagner, I. C., Grissmann, S., and Neuper, C. (2012). A hybrid ERD/SSVEP BCI for continuous simultaneous two dimensional cursor control. *J. Neurosci. Methods* 209, 299–307. doi: 10.1016/j.jneumeth.2012.06.022

Ang, K. K., and Guan, C. (2013). Brain-computer interface in stroke rehabilitation. *J. Comput. Sci. Eng.* 7, 139–146. doi: 10.5626/JCSE.2013.7.2.139

Blankertz, B., Dornhege, G., Krauledat, M., Müller, K.-R., and Curio, G. (2007). The non-invasive berlin brain–computer interface: fast acquisition of effective performance in untrained subjects. *Neuroimage* 37, 539–550. doi: 10.1016/j.neuroimage.2007.01.051

Bradberry, T. J., Rong, F., and Contreras-Vidal, J. L. (2009). Decoding center-out hand velocity from MEG signals during visuomotor adaptation. *Neuroimage* 47, 1691–1700. doi: 10.1016/j.neuroimage.2009.06.023

Busch, N. A., Dubois, J., and VanRullen, R. (2009). The phase of ongoing EEG oscillations predicts visual perception. *J. Neurosci.* 29, 7869–7876. doi: 10.1523/JNEUROSCI.0113-09.2009

Camus, M., Ragert, P., Vandermeeren, Y., and Cohen, L. G. (2009). Mechanisms controlling motor output to a transfer hand after learning a sequential pinch force skill with the opposite hand. *Clin. Neurophysiol.* 120, 1859–1865. doi: 10.1016/j.clinph.2009.08.013

Castaño-Candamil, S., Höhne, J., Martínez-Vargas, J.-D., An, X.-W., Castellanos-Domínguez, G., et al. (2015b). Solving the EEG inverse problem based on space-time-frequency structured sparsity constraints. *Neuroimage* 118, 598–612. doi: 10.1016/j.neuroimage.2015.05.052

Castaño-Candamil, S., Meinel, A., Dähne, S., and Tangermann, M. (2015a). "Probing meaningfulness of oscillatory EEG components with bootstrapping, label noise and reduced training sets," in *Engineering in Medicine and Biology Society (EMBC), 2015 37th Annual International Conference of the IEEE*, (Milan: IEEE), 5159–5162.

Castaño-Candamil, S., Meinel, A., Reis, J., and Tangermann, M. (2015c). P186. correlates to influence user performance in a hand motor rehabilitation task. *Clin. Neurophysiol.* 126, e166–e167. doi: 10.1016/j.clinph.2015.04.282

Chaisanguanthum, K. S., Shen, H. H., and Sabes, P. N. (2014). Motor variability arises from a slow random walk in neural state. *J. Neurosci.* 34, 12071–12080. doi: 10.1523/JNEUROSCI.3001-13.2014

Churchland, M. M., Byron, M. Y., Ryu, S. I., Santhanam, G., and Shenoy, K. V. (2006). Neural variability in premotor cortex provides a signature of motor preparation. *J. Neurosci.* 26, 3697–3712. doi: 10.1523/JNEUROSCI.3762-05.2006

Cohen, R., and Sternad, D. (2009). Variability in motor learning: relocating, channeling and reducing noise. *Exp. Brain Res.* 193, 69–83. doi: 10.1007/s00221-008-1596-1

Coupar, F., Pollock, A., Van Wijck, F., Morris, J., and Langhorne, P. (2010). Simultaneous bilateral training for improving arm function after stroke. *Cochrane Database Syst. Rev.* 4:CD006432. doi: 10.1002/14651858.CD006432.pub2

Dähne, S., Meinecke, F. C., Haufe, S., Höhne, J., Tangermann, M., Müller, K.-R., et al. (2014). SPoC: a novel framework for relating the amplitude of neuronal oscillations to behaviorally relevant parameters. *Neuroimage* 86, 111–122. doi: 10.1016/j.neuroimage.2013.07.079

Daly, I., Scherer, R., Billinger, M., and Muller-Putz, G. (2015). FORCe: Fully online and automated artifact removal for brain-computer interfacing. *IEEE Trans. Neural Syst. Rehabil. Eng.* 23, 725–736. doi: 10.1109/TNSRE.2014.2346621

Dobkin, B. H. (2004). Strategies for stroke rehabilitation. *Lancet Neurol.* 3, 528–536. doi: 10.1016/S1474-4422(04)00851-8

Faisal, A. A., Selen, L. P., and Wolpert, D. M. (2008). Noise in the nervous system. *Nat. Rev. Neurosci.* 9, 292–303. doi: 10.1038/nrn2258

Fawcett, T. (2006). An introduction to ROC analysis. *Pattern Recogn. Lett.* 27, 861–874. doi: 10.1016/j.patrec.2005.10.010

French, B., Thomas, L. H., Leathley, M. J., Sutton, C. J., McAdam, J., Forster, A., et al. (2007). Repetitive task training for improving functional ability after stroke. *Cochrane Database Syst. Rev.* 4:CD006073. doi: 10.1002/14651858.CD006073.pub2

Fritsch, B., Reis, J., Martinowich, K., Schambra, H. M., Ji, Y., Cohen, L. G., et al. (2010). Direct current stimulation promotes BDNF-dependent synaptic plasticity: potential implications for motor learning. *Neuron* 66, 198–204. doi: 10.1016/j.neuron.2010.03.035

Gonzalez Andino, S. L., Michel, C. M., Thut, G., Landis, T., and Grave de Peralta, R. (2005). Prediction of response speed by anticipatory high-frequency (gamma band) oscillations in the human brain. *Hum. Brain Mapp.* 24, 50–58. doi: 10.1002/hbm.20056

Grech, R., Cassar, T., Muscat, J., Camilleri, K., Fabri, S., Zervakis, M., et al. (2008). Review on solving the inverse problem in EEG source analysis. *J. Neuroengineering Rehabil.* 5, 792–800. doi: 10.1186/1743-0003-5-25

Grosse-Wentrup, M., Harmeling, S., Zander, T., Hill, J., and Scholkopf, B. (2013). "How to test the quality of reconstructed sources in independent component analysis (ICA) of EEG/MEG data," in *International Workshop on Pattern Recognition in Neuroimaging (PRNI)* (IEEE), 102–105. doi: 10.1109/PRNI.2013.35

Hadjiosif, A. M., and Smith, M. A. (2015). Flexible control of safety margins for action based on environmental variability. *J. Neurosci.* 35, 9106–9121. doi: 10.1523/JNEUROSCI.1883-14.2015

Hammer, E. M., Halder, S., Blankertz, B., Sannelli, C., Dickhaus, T., Kleih, S., et al. (2012). Psychological predictors of SMR-BCI performance. *Biol. Psychol.* 89, 80–86. doi: 10.1016/j.biopsycho.2011.09.006

Hammon, P. S., Makeig, S., Poizner, H., Todorov, E., and Sa, V. D. (2008). Predicting reaching targets from human EEG. *Signal Proces. Mag. IEEE* 25, 69–77. doi: 10.1109/MSP.2008.4408443

Hanslmayr, S., Aslan, A., Staudigl, T., Klimesch, W., Herrmann, C. S., and Bäuml, K.-H. (2007). Prestimulus oscillations predict visual perception performance between and within subjects. *NeuroImage* 37, 1465–1473. doi: 10.1016/j.neuroimage.2007.07.011

Haufe, S., Meinecke, F., Görgen, K., Dähne, S., Haynes, J.-D., Blankertz, B., et al. (2014). On the interpretation of weight vectors of linear models in multivariate neuroimaging. *NeuroImage* 87, 96–110. doi: 10.1016/j.neuroimage.2013.10.067

Hoogenboom, N., Schoffelen, J.-M., Oostenveld, R., and Fries, P. (2010). Visually induced gamma-band activity predicts speed of change detection in humans. *NeuroImage* 51, 1162–1167. doi: 10.1016/j.neuroimage.2010.03.041

Horschig, J. M., Jensen, O., van Schouwenburg, M. R., Cools, R., and Bonnefond, M. (2014a). Alpha activity reflects individual abilities to adapt to the environment. *NeuroImage* 89, 235–243. doi: 10.1016/j.neuroimage.2013.12.018

Horschig, J. M., Oosterheert, W., Oostenveld, R., and Jensen, O. (2014b). Modulation of posterior alpha activity by spatial attention allows for controlling a continuous brain–computer interface. *Brain Topogr.* 28, 852–864. doi: 10.1007/s10548-014-0401-7

Horschig, J. M., Zumer, J. M., and Bahramisharif, A. (2014c). Hypothesis-driven methods to augment human cognition by optimizing cortical oscillations. *Front. Syst. Neurosci.* 8:119. doi: 10.3389/fnsys.2014.00119

Hsu, S.-H., Mullen, T., Jung, T.-P., and Cauwenberghs, G. (2015). "Validating online recursive independent component analysis on EEG data," in *Neural Engineering (NER), 2015 7th International IEEE/EMBS Conference on*, (Montpellier: IEEE), 918–921. doi: 10.1109/NER.2015.7146775

Jensen, O., Bahramisharif, A., Oostenveld, R., Klanke, S., Hadjipapas, A., Okazaki, Y. O., et al. (2011). Using brain–computer interfaces and brain-state dependent stimulation as tools in cognitive neuroscience. *Front. Psychol.* 2:100. doi: 10.3389/fpsyg.2011.00100

Jerbi, K., Vidal, J., Mattout, J., Maby, E., Lecaignard, F., Ossandon, T., et al. (2011). Inferring hand movement kinematics from meg, EEG and intracranial EEG: from brain-machine interfaces to motor rehabilitation. *IRBM* 32, 8–18. doi: 10.1016/j.irbm.2010.12.004

Kindermans, P.-J., Tangermann, M., Müller, K.-R., and Schrauwen, B. (2014). Integrating dynamic stopping, transfer learning and language models in an adaptive zero-training erp speller. *J. Neural Eng.* 11:035005. doi: 10.1088/1741-2560/11/3/035005

Krauledat, M., Tangermann, M., Blankertz, B., and Müller, K.-R. (2008). Towards zero training for brain-computer interfacing. *PLoS ONE* 3:e2967. doi: 10.1371/journal.pone.0002967

Kwakkel, G., Kollen, B. J., and Krebs, H. I. (2008). Effects of robot-assisted therapy on upper limb recovery after stroke: a systematic review. *Neurorehabil. Neural Rep.* 22, 111–121. doi: 10.1177/1545968307305457

Lage, G. M., Ugrinowitsch, H., Apolinário-Souza, T., Vieira, M. M., Albuquerque, M. R., and Benda, R. N. (2015). Repetition and variation in motor practice: a review of neural correlates. *Neurosci. Biobehav. Rev.* 57, 132–141. doi: 10.1016/j.neubiorev.2015.08.012

Langhorne, P., Bernhardt, J., and Kwakkel, G. (2011). Stroke rehabilitation. *Lancet* 377, 1693–1702. doi: 10.1016/S0140-6736(11)60325-5

Lemm, S., Blankertz, B., Dickhaus, T., and Müller, K.-R. (2011). Introduction to machine learning for brain imaging. *NeuroImage* 56, 387–399. doi: 10.1016/j.neuroimage.2010.11.004

Lew, E. Y., Chavarriaga, R., Silvoni, S., and Millán, J. D. R. (2014). Single trial prediction of self-paced reaching directions from EEG signals. *Front. Neurosci.* 8:222. doi: 10.3389/fnins.2014.00222

Lodha, N., Naik, S. K., Coombes, S. A., and Cauraugh, J. H. (2010). Force control and degree of motor impairments in chronic stroke. *Clin. Neurophysiol.* 121, 1952–1961. doi: 10.1016/j.clinph.2010.04.005

Logar, V., Škrjanc, I., Belič, A., Karba, R., Brežan, S., Koritnik, B., et al. (2008). Gripping-force identification using EEG and phase-demodulation approach. *Neurosci. Res.* 60, 389–396. doi: 10.1016/j.neures.2007.12.009

Maeder, C. L., Sannelli, C., Haufe, S., and Blankertz, B. (2012). Pre-stimulus sensorimotor rhythms influence brain–computer interface classification performance. *Neural Syst. Rehabil. Eng. IEEE Trans.* 20, 653–662. doi: 10.1109/TNSRE.2012.2205707

Makeig, S., Kothe, C., Mullen, T., Bigdely-Shamlo, N., Zhang, Z., and Kreutz-Delgado, K. (2012). Evolving signal processing for brain–computer interfaces. *Proc. IEEE* 100, 1567–1584. doi: 10.1109/JPROC.2012.2185009

Meinel, A., Castaño-Candamil, J. S., Dähne, S., Reis, J., and Tangermann, M. (2015). "EEG band power predicts single-trial reaction time in a hand motor task," in *Proceedings of International IEEE Conference on Neural Engineering (NER)*, (Montpellier: IEEE), 182–185. doi: 10.1109/ner.2015.71 46590

Meyer, T., Peters, J., Zander, T. O., Schölkopf, B., and Grosse-Wentrup, M. (2014). Predicting motor learning performance from electroencephalographic data. *J. NeuroEng. Rehabil.* 11, 24. doi: 10.1186/1743-0003-11-24

Millán, J. D. R., Rupp, R., Müller-Putz, G. R., Murray-Smith, R., Giugliemma, C., et al. (2010). Combining brain–computer interfaces and assistive technologies: state-of-the-art and challenges. *Front. Neurosci.* 4:161. doi: 10.3389/fnins.2010.00161

Müller, K.-R., Tangermann, M., Dornhege, G., Krauledat, M., Curio, G., and Blankertz, B. (2008). Machine learning for real-time single-trial EEG-analysis: from brain–computer interfacing to mental state monitoring. *J. Neurosci. Methods* 167, 82–90. doi: 10.1016/j.jneumeth.2007.09.022

Müller-Putz, G. R., Leeb, R., Tangermann, M., Höhne, J., Kübler, A., Cincotti, F., et al. (2015). Towards non-invasive hybrid brain-computer interfaces: framework, practice, clinical application and beyond. *Proc. IEEE* 103, 926–943. doi: 10.1109/JPROC.2015.2411333

Osu, R., Morishige, K.-i., Nakanishi, J., Miyamoto, H., and Kawato, M. (2015). Practice reduces task relevant variance modulation and forms nominal trajectory. *Sci. Rep.* 5:17659. doi: 10.1038/srep17659

Ovbiagele, B., and Nguyen-Huynh, M. N. (2011). Stroke epidemiology: advancing our understanding of disease mechanism and therapy. *Neurotherapeutics* 8, 319–329. doi: 10.1007/s13311-011-0053-1

Pichiorri, F., Morone, G., Petti, M., Toppi, J., Pisotta, I., Molinari, M., et al. (2015). Brain–computer interface boosts motor imagery practice during stroke recovery. *Ann. Neurol.* 77, 851–865. doi: 10.1002/ana.24390

Pistohl, T., Ball, T., Schulze-Bonhage, A., Aertsen, A., and Mehring, C. (2008). Prediction of arm movement trajectories from ecog-recordings in humans. *J. Neurosci. Methods* 167, 105–114. doi: 10.1016/j.jneumeth.2007.10.001

Ramos-Murguialday, A., Broetz, D., Rea, M., Läer, L., Yilmaz, Ö., Brasil, F. L., et al. (2013). Brain–machine interface in chronic stroke rehabilitation: a controlled study. *Ann. Neurol.* 74, 100–108. doi: 10.1002/ana.23879

Ramoser, H., Muller-Gerking, J., and Pfurtscheller, G. (2000). Optimal spatial filtering of single trial EEG during imagined hand movement. *Rehabil. Eng. IEEE Trans.* 8, 441–446. doi: 10.1109/86.895946

Reis, J., Schambra, H. M., Cohen, L. G., Buch, E. R., Fritsch, B., Zarahn, E., et al. (2009). Noninvasive cortical stimulation enhances motor skill acquisition over multiple days through an effect on consolidation. *Proc. Natl. Acad. Sci. U.S.A.* 106, 1590-1595. doi: 10.1073/pnas.0805413106

Sannelli, C., Dickhaus, T., Halder, S., Hammer, E. M., Müller, K.-R., and Blankertz, B. (2010). On optimal channel configurations for SMR-based brain-computer interfaces. *Brain Topogr.* 23, 186–193. doi: 10.1007/s10548-010-0135-0

Schubert, R., Haufe, S., Blankenburg, F., Villringer, A., and Curio, G. (2009). Now you'll feel it, now you won't: EEG rhythms predict the effectiveness of perceptual masking. *J. Cogn. Neurosci.* 21, 2407–2419. doi: 10.1162/jocn.2008.21174

Tangermann, M., Reis, J., and Meinel, A. (2015). "Commonalities of motor performance metrics are revealed by predictive oscillatory EEG components," in *Proceedings of the 3rd International Congress on Neurotechnology, Electronics and Informatics (NEUROTECHNIX 2015)* (Lisbon), 32–38. doi: 10.5220/0005663100320038

Timmermans, A. A., Seelen, H. A., Willmann, R. D., and Kingma, H. (2009). Technology-assisted training of arm-hand skills in stroke: concepts on reacquisition of motor control and therapist guidelines for rehabilitation technology design. *J. Neuroeng. Rehabil.* 6:1. doi: 10.1186/1743-0003-6-1

Tonin, L., Leeb, R., Sobolewski, A., and del R Millán, J. (2013). An online EEG BCI based on covert visuospatial attention in absence of exogenous stimulation. *J. Neural Eng.* 10:056007. doi: 10.1088/1741-2560/10/5/056007

van Beers, R. J., van der Meer, Y., and Veerman, R. M. (2013). What autocorrelation tells us about motor variability: insights from dart throwing. *PLoS ONE* 8:e64332. doi: 10.1371/journal.pone.0064332

van Dijk, H., Schoffelen, J.-M., Oostenveld, R., and Jensen, O. (2008). Prestimulus oscillatory activity in the alpha band predicts visual discrimination ability. *J. Neurosci.* 28, 1816–1823. doi: 10.1523/JNEUROSCI.1853-07.2008

van Ede, F., Köster, M., and Maris, E. (2012). Beyond establishing involvement: Quantifying the contribution of anticipatory α-and β-band suppression to perceptual improvement with attention. *J. Neurophysiol.* 108, 2352–2362. doi: 10.1152/jn.00347.2012

Waldert, S., Preissl, H., Demandt, E., Braun, C., Birbaumer, N., Aertsen, A., et al. (2008). Hand movement direction decoded from MEG and EEG. *J. Neurosci.* 28, 1000–1008. doi: 10.1523/JNEUROSCI.5171-07.2008

Winkler, I., Brandl, S., Horn, F., Waldburger, E., Allefeld, C., and Tangermann, M. (2014). Robust artifactual independent component classification for bci practitioners. *J. Neural Eng.* 11:035013. doi: 10.1088/1741-2560/11/3/0 35013

Wolf, S. L., Blanton, S., Baer, H., Breshears, J., and Butler, A. J. (2002). Repetitive task practice: a critical review of constraint-induced movement therapy in stroke. *Neurologist* 8, 325. doi: 10.1097/01.nrl.0000031014.85777.76

Wu, H. G., Miyamoto, Y. R., Castro, L. N. G., Ölveczky, B. P., and Smith, M. A. (2014). Temporal structure of motor variability is dynamically regulated and predicts motor learning ability. *Nat. Neurosci.* 17, 312–321. doi: 10.1038/nn.3616

Yang, L., Leung, H., Plank, M., Snider, J., and Poizner, H. (2014). "Alpha and beta band power changes predict reaction time and endpoint error during planning reaching movements," in *Biomedical Engineering and Informatics (BMEI), 2014 7th International Conference on*, (IEEE), 264–268.

Zaepffel, M., Trachel, R., Kilavik, B. E., and Brochier, T. (2013). Modulations of EEG beta power during planning and execution of grasping movements. *PLoS ONE* 8:e60060. doi: 10.1371/journal.pone.0060060

13

Does a Combination of Virtual Reality, Neuromodulation and Neuroimaging Provide a Comprehensive Platform for Neurorehabilitation?

Wei-Peng Teo[1], Makii Muthalib[2,3], Sami Yamin[4,5], Ashlee M. Hendy[6], Kelly Bramstedt[4], Eleftheria Kotsopoulos[4,7], Stephane Perrey[2] and Hasan Ayaz[8,9,10]*

[1] *Institute for Physical Activity and Nutrition (IPAN), Deakin University, Burwood, VIC, Australia,* [2] *EuroMov, University of Montpellier, Montpellier, France,* [3] *Cognitive Neuroscience Unit, Deakin University, Burwood, VIC, Australia,* [4] *Liminal Pty Ltd., Melbourne, VIC, Australia,* [5] *Adult Mental Health, Monash Health, Dandenong, VIC, Australia,* [6] *School of Exercise and Nutrition Sciences, Deakin University, Burwood, VIC, Australia,* [7] *Aged Persons Mental Health Service, Monash Health, Cheltenham, VIC, Australia,* [8] *School of Biomedical Engineering, Science and Health Systems, Drexel University, Philadelphia, PA, USA,* [9] *Department of Family and Community Health, University of Pennsylvania, Philadelphia, PA, USA,* [10] *The Division of General Pediatrics, Children's Hospital of Philadelphia, Philadelphia, PA, USA*

***Correspondence:**
Wei-Peng Teo
weipeng.teo@deakin.edu.au

In the last decade, virtual reality (VR) training has been used extensively in video games and military training to provide a sense of realism and environmental interaction to its users. More recently, VR training has been explored as a possible adjunct therapy for people with motor and mental health dysfunctions. The concept underlying VR therapy as a treatment for motor and cognitive dysfunction is to improve neuroplasticity of the brain by engaging users in multisensory training. In this review, we discuss the theoretical framework underlying the use of VR as a therapeutic intervention for neurorehabilitation and provide evidence for its use in treating motor and mental disorders such as cerebral palsy, Parkinson's disease, stroke, schizophrenia, anxiety disorders, and other related clinical areas. While this review provides some insights into the efficacy of VR in clinical rehabilitation and its complimentary use with neuroimaging (e.g., fNIRS and EEG) and neuromodulation (e.g., tDCS and rTMS), more research is needed to understand how different clinical conditions are affected by VR therapies (e.g., stimulus presentation, interactivity, control and types of VR). Future studies should consider large, longitudinal randomized controlled trials to determine the true potential of VR therapies in various clinical populations.

Keywords: neurorehabilitation, neuroplasticity, tDCS, fNIRS, EEG, virtual reality therapy

INTRODUCTION

In the last two decades, the application of VR training has become increasingly popular, not only as a means to enhance gaming experiences, but also in the education and healthcare settings to improve learning and rehabilitation outcomes. Particularly in the area of neurorehabilitation, the use of VR technology has shown great promise by providing a sense of realism during training, thereby promoting skill acquisition and retention, and inducing functional recovery (**Figure 1**; for review, see Adamovich et al., 2009).

In the context of neurorehabilitation, VR therapy can be described as a method of brain–computer interaction that involves real-time simulation of an environment, scenario or activity that allows for user interaction and targets multiple senses. In particular, the combination of VR and recent technological advances in robotic and haptic interfaces allow users a seemingly life-like interactional experience in a VE (Jung et al., 2012; Yeh et al., 2014). For example, VR has been used in clinical settings as a training tool for surgeons to learn intricate fine motor skills associated with precision surgery (Wang, 2012; Fang et al., 2014), and as a tool to deliver cognitive-based therapies (Kim et al., 2011; Kandalaft et al., 2013). More complex forms of VR presentation such as augmented VR (whereby VR is superimposed on the actual environment) and immersive VR (first-person interaction in a VR environment) brings the immersive experience to another level with technology such as head-mounted displays (i.e., Oculus® Rift and Microsoft® Hololens) or screens. It is through this naturalistic environment, and allowing for interactive behaviors while being monitored and recorded, that is the primary advantage of implementing VR technology. This means that VR technology can be used to deliver meaningful and relevant stimulation to an individual's nervous system and thereby capitalize on neuroplasticity to promote both cognitive and motor rehabilitation.

In this review, we will discuss the theoretical framework for the use of VR in the context of neurorehabilitation. We will provide evidence for the use of VR in motor rehabilitation for neurological disorders such as PD, CP and stroke and in mood and mental health disorders such as anxiety, PTSD and schizophrenia. We will also review the concurrent use of non-invasive brain stimulation and neuroimaging techniques during VR, discussing how these combined techniques may augment the benefits and complement current VR training protocols.

THEORETICAL FRAMEWORK FOR VR AND LEARNING

Experiential Learning

The most important aspect of using VR is to provide new experiences by allowing users to interact physically and emotionally within a VE that is almost identical to the real world. The combination of physical, mental and emotional interaction encourages active participation and involvement of the user. In this sense, users of VR assimilate knowledge more effectively when they have the freedom to engage in self-directed activities within their learning context. By finding solutions and learning new skills autonomously, users of VR invest mental effort by constructing conceptual models that are both consistent with what they already understand and with the new content that is presented (Garrison and Garrison, 1997). Another key feature of VR training is that it offers users the opportunity to acquire skills in the context where they need to be applied. This results in more meaningful and effective learning, as compared with learning out of context (Nieuwenhuijsen et al., 2006). In physical rehabilitation for example, rehabilitation of fine motor control of the hands and wrists can be "re-trained" by simulating a VE where a stroke patient needs to pour him or herself a glass of water in the kitchen. In this way, patients practice and refine fine motor control of muscles controlling the hands and wrists through manipulating a virtual object that allows the same kind of natural interaction with objects that patients would engage in the real world.

Augmented Feedback: Knowledge of Results and Performance

Another important aspect of VR therapy is the ability to provide augmented feedback to its users. Augmented feedback is additional information provided through any means (e.g., visual, auditory or kinesthetic) that is complimentary to the inherent feedback received via the sensory systems. There is no hard and fast rule as to how or what kinds of information augmented feedback should provide, however, VR therapy offers two vital pieces of information that is essential for learning (Winstein, 1991; Lauber and Keller, 2014); (1) knowledge of performance - information on how the participant performs during movement (i.e., movement sequences, joint angles, force outputs at each phase of movement etc.); (2) knowledge of results - information on the outcome of the performance (i.e., overall quality and quantity of movement). Currently, most commercially available VR games would incorporate visual, auditory and even kinesthetic feedback that can be provided either during or after the game. Very often, these VR games are designed in a manner that users have to maintain or achieve a pre-determined score or level in order for the game to progress. For example, VR applications can provide knowledge of performance throughout gameplay in the form of movement kinematics (i.e., joint angles, velocity, and speed), kinetics (i.e., ground reaction forces and torque) or even the level of activation in specific brain regions during a particular task. In order for users to progress to the next level, users must maintain or exceed a threshold that has been set based on previous trials or specific performance outcomes. Upon task completion, knowledge of results and performance can be provided, allowing both clinicians and users to understand deficiencies in movement patterns that are associated with specific dysfunctional movement outcomes, apply progressions

Abbreviations: BCI, brain computer interface; CP, cerebral palsy; EEG, electroencephalography; fMRI, functional magnetic resonance imaging; fNIRS, functional near-infrared spectroscopy; PD, Parkinson's disease; PTSD, post-traumatic stress disorder; tDCS, transcranial direct current stimulation; VE, virtual environment; VR, virtual reality.

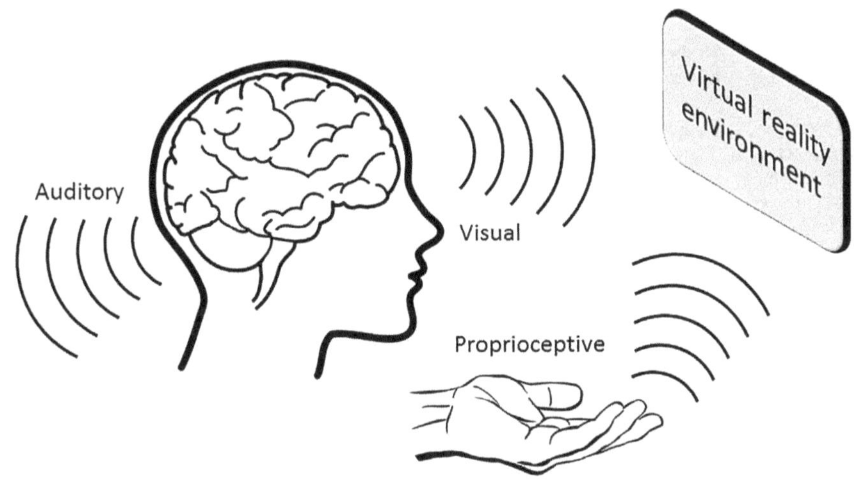

FIGURE 1 | A VR environment induces multisensory feedback that contributes toward greater memory consolidation and retention.

appropriately, and address those deficiencies with a targeted rehabilitation approach.

Observational Learning

Apart from providing feedback that is necessary for learning, another aspect of VR training is the enhancement of observational learning. The basis for learning, or at least its intended outcome, is to mimic or replicate an ideal response that brings about a desired result and induce a lasting change in behavior. In terms of neurorehabilitation, observation of goal-oriented movements or processes provides sensory feedback about the movement, behavior or emotional state, which contributes to learning (Oouchida et al., 2013; Williams and Carnahan, 2014). These observations preferentially activate parts of the brain that are involved with the physical performance itself allowing a motor program to be developed based upon the observed movements (Burke et al., 2010). Training in a VE may facilitate observational learning in four different ways; (1) VR applications can provide an accurate visual representation of the user's body and limb position using motion capture technology; (2) VR applications commonly use an avatar to mimic the movement of users, or conversely, the user could mimic the movements of the avatar; (3) accurate guides or a correct movement pattern can be produced for which users can follow; (4) VR applications can facilitate mental imagery by inducing optimal mood states and instructions for mental imagery.

Motivation

Importantly, the goal-oriented nature of VR tasks may support the maintenance and adherence of neurorehabilitation programs. Unlike traditional therapist-led sessions, where improvements in physical or cognitive function may be subjective or difficult for patients to identify (Van den Broek, 2005), VR programs can provide an objective, quantitative measure of session outcomes and objectives. Furthermore, VR applications can provide both users and clinicians the ability to individualize training programs or alter the progression of a training session based upon the user's personal performance. The capacity to individualize therapy intensity may enhance motivation by allowing users to select practice sessions that are catered to their individual time and need, and more importantly, to manipulate treatment parameters to create optimal learning conditions. Another important consideration for VR to improve motivation is by incorporating competition or co-operation between other players during therapy sessions. Engaging users in a group environment either competing against each other or working in teams promotes an element of enjoyment through increased social interaction, particularly amongst people suffering with similar conditions (Van den Broek, 2005).

EVIDENCE OF VR THERAPY IN MOVEMENT NEUROREHABILITATION

Stroke

The use of motion-controlled VR game consoles, including the Nintendo® Wii and Xbox® Kinect, have been explored as adjuncts to conventional physical therapy (see **Table 1**), specifically for improving upper limb function (Thomson et al., 2014; Laver et al., 2015). VR programs for stroke neurorehabilitation are based on the potential for brain neuroplasticity after neurological injury to support acquisition and retention of new motor skills to recover motor function. The goal of VR therapy in stroke is to apply these motor learning principles for stroke neurorehabilitation, such as providing repetitive, graded intensity, and motivating task-specific training with real time multimodal feedback of movements and performance (Saposnik et al., 2011). Thus, VR systems are designed to enhance conventional therapy by providing a tool to deliver more specific, intensive and enjoyable therapy with real time feedback of performance (Levin et al., 2015).

TABLE 1 | Examples of recent systematic reviews and meta-analyses demonstrating the effects of VR in neurorehabilitation of stroke, PD and CP.

Author and year	Study aims	Studies included and sample (*n*)	Study outcomes	Points of discussion
Stroke				
Laver et al. (2015)	Compared the effects of virtual reality on arm function, walking speed and independence in managing daily activities after stroke versus an alternative intervention or no intervention.	37 studies ($n = 1019$)	12 studies found improved arm function. 4 studies found improved walking speed. 8 studies found slight improvements in activities of daily living.	Low sample size in most studies. Some studies reported pain, headaches or dizziness in small number of participants, but no adverse events overall. Low quality evidence for arm function. Very low quality evidence for walking ability, global motor function and independence in performing daily activities. The quality of the evidence for each outcome was limited due to small numbers of study participants, inconsistent results across studies and poor reporting of study details.
Corbetta et al. (2015)	Compared the effects of VR-based rehabilitation on gait, balance and mobility versus standard therapy.	15 studies ($n = 341$)	Significant improvements in walking speed, balance, and mobility. Significant improvements in mobility if VR training was combined with standard therapy. Insufficient evidence to support to use of combined VR and standard therapy on balance and walking speed.	Substituting some or all of a standard rehabilitation regimen with VR training provides greater benefits in walking speed, balance, and mobility. Although the benefits are small, the cost of administering VR is also small particularly when patient demand is high in a clinic setting.
Luque-Moreno et al. (2015)	Compared the effects of VR interventions on lower extremity rehabilitation.	11 studies ($n = 231$)	High heterogeneity in study designs. Small sample sizes. Mean sample size of 20 per study. Studies were ranked between 4 and 7 points (out of 10) on the PEDro scale.	VR interventions (more than 10 sessions) may have a positive impact on lower limb function. Multimodal approach (i.e., a combination of VR and conventional therapy) may elicit greater results. Adaptability of software seemed to adapt better to patient's requirements, allowing for individualized treatments.
Lohse et al. (2014)	Compared the effects of custom built virtual games and commercially available gaming systems.	26 studies ($n = ?$)	Only 4 studies used commercial games while 20 studies used custom built virtual games. Mean PEDro score for all studies was 5.42 ± 1.6 (out of 10). Methodological limitations of studies include subject, experimenter and therapist blinding, small sample size, and difficulty in determining a dose-response effect. Significant improvements in body function and activity outcomes.	VR intervention improves outcomes compared to conventional therapies. Small samples and few number of studies in commercial games limits the assessment of potential benefits.
Parkinson's disease				
Harris et al. (2015)	Compared the effects of exergaming on static and dynamic balance in older adults and PD.	11 studies ($n = 325$ healthy older adults, 56 PD)	9 studies showed a significant improvement in static balance and postural control in healthy aging individuals. 2 studies found a significant improvement in static balance and postural control people with PD. Studies were ranked between 4 and 8 points (out of 10) on the PEDro scale.	Few studies in PD and small sample size limits the interpretation of the effectiveness of exergaming in PD. Evidence found in this meta-analysis supports the use of exergaming as an adjunctive tool to improve balance and postural control.

(Continued)

TABLE 1 | Continued

Author and year	Study aims	Studies included and sample (n)	Study outcomes	Points of discussion
Barry et al. (2014)	Examined the safety, feasibility and effectiveness of exergaming in people with PD.	7 studies ($n = 110$)	Only 2 studies addressed patient safety. No objective measures (such as falls or near falls) or subjective measures (patient's perception) were recorded in any studies. Only 1 study recorded gameplay experience. Good levels of motivation during game play were reported although difficulties with the fast pace and cognitive complexity of some games were raised. Exergaming was found to be just as effective as standard physical therapy for improving clinical measures of balance and cognition even up to 60 days post-intervention.	While the effectiveness and feasibility are often measured, more research is required to establish the safety, particularly in home-based VR therapy. The use of commercial games may be too difficult for some people with PD, and exergames that tailor specifically to the needs and capabilities of patients may be more effective.
Cerebral Palsy				
Dewar et al. (2015)	Systematic review of various interventions to improve postural control in children with CP	45 studies ($n = ?$)	4 studies investigated the use of VR on postural control. 2 studies were rated weak in study conduct while 2 had a strong study design. 3 studies showed improvements in balance, while 2 study showed improvements in walking capacity.	The systematic review provided conflicting evidence of VR on postural control and gait. Due to the preliminary nature of these studies, it is difficult to truly ascertain if indeed the use of VR had any effects on postural control and gait.
Chen et al. (2014)	Examined the effects of virtual gaming on upper extremity function in children with CP	14 studies ($n = 122$)	3 RCTs, 2 cohort studies, 7 case studies and 2 single-subject design studies. For 3 RCTs, no difference was found between VR therapy and conventional therapy. Overall upper extremity function was significantly improved after VR therapy. Strongest effects of VR was shown in younger children, custom-built systems in the home or laboratory setting.	The use of VR may be highly applicable in a pediatric population. Small sample size and the lack of large RCT is a limiting factor in interpreting the results.

PEDro, physiotherapy evidence database (PEDro); RCT, Randomized controlled trials; PD, parkinson's disease; CP, cerebral palsy; VR, virtual reality.

Despite the potential utility of commercial VR game consoles for stroke neurorehabilitation, a number of limitations have been highlighted (Bower et al., 2015): (1) VR games designed for the general population can be too challenging for stroke patients with physical and cognitive deficits; (2) the difficulty levels and control of VR games are often not readily adjustable to rehabilitation targets, and the tasks may lack functional relevance; (3) feedback and scoring provided can be negative and frustrating for the user; (4) current VR games do not include neurological assessment; (5) VR does not integrate multiple environmental factors that connect to motor performance. In response to some of these limitations, there has been an emergence of research and development of modified VR programs specifically designed for stroke neurorehabilitation using adaptable software and hardware components of commercial VR systems (e.g., Kinect system) and guidance from clinicians in their development (Laffont et al., 2014; Bower et al., 2015). These adapted VR systems are progressively optimized with new functions including: (1) allowing automatic adaptation/intensity grading of the activity to the patient's own achievements; (2) allowing the therapist to adapt online the task's characteristics to the patient's needs; (3) allowing multiplayer VR systems via a web-service platform to enhance interactivity; (4) automatic recording of the patient's movements to provide therapists with data describing the quality and quantity of motor function recovery/progression, including the level of compensatory movements (Laffont et al., 2014).

While there is some evidence to suggest that VR may be highly applicable for stroke rehabilitation, the evidence from recent systematic reviews and meta-analyses indicate that current studies are limited by sample size issues and study designs (see **Table 1**). Early VR interventions used commercial applications such as the Nintendo Wii that controls an avatar, however, more recently customized systems have focused on interactive platforms to target activities of everyday living (i.e., reaching and grasping tasks). However, a major challenge with stroke is that no one stroke patient will present with the same motor deficit and therefore an individualized approach to therapy, including VR therapy, is needed. In this sense, future systems must be adaptive and customizable to manage the heterogenous nature of stroke for patients to gain greater benefits.

Parkinson's Disease

Emerging VR therapies presents as an attractive option for delivering neurorehabilitation therapies to manage the cognitive-motor symptoms in people with PD, as it can be employed at any stage as an adjunct to standard pharmacological (Levodopa therapy) and/or surgical (ablation, deep brain stimulation) treatment (see **Table 1**). This new possibility in the field of neurorehabilitation aims to provide PD patients with a motivating way to perform multiple motor neurorehabilitation exercises with the rationale that the VR system might promote balance training, and cognitive-motor practice. Some commercial VR systems, such as the Nintendo® Wii system using a balance board, has drawn considerable attention from both the research and clinical communities as effective and feasible neurorehabilitation interventions to enhance gait and balance for people with PD (Barry et al., 2014; Harris et al., 2015). More recent studies have implemented custom programming and hardware to their VR systems to specifically improve balance and gait in PD (Mirelman et al., 2011).

It has been demonstrated that a VR neurorehabilitation program of 6–8 weeks involving 40–60 min a day, three times per week appears to be a viable option for significantly improving balance in a clinical population of individuals with PD (Esculier et al., 2012). The intensity/difficulty load of interventions used across existing studies appears a key contributing factor for the discordant findings reported in the literature (Esculier et al., 2012). In addition, activity selection could have contributed to some differential findings among studies. Some studies targeted static slow controlled movements in a closed environment such as the Wii Fit with balance board (dos Santos Mendes et al., 2012; Esculier et al., 2012), while others involve dynamic movements in an open environment such as Wii Sports (Herz et al., 2013).

Despite some evidence for performance improvement in balance, there are still limitations inherent in commercial VR systems that may not directly apply to realistic everyday settings for PD neurorehabilitation. Additionally, the programs are not very scalable, or modifiable, to each individual's needs or progress for all stages of disease. Mirelman et al. (2011, 2013) utilized a custom-made VR system to incorporate virtual obstacles presented on a screen during treadmill walking (18 sessions over 6 weeks). During the gait training they used a novel method (V-TIME) for tracking foot position based on the X-box Kinect technology. Interestingly, Mirelman et al. (2011) observed significant elevated gait speed with and without a cognitive dual-task upon completion of training and 4 weeks post-training. However, this VR gait training protocol confines participants to straight-walking, a gait pattern that is relatively uncommon in real-life environments. Perhaps a more viable approach may be the development of a VR system that may be used in conjunction with activities of daily living. People with PD are known to use visual and/or auditory cues to improve physical performance (Lee et al., 2012), and perhaps the use of augmented VR, via goggles or smart glasses, may be used to provide sensory cues as a feedforward or feedback mechanism to improve physical performance.

Cerebral Palsy

Cerebral Palsy (CP) is the most common pediatric physical disability, thought to affect three to four individuals per 1000 of the population (Aisen et al., 2011; Oskoui et al., 2013) characterized as a spectrum of disorders of motor and postural development that cause limited functionality or dysfunction (Monge Pereira et al., 2015). Studies investigating exercise-based treatments for children with CP has provided growing evidence in the last decades for effectiveness in improving postural control (see **Table 1**). Although effective, traditional physical exercise in the clinical settings consists of repetitive tasks that limits the enthusiasm over regular periodic application.

While the study of VR in children with CP is still at its infancy, Denise Reid at the University of Toronto's Virtual Reality Laboratory (Reid, 2002a,b, 2004) has provided preliminary evidence to support its use. In these studies, children with CP were engaged with VR based exercises for upper extremity and postural control. The self-reported effect of VR on perceived self-efficacy to perform given tasks was tested in an uncontrolled study, before and after intervention (Reid, 2002a). Based on the self-efficacy theory, Reid (2002b) attempted to identify if use of VR could increase the motivation for exercise in children with CP. The pilot study yielded encouraging results for VR use with improvement in perceived performance abilities and satisfaction with performance. In a follow up study on upper-extremity efficiency, improvement was also reported with VR use (Reid, 2002b). Similarly, Reid (2004) later investigated the effect of VR intervention on playfulness and found that VR environments stimulated playfulness in children, specifically the VR tasks that allowed creativity, expression, and choice of activity. You et al. (2005) used fMRI in a case report to investigate cortical reorganization and associated motor function improvement after a VR therapy. Neuroplastic changes were observed in the primary sensorimotor cortex and supplementary motor area following VR therapy, together with enhanced functional motor skills. A later study by Bryanton et al. (2006) compared the VR therapy with conventional exercises in children and found that although children completed more repetitions of the conventional exercises, the range of motion and hold time in stretched position was greater during VR tasks.

While the current research for VR in children is still in the early stages, VR therapies represent a viable option to increase exercise adherence and physical activity as they are both engaging and rewarding particularly in an adolescent population. The process of gamification, one that entails an interactive dynamic storyline and an overall goal, is likely to better capture and retain the attention of children over traditional physical training (Lister et al., 2014). The challenge, particularly in children with CP, will be to incorporate a diversity of activities performed during the game to train a repertoire of fundamental skills so as to further develop their motor and cognitive skills.

EVIDENCE FOR VR THERAPY IN COGNITIVE REHABILITATION AND MENTAL HEALTH

Anxiety, Phobias and Post-traumatic Stress Disorder

Anxiety can be generalized in nature [i.e., generalized anxiety disorder (GAD)], characterized by long-lasting anxiety that is not focused on a specific object, or may be more focal (i.e., phobias) occurring in the presence of, or in anticipation of, a specific object or situation. Preliminary evidence on the use of VR in GAD indicate that a combination of relaxation, controlled exposure and stress inoculation may help patients to cope with various stressors and sources of worry (Gorini et al., 2010; Repetto and Riva, 2011). Additionally, the combination of biofeedback (e.g., heart rate and electro-dermal skin response) may potentially help to identify particular sources of worry and emotion that can be used to modify specific features of the VR environment (Gorini et al., 2010; Repetto and Riva, 2011).

Despite the limited evidence for the use of VR therapy in GAD, there is some support for the use of VR in a range of other anxiety disorders (see **Table 2**) including specific phobias (Cote and Bouchard, 2005; Maskey et al., 2014), panic disorder (Vincelli et al., 2002) and social phobia (Klinger et al., 2004, 2005). Current VR therapies, particularly for phobias, use controlled exposure therapy that allows the patient to experience a sense of presence in an immersive, interactive VE that minimizes avoidance behavior and facilitates emotional involvement. This VE also allows controlled delivery of sensory stimulation via the therapist, for which the patient confronts the feared stimuli in a progressive manner. Another advantage of VR therapy is being able to recreate situations that cannot be re-experienced *in vivo* (i.e., combat situation or terrorist attack). VR therapy may be used as an alternative to imaginal exposure, meaning that patients with PTSD need not rely on internal imagery to visualize an event. A potential limitation in imaginal exposure therapy is that the therapist has no control over, or even knowledge of, what imagery the patient actually evokes (Strosahl and Ascough, 1981). Whereas in the VE, the stimuli presented can be carefully controlled and monitored. As with phobic patients, VR-based exposure therapy may be particularly useful for patients with PTSD for whom avoidance and failure to engage with therapy may hinder the therapeutic process. The efficacy of VR therapy for the treatment of PTSD has predominantly been examined in military populations (Cukor et al., 2009; Goncalves et al., 2012). A systematic review found that VR therapy was just as efficacious as traditional exposure treatment for PTSD (Goncalves et al., 2012). Seven of the 10 studies included in Goncalves's review found that VR environments significantly reduced PTSD symptoms in comparison to control, however, no significant differences in symptoms were observed between VR therapy and traditional exposure treatment.

Whilst the existing literature on the use of VR therapy for phobias, panic disorder, and PTSD were promising, several limitations must be considered (Powers and Emmelkamp, 2008; Meyerbroker and Emmelkamp, 2010; Opris et al., 2012). Meyerbroker and Emmelkamp (2010) noted that VR as a therapeutic tool is difficult to assess as it is often combined with other techniques. This potentially masks any underlying benefits of VR therapy on the patient. Furthermore, most studies do not include behavioral avoidance tasks, which would help to determine how transferable the results are to the real world.

Schizophrenia

As an assessment tool, VR offers the possibility of creating unique environments allowing researchers to better identify and understand specific areas of the brain commonly effected in schizophrenia. It is proposed that binding errors during the memory encoding process are responsible for the episodic memory impairments reported in schizophrenia (Waters et al., 2004). In this sense, VR is able to tease out areas of the brain responsible for binding impairments by providing specific situations or tasks for which patients have to perform. For example, a study by Ledoux et al. (2013) examined contextual binding in schizophrenia using fMRI during a navigation task in a virtual town (i.e., find the grocery store from the school). Their results showed significantly less activation among patients relative to controls in the left middle frontal gyrus, and right and left hippocampi. Ledoux et al. (2013) further suggested that the reduced activation was indicative of context and content not being appropriately linked, therefore affecting the formation of a cognitive map representation in the patient group and eliciting a contextual binding deficit.

As a rehabilitation tool, VR offers a unique potential to expose individuals to controlled rehabilitation environments and allow for interaction within a VE. Indeed, VEs may be perceived as less intimidating for patients as it allows for more gradual increase in task difficulty and may therefore enhance participation with rehabilitation (Rizzo et al., 1998). In particular, VR therapy has been explored as an alternative option to improve cognitive function (Marques et al., 2008) and vocational skills (Tsang and Man, 2013) in schizophrenic patients with some success. However, perhaps one of the most important roles of VR therapy may be to attenuate the deficit in social skills associated with schizophrenia. Traditionally, social skills training using role-play has been effective in remediating these deficits (Benton and Schroeder, 1990), however, role-playing of social skills training are limited in that they require appropriately matched groups, and may produce social anxiety, negative symptoms and poor insight. VR-based techniques offer an alternative to traditional role playing techniques by providing a computer-generated but realistic three-dimensional world and human-like avatars that can provide emotional stimuli. These VR-based techniques may be highly beneficial to re-train conversational skills (i.e., beginning a conversation, breaking silences, and differentiating facial expressions; Ku et al., 2007; Park et al., 2011).

While there is great potential for the role of VR in the treatment of schizophrenia, the evidence for its use remains contentious. Questions still remain if the effects of VR directly affects the condition itself, or perhaps the effects of VR may attenuate other psychiatric comorbidities such as anxiety or

TABLE 2 | Examples of systematic reviews and meta-analyses demonstrated the use of VR in treating PTSD and anxiety disorders.

Author and year	Study aims	Studies included and sample (n)	Study outcomes	Points of discussion
PTSD				
Kuester et al. (2016)	Examined the efficacy of internet-based CBT and expressive writing in people with PTSD vs. waitlist or active controls.	20 studies (n = 973 intervention, 805 controls)	Internet-based CBT are showed medium to large effect sizes compared to passive controls, but not against active controls receiving face-to-face CBT with therapist.	Internet-based CBT may be just as beneficial as conventional CBT. Due to large variability in outcome measures of included studies, subgroup analyses was limited.
Goncalves et al. (2012)	A systematic review of the efficacy of VR exposure therapy in the treatment of PTSD vs. waitlist or active controls.	10 studies (n = ?)	Patients in VR exposure therapy showed insignificantly better results compared to waitlist controls, but no differences was observed when compared to exposure therapy. Majority of VR exposure therapy used head-mounted displays and customized virtual environment specific to the condition. No difference in dropout rates between VR therapy and conventional CBT.	Preliminary evidence suggests that VR exposure therapy is just as efficacious as conventional CBT. Studies included did not use intent-to-treat analysis or did not state concomitant treatments and/or comorbidities.
Anxiety disorder				
Opris et al. (2012)	Treatment efficacy of VR exposure therapy vs. conventional CBT in anxiety disorders vs. active controls.	23 studies (n = 608)	VR therapy was significantly better than waitlist controls. Similar improvements were observed between VR and conventional CBT therapy. Similar improvements in outcome measures were maintained over time in both the VR and conventional CBT groups.	The use of VR exposure therapy may be a viable option. There is a future need to determine the use of VR exposure therapy to other forms of VR therapies targeted at anxiety disorders. No measure of dropout rates in studies reviewed.
Powers and Emmelkamp (2008)	Examined the effects of VR in anxiety disorders vs. waitlist or conventional CBT controls.	13 studies (n = 397)	VR therapy was more efficacious that waitlist or active control. Significant improvements were observed in subjective distress, cognitive and behavioral measures, and psychophysiological measures. VR therapy was more effective than *in vivo* exposures. Non-significant trend toward a dose-response relationship was observed between number of sessions and outcome measures.	VR exposure therapy was highly effective in treating anxiety disorders. Behavioral avoidance tests should be administered to assess the impact of treatment on anxiety-provoking situations and generalization to the real world.

CBT, cognitive behavioral Therapy; PTSD, post-traumatic stress disorder; VR, virtual reality.

depression that may trigger visual or auditory hallucinations in sufferers of schizophrenia. As these are still early days for VR therapy in general, there is a need to determine the precise role of VR in treatment therapies for schizophrenia and its limitations.

FUTURE OUTLOOK TO THE MOST PROMISING RESEARCH AVENUES - COMPLEMENTING VR THERAPY USING NON-INVASIVE NEUROMODULATION AND NEUROIMAGING TECHNOLOGIES

This review so far has provided evidence for the use of VR therapy in various clinical populations as a standalone or adjunctive tool with mainstream neurorehabilitation treatment modalities. However, the question remains as to whether the beneficial effects of VR can be augmented via neuromodulation techniques such as tDCS, or if it is possible for a more targeted approach to monitor the effects of VR via non-invasive and portable neuroimaging methods such as fNIRS and EEG.

Augmenting VR Therapy with tDCS

Transcranial direct current stimulation is an emerging non-invasive brain stimulation technique that uses low-intensity constant direct electrical currents to modulate the excitability of cortical neurons and related networks (Nitsche and Paulus, 2000; Lang et al., 2005). By placing either a positive anode or negative cathode electrode over the scalp of the head, tDCS is able to facilitate (anodal tDCS) or inhibit (cathodal tDCS) excitability of the underlying cortical neurons in a polarity-specific manner. Due to this robust neuromodulatory effect, tDCS has often been used in conjunction either before (offline) or during (online) rehabilitation therapy to improve motor and cognitive performance in healthy and clinical populations (for a recent reviews, see Coffman et al., 2014 and Floel, 2014).

In theory, the application of tDCS with VR therapy to augment neurorehabilitation appear complimentary. A study by Lee and Chun (2014) showed an improvement in stroke-specific clinical measures, manual muscle test and the Korean-modified Barthel Index in subacute stroke patients after 15 sessions of VR therapy with online cathodal tDCS to the unaffected motor cortex compared to sham. Kim et al. (2014) further demonstrated that the addition of online anodal tDCS to the affected motor cortex with VR therapy not only improved upper arm function, but also increased corticospinal excitability in subacute stroke patients.

In contrast to the aforementioned findings, mixed results were reported by Viana et al. (2014) that compared the effects of combining VR with offline anodal tDCS over the affected motor cortex of stroke patients, across 15 1-h VR therapy sessions. While the results showed no statistical differences in stroke-specific clinical measures (i.e., Fugl-Meyer assessment, Wolf motor assessment, and modified Ashworth scale) of upper arm function between patients receiving real tDCS compared to sham, it is important to note that more than 50% of participants receiving anodal tDCS and VR therapy had clinically significant improvements in wrist spasticity following treatment. Based on these limited combined VR and tDCS findings, it can be seen that performing tDCS during the VR therapy is a significant factor for enhancing the effects of VR therapy alone, which is also the case for combining tDCS with neurorehabilitation (Rothwell, 2012). Although combined VR and neuromodulation (tDCS) has been primarily applied in movement disorders, to the best of our knowledge, there are currently no known studies that have investigated this combination in cognitive and mood disorders. Thus therapists that are currently adopting the use of VR therapy in mental and mood disorders can potentially exploit the concurrent use of both VR and tDCS to augment therapy benefits above and beyond VR therapy alone.

It is likely that the combined effects of VR and tDCS is influenced by a combination of several factors, namely (1) general patient characteristics (e.g., brain region affected, and structural/functional reserve) and (2) tDCS parameters including electrode placement (affected or unaffected brain region), polarity (anodal or cathodal) and timing of tDCS application (online or offline). In such circumstances, where the efficacy of combined VR and tDCS interventions are both timing and location dependent (i.e., when and where to stimulate), a method of detecting and monitoring changes to neurophysiological function as patients receive treatment is crucial for optimizing intervention effects. In this regard, neuroimaging methods could be applied to monitor treatment VR progression, which will be discussed in the subsequent section.

Monitoring VR Therapy with Neuroimaging

Neurophysiological changes associated with VR neurorehabilitation can be measured by non-invasive and portable neuroimaging techniques including fNIRS and/or EEG, to ascertain changes in cerebral hemodynamic responses or oscillatory brainwaves, respectively. In particular, the use of fNIRS as a tool to measure online cerebral hemodynamic responses during neurorehabilitation has received attention (for review see Irani et al., 2007; Ferrari and Quaresima, 2012). The use of fNIRS as a neuroimaging method relies on the principle of neurovascular coupling that measures the increase in regional cerebral blood flow (i.e., increase in oxygenated and decrease in deoxygenated hemoglobin) induced by neuronal activation, which is analogous to the blood-oxygenation-level-dependent responses measured by fMRI (Ferrari et al., 2004). Cortical activation measurements by fMRI and fNIRS techniques show highly correlated results in both motor and cognitive tasks (Huppert et al., 2006; Cui et al., 2011; Muthalib et al., 2013). While the application of fNIRS techniques is gaining popularity, EEG has long been used to measure online brain activity during a cognitive or motor task, and in various clinical populations (Bonanni et al., 2008; Gosselin et al., 2011). Of particular importance, EEG is used to detect changes in various brainwaves (i.e., Gamma, Alpha, Beta, Theta, and Delta) which are differentially affected by changes in mood (Huang and Lo, 2009), wakefulness (De Gennaro et al., 2001), neurological diseases (Bonanni et al., 2008), and brain injury (Gosselin et al., 2011). Both fNIRS and EEG have several advantages over fMRI, as they are portable, relatively inexpensive to use, and easy to operate with high temporal resolution. Furthermore, new generation systems are battery operated, wireless and further miniaturized to the size of a smartphone, ideal for ambulatory and untethered measurements consistent with a neuroergonomics approach (Ayaz et al., 2013; de Lissa et al., 2015).

As the use of fNIRS and EEG techniques in VR therapy is still relatively new, most studies to date have focused on healthy individuals (Bayliss and Ballard, 2000; Mingyu et al., 2005; Holper et al., 2010; Seraglia et al., 2011; Basso Moro et al., 2014), with the potential for more studies in clinical populations emerging as the popularity of these portable neuroimaging technologies increases. The current use of fNIRS and EEG in VR therapy has two proposed roles; (1) to monitor and provide augmented feedback regarding regions of cortical activation during therapy and (2) to use fNIRS or EEG as part of a BCI paradigm for therapy. In support of the first role, several studies have investigated the efficacy of fNIRS and EEG to record cortical hemodynamic and oscillatory changes during actual motor tasks and motor imagery in a VR environment. These studies demonstrated the efficacy of fNIRS and EEG to detect task-specific changes in cortical hemodynamics (Holper et al., 2010; Seraglia et al., 2011; Basso Moro et al., 2014) and oscillatory patterns (Bayliss and Ballard, 2000; Mingyu et al., 2005).

The ability of fNIRS and EEG to detect changes in these neurophysiological measures can provide both feedback on

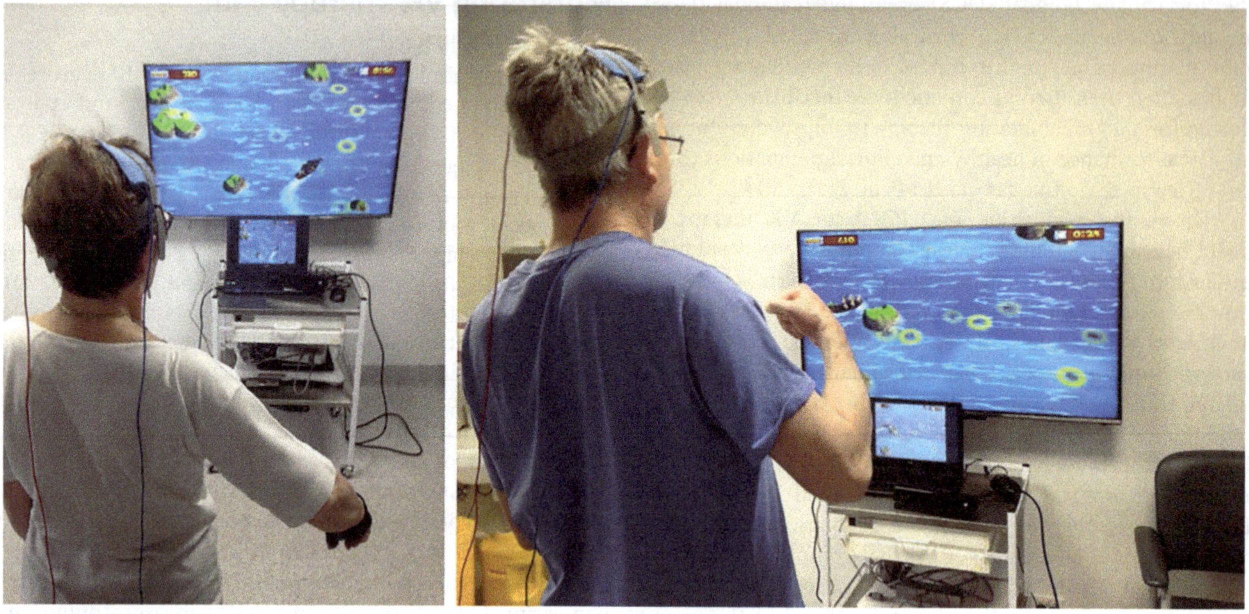

FIGURE 2 | Stroke participants engaged in VR therapy using an X-Box Kinect motion capture system while receiving tDCS.

location and level of activation, for which clinicians and users can use to set intensity and progression of therapy. Furthermore, feedback on cortical activation can also be used to identify areas of hypo- or hyperactivity, which can be modulated using neuromodulatory techniques such as tDCS (see Prospective Integration of Neuromodulation-Neuroimaging with VR Therapy). In support of the second role, identifying cortical areas of activation, patterns and timing of cortical activation associated with various movements or mood states may also be recorded as classifiers for BCI training. Indeed, most BCI studies to date have employed the use of EEG as a measure for cortical activation for which to control a robotic limb or avatar in a VR environment (Lin et al., 2007; Formaggio et al., 2013, 2015). Although relatively new, there are also fNIRS-based BCI approaches demonstrating feasibility for future integration with VR and neurorehabilitation (Sitaram et al., 2007; Hong et al., 2015). Moreover, joint use of fNIRS- and EEG-based BCI approaches have also been demonstrated (Koo et al., 2015; Xuxian et al., 2015). This shows the potential to adopt fNIRS in a similar manner, whereby appropriate cortical hemodynamic responses can be classified to control a robotic or computer interface.

Prospective Integration of Neuromodulation-Neuroimaging with VR Therapy

In the last 5 years, new research suggests that the combination of VR therapy with neuromodulation and neuroimaging techniques may help to improve the effects and delivery of VR therapies. Neuromodulation techniques such as tDCS (**Figure 2**) and neuroimaging methods such as fNIRS (**Figure 3**) and EEG have already been combined and have shown some success (Ang et al., 2015; Dutta et al., 2015; Muthalib et al., 2016). While the use of these techniques in combination with VR is still in its infancy, the available evidence suggests highly complementary effects when combining neuromodulation and neuroimaging with VR therapy.

As both neuroimaging (fNIRS/EEG) and neuromodulation (tDCS) techniques have complimentary capabilities, and they both can be built as wearable and wireless systems, integration of the two presents as a natural avenue for applications in natural environments and real world settings (McKendrick et al., 2015). One potential use is enhancing BCI applications. In its most general form, BCI provides a route for neural output that does not involve the neuromuscular system (Wolpaw et al., 2002). Almost all current non-invasive BCI systems are read-only, that is, brain signals are read directly to the system (via neuroimaging) and the system can provide an output or feedback that relies on sensory input mechanisms and peripheral nervous system to reach back to the brain. A more direct BCI could eliminate the need for sensory input with the use of neuromodulation, and hence provide feedback directly to the brain for a read-write BCI.

Integration of VR therapy for such a read/write BCI hold potential for enhanced or accelerated therapeutical processes in neurorehabilitation. A study by Ang et al. (2015) was one of the first studies that combined VR with both tDCS and EEG to investigate the additive effect of offline anodal tDCS on BCI haptic training with chronic stroke patients. Although this study reported no difference in the Fugl-Meyer assessment and block-and-box test between groups that received real tDCS prior to BCI training, compared to sham, the study did demonstrate an increased state of EEG mu rhythm suppression in the real tDCS group. Thus indicating improved neurophysiological responses in motor preparation. Future studies are necessary to determine

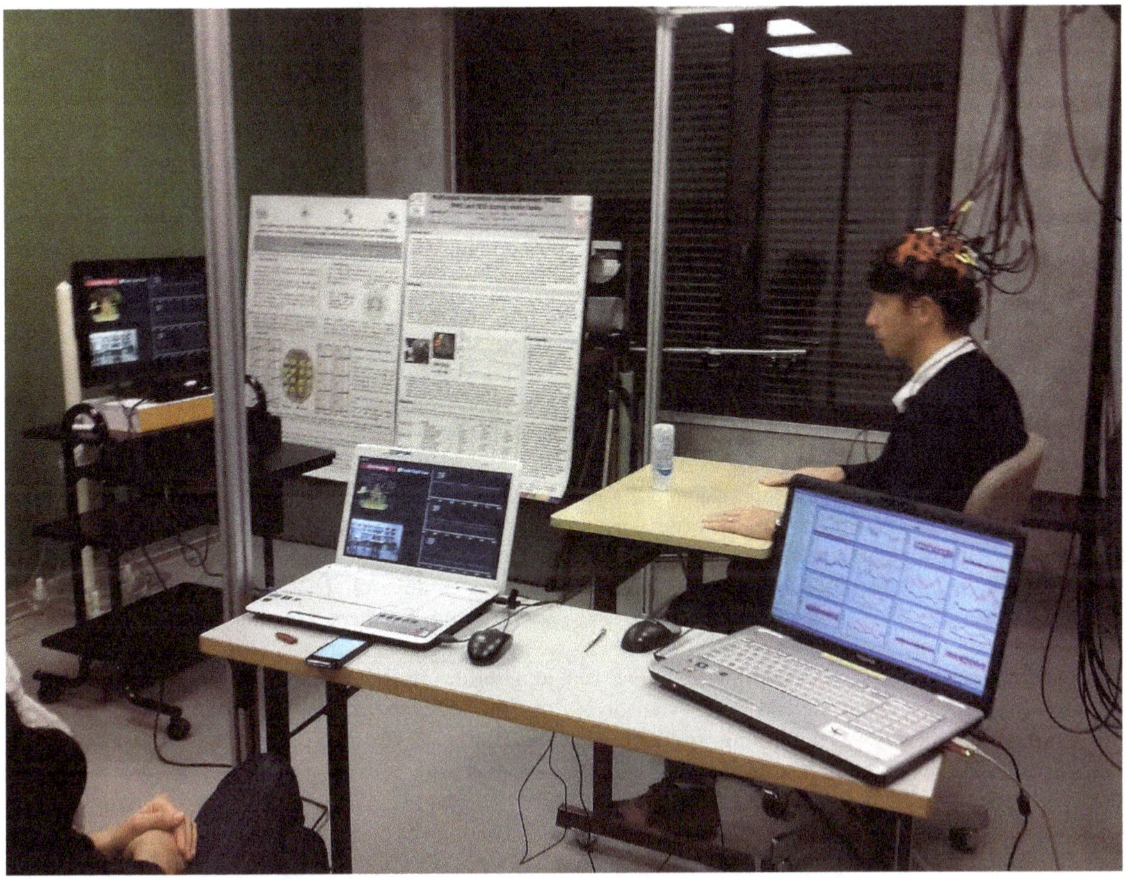

FIGURE 3 | The use of a semi-immersive VR environment and fNIRS system.

the significance of these neurophysiological improvements to clinical outcomes.

Neuroimaging guided tDCS and VR therapy can be applied to neurorehabilitation in general. The optimal location for applying tDCS electrodes to modulate a target cortical region and connected networks is a debated point in the field. Modeling studies of current flow between the tDCS electrodes have provided some guidance to the placement of electrodes to stimulate a specific brain region; however, whether these models predict the actual current flow and polarization of the targeted brain networks is not known. Simultaneous tDCS-neuroimaging could provide a solution to confirming the modeling predictions and/or to guide the direction of current flow between multi-electrode tDCS montages (Ruffini et al., 2014). For example, a motor task could be used to activate a broad network of cortical regions of interest that can be measured using fNIRS/EEG neuroimaging. Once the locations of the tDCS electrodes have been determined using neuroimaging guidance, neuroimaging and tDCS could be simultaneously or independently used to guide and modulate VR therapy. In this scenario, neuroimaging during VR tasks can be used to adapt the intensity based on the level of activation, such as the attentional hub of the dorsolateral prefrontal cortex (DLPFC). The level of DLPFC activation during the initial task would be expected to be high due to the novelty of the activity, however, as the activity progresses the learning of task requirements become automatic and performance improves, less attentional resources would be required, and the level of DLPFC would be expected to decrease (Ayaz et al., 2012; McKendrick et al., 2014). In such a scenario, the VR task can be adapted online to modulate the intensity level and maintain optimal DLPFC activation. Also, if the levels of DLPFC activation remain at high levels and/or performance is stagnant, then tDCS could potentially be applied online to upregulate neuronal networks required to perform the task. Preliminary evidence using a modeling approach to locate tDCS electrodes was provided by McKendrick et al. (2015) using a spatial memory task with concurrent fNIRS and tDCS. They showed that when task performance declined rapidly following baseline, the application of tDCS almost immediately eliminated the performance decrement. Furthermore, they showed that tDCS can modulate the neural activity of specific brain regions near the site of stimulation. However, they cautioned that current models and protocols for determining tDCS montages are lacking, due to complex interactions between stimulation montage, task performance and underlying hemodynamics that are not fully understood. Therefore, additional joint tDCS and fNIRS/EEG studies are required to further unravel these complexities and to better define the pattern of cortical excitation induced by tDCS during the performance of cognitive and motor tasks.

CURRENT LIMITATIONS OF VR THERAPY

While using a VE offers many unique advantages to traditional treatment and neurorehabilitation approaches, limitations to their efficacy and practicality must be acknowledged. Firstly, larger clinical studies are required to establish the efficacy of using VR in physical and cognitive rehabilitation in different clinical populations. Much of the existing literature report mixed findings from small sample sizes, and often lack appropriate control comparisons (see **Tables 1** and **2**). Secondly, there is little information on the transfer of the training effects of VR into the corresponding physical environment in general, and the VR training parameters associated with optimal transfer to real-world functional improvements are yet to be elucidated. Thirdly, in many clinical populations it is unclear whether advantages of VR over real-world training exist, and if so, precisely what these advantages are (see **Tables 1** and **2** for study limitations). Furthermore, because this literature is extremely vulnerable to selective reporting and Type-I statistical error, there is an inherent bias of publishing results that show correlation between rehabilitation improvements and the application of VR. Therefore to potentially limit any bias in future studies, it may be useful for future studies to adopt a double-blinded protocol for the evaluation of the effectiveness of the use of VR. Lastly, it is important to investigate any unique rehabilitative effects of VR that may be exploited, or whether the benefits of VR can be attributed to the enjoyment of gaming platforms associated with VR themselves (i.e., VR therapies may only present as more effective because they engage and motivate participants throughout their training session, providing increased adherence). While limitations in VR technology exist, the potential for favorable neuroplasticity afforded by such technology undoubtedly warrants further investigation.

CONCLUSION

In summary, this review has discussed the strengths and limitations for the use of VR therapies in motor and mental health neurorehabilitation. The current evidence suggest that a combination of VR and conventional therapies are safe and likely to be more efficacious compared to just traditional or VR therapy alone. However, it is not known if the use of VR therapies can lead to cost-saving benefits (i.e., reduced financial and manpower cost) or even if current commercial or customized systems will be applicable by patients that are living within the community. More importantly, there is a need to elucidate the aspects of VR that are most effective for rehabilitation. While this is not apparent in the current review, future studies should attempt to systematically determine the role of self-projection, sensory feedback or motivation on rehabilitation in relation to specific diseases or impairments. Furthermore, we have discussed the potential for VR therapy to be complemented by other forms of technologies such as neuromodulation (tDCS) and neuroimaging (fNIRS/EEG) in order to augment training benefits of VR, and provide a more targeted approach to neurorehabilitation. Large-scale longitudinal studies will also be required to determine the effects of VR therapy (in combination with tDCS/fNIRS/EEG) and the translation of VR therapy in a non-clinical environment (i.e., home setting).

AUTHOR CONTRIBUTIONS

All authors listed, have made substantial, direct and intellectual contribution to the work, and approved it for publication.

ACKNOWLEDGMENTS

W-PT is supported by an Alfred Deakin Postdoctoral Research Fellowship. MM is supported by a Postdoctoral Research Fellowship of the University of Montpellier.

REFERENCES

Adamovich, S. V., Fluet, G. G., Tunik, E., and Merians, A. S. (2009). Sensorimotor training in virtual reality: a review. *NeuroRehabilitation* 25, 29–44. doi: 10.3233/NRE-2009-0497

Aisen, M. L., Kerkovich, D., Mast, J., Mulroy, S., Wren, T. A., Kay, R. M., et al. (2011). Cerebral palsy: clinical care and neurological rehabilitation. *Lancet Neurol.* 10, 844–852. doi: 10.1016/S1474-4422(11) 70176-4

Ang, K. K., Guan, C., Phua, K. S., Wang, C., Zhao, L., Teo, W. P., et al. (2015). Facilitating effects of transcranial direct current stimulation on motor imagery brain-computer interface with robotic feedback for stroke rehabilitation. *Arch. Phys. Med. Rehabil.* 96, S79–S87. doi: 10.1016/j.apmr.2014. 08.008

Ayaz, H., Onaral, B., Izzetoglu, K., Shewokis, P. A., Mckendrick, R., and Parasuraman, R. (2013). Continuous monitoring of brain dynamics with functional near infrared spectroscopy as a tool for neuroergonomic research: empirical examples and a technological development. *Front. Hum. Neurosci.* 7:871. doi: 10.3389/fnhum.2013.00871

Ayaz, H., Shewokis, P. A., Bunce, S., Izzetoglu, K., Willems, B., and Onaral, B. (2012). Optical brain monitoring for operator training and mental workload assessment. *Neuroimage* 59, 36–47. doi: 10.1016/j.neuroimage.2011.06.023

Barry, G., Galna, B., and Rochester, L. (2014). The role of exergaming in Parkinson's disease rehabilitation: a systematic review of the evidence. *J. Neuroeng. Rehabil.* 11:33. doi: 10.1186/1743-0003-11-33

Basso Moro, S., Bisconti, S., Muthalib, M., Spezialetti, M., Cutini, S., Ferrari, M., et al. (2014). A semi-immersive virtual reality incremental swing balance task activates prefrontal cortex: a functional near-infrared spectroscopy study. *Neuroimage* 85, 451–460. doi: 10.1016/j.neuroimage.2013.05.031

Bayliss, J. D., and Ballard, D. H. (2000). A virtual reality testbed for brain-computer interface research. *IEEE Trans. Rehabil. Eng.* 8, 188–190. doi: 10.1109/86.847811

Benton, M. K., and Schroeder, H. E. (1990). Social skills training with schizophrenics: a meta-analytic evaluation. *J. Consult. Clin. Psychol.* 58, 741–747. doi: 10.1037/0022-006X.58.6.741

Bonanni, L., Thomas, A., Tiraboschi, P., Perfetti, B., Varanese, S., and Onofrj, M. (2008). EEG comparisons in early Alzheimer's disease, dementia with Lewy bodies and Parkinson's disease with dementia patients with a 2-year follow-up. *Brain* 131, 690–705. doi: 10.1093/brain/awm322

Bower, K. J., Louie, J., Landesrocha, Y., Seedy, P., Gorelik, A., and Bernhardt, J. (2015). Clinical feasibility of interactive motion-controlled games for stroke rehabilitation. *J. Neuroeng. Rehabil.* 12:63. doi: 10.1186/s12984-015-0057-x

Bryanton, C., Bosse, J., Brien, M., Mclean, J., Mccormick, A., and Sveistrup, H. (2006). Feasibility, motivation, and selective motor control: virtual reality compared to conventional home exercise in children with cerebral palsy. *Cyberpsychol. Behav.* 9, 123–128. doi: 10.1089/cpb.2006.9.123

Burke, C. J., Tobler, P. N., Baddeley, M., and Schultz, W. (2010). Neural mechanisms of observational learning. *Proc. Natl. Acad. Sci. U.S.A.* 107, 14431–14436. doi: 10.1073/pnas.1003111107

Chen, Y. P., Lee, S. Y., and Howard, A. M. (2014). Effect of virtual reality on upper extremity function in children with cerebral palsy: a meta-analysis. *Pediatr. Phys. Ther.* 26, 289–300. doi: 10.1097/PEP.0000000000000046

Coffman, B. A., Clark, V. P., and Parasuraman, R. (2014). Battery powered thought: enhancement of attention, learning, and memory in healthy adults using transcranial direct current stimulation. *Neuroimage* 85, 895–908. doi: 10.1016/j.neuroimage.2013.07.083

Corbetta, D., Imeri, F., and Gatti, R. (2015). Rehabilitation that incorporates virtual reality is more effective that standard rehabilitation for improving walking speed, balance and mobility after stroke: a systematic review. *J. Physiother.* 61, 117–124. doi: 10.1016/j.jphys.2015.05.017

Cote, S., and Bouchard, S. (2005). Documenting the efficacy of virtual reality exposure with psychophysiological and information processing measures. *Appl. Psychophysiol. Biofeedback* 30, 217–232. doi: 10.1007/s10484-005-6379-x

Cui, X., Bray, S., Bryant, D. M., Glover, G. H., and Reiss, A. L. (2011). A quantitative comparison of NIRS and fMRI across multiple cognitive tasks. *Neuroimage* 54, 2808–2821. doi: 10.1016/j.neuroimage.2010.10.069

Cukor, J., Spitalnick, J., Difede, J., Rizzo, A., and Rothbaum, B. O. (2009). Emerging treatments for PTSD. *Clin. Psychol. Rev.* 29, 715–726. doi: 10.1016/j.cpr.2009.09.001

De Gennaro, L., Ferrara, M., Curcio, G., and Cristiani, R. (2001). Antero-posterior EEG changes during the wakefulness-sleep transition. *Clin. Neurophysiol.* 112, 1901–1911. doi: 10.1016/S1388-2457(01)00649-6

de Lissa, P., Sorensen, S., Badcock, N., Thie, J., and Mcarthur, G. (2015). Measuring the face-sensitive N170 with a gaming EEG system: a validation study. *J. Neurosci. Methods* 253, 47–54. doi: 10.1016/j.jneumeth.2015.05.025

Dewar, R., Love, S., and Johnston, L. M. (2015). Exercise interventions improve postural control in children with cerebral palsy: a systematic review. *Dev. Med. Child Neurol.* 57, 504–520. doi: 10.1111/dmcn.12660

dos Santos Mendes, F. A., Pompeu, J. E., Modenesi Lobo, A., Guedes da Silva, K., Oliveira Tde, P., Peterson Zomignani, A., et al. (2012). Motor learning, retention and transfer after virtual-reality-based training in Parkinson's disease–effect of motor and cognitive demands of games: a longitudinal, controlled clinical study. *Physiotherapy* 98, 217–223. doi: 10.1016/j.physio.2012.06.001

Dutta, A., Jacob, A., Chowdhury, S. R., Das, A., and Nitsche, M. A. (2015). EEG-NIRS based assessment of neurovascular coupling during anodal transcranial direct current stimulation–a stroke case series. *J. Med. Syst.* 39:205. doi: 10.1007/s10916-015-0205-7

Esculier, J. F., Vaudrin, J., Bériault, P., Gagnon, K., and Tremblay, L. E. (2012). Home-based balance training programme using Wii Fit with balance board for Parkinsons's disease: a pilot study. *J. Rehabil. Med.* 44, 144–150. doi: 10.2340/16501977-0922

Fang, T. Y., Wang, P. C., Liu, C. H., Su, M. C., and Yeh, S. C. (2014). Evaluation of a haptics-based virtual reality temporal bone simulator for anatomy and surgery training. *Comput. Methods Programs* 113, 674–681. doi: 10.1016/j.cmpb.2013.11.005

Ferrari, M., Mottola, L., and Quaresima, V. (2004). Principles, techniques, and limitations of near infrared spectroscopy. *Can. J. Appl. Physiol.* 29, 463–487. doi: 10.1139/h04-031

Ferrari, M., and Quaresima, V. (2012). A brief review on the history of human functional near-infrared spectroscopy (fNIRS) development and fields of application. *Neuroimage* 63, 921–935. doi: 10.1016/j.neuroimage.2012.03.049

Floel, A. (2014). tDCS-enhanced motor and cognitive function in neurological diseases. *Neuroimage* 85, 934–947. doi: 10.1016/j.neuroimage.2013.05.098

Formaggio, E., Storti, S. F., Boscolo Galazzo, I., Gandolfi, M., Geroin, C., Smania, N., et al. (2013). Modulation of event-related desynchronization in robot-assisted hand performance: brain oscillatory changes in active, passive and imagined movements. *J. Neuroeng. Rehabil.* 10:24. doi: 10.1186/1743-0003-10-24

Formaggio, E., Storti, S. F., Boscolo Galazzo, I., Gandolfi, M., Geroin, C., Smania, N., et al. (2015). Time-frequency modulation of ERD and EEG coherence in robot-assisted hand performance. *Brain Topogr.* 28, 352–363. doi: 10.1007/s10548-014-0372-8

Garrison, D. R., and Garrison, D. R. (1997). Self-directed learning: toward a comprehensive model. *Adult Educ. Q.* 48, 18–33. doi: 10.1177/074171369704800103

Goncalves, R., Pedrozo, A. L., Coutinho, E. S., Figueira, I., and Ventura, P. (2012). Efficacy of virtual reality exposure therapy in the treatment of PTSD: a systematic review. *PLoS ONE* 7:e48469. doi: 10.1371/journal.pone.0048469

Gorini, A., Pallavicini, F., Algeri, D., Repetto, C., Gaggioli, A., and Riva, G. (2010). Virtual reality in the treatment of generalized anxiety disorders. *Stud. Health Technol. Inform.* 154, 39–43.

Gosselin, N., Bottari, C., Chen, J. K., Petrides, M., Tinawi, S., De Guise, E., et al. (2011). Electrophysiology and functional MRI in post-acute mild traumatic brain injury. *J. Neurotrauma* 28, 329–341. doi: 10.1089/neu.2010.1493

Harris, D. M., Rantalainen, T., Muthalib, M., Johnson, L., and Teo, W. P. (2015). Exergaming as a viable therapeutic tool to improve static and dynamic balance among older adults and people with idiopathic Parkinson's disease: a systematic review and meta-analysis. *Front. Aging Neurosci.* 7:167. doi: 10.3389/fnagi.2015.00167

Herz, N. B., Herz, N. B., Mehta, S. H., Sethi, K. D., Jackson, P., Hall, P., et al. (2013). Nintendo Wii rehabilitation ('Wii-hab') provides benefits in Parkinson's disease. *Parkinsonism. Relat. Disord.* 19, 1039–1042. doi: 10.1016/j.parkreldis.2013.07.014

Holper, L., Muehlemann, T., Scholkmann, F., Eng, K., Kiper, D., and Wolf, M. (2010). Testing the potential of a virtual reality neurorehabilitation system during performance of observation, imagery and imitation of motor actions recorded by wireless functional near-infrared spectroscopy (fNIRS). *J. Neuroeng. Rehabil.* 7:57. doi: 10.1186/1743-0003-7-57

Hong, K. S., Naseer, N., and Kim, Y. H. (2015). Classification of prefrontal and motor cortex signals for three-class fNIRS-BCI. *Neurosci. Lett.* 587, 87–92. doi: 10.1016/j.neulet.2014.12.029

Huang, H. Y., and Lo, P. C. (2009). EEG dynamics of experienced Zen meditation practitioners probed by complexity index and spectral measure. *J. Med. Eng. Technol.* 33, 314–321. doi: 10.1080/03091900802602677

Huppert, T. J., Hoge, R. D., Diamond, S. G., Franceschini, M. A., and Boas, D. A. (2006). A temporal comparison of BOLD, ASL, and NIRS hemodynamic responses to motor stimuli in adult humans. *Neuroimage* 29, 368–382. doi: 10.1016/j.neuroimage.2005.08.065

Irani, F., Platek, S. M., Bunce, S., Ruocco, A. C., and Chute, D. (2007). Functional near infrared spectroscopy (fNIRS): an emerging neuroimaging technology with important applications for the study of brain disorders. *Clin. Neuropsychol.* 21, 9–37. doi: 10.1080/13854040600910018

Jung, E. Y., Park, D. K., Lee, Y. H., Jo, H. S., Lim, Y. S., and Park, R. W. (2012). Evaluation of practical exercises using an intravenous simulator incorporating virtual reality and haptics device technologies. *Nurse Educ. Today* 32, 458–463. doi: 10.1016/j.nedt.2011.05.012

Kandalaft, M. R., Didehbani, N., Krawczyk, D. C., Allen, T. T., and Chapman, S. B. (2013). Virtual reality social cognition training for young adults with high-functioning autism. *J. Autism. Dev. Disord.* 43, 34–44. doi: 10.1007/s10803-012-1544-6

Kim, B. R., Chun, M. H., Kim, L. S., and Park, J. Y. (2011). Effect of virtual reality on cognition in stroke patients. *Ann. Rehabil. Med.* 35, 450–459. doi: 10.5535/arm.2011.35.4.450

Kim, Y. J., Ku, J., Cho, S., Kim, H. J., Cho, Y. K., Lim, T., et al. (2014). Facilitation of corticospinal excitability by virtual reality exercise following anodal transcranial direct current stimulation in healthy volunteers and subacute stroke subjects. *J. Neuroeng. Rehabil.* 11:124. doi: 10.1186/1743-0003-11-124

Klinger, E., Bouchard, S., Legeron, P., Roy, S., Lauer, F., Chemin, I., et al. (2005). Virtual reality therapy versus cognitive behavior therapy for social phobia: a preliminary controlled study. *Cyberpsychol. Behav.* 8, 76–88. doi: 10.1089/cpb.2005.8.76

Klinger, E., Legeron, P., Roy, S., Chemin, I., Lauer, F., and Nugues, P. (2004). Virtual reality exposure in the treatment of social phobia. *Stud. Health Technol. Inform.* 99, 91–119.

Koo, B., Lee, H. G., Nam, Y., Kang, H., Koh, C. S., Shin, H. C., et al. (2015). A hybrid NIRS-EEG system for self-paced brain computer interface with online motor imagery. *J. Neurosci. Methods* 244, 26–32. doi: 10.1016/j.jneumeth.2014.04.016

Ku, J., Han, K., Lee, H. R., Jang, H. J., Kim, K. U., Park, S. H., et al. (2007). VR-based conversation training program for patients with schizophrenia: a preliminary clinical trial. *Cyberpsychol. Behav.* 10, 567–574. doi: 10.1089/cpb.2007.9989

Kuester, A., Niemeyer, H., and Knaevelsrud, C. (2016). Internet-based interventions for posttramatic stress: a meta-analysis of randomized controlled trials. *Clin. Psychol. Rev.* 43, 1–16. doi: 10.1016/j.cpr.2015.11.004

Laffont, I., Bakhti, K., Coroian, F., Van Dokkum, L., Mottet, D., Schweighofer, N., et al. (2014). Innovative technologies applied to sensorimotor rehabilitation after stroke. *Ann. Phys. Rehabil. Med.* 57, 543–551. doi: 10.1016/j.rehab.2014.08.007

Lang, N., Siebner, H. R., Ward, N. S., Lee, L., Nitsche, M. A., Paulus, W., et al. (2005). How does transcranial DC stimulation of the primary motor cortex alter regional neuronal activity in the human brain? *Eur. J. Neurosci.* 22, 495–504. doi: 10.1111/j.1460-9568.2005.04233.x

Lauber, B., and Keller, M. (2014). Improving motor performance: selected aspects of augmented feedback in exercise and health. *Eur. J. Sport Sci.* 14, 36–43. doi: 10.1080/17461391.2012.725104

Laver, K., George, S., Thomas, S., Deutsch, J. E., and Crotty, M. (2015). Virtual reality for stroke rehabilitation: an abridged version of a Cochrane review. *Eur. J. Phys. Rehabil. Med.* 51, 497–506.

Ledoux, A. A., Phillips, J. L., Labelle, A., Smith, A., Bohbot, V. D., and Boyer, P. (2013). Decreased fMRI activity in the hippocampus of patients with schizophrenia compared to healthy control participants, tested on a wayfinding task in a virtual town. *Psychiatry Res.* 211, 47–56. doi: 10.1016/j.pscychresns.2012.10.005

Lee, S. J., and Chun, M. H. (2014). Combination transcranial direct current stimulation and virtual reality therapy for upper extremity training in patients with subacute stroke. *Arch. Phys. Med. Rehabil.* 95, 431–438. doi: 10.1016/j.apmr.2013.10.027

Lee, S. J., Yoo, J. Y., Ryu, J. S., Park, H. K., and Chung, S. J. (2012). The effects of visual and auditory cues on freezing of gait in patients with Parkinson's disease. *Am. J. Phys. Med. Rehabil.* 91, 2–11. doi: 10.1097/PHM.0b013e31823c7507

Levin, M., Magdalon, E. C., Michaelsen, S. M., and Quevedo, A. (2015). Quality of grasping and the role of haptics in a 3D immersive virtual reality environment in individuals with stroke. *IEEE Trans. Neural Syst. Rehabil. Eng.* 23, 1047–1055. doi: 10.1109/TNSRE.2014.2387412

Lin, C. T., Chung, I. F., Ko, L. W., Chen, Y. C., Liang, S. F., and Duann, J. R. (2007). EEG-based assessment of driver cognitive responses in a dynamic virtual-reality driving environment. *IEEE Trans. Biomed. Eng.* 54, 1349–1352. doi: 10.1109/TBME.2007.891164

Lister, C., West, J. H., Cannon, B., Sax, T., and Brodegard, D. (2014). Just a fad. Gamification in health and fitness apps. *JIMR Serious Games* 2:e9. doi: 10.2196/games.3413

Lohse, K. R., Hilderman, C. G., Cheung, K. L., Tatla, S., and Van Der Loos, H. F. (2014). Virtual reality therapy for adults post-stroke: a systematic review and meta-analysis exploring virtual environments and commercial games in therapy. *PLoS ONE* 9:e93318. doi: 10.1371/journal.pone.0093318

Luque-Moreno, C., Ferragut-Garcías, A., Rodríguez-Blanco, C., Heredia-Rizo, A. M., Oliva-Pascual-Vaca, J., Kiper, P., et al. (2015). A decade of progress using virtual reality for poststroke lower extremity rehabilitation: systematic review of the intervention methods. *Biomed. Res. Int.* 2015:7. doi: 10.1155/2015/342529

Marques, A., Queirós, C., and Rocha, N. (2008). "Virtual reality and neuropsychology: a cognitive rehabilitation approach for people with psychiatric disabilities," in *ICDVRAT-Proceedings of 7th International Conference on Disability Virtual Reality and Associated Technologies (Sep 8-11 2008)* (Maia: Citeseer), 39–46.

Maskey, M., Lowry, J., Rodgers, J., Mcconachie, H., and Parr, J. R. (2014). Reducing specific phobia/fear in young people with autism spectrum disorders (ASDs) through a virtual reality environment intervention. *PLoS ONE* 2:e100374. doi: 10.1371/journal.pone.0100374

McKendrick, R., Ayaz, H., Olmstead, R., and Parasuraman, R. (2014). Enhancing dual-task performance with verbal and spatial working memory training: continuous monitoring of cerebral hemodynamics with NIRS. *Neuroimage* 85, 1014–1026. doi: 10.1016/j.neuroimage.2013.05.103

McKendrick, R., Parasuraman, R., and Ayaz, H. (2015). Wearable functional near infrared spectroscopy (fNIRS) and transcranial direct current stimulation (tDCS): expanding vistas for neurocognitive augmentation. *Front. Syst. Neurosci.* 9:27. doi: 10.3389/fnsys.2015.00027

Meyerbroker, K., and Emmelkamp, P. M. (2010). Virtual reality exposure therapy in anxiety disorders: a systematic review of process-and-outcome studies. *Depress. Anxiety* 27, 933–944. doi: 10.1002/da.20734

Mingyu, L., Jue, W., Nan, Y., and Qin, Y. (2005). "Development of EEG biofeedback system based on virtual reality environment," in *Proceedings of the 27th Annual Conference on IEEE Engineering in Medicine and Biology, Shanghai* (Rome: IEEE), 5362–5364. doi: 10.1109/IEMBS.2005.1615693

Mirelman, A., Maidan, I., Herman, T., Deutsch, J. E., Giladi, N., and Hausdorff, J. M. (2011). Virtual reality for gait training: can it induce motor learning to enhance complex walking and reduce fall risk in patients with Parkinson's disease? *J. Gerontol. A Biol. Sci. Med. Sci.* 66, 234–240. doi: 10.1093/gerona/glq201

Mirelman, A., Rochester, L., Reelick, M., Nieuwhof, F., Pelosin, E., Abbruzzese, G., et al. (2013). V-TIME: a treadmill training program augmented by virtual reality to decrease fall risk in older adults: study design of a randomized controlled trial. *BMC Neurol.* 13:15. doi: 10.1186/1471-2377-13-15

Monge Pereira, E., Molina Rueda, F., Alguacil Diego, I. M., Cano de la Cuerda, R., De Mauro, A., and Miangolarra Page, J. C. (2015). Use of virtual reality systems as proprioception method in cerebral palsy: clinical practice guideline. *Neurologia* 30, 550–559. doi: 10.1016/j.nrl.2011.12.004

Muthalib, M., Anwar, A. R., Perrey, S., Dat, M., Galka, A., Wolff, S., et al. (2013). Multimodal integration of fNIRS, fMRI and EEG neuroimaging. *Clin. Neurophysiol.* 124, 2060–2062. doi: 10.1016/j.clinph.2013.03.018

Muthalib, M., Besson, P., Rothwell, J. C., Ward, T. E., and Perrey, A. (2016). Effects of anodal high-definition transcranial direct current stimulation on bilateral sensorimotor cortex activation during sequential finger movements: an fNIRS study. *Adv. Exp. Med. Biol.* 876, 351–359. doi: 10.1007/978-1-4939-302 3-4_44

Nieuwenhuijsen, E. R., Zemper, E., Miner, K. R., and Epstein, M. (2006). Health behavior change models and theories: contributions to rehabilitation. *Disabil. Rehabil.* 28, 245–256. doi: 10.1080/09638280500197743

Nitsche, M. A., and Paulus, W. (2000). Excitability changes induced in the human motor cortex by weak transcranial direct current stimulation. *J. Physiol.* 527(Pt 3), 633–639. doi: 10.1111/j.1469-7793.2000.t01-1-00633.x

Oouchida, Y., Suzuki, E., Aizu, N., Takeuchi, N., and Izumi, S. (2013). Application of observational learning in neurorehabilitation. *Int. J. Phys. Med. Rehabil.* 1:5.

Opris, D., Pintea, S., Garcia-Palacios, A., Botella, C., Szamoskozi, S., and David, D. (2012). Virtual reality exposure therapy in anxiety disorders: a quantitative meta-analysis. *Depress. Anxiety* 29, 85–93. doi: 10.1002/da.20910

Oskoui, M., Coutinho, F., Dykeman, J., Jette, N., and Pringsheim, T. (2013). An update on the prevalence of cerebral palsy: a systematic review and meta-analysis. *Dev. Med. Child Neurol.* 55, 509–519. doi: 10.1111/dmcn.12080

Park, K. M., Ku, J., Choi, S. H., Jang, H. J., Park, J. Y., Kim, S. I., et al. (2011). A virtual reality application in role-plays of social skills training for schizophrenia: a randomized, controlled trial. *Psychiatry Res.* 189, 166–172. doi: 10.1016/j.psychres.2011.04.003

Powers, M. B., and Emmelkamp, P. M. (2008). Virtual reality exposure therapy for anxiety disorders: a meta-analysis. *J. Anxiety Disord.* 22, 561–569. doi: 10.1016/j.janxdis.2007.04.006

Reid, D. (2004). The influence of virtual reality on playfulness in children with cerebral palsy: a pilot study. *Occup. Ther. Int.* 11, 131–144. doi: 10.1002/oti.202

Reid, D. T. (2002a). Benefits of a virtual play rehabilitation environment for children with cerebral palsy on perceptions of self-efficacy: a pilot study. *Pediatr. Rehabil.* 5, 141–148. doi: 10.1080/1363849021000039344

Reid, D. T. (2002b). The use of virtual reality to improve upper-extremity efficiency skills in children with cerebral palsy: a pilot study. *Technol. Disabil.* 14, 53–62.

Repetto, C., and Riva, G. (2011). From virtual reality to interreality in the treatment of anxiety disorders. *Neuropsychiatry* 1, 31–43. doi: 10.2196/jmir.3235

Rizzo, A., Buckwalter, G., Neumann, U., Kesselman, C., and Thiebaux, M. (1998). Basic issues in the application of virtual reality for the assessment and rehabilitation of cognitive impairments and functional disabilities. *Cyberpsychol. Behav.* 1, 59–78. doi: 10.1089/cpb.1998.1.59

Rothwell, J. C. (2012). Clinical applications of noninvasive electrical stimulation: problems and potentials. *Clin. EEG Neurosci.* 43, 209–214. doi: 10.1177/1550059412444973

Ruffini, G., Fox, M. D., Ripolles, O., Miranda, P. C., and Pascual-Leone, A. (2014). Optimization of multifocal transcranial current stimulation for weighted cortical pattern targeting from realistic modeling of electric fields. *Neuroimage* 89, 216–225. doi: 10.1016/j.neuroimage.2013.12.002

Saposnik, G., Levin, M., and Outcome Research Canada (SORCan) Working Group (2011). Virtual reality in stroke rehabilitation: a meta-analysis and implications for clinicians. *Stroke* 42, 1380–1386. doi: 10.1161/STROKEAHA.110.605451

Seraglia, B., Gamberini, L., Priftis, K., Scatturin, P., Martinelli, M., and Cutini, S. (2011). An exploratory fNIRS study with immersive virtual reality: a new method for technical implementation. *Front. Hum. Neurosci.* 5:176. doi: 10.3389/fnhum.2011.00176

Sitaram, R., Zhang, H., Guan, C., Thulasidas, M., Hoshi, Y., Ishikawa, A., et al. (2007). Temporal classification of multichannel near-infrared spectroscopy signals of motor imagery for developing a brain-computer interface. *Neuroimage* 34, 1416–1427. doi: 10.1016/j.neuroimage.2006.11.005

Strosahl, K. D., and Ascough, J. C. (1981). Clinical uses of mental imagery: experimental foundations, theoretical misconceptions, and research issues. *Psychol. Bull.* 89, 422–438. doi: 10.1037/0033-2909.89.3.422

Thomson, K., Pollock, A., Bugge, C., and Brady, M. (2014). Commercial gaming devices for stroke upper limb rehabilitation: a systematic review. *Int. J. Stroke* 9, 479–488. doi: 10.1111/ijs.12263

Tsang, M. M., and Man, D. W. (2013). A virtual reality-based vocational training system (VRVTS) for people with schizophrenia in vocational rehabilitation. *Schizophr. Res.* 144, 51–62. doi: 10.1016/j.schres.2012.12.024

Van den Broek, M. D. (2005). Why does neurorehabilitation fail? *J. Head Trauma Rehabil.* 20, 464–473. doi: 10.1097/00001199-200509000-00007

Viana, R. T., Viana, R. T., Laurentino, G. E. C., Souza, R. J. P., Fonseca, J. B., Silva Filho, E. M., et al. (2014). Effects of the addition of transcranial direct current stimulation to virtual reality therapy after stroke: a pilot randomized controlled trial. *NeuroRehabilitation* 34, 437–446. doi: 10.3233/NRE-141065

Vincelli, F., Choi, H., Molinari, E., Wiederhold, B. K., Bouchard, S., and Riva, G. (2002). Virtual reality assisted cognitive behavioral therapy for the treatment of panic disorders with Agoraphobia. *Stud. Health Technol. Inform.* 85, 552–559.

Wang, C. T. (2012). [Research and application of a haptics-based virtual-reality training system for craniomaxillofacial surgery]. *Zhonghua Kou Qiang Yi Xue Za Zhi* 47, 458–462. doi: 10.3760/cma.j.issn.1002-0098.2012.08.003

Waters, F. A., Maybery, M. T., Badcock, J. C., and Michie, P. T. (2004). Context memory and binding in schizophrenia. *Schizophr. Res.* 68, 119–125. doi: 10.1016/S0920-9964(03)00221-4

Williams, C. K., and Carnahan, H. (2014). Motor learning perspectives on haptic training for the upper extremities. *IEEE Trans. Haptics* 7, 240–250. doi: 10.1109/TOH.2013.2297102

Winstein, C. J. (1991). Knowledge of results and motor learning–implications for physical therapy. *Phys. Ther.* 71, 140–149.

Wolpaw, J. R., Birbaumer, N., Mcfarland, D. J., Pfurtscheller, G., and Vaughan, T. M. (2002). Brain-computer interfaces for communication and control. *Clin. Neurophysiol.* 113, 767–791. doi: 10.1016/S1388-2457(02)00057-3

Xuxian, Y., Baolei, X., Changhao, J., Yunfa, F., Zhidong, W., Hongyi, L., et al. (2015). A hybrid BCI based on EEG and fNIRS signals improves the performance of decoding motor imagery of both force and speed of hand clenching. *J. Neural. Eng.* 12, 036004. doi: 10.1088/1741-2560/12/3/036004

Yeh, S. C., Lee, S. H., Chan, R. C., Chen, S., and Rizzo, A. (2014). A virtual reality system integrated with robot-assisted haptics to simulate pinch-grip task: motor ingredients for the assessment in chronic stroke. *NeuroRehabilitation* 35, 435–449. doi: 10.3233/NRE-141134

You, S. H., Jang, S. H., Kim, Y. H., Kwon, Y. H., Barrow, I., and Hallett, M. (2005). Cortical reorganization induced by virtual reality therapy in a child with hemiparetic cerebral palsy. *Dev. Med. Child Neurol.* 47, 628–635. doi: 10.1017/S0012162205001234

14

From Trust in Automation to Decision Neuroscience: Applying Cognitive Neuroscience Methods to Understand and Improve Interaction Decisions Involved in Human Automation Interaction

Kim Drnec[1], Amar R. Marathe[1], Jamie R. Lukos[2] and Jason S. Metcalfe[1]*

[1] Human Research and Engineering Directorate, U.S. Army Research Laboratory, Aberdeen, MD, USA, [2] Advanced Concepts and Applied Research Branch, Space and Naval Warfare Systems Center Pacific, San Diego, CA, USA

***Correspondence:**
Kim Drnec
kdrnec@gmail.com;
kim.a.drnec2.ctr@mail.mil

Human automation interaction (HAI) systems have thus far failed to live up to expectations mainly because human users do not always interact with the automation appropriately. Trust in automation (TiA) has been considered a central influence on the way a human user interacts with an automation; if TiA is too high there will be overuse, if TiA is too low there will be disuse. However, even though extensive research into TiA has identified specific HAI behaviors, or trust outcomes, a unique mapping between trust states and trust outcomes has yet to be clearly identified. Interaction behaviors have been intensely studied in the domain of HAI and TiA and this has led to a reframing of the issues of problems with HAI in terms of reliance and compliance. We find the behaviorally defined terms reliance and compliance to be useful in their functionality for application in real-world situations. However, we note that once an inappropriate interaction behavior has occurred it is too late to mitigate it. We therefore take a step back and look at the interaction decision that precedes the behavior. We note that the decision neuroscience community has revealed that decisions are fairly stereotyped processes accompanied by measurable psychophysiological correlates. Two literatures were therefore reviewed. TiA literature was extensively reviewed in order to understand the relationship between TiA and trust outcomes, as well as to identify gaps in current knowledge. We note that an interaction decision precedes an interaction behavior and believe that we can leverage knowledge of the psychophysiological correlates of decisions to improve joint system performance. As we believe that understanding the interaction decision will be critical to the eventual mitigation of inappropriate interaction behavior, we reviewed the decision making literature and provide a synopsis of the state of the art understanding of the decision process from a decision neuroscience perspective. We forward hypotheses based on this understanding that could shape a research path toward the ability to mitigate interaction behavior in the real world.

Keywords: trust in automation, interaction decisions, decision making, human automation interaction, neuroergonomics

INTRODUCTION

The purpose of this review is to address a largely unexplored aspect of human automation interaction (HAI); that is, the human decision that leads to interaction behavior, traditionally considered a manifestation of the user's level of Trust in Automation (TiA). The extension of this concept has been that, if HAI is to be actively managed in joint human-automation systems, one must calibrate the TiA of the user so that decisions about interactions with automation are appropriate. Further, it has been considered that if one could measure instantaneous levels of TiA, inappropriate interaction decisions could be predicted and mitigated. Research interest in HAI systems is motivated in large part because of observations that even the most advanced HAI systems have not yet fully realized the ultimate vision of both safe and seamless integration of the human into the system that would lead to improved task performance. Specifically, successful applications of automation within task spaces involving human operators have not yet been realized without simultaneous definition of significant context-specific design constraints that delineate human and automation responsibilities. Such constraints may improve focused aspects of performance, but also increase the risk in other ways, particularly in circumstances and moments involving handoff of control authority, and these constraints limit more generalized application of HAI concepts and methods, particularly in terms of improving joint system efficiency (Parasuraman and Riley, 1997; Dekker and Woods, 2002; Dzindolet et al., 2003; Jamieson and Vicente, 2005; Parasuraman and Manzey, 2010).

Decades of human factors research have resulted in an understanding of what factors affect TiA, but as of yet, it remains unclear how specific levels of TiA translate into specific human decisions regarding interaction with a given automation. This knowledge gap may exist because human behavior and joint system performance can be thought of as the result of a combination of many factors only one of which is TiA (Hancock et al., 2011; Schaefer et al., 2014). Research aimed at predicting interaction behaviors has previously met with some success, particularly with respect to decision aid systems (Bliss et al., 1995; Meyer and Bitan, 2002; Meyer et al., 2014) and automated driving aids (Kumagai et al., 2003; Gold et al., 2015; Terai et al., 2015). We consider such results to suggest that understanding the interaction behavior may be a more fruitful and immediate route toward active, online mitigation of problems thought to arise from mis-calibrated TiA. This idea is developed with the appreciation that interaction behaviors result from decisions about how and when to interact, and any individual interaction decision may or may not be motivated by a change in TiA.

Our specific proposal is that, as much as behavior is a key to managing HAI, understanding the process of decision-making in the context of HAI is critical for understanding and predicting interaction behaviors. It is an important step that is implicitly necessary for eventual online mitigation of inappropriate interaction behavior. This is especially applicable in our discussion inasmuch as we believe that TiA reflects changing degrees of perceived risk and uncertainty and is an instance of value based decision making in dynamic contexts. We further suggest that physiological correlates of value based decisions could be measured and leveraged to provide valuable data that may increase the likelihood of predicting a consequent interaction. To develop the connection between TiA and value based decision making, the discussion begins by reviewing extant human factors literature to demonstrate that, while TiA is one of many important factors influencing HAI performance, it is ultimately the interaction behavior that is of interest. It is then argued that this behavior, if intentional, is the result of a decision, and thus understanding the decision process leading to the behavior may facilitate near- to medium-term solutions for active mitigation strategies while understanding of the nuances and complexities of TiA continues to evolve over the long term. The discussion then turns towards a synthesis of selected cognitive neuroscience literature that focuses particularly on value based decision making. We conclude with future research directions that would be necessary to enable decision based monitoring and prediction of interaction behaviors and the eventual development of active mitigations for the types of HAI problems currently believed to be brought about by mis-calibrated TiA.

THE IMPORTANCE OF TiA IN JOINT SYSTEM PERFORMANCE

The term automation, or automated system, as used here is best defined by Parasuraman et al. (2000) as a "machine execution of functions". This definition includes automation with capabilities as diverse as controlling a sophisticated cockpit system or as simple as an automated coffee maker. Because automation is not yet fully "intelligent" it has no agency for adapting to unexpected circumstances, and therefore often requires the supervision and/or occasional intervention of humans. Part of this supervisory role requires that there be HAIs, but these interactions need to be appropriate, or the joint system performance will suffer. Decades of HAI system research have indicated that appropriate interactions are the result of decisions subsequent to calibrated TiA. An established conceptual model of factors influencing HAI performance is provided in **Figure 1**. As the model suggests, TiA has traditionally been considered to be the critical component driving human user decisions about interactions such as intervening in an automated task. Given the importance that TiA has been accorded to overall joint system performance, in this section we provide a brief review of important aspects of TiA and its dynamics. We aim to highlight the complex relationship between TiA and human user behavior, and implications arising from this relationship that imply that even if moment to moment levels of TiA were to be measured, it is unclear how such information could be leveraged to predict an interaction behavior.

Early theories about the construct of TiA were developed from the psychological construct of interpersonal trust, and they posited that calibrated TiA was critical for successful HAI system performance (Sheridan, 1980; Sheridan and Hennessy, 1984). There are aspects of interpersonal trust that are analogous to TiA,

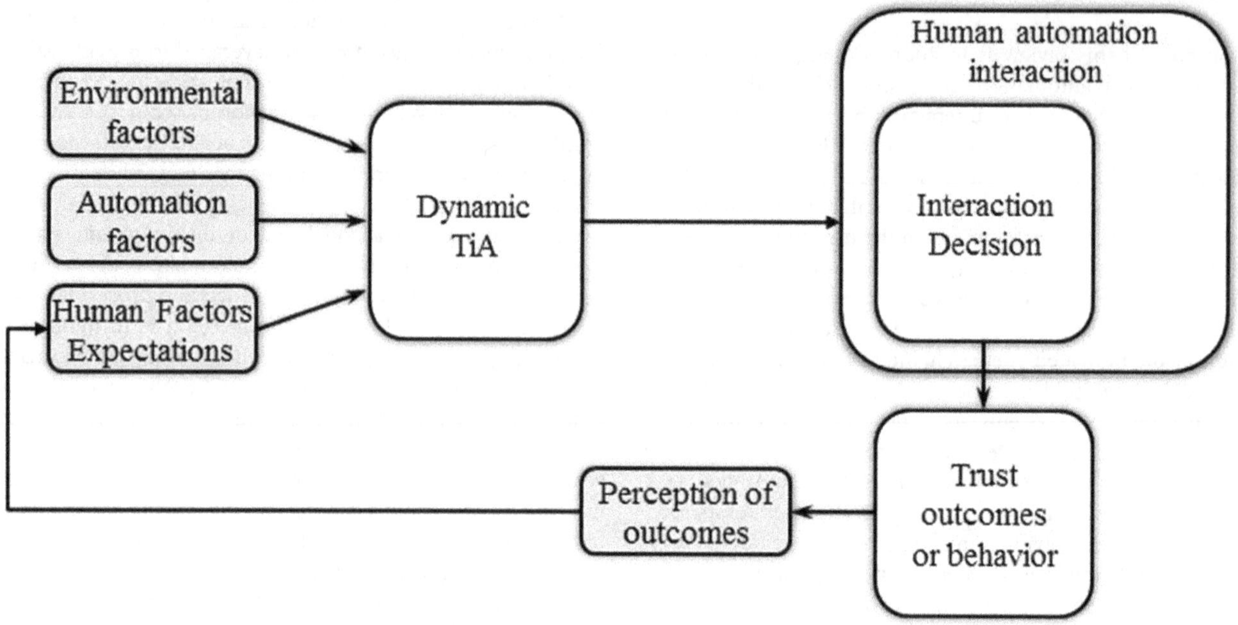

FIGURE 1 | A conceptual organization of trust and human user-automation interaction (Adapted from Hancock et al., 2011 with permission from Sage Publishing). This article focuses on interaction decisions that are part of the overall human automation interaction (HAI).

in particular that there needs to be a sense of risk or vulnerability on the part of the trustor for trust to develop (Lee and Moray, 1994; Muir, 1994; Corritore et al., 2003; Lee and See, 2004; Evans and Krueger, 2011). However, it has been debated whether the two constructs are homologous (Madhavan and Wiegmann, 2007), and so trust as it specifically applies to automation became a central point of interest in human factors research aimed at improving joint system performance (Lee and Moray, 1992; Muir, 1994; Muir and Moray, 1996; Lee and See, 2004). Myriad definitions of TiA imply that it is the result of a feeling of trustworthiness towards the automation such that a human user can depend on the automation to perform the task for which it was designed. It is worth noting that if the consequence of the task to the human user is small, if TiA develops at all, its level becomes irrelevant because the outcome of the joint system fails to be important. Therefore, much like interpersonal trust (Lee and Moray, 1994; Muir, 1994), TiA develops in the face of a sense of risk. In these situations, TiA then develops and shows dynamic changes from the ongoing comparison of the expectations about the automation's behavior and observations by the human user about the automation's performance weighted heavily on the risk borne by the human user (Sheridan and Hennessy, 1984; Muir, 1994; Muir and Moray, 1996).

Determinants and Dynamics of Trust in Automation: Expectations and Observations

One of the first explicit theories of TiA (Muir, 1994) stated that appropriate levels of TiA would develop if three expectations were met during the course of automation interaction. These expectations are technical competence, persistence, and fiduciary responsibility, but they play differential roles in TiA development and dynamics throughout the course of automation use. For example, perceptions of competence might be more important in the early stages of automation use than later in time. The expectation of technical competence is the expectation that the automation will accurately and successfully perform the functions for which it was designed. Persistence, perhaps here better conceived of as predictability, relates to the issue of reliability in that an automation that performs in a particular manner now will be expected to perform in a same or similar manner when it encounters similar circumstances in the future. Finally, fiduciary responsibility addresses the notion that a given human user will hold expectations of an automation of a particular type that will impact role allocation. That is, the human user will expect that the automation will necessarily be responsible for its designed functions as they understand them and thus fewer personal resources need to be allocated to carrying out those functions. The importance of these expectations related to TiA dynamics differ depending on the stage of the interaction with the automation.

When first presented with an automated system there is limited information available for the human user to observe, and thus little with which to evaluate the trustworthiness of the automation. Some key elements that significantly affect early levels of TiA include initial expectations borne from biases toward automations in general, and initial observations about the design of the automation (Muir and Moray, 1996; Nass et al., 1996; Dzindolet et al., 2002; Lee and See, 2004; Parasuraman and Miller, 2004; Miller, 2005; Merritt and Ilgen, 2008; Merritt, 2011; Merritt et al., 2012; Pak et al., 2012). After having been introduced to an automation, human users tend to explore different strategies for subsequent interaction (Lee and Moray, 1992) and thus learn more about the automation's behavior. This experimentation arguably helps the human user gauge competence, which emerges as one of the most important predictors of TiA at this early stage. However, it is worth noting that for various reasons, human users are notoriously poor at making accurate judgments of competence (Sheridan and Hennessy, 1984; Lee and Moray, 1992; Dzindolet et al., 2002, 2003; Madhavan et al., 2006; Verberne et al., 2012; Merritt et al., 2014). Once automation competence has been judged, whether correct or not, the most important factor driving levels of TiA is persistence or predictability of performance over time (Lee and Moray, 1992). Persistence of performance is important enough that as long as errors are predictable and the automation error rate is at a consistent rate of approximately 30% or less, most human users will decide to continue to use and benefit from the automation (Parasuraman et al., 2000; Wickens and Dixon, 2007; Wang et al., 2009). As levels of TiA dynamically change throughout the course of observations about the automation's behavior, theory posits that interaction decisions, and consequent behaviors, should reflect the extant level of TiA. If there is too much or too little TiA, as it goes, a human user may decide to overuse or underuse the automation, respectively. Specific patterns of behaviors resulting from decisions about how to interact with the automation have been well documented and are commonly referred to as trust outcomes as they are believed to directly reflect certain levels of TiA.

Trust Outcomes and their Relationship to TiA

The trust outcomes most commonly discussed are misuse and disuse and are described in detail by Parasuraman and Riley (1997). Misuse refers to instances when the automation is used without undo skepticism, tending to result in overuse (Parasuraman and Riley, 1997; Bahner et al., 2008; Parasuraman and Manzey, 2010). Misuse has two related causes; automation bias and complacency (Manzey et al., 2006; Parasuraman and Manzey, 2010). They are related in that they both result in a lack of monitoring where lack of attention plays a central role (Parasuraman and Manzey, 2010). Automation bias arises through the mere presence of an automated system, possibly because humans demonstrate a tendency to choose the route of least cognitive effort, making it easier, or at least preferable, to accept that feedback from an automation as correct (Dzindolet et al., 1999, 2001; Skitka et al., 1999, 2000; Wang et al., 2008; Parasuraman and Manzey, 2010; Goddard et al., 2014; Mosier and Skitka, 1996). Complacency, less well understood, can be said to occur when monitoring is less than optimal and joint system performance suffers (Parasuraman and Manzey, 2010). However, both automation bias and complacency tend to increase in cases of high workload and high consequence environments wherein users often make conscious decisions to rely on even imperfect automation (Dixon et al., 2007; Wickens and Dixon, 2007). Disuse describes a continuum that spans from the user underutilizing the automation to entirely abandoning the automation in favor of a manual mode. Disuse tends to occur if a human user has a high expectation of automation performance and then observes unexpected errors or has more self confidence in her ability to perform the task than confidence in the efficacy of the automation for the same task (Lee and Moray, 1994; Parasuraman and Riley, 1997; Moray et al., 2000; Dzindolet et al., 2003).

Although trust outcomes have been well defined, a synthesis of the literature, and recent experimental evidence (Wiczorek and Manzey, 2010; Chancey et al., 2015) indicate a far more complex relationship between TiA and trust outcomes than is implied in the above discussion, and this implies that predicting interactions based on extant TiA levels is problematic. Such complex interactions involve perceived risk, self-confidence, workload, and even personality type (Lee and Moray, 1994; Muir, 1994; Parasuraman and Riley, 1997; Lee and See, 2004; Merritt and Ilgen, 2008; Hancock et al., 2011; Schaefer et al., 2012; Merritt et al., 2014). For instance, human users have been documented as reporting a high level of TiA and then, paradoxically choosing a manual operation mode, demonstrating disuse (Lee and Moray, 1992). Conversely, even when low TiA has been reported, human users may misuse even a poorly competent automation, particularly under high workload conditions (Daly, 2002; Biros et al., 2004). Clearly levels of TiA do not map uniquely onto trust outcomes, regardless of how they are represented (i.e., attention, intervention rate, etc.). Therefore, they are not predictive of the way a human user will decide to interact with an automation, limiting the use of measuring TiA for real world applications to improve HAI. We suggest that this is because TiA is far more complex than may be useful for those with more immediate concerns regarding actively managing HAI. However, it is important to note that when TiA is studied it is the interaction behavior that is of interest most often. Therefore, regardless of the manageability of trust, what might be learned if we focus more simply and exclusively on the behavior?

TiA as Predictable Behavior

The present discussion is not the first to offer that a shift in focus from trust to behavior is well justified. In fact, a number of researchers in this domain have re-framed the problem space of TiA into one of reliance and compliance, which are defined exclusively in terms of observable behavior, and are not intended to imply specific psychological cause such as trust (Meyer, 2001, 2004; Parasuraman et al., 2008; Rice, 2009; Meyer et al., 2014). Indeed, there is a non-unique mapping of reliance and compliance to traditional trust outcomes such that an observation of inappropriate amounts of either may alternately signal disuse or misuse and possibly motivate conflicting interpretations of TiA. We find these behaviorally defined terms to be useful in their functionality for application in real world situations. That is, objectively defined and observable behaviors are especially valuable for the purposes of modeling and prediction because they obviate the need for drawing inferences to and making assumptions about manifestations of more subjectively defined constructs, such as TiA, automation bias or complacency that are difficult to measure objectively and thus unsuitable for use in attempts at active optimization and/or mitigation.

Reliance is the tendency of the human user to accept the lack of an alarm, alert, warning, or prompt as a true reflection of the state of the world (Lee and Moray, 1994; Singh et al., 1997; Parasuraman et al., 2000; Yeh and Wickens, 2000; Moray, 2003; Dixon et al., 2006). That is, in the absence of an alarm or warning, the human user accepts, often tacitly, that all is well and there is no reason for possible intervention. Compliance, on the other hand, is defined when the user responds to, putatively agrees with, and ultimately takes the action specified by an alarm or recommendation from the automation (Meyer, 2001, 2004). Though reliance and compliance are often discussed in terms of optimal behavior, too much of either in the wrong context is detrimental to system performance. For instance, if an alarm is absent and the human user assumes that no circumstances warranting an alarm exist and thus fails to monitor the automation over significant time, he or she is at risk of over-reliance and the consequences thereof. Conversely, over-compliance occurs when the human accepts all suggestions from the automation (when present) without confirming their validity.

Beyond observation of general behavioral patterns, the greater benefit of defining compliance and reliance behaviors has been in providing an avenue towards greater precision in understanding the factors that affect automation use during HAI, which might eventually lead to prediction of an interaction. For instance, some have observed that reliance and compliance are differentially affected by error type, i.e., false alarms vs. misses in target detection tasks (Meyer, 2004; Rice and Geels, 2010; Wiczorek and Manzey, 2014), and by the predictive value of the alarm (Meyer and Bitan, 2002; Manzey et al., 2014). If a human user observes frequent failures to trigger alarms, the frequency of monitoring the automation will increase, thereby reducing reliance on the automated agent (Masalonis and Parasuraman, 1999; Bagheri and Jamieson, 2004; Meyer, 2004; Madhavan and Wiegmann, 2007; Parasuraman and Manzey, 2010; Geels-Blair et al., 2013). Compliance, however, is degraded by higher rates of false alarms. In particular, when higher rates of false alarms are observed, users tend to consume critical time and attentional resources to verify alarms before choosing a response. Further progress in this line of inquiry has resulted in more general characterization of how interaction behaviors change with the positive and negative predictive value of an alarm. Positive predictive value is derived from a Bayesian calculation of the likely existence of a hazard given an alarm and, likewise, the probability of an alarm given no existing hazard (Meyer et al., 2014). Negative predictive value is calculated similarly, but in the absence of an alarm. Therefore, positive predictive value decreases as false alarm rate goes up and negative predictive value decreases with more frequent misses (no alarm in the presence of a hazard). Interaction behavior is thus differentially affected by changing positive vs. negative predictive value. Positive predictive value has been shown to have strong effects on reliance, but only for values less than 0.75 (Meyer et al., 2014), where values below this threshold have been associated with excessive time spent monitoring the automation. Research in HAI domains has thus befitted considerably from the use of these narrowly and objectively defined behavioral terms.

We advocate here for shifting research towards more clearly defined behaviors and the factors that affect them because of how this shift creates important opportunities for systematic research into HAI. The domain of application for such a shifted focus would include contexts where TiA may be involved, at least inasmuch as TiA reflects assessments of the relative value of specific behavioral options defined in terms of probable risk versus reward. We argue that such behavior-based understandings are important for progress on multiple levels from phenomenology to predictive modeling. The extant work discussed above has provided an essential corpus of knowledge regarding the relationship between automation performance characteristics (i.e., error rate, type, and predictive value) and human user interaction behaviors. However, we also suggest that in order to be useful down the road for real-world mitigation of inappropriate interactions, this shift from trust to behavior does not go quite far enough for two important reasons. First, to mitigate a potentially detrimental interaction behavior in a dynamic context, prediction is necessary. This is because a behavior that has already occurred cannot be changed and the consequences are likely to be too immediate to offset in *post hoc* fashion. Moreover, the predictive power required must occur on a time-scale that allows a reasonable opportunity to enact a mitigation when an inappropriate behavior is expected. Second, the current understanding of reliance and compliance is tied to automation design; an automation that frequently misses events reduces reliance, and an automation that frequently produces false alarms reduces compliance. This understanding, then, usefully provides an improved framework for HAI, but has yet to account for variability in individual instances of HAI. Therefore, the predictive power of the current understanding of interaction behaviors based on population averages remains limited to overall design strategies whereas we are interested in building towards eventual prediction and mitigation of reliance and compliance at the level of individual instances of interaction behavior. In order to improve the ability to predict an interaction behavior we thus believe it is necessary to consider not only the effects of automation design on interaction behaviors such as compliance and reliance, but also the individual internal phenomena that precedes the behavior.

INTERACTION BEHAVIOR REFRAMED AS A DECISION TO INTERACT WITH AN AUTOMATION

Before an intentional behavior occurs, the human user must make a decision as to which among a limited array of options will be selected. Here we argue that research concerned with improving HAI would benefit greatly from studying the decisions that precede interaction behaviors. Such an approach satisfies the need for focus on individual interactions in a manner that affords prediction on a time-scale that is useful for active mitigation. We define such decisions as interaction decisions, given as specific to the intention to interact with an automation.

While TiA has often been considered to motivate interaction decisions, the richness of the decision process itself, as well as accompanying stereotypical psychophysiological indicators thereof, has not been thoroughly investigated as a source of information that could be applied to the prediction of a consequent interaction behavior. Our starting point in this pursuit is to understand the underlying psychological and physiological processes of decision making, with a particular focus on value based decision making. This understanding can provide a cornerstone for the advancement of scientifically based hypotheses about how interaction behaviors may eventually be predicted for the sake of active mitigation. Predicting decision outcomes, or the interaction behavior in a real-world HAI context, is of course not trivial, but laboratory-based research in decision neuroscience has established decision making as a reasonably stereotyped process with clear behavioral and physiological precursors. Further, the ability to predict decision outcomes has been pursued by both the cognitive neuroscience (Soon et al., 2008; Haynes, 2011; Perez et al., 2015) and brain computer interface (Musallam et al., 2004) communities. Indeed, attempts at predicting some types of decision outcome behaviors have already met with success in a laboratory environment, possibly because the specifics of a decision process in the brain begin even before there is conscious awareness of the impending decision (Soon et al., 2008, 2013; Haynes, 2011; Perez et al., 2015). Some of these studies have been criticized because there lacks a sense of risk or value to the decision maker in a controlled experiment, and therefore, the assumption is that the decision outcomes that are being predicted are trivial (Gold and Shadlen, 2007; Lavazza and De Caro, 2010).

The lack of risk, value, or reward in these controlled laboratory environments is in contrast to interaction decisions that inherently involve some type of personal risk or reward. For example, over relying on an automation can compromise joint system performance, and therefore causes degradations in joint system performance. Thus, we are chiefly concerned with decisions that are based on expected value and risk, or value based decisions (Rangel et al., 2008; Wallis, 2012). Value based decisions are particularly relevant to the HAI context because it is often required that a human user continuously weigh the expected personal value of allowing the automation to complete the task versus performing it manually or, rather, whether to comply with the recommendation of an automated system. Importantly, this assessment and subsequent judgment of value to the user must be made against the backdrop of risk that the decision may compromise joint system performance. Thus, through the common elements of risk, reward, and expected value, we believe interaction decisions during HAI to be an instance of value based decision making. We believe that understanding the value based decision process is important to improving HAI and, therefore, we briefly discuss results of value based decision making research as it relates to HAI in order to support hypotheses forwarded in the discussion, aimed at establishing a research path that will allow the eventual prediction of HAI interaction behaviors.

The Importance of Considering the Decision Process

An important argument in favor of studying the decision process in order to improve HAI is that significant efforts in cognitive neuroscience have revealed decision making as fairly stereotyped, and therefore, a potentially predictable process. Moreover, this body of research has identified a number of psychophysiological correlates that unfold in advance of, and during a decision. Critically, these correlates are measurable, and therefore useful for understanding the decision process, at least in laboratory settings. Some have observed that these correlates unfold in predictable ways through defined cognitive stages, and therefore measuring them has potential use for active mitigations of inappropriate interaction decisions and behavior. This approach is fundamentally different than attempting to measure and calibrate TiA because the psychophysiological correlates of a decision are measurable whereas the construct of TiA is yet to be defined in a way that is equally useful for active monitoring. In general, many cognitive neuroscientists model decisions as comprising three cognitive stages (Fellows, 2004; Bogacz, 2007). However, five cognitive processes, some analogous to stages of the cognitive models of general decisions, have been described in value based decision making (Rangel et al., 2008) and are therefore relevant to our discussion of interaction decisions. These processes, which are not discrete stages *per se*, are: (1) representation of the problem, i.e., identification of alternative choices, and of internal and external states that affect the value of the choices; (2) evaluation of gathered evidence that allows the assignment of a value to the alternatives; (3) comparison of these values in order to make a decision; (4) accumulation of the comparative value for each alternative and making the decision; and (5) generation of prediction errors that provide feedback in order for learning to occur. The psychophysiological processes that unfold within the first four processes will be discussed as they relate to HAI contexts such as risk and reward. The fifth process, generating feedback on the decision has been studied in the context of learning, and may be useful for later development of adaptive mitigation strategies, but is beyond the scope of the current review (Nieuwenhuis et al., 2005; Christie and Tata, 2009; Cohen et al., 2011; van de Vijver et al., 2011). We note that we discuss these processes sequentially mainly for organizational purposes, however, during the decision process they may overlap or even occur in parallel (Rangel et al., 2008).

The Value Based Decision Process

In order for the need to identify alternatives to arise, there must be some recognition of the need for a decision; in a sense it is the motivation to perform a task (Gold and Shadlen, 2007). Decisions must be initiated by either salient external or internal stimuli. These stimuli will often produce an orienting response (Sokolov et al., 2002; Glimcher and Rustichini, 2004; Delgado et al., 2005), characterized in humans by a measurable increase in tonic skin conductance (SC) levels and a decrease in heart rate variability (Figner and Murphy, 2011). In an HAI domain, relevant stimuli typically include those specifying alerts from the automation, acute changes in environment, or internal feelings that the current behavior is inappropriate (typically seen as an error-related potential in the brain or a gradual shift in peripheral physiology). Once the need for a decision has been established, however, decision alternatives are identified. As alternatives are identified, in the case of interaction decisions, the human user will also identify, if not consciously, a representation of internal and external states (Rangel et al., 2008). These representations play an important part during the process of assigning values to individual alternatives. For example, a human user is more likely to take control from the automation if they detect that the automation is malfunctioning and they perceive an associated risk. The neural basis of this early stage in the decision process is not well understood. For example, it is unclear how the brain decides which alternatives should be considered, and if there is a functional limit to the number that can be assessed at one time (Rangel et al., 2008). Nevertheless, such questions are important for determining how to leverage physiological indicators into models of decision making during HAI.

Once the possible alternatives are identified evidence for or against each alternative must be evaluated in order to make an optimal decision. In the case of interaction decisions, which due to the presence of risk are analogous to value based decisions, it has been hypothesized by some (Rangel et al., 2008; Glimcher and Fehr, 2013) Reading hidden intentions in the human brain cognitive valuation systems that the brain might use; the Pavlovian, Habitual, and Goal directed. We believe the goal directed system to be most relevant to our discussion because the goal directed system assigns values to potential actions by calculating action-outcome associations from previous experience and comparing this value to the perceived rewards associated with possible outcomes of the decision (Rangel et al., 2008). In the goal directed valuation system the value assigned to a piece of evidence is equivalent to the potential value of the alternative it supports, with the value assigned to an alternative being equal to the expected reward of the action. In the context of HAI, an important research question would be whether the probability of success is greater by relying on the automation or not and, moreover, how that probability scales with perceived risk to determine the direction of a given interaction decision.

When a person valuates a piece of evidence they will do so by observing the relevant data (e.g., visual scanning, sound or other stimulus), consulting their memory, and integrating this against a backdrop of expectations (Mulder et al., 2014). In the case of visual evidence, gaze fixation is thought to support evidence evaluation such that evidence about the value of an alternative is sampled at each fixation (Krajbich et al., 2010; Krajbich and Rangel, 2011). Memory consultation causes a person to compare past decision outcomes with the available alternatives. The brain creates a prediction error that would represent the difference between the expected value of choosing current decision alternatives from the value that has been experienced in the past by choosing alternatives that are similar in nature (Hare et al., 2008). For example, consider a human user who has previously experienced aberrant behavior from an automation, but there has been no decrement in joint system performance, and joint system performance continues to remain better than what would be expected from only one agent performing the task. Even in risky environments such as in the battlefield, or during a search and rescue operation, the experienced user is more likely to rely on an automation (Lyons and Stokes, 2012) than a user who has not experienced the aberrant behavior because the experienced user has realized the value in relying on the automation despite the probability of an error.

At a cellular level, data have suggested that the cognitive evaluation of evidence is supported by neural "evaluators" that store dynamic estimates of which decision alternative is supported by the evidence. For instance, studies using fMRI in risk reward scenarios have identified two candidate neural evaluators; the amygdala and ventral striatum. A reward based fMRI study indicated that the amygdala evaluates the cost or risk of acting on an alternative (Yacubian et al., 2006; Basten et al., 2010). In the same fMRI study the ventral striatum was implicated in the formation of representations of the expected value or reward of an alternative (Yacubian et al., 2006; Kable and Glimcher, 2007; Rangel et al., 2008; Basten et al., 2010; Lim et al., 2011). Other authors, however, have found that in addition to the amygdala and the ventral striatum that the lateral orbitofrontal cortex and the medial orbital frontal cortex also act as neural evaluators for risk and reward, respectively (Hare et al., 2008; Rangel et al., 2008; Rangel and Hare, 2010). The neural substrates that have been observed support value based decision making processes are detailed in **Table 1**.

The neural evaluators, then, form representations of the risks and rewards for each alternative; the benefit of relying or complying with an automation, as opposed to choosing to complete the task manually. As the risks and rewards of a potential interaction behavior are processed by the amygdala and ventral striatum, the value of these representations must be assessed relative to each other; they must be compared. Neural correlates of this third process involved in value based decision making, comparison of the values assigned to the evidence, have been observed in fMRI studies. That is, value based comparison has been suggested as supported by activation in the ventral medial prefrontal cortex (vmPFC; Chib et al., 2009; Gläscher et al., 2009; Basten et al., 2010), whereas the "comparator" function in perceptual decisions has been associated with increased activity in the dorsolateral prefrontal cortex (dlPFC; Basten et al., 2010; Philiastides et al., 2011). While the evidence comparison process unfolds, some have hypothesized that the comparative value, also known as the decision variable, is accumulated in the lateral intraparietal cortex (LIP) until a decision threshold is reached, bringing about a decision (Platt and Glimcher, 1999; Kiani and Shadlen, 2009; Mulder et al., 2014). Evidence to support this hypothesis has mainly been shown in primate studies of single cell recordings during cued saccade trials (Platt and Glimcher, 1999; Platt, 2002). However, there has been evidence from fMRI studies that the human parietal cortex is also involved in accumulating the decision variable (Ploran et al., 2007; Heekeren et al., 2008). It is interesting to note that the temporal integration of activity in the frontal-parietal regions, which are considered to be involved in comparing and accumulating compared value

TABLE 1 | Neural substrates and their putative role in decision making.

Neural substrate	Role in decision making	Reference
Amygdala	Processes/computes the value of negative stimuli	Yacubian et al. (2006) and Basten et al. (2010)
Ventral striatum	Processes/computes the value of positive stimuli	Yacubian et al. (2006), Basten et al. (2010) and Lim et al. (2011)
Ventral medial prefrontal cortex (vmPFC)	Calculates the difference of value signals from amygdala and ventral striatum in value based decisions	Basten et al. (2010) and Philiastides et al. (2011)
Dorsolateral prefrontal cortex (dlPFC)	Calculates the difference of signals from amygdala and ventral striatum in perceptual decisions	Basten et al. (2010) and Philiastides et al. (2011)
Lateral intraparietal cortex (LIP)	Accumulates and integrates the value of evidence processed by the vmPFC (evidence largely from monkeys)	Platt and Glimcher (1999); Platt (2002); Basten et al. (2010) and Rorie et al. (2010)
	A cortical area involved in gaze fixation, saccade, and attention, underlying evidence accumulation	Coe et al. (2002) and Goldberg et al. (2006)

signals, has been observed as preceeding the conscious decision to act (Gold and Shadlen, 2007; Soon et al., 2013; Perez et al., 2015).

The putative involvement of the parietal cortex in decision making is noteworthy because of its central role in the process. For example, gaze fixation, critical for evidence evaluation (Poole and Ball, 2006) in visually based decisions, is controlled by the LIP in monkeys (Coe et al., 2002). This region forms a "salience map" for the oculomotor system to saccade to a target, or maintain gaze fixation on a target (Goldberg et al., 2006). The LIP then, not only plays a role in accumulating the comparative value of the evidence as discussed above, but is critical for its initial evaluation. Brain computer interface research has also found that the medial intraparietal cortex in monkeys forms representations of the value of an alternative that has been encoded in the vmPFC (Musallam et al., 2004), such that the intent of the monkey to choose one alternative over an other can be decoded from intracellular electrodes. Although much evidence of the importance of the parietal cortex during decision making, and especially value based decision making, has come from primate research, there is evidence that analogs in the human parietal cortex are also central to decision making (Ploran et al., 2007; Heekeren et al., 2008).

Despite the hypothesized causal role of integrated frontal-parietal activity in the conscious decision to act, there are no measurable psychophysiological variables that allow an accurate determination of the exact time that a decision threshold is reached. However, psychophysiological correlates occurring hundreds of milliseconds before a conscious decision involving risk and reward (Cohen et al., 2009), inherent in value based decision making, have been identified. For instance, the readiness potential, a slow negativity in scalp recording of cortical activity precedes fully endogenous decisions by a few hundred milliseconds (Libet, 1993). Even more proximal to the decision spectral correlates have been observed. In a paradigm involving playing a competitive game against a computer, spectral decomposition of scalp-recorded EEG led to the finding that the decision process was accompanied by a general shift in power between lower bands (delta, 1–4 Hz and theta, 5–7 Hz) to higher frequency bands (alpha, 8–12 Hz and beta, 13–35 Hz), as well as a broadband increase in cross-trial phase coherence at about 220 ms post stimulus (Cohen and Donner, 2013). Similar indications were found during complex real world choice tasks and a two-choice forced-decision paradigm. In these cases, significant correlations of increased power were seen in delta, theta, beta, and gamma (36 + Hz) bands of EEG activity approximately 250–500 ms post-stimulus (Guggisberg et al., 2007; Davis et al., 2011). In decisions involving risk, risk is represented by an asymmetry in the alpha band such that there is an increased alpha power in the right frontal region (Gianotti et al., 2009). These spectral correlates of value based decision making are measurable in real time and available for current application outside a laboratory, which is encouraging in the context of improving HAI. However, these scalp recorded spectral correlates occur only hundreds of milliseconds before an interaction decision and therefore have limited use because they are so temporally proximal to the behavior itself.

The proximity of these value based decision correlates to the actual decision may be discouraging in the context of predicting and mitigating interaction behavior. Nonetheless, research efforts in decision neuroscience and in brain computer interface have found in fMRI studies that the correlates of an outcome of a decision to move at a time chosen by the subject are measurable up to 7 s before the conscious awareness of the decision is reached. Moreover, through analysis of these correlates, the intended goal of the decision can be decoded before conscious awareness of it arises (Haynes et al., 2007; Soon et al., 2008, 2013; Haynes, 2011; Perez et al., 2015). In two fMRI studies (Haynes, 2011; Soon et al., 2013) subjects were asked to decide at will when to either press a button on their left or right side, or add or multiply a set of numbers, and then to report when they were consciously aware of the decision. Spatial pattern analysis of the blood oxygen level dependent signal, a measure of neural activation in fMRI studies, revealed that the frontal polar cortex appeared to encode the intentions of the subjects before they reported having made the decision. In a driving study using implanted EEG electrodes in human epilepsy patients a modulation of gamma power in the posterior lateral cortex predicted whether the subjects would turn left or right at an intersection before they consciously made the decision

(Perez et al., 2015). These studies made use of technology such as fMRI that as yet is not available for real world applications, unlike EEG, because of the need for the subject to lie still in the large, importable fMRI equipment. Further, although EEG is portable, it cannot directly measure activity in deep cortical and subcortical areas, and these are exactly the areas that showed activity prior to a conscious decision. However, the results are encouraging for making use of the interaction decision process to improve HAI and, moreover, can be leveraged into research aimed at developing models that capture relations between cortical and subcortical brain activations during value based decision making. Identification of such relations is an important avenue for future research aimed at active mitigation during HAI.

Indeed, decision neuroscience and brain computer interface research have facilitated the development of precise understandings of decision making that could facilitate the development of methods for identifying an interaction decision within the contextual space of HAI. Efforts in decision neuroscience as well as in more applied domains, such as neuroergonomics, have shown that there are clear and measurable behavioral and psychophysiological correlates (fMRI activation patterns, EEG, SC, gaze fixation, heart rate, etc.) of component processes that are antecedent to the decision. In addition, decision neuroscience has begun to provide an understanding of the underlying cortical and sub-cortical processes involved in decision making. While many of these processes have as yet only been identified by fMRI, their understanding will allow meaningful hypotheses to be advanced about measures that can be recorded in real time.

DISCUSSION

HAI systems have as yet to live up to their expectations, and one critical reason is that human users often make inappropriate decisions about how and when to interact with an automation. These interaction decisions have traditionally been considered to be motivated by extant levels of TiA. Therefore, if TiA can be measured, it is expected that it can be managed and inappropriate interaction behaviors could be mitigated. Given that substantive theory, it was appreciated that TiA is an important construct that undoubtedly affects human user interaction behavior, and hence we reviewed and synthesized the TiA literature. From that exercise, we observed that the relationship between TiA and human behavior is complex and not fully understood. Further, relevant to immediate real world applications for improving HAI system performance, TiA cannot be readily measured, and even if it were measurable in real time it is unclear how certain levels of TiA map onto specific interaction behaviors. By contrast, specific behaviors such as reliance and compliance are readily observed and measured in real time and do not have the confounding effect of inferring psychological causality. Such cause-agnostic variables are particularly attractive in HAI research aimed at defining concrete methods for improving joint system performance, both in terms of initial system design as well as for ultimate real-time applications.

Reframing the problem space of HAI and TiA as a problem of behavior, rather than of TiA, has been successful in allowing general predictions of interaction behavior based on knowledge of system design given specific environmental and internal conditions such as increased risk or increased workload, respectively. For example, knowing that an automation is prone to false alarms will allow the general prediction that a human user will often fail to comply with alerts. This understanding allows a system designer to set thresholds for alarms that are appropriate to intended use. For example, in high risk environments it may be better to set an alarm threshold low so that critical cases are not missed. This predictive ability has been significant in designing systems, but the knowledge is unlikely to allow active mitigation of interaction behavior on an individual basis in real time application, an implicit goal of the aims of HAI focused research. This is the case for two important reasons. First, we argue that focusing attention on interaction behavior does not go far enough because once the behavior has occurred it is too late to mitigate it in an *post hoc* fashion in a timely manner. Second, behaviorally based predictions for automation use are by definition general because the predictive ability has been achieved through extensive observation of how human user behavior is affected by system design. The behaviorally based predictions, however, do not take into account individual variation and dynamic changes in environment. Therefore, they are unlikely to apply to individuals on a case by case basis. For example, it has been shown that a human user may continue to rely on an automation that persistently commits errors of omission, or "misses", due to automation independent reasons such as increasing workload. Therefore, an approach is needed that considers individual cognitive and behavioral aspects, as well as ensuring that there is time to not only mitigate behavior, but allow the prediction of the likelihood of an interaction behavior.

We note that antecedent to the interaction behavior is a decision, which has been characterized by the decision neuroscience community as fairly stereotyped and accompanied by measurable psychophysiological correlates. These properties of decisions suggest predictability, and importantly, as decisions are individual in nature, these properties also imply the likelihood of behavioral prediction at an individual level. We thus believe that understanding the interaction decision is a useful approach to improving HAI, and that with future research that the decision correlates can be leveraged to predict the likelihood of an individual's impending interaction behavior. This approach not only satisfies the problems just discussed, but takes into consideration the human and environmental variability that is found in real world situations in ways that research focused on reliance and compliance has yet to achieve. While it is true that many of the psychophysiological correlates of value based decisions are only measurable with fMRI, we consider that the discoveries afforded by fMRI studies provide a solid basis to form specific scientific hypotheses to guide future research aimed at understanding the interaction decision and consequent interaction behavior. We understand that the fruit of decision neuroscience research might be applied to any domain where it would be advantageous for one decision outcome over another. However, our domain of interest is HAI, and therefore, our focus is in leveraging what is known about value based decision making to understand interaction decisions in the hopes of eventually predicting the likelihood of one decision over another. This goal will require future research, and we begin by forwarding hypotheses to guide research efforts.

One of our first assumptions in this review is that interaction decisions are in fact a case of value based decisions, and that assumption guides our first hypothesis; interaction decisions are a special instance of value based decisions, and therefore the neural correlates accompanying value based decisions will be observable during interaction decisions. One of the first avenues of research is to demonstrate that value based decisions and interaction decisions are analogous in that the sense of risk and reward are inherent in both. This could be achieved by measuring bilateral frontal alpha power during an interaction decision to look for the characteristic asymmetry found in situations entailing risk. Further research to support this hypothesis should necessarily include observing the predicted vmPFC-parietal activation found in value based decision making, during an interaction decision. The strength of this evidence, if found, could be enhanced if concurrent with the parietal-vmPFC activation there is significantly less activation of the dlPFC.

If our first hypothesis is confirmed, we can begin to make more specific hypotheses. Our second hypothesis relates to the fact that there is little understanding of the first stage of value based decision making, the observation of alternatives and representation of internal and external states. Understanding this stage could be particularly important for mitigating inappropriate behavior because it is also accompanied by physiological changes (SC, decreased heart rate variability), which are readily observed. We believe that future research should be aimed at revealing neural correlates of this stage. We hypothesize that activity in the frontal polar cortex and in areas of the parietal cortex during, or just prior to a conscious decision to interact with an automation will occur along with or just prior to the physiological correlates. Evidence previously discussed, that activation patterns in the area of the frontal polar cortex in humans, and in the area of the mid-parietal in monkeys, can be decoded to reveal behavioral intention supports this hypothesis. Should this hypothesis be confirmed, it would add significant evidence that the approach of focusing on interaction decisions will provide an improved method to mitigate interaction behaviors on an individual level. For example, consider the fact that users tend to rely on an automation in the face of risk as demonstrated by traditional behavioral research. However, if this interaction behavior is inappropriate, but the decision to rely can be decoded, there is a chance to mitigate the inappropriate interaction behavior.

While not hypotheses, we believe that future research should also be focused on understanding the psychophysiological basis for, or correlates of, the interaction behaviors of relying or complying on an automation. One first step should include finding the psychophysiological correlates of the demonstrated tendencies of users to rely or comply with automations in circumstances such as workload and risk. For example, what psychophysiological processes drive a human user to perhaps over comply with an automation in conditions of increased cognitive workload, and are there measurable correlates that would suggest that this is the likely interaction behavior? Conversely, what psychophysiological correlates can be found, apart from alpha asymmetry, that appear to suggest the human user is perceiving increased risk, and therefore more likely to over rely on an automation? In order to mitigate disuse, potential psychophysiological correlates, such as particular levels of heart rate variability, SC and EEG power require future study.

Finally, though on a longer horizon, we suggest that it might ultimately be feasible to leverage the understanding of value based decisions in behavioral mitigations aimed at improving HAI system performance. Logically, management of a particular interaction between a human and an automated system requires a minimum of three elements. First, it is essential to understand the capabilities and vulnerabilities of both the particular operator and the particular automation as well as how these may vary under different task and contextual constraints. With such knowledge, one may be able to infer an optimal strategy for allocation of control or decision authority, such as has been done with behaviorally based predictions. Second, though the behavior of automated controls is relatively predictable with knowledge of how its control system was designed, establishing likelihood of human behaviors is a much more challenging task. Therefore, it is also critical to develop methods for prediction of likely changes in operator behavior on a time-scale that leaves room for active intervention through the understanding of the interaction decision. Third, an understanding of how to influence the decision process of humans in principled ways is necessary to ultimately define appropriate systems of actuation when inappropriate behaviors are expected. Of these three elements, it seems that the second may be the most challenging. This is because it is relatively trivial to establish baseline operational or performance characteristics of both humans and automated systems and it is already known that human behaviors and perceptions are subject to influence by a variety of factors, including workload, display properties, transparency, and may be amenable to influence by other task and contextual factors. However, predicting impending behavioral choices is particularly challenging because this requires methods to develop advance insight into the unfolding of the decision process that has largely been studied through the use of fMRI. Here, we offer one way of addressing this; by the application of modern techniques from cognitive neuroscience and psychophysiology.

CONCLUSION

The main purpose of this review is to explore the gap between the understanding of TiA and the actual human user interaction behavior which does not appear to have a clear mapping from TiA levels. We argue in this article that, in addition to understanding the influence of changing levels of TiA, understanding the antecedent decision of the human user's interaction behavior is critical for improving HAI system performance. Decisions have not been explicitly studied in the context of HAI and TiA specifically, but due to the importance of these interaction decisions we reviewed decision making literature and summarized findings that provide a basic understanding of the psychophysiological processes involved in decision making. We are particularly interested in value based decision making because, just as in the case of TiA, if there is no risk, the behavior ceases to be important. While the value based decision process is not yet fully understood as it relates to interaction behaviors, there is a significant understanding of the underlying psychophysiological processes and correlates. This knowledge can be used to advance hypotheses that define a research path aimed at achieving mitigation of human user interaction behaviors.

AUTHOR CONTRIBUTIONS

KD: completed literature review and steered review towards current domain; main contributing author. JSM: final approval authority, guided literature review, advanced concepts germane to content, significant contribution to authorship. ARM: advised in fundamental concepts regarding BCI, HCI, and HAI; also reviewed, edited, and approved successive steps in the process. JRL: provided expertise in the cognitive neuroscience of trust in automation; also reviewed, edited and approved successive review and writing processes.

ACKNOWLEDGMENTS

This research was supported by the U.S. Office of the Secretary of Defense through the Autonomy Research Pilot Initiative (MIPR DWAM31168) as well as by an appointment to the US Army Research Laboratory Postdoctoral Fellowship program administered by the Oak Ridge Associated Universities through a cooperative agreement with the US Army Research Laboratory. We would also like to acknowledge Dr. Kristin Schaefer for her insights and guidance regarding understanding the complex set of human factors that influence trust in automation. The authors are also very grateful for the feedback and guidance of two reviewers whose suggestions have proven rather valuable in improving the quality of the final work.

REFERENCES

Bagheri, N., and Jamieson, G. A. (2004). "Considering subjective trust and monitoring behavior in assessing automation-induced complacency," in *Human Performance, Situation Awareness and Automation: Current Research and Trends*, eds D. A. Vicenzi, M. Mouloua, and P. A. Hancock (Mahwah, NJ: Erlbaum), 54–59.

Bahner, J. E., Hüper, A.-D., and Manzey, D. (2008). Misuse of automated decision aids: complacency, automation bias and the impact of training experience. *Int. J. Hum. Comput. Stud.* 66, 688–699. doi: 10.1016/j.ijhcs.2008.06.001

Basten, U., Biele, G., Heekeren, H. R., and Fiebach, C. J. (2010). How the brain integrates costs and benefits during decision making. *Proc. Natl. Acad. Sci. U S A* 107, 21767–21772. doi: 10.1073/pnas.0908104107

Biros, D., Daly, M., and Gunsch, G. (2004). The influence of task load and automation trust on deception detection. *Group Decis. Negot.* 13, 173–189. doi: 10.1023/b:grup.0000021840.85686.57

Bliss, J. P., Gilson, R. D., and Deaton, J. E. (1995). Human probability matching behaviour in response to alarms of varying reliability. *Ergonomics* 38, 2300–2312. doi: 10.1080/00140139508925269

Bogacz, R. (2007). Optimal decision-making theories: linking neurobiology with behaviour. *Trends Cogn. Sci.* 11, 118–125. doi: 10.1016/j.tics.2006.12.006

Chancey, E. T., Bliss, J. P., Proaps, A. B., and Madhavan, P. (2015). The role of trust as a mediator between system characteristics and response behaviors. *Hum. Factors* 57, 947–958. doi: 10.1177/0018720815582261

Chib, V. S., Rangel, A., Shimojo, S., and O'Doherty, J. P. (2009). Evidence for a common representation of decision values for dissimilar goods in human ventromedial prefrontal cortex. *J. Neurosci.* 29, 12315–12320. doi: 10.1523/JNEUROSCI.2575-09.2009

Christie, G. J., and Tata, M. S. (2009). Right frontal cortex generates reward-related theta-band oscillatory activity. *Neuroimage* 48, 415–422. doi: 10.1016/j.neuroimage.2009.06.076

Coe, B., Tomihara, K., Matsuzawa, M., and Hikosaka, O. (2002). Visual and anticipatory bias in three cortical eye fields of the monkey during an adaptive decision-making task. *J. Neurosci.* 22, 5081–5090.

Cohen, M. X., and Donner, T. H. (2013). Midfrontal conflict-related theta-band power reflects neural oscillations that predict behavior. *J. Neurophysiol.* 110, 2752–2763. doi: 10.1152/jn.00479.2013

Cohen, M. X., Elger, C. E., and Fell, J. (2009). Oscillatory activity and phase-amplitude coupling in the human medial frontal cortex during decision making. *J. Cogn. Neurosci.* 21, 390–402. doi: 10.1162/jocn.2008.21020

Cohen, M. X., Wilmes, K. A., and van de Vijver, I. (2011). Cortical electrophysiological network dynamics of feedback learning. *Trends Cogn. Sci.* 15, 558–566. doi: 10.1016/j.tics.2011.10.004

Corritore, L., Kracher, B., and Wiedenbeck, S. (2003). On-line trust: concepts, evolving themes, a model. *Int. J. Hum. Comput. Stud.* 58, 737–758. doi: 10.1016/s1071-5819(03)00041-7

Daly, M. A. (2002). *Task Load and Automation Use in an Uncertain Environment.* No. AFIT/GAQ/ENV/02M-05. Wright-Patterson AFB, OH: Air Force Institute of Technology, School of Engineering and Management.

Davis, C. E., Hauf, J. D., Wu, D. Q., and Everhart, D. E. (2011). Brain function with complex decision making using electroencephalography. *Int. J. Psychophysiol.* 79, 175–183. doi: 10.1016/j.ijpsycho.2010.10.004

Dekker, S. W., and Woods, D. D. (2002). Maba-maba or abracadabra? Progress on human-automation co-ordination. *Cogn. Technol. Work* 4, 240–244. doi: 10.1007/s101110200022

Delgado, M. R., Frank, R. H., and Phelps, E. A. (2005). Perceptions of moral character modulate the neural systems of reward during the trust game. *Nat. Neurosci.* 8, 1611–1618. doi: 10.1038/nn1575

Dixon, S. R., Wickens, C. D., and McCarley, J. S. (2006). "How do automation false alarms and misses affect operator compliance and reliance?," in Paper presented at the *Proceedings of the Human Factors and Ergonomics Society 50th Annual Meeting* (Champaign, IL), 25–29.

Dixon, S. R., Wickens, C. D., and McCarley, J. S. (2007). On the independence of compliance and reliance: are automation false alarms worse than misses? *Hum. Factors* 49, 564–572. doi: 10.1518/001872007x215656

Dzindolet, M. T., Pierce, L. G., Beck, H. P., Dawe, L. A. and Anderson, B. W. (2001). Predicting misuse and disuse of combat identification systems. *Mil. Psychol.* 13, 147–164. doi: 10.1207/s15327876mp1303_2

Dzindolet, M. T., Pierce, L. G., Beck, H. P., and Dawe, L. A. (1999). "Misuse and disuse of automated aids.," in *Proceedings of the 43rd Annual Meeting of the Human Factors and Ergonomics Society* (Santa Monica, CA), 339–343.

Dzindolet, M. T., Pierce, L. G., Beck, H. P., and Dawe, L. A. (2002). The perceived utility of human and automated aids in a visual detection task. *Hum. Factors* 44, 79–94. doi: 10.1518/0018720024494856

Dzindolet, M., Peterson, S., Pomranky, T., and Beck, P. (2003). The role of trust in automation reliance. *Int. J. Hum. Comput. Stud.* 58, 697–718. doi: 10.1016/s1071-5819(03)00038-7

Evans, A. M., and Krueger, J. I. (2011). Elements of trust: risk and perspective-taking. *J. Exp. Soc. Psychol.* 47, 171–177. doi: 10.1016/j.jesp.2010.08.007

Fellows, L. K. (2004). The cognitive neuroscience of human decision making: a review and conceptual framework. *Behav. Cogn. Neurosci. Rev.* 3, 159–172. doi: 10.1177/1534582304273251

Figner, B., and Murphy, R. O. (2011). "Using skin conductance in judgment and decision making research," in *A Handbook of Process Tracing Methods for Decision Research*, eds M. Schulte-Mecklenbeck, A. Kuehberger, and R. Ranyard (New York, NY: Psychology Press), 163–184.

Geels-Blair, K., Rice, S., and Schwark, J. (2013). Using system-wide trust theory to reveal the contagion effects of automation false alarms and misses on compliance and reliance in a simulated aviation task. *Int. J. Aviat. Psychol.* 23, 245–266. doi: 10.1080/10508414.2013.799355

Gianotti, L. R., Knoch, D., Faber, P. L., Lehmann, D., Pascual-Marqui, R. D., Diezi, C., et al. (2009). Tonic activity level in the right prefrontal cortex predicts individuals' risk taking. *Psychol. Sci.* 20, 33–38. doi: 10.1111/j.1467-9280.2008.02260.x

Gläscher, J., Hampton, A. N., and O'Doherty, J. P. (2009). Determining a role for ventromedial prefrontal cortex in encoding action-based value signals during reward-related decision making. *Cereb. Cortex* 19, 483–495. doi: 10.1093/cercor/bhn098

Glimcher, P. W., and Fehr, E. (2013). Neuroeconomics: Decision Making and the Brain. (New York, NY: Academic Press).

Glimcher, P. W., and Rustichini, A. (2004). Neuroeconomics: the consilience of brain and decision. *Science* 306, 447–452. doi: 10.1126/science.1102566

Goddard, K., Roudsari, A., and Wyatt, J. C. (2014). Automation bias: empirical results assessing influencing factors. *Int. J. Med. Inform.* 83, 368–375. doi: 10.1016/j.ijmedinf.2014.01.001

Gold, C., Körber, M., Hohenberger, C., Lechner, D., and Bengler, K. (2015). Trust in automation-Before and after the experience of take-over scenarios in a highly automated vehicle. *Procedia Manuf.* 3, 3025–3032. doi: 10.1016/j.promfg.2015.07.847

Gold, J. I., and Shadlen, M. N. (2007). The neural basis of decision making. *Annu. Rev. Neurosci.* 30, 535–574. doi: 10.1146/annurev.neuro.29.051605.113038

Goldberg, M. E., Bisley, J. W., Powell, K. D., and Gottlieb, J. (2006). Saccades, salience and attention: the role of the lateral intraparietal area in visual behavior. *Prog. Brain Res.* 155, 157–175. doi: 10.1016/s0079-6123(06)55010-1

Guggisberg, A. G., Dalal, S. S., Findlay, A. M., and Nagarajan, S. S. (2007). High-frequency oscillations in distributed neural networks reveal the dynamics of human decision making. *Front. Hum. Neurosci.* 1:14. doi: 10.3389/neuro.09.014.2007

Hancock, P. A., Billings, D. R., Schaefer, K. E., Chen, J. Y., de Visser, E. J., and Parasuraman, R. (2011). A meta-analysis of factors affecting trust in human-robot interaction. *Hum. Factors* 53, 517–527. doi: 10.1177/0018720811417254

Hare, T. A., O'Doherty, J., Camerer, C. F., Schultz, W., and Rangel, A. (2008). Dissociating the role of the orbitofrontal cortex and the striatum in the computation of goal values and prediction errors. *J. Neurosci.* 28, 5623–5630. doi: 10.1523/JNEUROSCI.1309-08.2008

Haynes, J. D. (2011). Decoding and predicting intentions. *Ann. N Y Acad. Sci.* 1224, 9–21. doi: 10.1111/j.1749-6632.2011.05994.x

Haynes, J. D., Sakai, K., Rees, G., Gilbert, S., Frith, C., and Passingham, R. E.. (2007). Reading hidden intentions in the human brain. *Curr. Biol.* 17, 323–328. doi: 10.1016/j.cub.2006.11.072

Heekeren, H. R., Marrett, S., and Ungerleider, L. G. (2008). The neural systems that mediate human perceptual decision making. *Nat. Rev. Neurosci.* 9, 467–479. doi: 10.1038/nrn2374

Jamieson, G. A., and Vicente, K. J. (2005). Designing effective human-automation-plant interfaces: a control-theoretic perspective. *Hum. Factors* 47, 12–34. doi: 10.1518/0018720053653820

Kable, J. W., and Glimcher, P. W. (2007). The neural correlates of subjective value during intertemporal choice. *Nat. Neurosci.* 10, 1625–1633. doi: 10.1038/nn2007

Kiani, R., and Shadlen, M. N. (2009). Representation of confidence associated with a decision by neurons in the parietal cortex. *Science* 324, 759–764. doi: 10.1126/science.1169405

Krajbich, I., Armel, C., and Rangel, A. (2010). Visual fixations and the computation and comparison of value in simple choice. *Nat. Neurosci.* 13, 1292–1298. doi: 10.1038/nn.2635

Krajbich, I., and Rangel, A. (2011). Multialternative drift-diffusion model predicts the relationship between visual fixations and choice in value-based decisions. *Proc. Natl. Acad. Sci. U S A* 108, 13852–13857. doi: 10.1073/pnas.1101328108

Kumagai, T., Sakaguchi, Y., Owuwa, M., and Akamatsu, M. (2003). "Prediction of driving behavior through probabilistic inference.," in Paper presented at the *Proceedings of the Eighth International Conference On Engineering Applications of Neural Networks (EANN'03)* (Torremolinos, Malaga, Spain), 117–123.

Lavazza, A., and De Caro, M. (2010). Not so fast. On some bold neuroscientific claims concerning human agency. *Neuroethics* 3, 23–41. doi: 10.1007/s12152-009-9053-9

Lee, J., and Moray, N. (1992). Trust, control strategies and allocation of function in human-machine systems. *Ergonomics* 35, 1243–1270. doi: 10.1080/00140139208967392

Lee, J. D., and Moray, N. (1994). Trust, self-confidence and operators' adaptation to automation. *Int. J. Hum. Comput. Stud.* 40, 153–184. doi: 10.1006/ijhc.1994.1007

Lee, J. D., and See, K. A. (2004). Trust in automation: designing for appropriate reliance. *Hum. Factors* 46, 50–80. doi: 10.1518/hfes.46.1.50.30392

Libet, B. (1993). Unconscious cerebral initiative and the role of conscious will in voluntary action. . *Neurophysiol. Conscious.*, (Boston: Birkhäuser), 269–306. doi: 10.1007/978-1-4612-0355-1_16

Lim, S.-L., O'Doherty, J. P., and Rangel, A. (2011). The decision value computations in the vmPFC and striatum use a relative value code that is guided by visual attention. *J. Neurosci.* 31, 13214–13223. doi: 10.1523/JNEUROSCI.1246-11.2011

Lyons, J. B., and Stokes, C. K. (2012). Human-human reliance in the context of automation. *Hum. Factors* 54, 112–121. doi: 10.1177/0018720811427034

Madhavan, P., and Wiegmann, D. (2007). Similarities and differences between human-human and human-automation trust: an integrative review. *Theor. Issues Ergon. Sci.* 8, 277–301. doi: 10.1080/14639220500337708

Madhavan, P., Wiegmann, D. A., and Lacson, F. C. (2006). Automation failures on tasks easily performed by operators undermine trust in automated aids. *Hum. Factors* 48, 241–256. doi: 10.1518/001872006777724408

Manzey, D., Bahner, J. E., and Hueper, A.-D. (2006). Misuse of automated aids in process control: complacency, automation bias and possible training interventions. *Proc. Hum. Factors Ergon. Soc. Annu. Meeting*, 50, 220–224. doi: 10.1177/154193120605000303

Manzey, D., Gérard, N., and Wiczorek, R. (2014). Decision-making and response strategies in interaction with alarms: the impact of alarm reliability, availability of alarm validity information and workload. *Ergonomics* 57, 1833–1855. doi: 10.1080/00140139.2014.957732

Masalonis, A. J., and Parasuraman, R. (1999). Trust as a construct for evaluation of automated aids: past and future theory and research. *Proc. Hum. Factors Ergon. Soc. Annu. Meeting*, 43, 184–187. doi: 10.1177/154193129904300312

Merritt, S. M. (2011). Affective processes in human automation interactions. *Hum. Factors* 53, 356–370. doi: 10.1177/0018720811411912

Merritt, S. M., Heimbaugh, H., LaChapell, J., and Lee, D. (2012). I trust it, but I don't know why effects of implicit attitudes toward automation on trust in an automated system. *Hum. Factors* 55, 520–534. doi: 10.1177/0018720812465081

Merritt, S. M., Huber, K., LaChapell-Unnerstall, J., and Lee, D. (2014). *Continuous Calibration of Trust in Automated Systems.* St. Louis, MO: University of Missouri-St. Louis.

Merritt, S. M., and Ilgen, D. R. (2008). Not all trust is created equal: dispositional and history-based trust in human-automation interactions. *Hum. Factors* 50, 194–210. doi: 10.1518/001872008x288574

Meyer, J. (2001). Effects of warning validity and proximity on responses to warnings. *Hum. Factors* 43, 563–572. doi: 10.1518/001872001775870395

Meyer, J. (2004). Conceptual issues in the study of dynamic hazard warnings. *Hum. Factors* 46, 196–204. doi: 10.1518/hfes.46.2.196.37335

Meyer, J., and Bitan, Y. (2002). Why better operators receive worse warnings. *Hum. Factors* 44, 343–353. doi: 10.1518/0018720024497754

Meyer, J., Wiczorek, R., and Günzler, T. (2014). Measures of reliance and compliance in aided visual scanning. *Hum. Factors* 56, 840–849. doi: 10.1177/0018720813512865

Miller, C. A. (2005). "Trust in adaptive automation: the role of etiquette in tuning trust via analogic and affective methods," in Paper Presented at the

Proceedings of the 1st International Conference on Augmented Cognition (Las Vegas, NV).

Moray, N. (2003). Monitoring, complacency, scepticism and eutactic behaviour. *Int. J. Ind. Ergon.* 31, 175–178. doi: 10.1016/s0169-8141(02)00194-4

Moray, N., Inagaki, T., and Itoh, M. (2000). Adaptive automation, trust and self-confidence in fault management of time-critical tasks. *J. Exp. Psychol. Appl.* 6, 44–58. doi: 10.1037/1076-898x.6.1.44

Mosier, K. L., and Skitka, L. J. (1996). Human decision makers and automated decision aids: made for each other. *Autom. Hum. Perform. Theory Appl.* 40, 201–220.

Muir, B. M. (1994). Trust in automation: Part I. Theoretical issues in the study of trust and human intervention in automated systems. *Ergonomics* 37, 1905–1922. doi: 10.1080/00140139408964957

Muir, B. M., and Moray, N. (1996). Trust in automation. Part II. Experimental studies of trust and human intervention in a process control simulation. *Ergonomics* 39, 429–460. doi: 10.1080/00140139608964474

Mulder, M., van Maanen, L., and Forstmann, B. (2014). Perceptual decision neurosciences-a model-based review. *Neuroscience* 277, 872–884. doi: 10.1016/j.neuroscience.2014.07.031

Musallam, S., Corneil, B., Greger, B., Scherberger, H., and Andersen, R. (2004). Cognitive control signals for neural prosthetics. *Science* 305, 258–262. doi: 10.1126/science.1097938

Nass, C., Fogg, B., and Moon, Y. (1996). Can computers be teammates? *Int. J. Hum. Comput. Stud.* 45, 669–678. doi: 10.1006/ijhc.1996.0073

Nieuwenhuis, S., Aston-Jones, G., and Cohen, J. D. (2005). Decision making, the P3, and the locus coeruleus-norepinephrine system. *Psychol. Bull.* 131, 510–532. doi: 10.1037/0033-2909.131.4.510

Pak, R., Fink, N., Price, M., Bass, B., and Sturre, L. (2012). Decision support aids with anthropomorphic characteristics influence trust and performance in younger and older adults. *Ergonomics* 55, 1059–1072. doi: 10.1080/00140139.2012.691554

Parasuraman, R., and Manzey, D. (2010). Complacency and bias in human use of automation: an attentional integration. *Hum. Factors* 52, 381–410. doi: 10.1177/0018720810376055

Parasuraman, R., and Miller, C. A. (2004). Trust and etiquette in high-criticality automated systems. *Commun. ACM* 47, 51–55. doi: 10.1145/975817.975844

Parasuraman, R., and Riley, V. (1997). Humans and automation; use misuse, disuse, abuse. *Hum. Factors* 39, 230–253. doi: 10.1518/001872097778543886

Parasuraman, R., Sheridan, T. B., and Wickens, C. D. (2000). A model for types and levels of human interaction with automation. *IEEE Trans. Syst. Man Cybern. A Syst. Hum.* 30, 286–297. doi: 10.1109/3468.844354

Parasuraman, R., Sheridan, T. B., and Wickens, C. D. (2008). Situation awareness, mental workload and trust in automation: viable, empirically supported cognitive engineering constructs. *J. Cogn. Eng. Decis. Mak.* 2, 140–160. doi: 10.1518/155534308x284417

Perez, O., Mukamel, R., Tankus, A., Rosenblatt, J. D., Yeshurun, Y., and Fried, I. (2015). Preconscious prediction of a driver's decision using intracranial recordings. *J. Cogn. Neurosci.* 27, 1492–1502. doi: 10.1162/jocn_a1004_00799

Philiastides, M. G., Auksztulewicz, R., Heekeren, H. R., and Blankenburg, F. (2011). Causal role of dorsolateral prefrontal cortex in human perceptual decision making. *Curr. Biol.* 21, 980–983. doi: 10.1016/j.cub.2011.04.034

Platt, M. L. (2002). Neural correlates of decisions. *Curr. Opin. Neurobiol.* 12, 141–148. doi: 10.1016/s0959-4388(02)00302-1

Platt, M. L., and Glimcher, P. W. (1999). Neural correlates of decision variables in parietal cortex. *Nature* 400, 233–238. doi: 10.1038/22268

Ploran, E. J., Nelson, S. M., Velanova, K., Donaldson, D. I., Petersen, S. E., and Wheeler, M. E. (2007). Evidence accumulation and the moment of recognition: dissociating perceptual recognition processes using fMRI. *J. Neurosci.* 27, 11912–11924. doi: 10.1523/jneurosci.3522-07.2007

Poole, A., and Ball, L. J. (2006). Eye tracking in HCI and usability research. *Encyclopedia Hum. Comput. Interact.* 1, 211–219. doi: 10.4018/978-1-59140-562-7.ch034

Rangel, A., Camerer, C., and Montague, P. R. (2008). A framework for studying the neurobiology of value-based decision making. *Nat. Rev. Neurosci.* 9, 545–556. doi: 10.1038/nrn2357

Rangel, A., and Hare, T. (2010). Neural computations associated with goal-directed choice. *Curr. Opin. Neurobiol.* 20, 262–270. doi: 10.1016/j.conb.2010.03.001

Rice, S. (2009). Examining single-and multiple-process theories of trust in automation. *J. Gen. Psychol.* 136, 303–322. doi: 10.3200/GENP.136.3.303–322

Rice, S., and Geels, K. (2010). Using system-wide trust theory to make predictions about dependence on four diagnostic aids. *J. Gen. Psychol.* 137, 362–375. doi: 10.1080/00221309.2010.499397

Rorie, A. E., Gao, J., McClelland, J. L., and Newsome, W. T. (2010). Integration of sensory and reward information during perceptual decision-making in lateral intraparietal cortex (LIP) of the macaque monkey. *PLoS One* 5:e9308. doi: 10.1371/journal.pone.0009308

Schaefer, K. E., Billings, D. R., Szalma, J. L., Adams, J. K., Sanders, T. L., Chen, J. Y., et al. (2014). *A Meta-Analysis of Factors Influencing the Development of Trust in Automation: Implications for Human-Robot Interaction.* No. ARL-TR-6984. Aberdeen, MD: Army Research Laboratory's, Human Research and Engineering Directorate.

Schaefer, K. E., Sanders, T. L., Yordon, R. E., Billings, D. R., and Hancock, P. (2012). "Classification of robot form: factors predicting perceived trustworthiness," in Paper Presented at the *Proceedings of the Human Factors and Ergonomics Society 56th Annual Meeting* (Boston, MA).

Sheridan, T. (1980). "Theory of man-machine interaction as related to computerized automation," in *Paper Presented at the Proceedings of the Sixth Annual Advanced Control Conference*, (Cambridge, MA: MIT Press).

Sheridan, T. B., and Hennessy, R. T. (1984). *Research and Modeling of Supervisory Control Behavior. Report of a Workshop.* Washington, DC: National Research Council, Committee on Human Factors.

Singh, I. L., Molloy, R., and Parasuraman, R. (1997). Automation-induced monitoring inefficiency: role of display location. *Int. J. Hum. Comput. Stud.* 46, 17–30. doi: 10.1006/ijhc.1996.0081

Skitka, L. J., Mosier, K. L., and Burdick, M. (1999). Does automation bias decision-making? *Int. J. Hum. Comput. Stud.* 51, 991–1006. doi: 10.1006/ijhc.1999.0252

Skitka, L. J., Mosier, K. L., Burdick, M., and Rosenblatt, B. (2000). Automation bias and errors: are crews better than individuals? *Int. J. Aviat. Psychol.* 10, 85–97. doi: 10.1207/s15327108ijap1001_5

Sokolov, E., Spinks, J., Naatanen, R., and Risto-Ktttubebm, G. (2002). *The Orienting Response in Information Processing.* Mahwah, NJ: Lawrence Erlbaum Associates Publishers.

Soon, C. S., Brass, M., Heinze, H.-J., and Haynes, J.-D. (2008). Unconscious determinants of free decisions in the human brain. *Nat. Neurosci.* 11, 543–545. doi: 10.1038/nn.2112

Soon, C. S., He, A. H., Bode, S., and Haynes, J.-D. (2013). Predicting free choices for abstract intentions. *Proc. Natl. Acad. Sci. U S A* 110, 6217–6222. doi: 10.1073/pnas.1212218110

Terai, H., Okuda, H., Hitomi, K., Bando, T., Miyajima, C., Hirayama, Y., et al. (2015). An experimental study on the difference in drivers' decision making behavior during manual and supported driving. *Procedia Manuf.* 3, 3136–3141. doi: 10.1016/j.promfg.2015.07.974

van de Vijver, I., Ridderinkhof, K. R., and Cohen, M. X. (2011). Frontal oscillatory dynamics predict feedback learning and action adjustment. *J. Cogn. Neurosci.* 23, 4106–4121. doi: 10.1162/jocn_a_00110

Verberne, F. M. F., Ham, J., and Midden, C. J. H. (2012). Trust in smart systems: sharing driving goals and giving information to increase trustworthiness and acceptability of smart systems in cars. *Hum. Factors* 54, 799–810. doi: 10.1177/0018720812443825

Wallis, J. D. (2012). Cross-species studies of orbitofrontal cortex and value-based decision-making. *Nat. Neurosci.* 15, 13–19. doi: 10.1038/nn.2956

Wang, L., Jamieson, G. A., and Hollands, J. G. (2008). "Selecting methods for the analysis of reliance on automation," in Paper Presented at the *Proceedings of the Human Factors and Ergonomics Society 52nd Annual Meeting* (Santa Monica, CA), 287–291.

Wang, L., Jamieson, G. A., and Hollands, J. G. (2009). Trust and reliance on an automated combat identification system. *Hum. Factors* 51, 281–291. doi: 10.1177/0018720809338842

Wickens, C. D., and Dixon, S. R. (2007). The benefits of imperfect diagnostic automation: a synthesis of the literature. *Theor. Issues Ergon. Sci.* 8, 201–212. doi: 10.1080/14639220500370105

Wiczorek, R., and Manzey, D. (2010). "Is operators' compliance with alarm systems a product of rational consideration?," in Paper presented at the *Proceedings of the Human Factors and Ergonomics Society 54th Annual Meeting* (San Francisco, CA), pp. 1722–1726

Wiczorek, R. and Manzey, D. (2014). Supporting attention allocation in multitask environments: effects of likelihood alarm systems on trust, behavior, and performance. *Hum. Factors* 56, 1209–1221. doi: 10.1177/0018720814528534

Yacubian, J., Gläscher, J., Schroeder, K., Sommer, T., Braus, D. F., and Büchel, C. (2006). Dissociable systems for gain-and loss-related value predictions and errors of prediction in the human brain. *J. Neurosci.* 26, 9530–9537. doi: 10.1523/jneurosci.2915-06.2006

Yeh, M., and Wickens, C. D. (2000). Effects of cue reliability, realism and interactivity on biases of attention and trust in augmented reality. *Proc Hum. Factors Ergon. Soc. Annu. Meeting*, 44, 511–514. doi: 10.1177/154193120004400507

Establishing Shot Type Affects Arousal and Cognitive Load During Transitions Between Novel Interior Locations in Films

Grant Brighter[1]* *and Nancy Rader*[2]

[1] *Mind-Body Laboratory, Department of Psychology, Ithaca College, Ithaca, NY, United States,* [2] *Cognition Laboratory, Department of Psychology, Ithaca College, Ithaca, NY, United States*

***Correspondence:**
Grant Brighter
gbrighter@ithaca.edu;
gmb1001@gmail.com

An "establishing shot" prefaces a scene in a movie with a wide shot of the scene's location. It is meant to help viewers process a shift to a new location. Establishing shots can depict the actors in the space in which they will be acting, the exterior of a building, or the larger geographic context of the scene. While use of an establishing shot is standard filmmaking practice, some argue that establishing shots are unnecessary. This study sought to investigate how effective four types of establishing shots are at helping viewers process location shifts. Pupil diameter was recorded using a MangoldVision eye tracking system as a measure of arousal and cognitive load. Oxygenation levels in the prefrontal cortex provided an additional measure of cognitive load assessed through functional near infrared spectroscopy (fNIRS). We expected scene transitions to be followed by transient increases in pupil diameter and oxygenation levels, suggesting increased cognitive load and arousal. We predicted that participants should experience less cognitive load and arousal after a transition to a new scene when that scene has been prefaced with an establishing shot and that these effects would be greatest for establishing shots that depict actors. We found that geographic establishing shots produced significantly lower average pupil diameter than all other establishing shot types and the use of no establishing shot. Actors establishing shots elicited significantly lower average pupil diameter values than the use of no establishing shot. Maximum and average oxygenation values for the actors establishing shot condition were significantly higher than for the exterior establishing shot condition. An alpha level of 0.05 was used for all analyses. These results suggest differences between pupil diameter and fNIRS in terms of the psychological phenomenon they measure, and may inform the design of future films.

Keywords: establishing shot, fNIRS, cognitive load, arousal, pupil diameter, continuity editing, functional near-infrared spectroscopy

INTRODUCTION

A standard practice in commercial, narrative filmmaking is the use of establishing shots. An establishing shot is a long[1], wide shot that prefaces a scene and depicts the location in which the scene will take place. A scene "takes place in one location over a continuous but relatively small amount of time" (Cutting et al., 2012, p. 3); thus, a change in scene is generally linked to a change in location. Pincus and Ascher (2012) succinctly describe an establishing shot as "a long shot that defines the basic space or locale where events will take place" (p. 323).

The present study makes use of three different types of establishing shots. The first is an establishing shot where actors are depicted in a long shot within the space in which they will be acting during the scene. This type of establishing shot, in theory, helps the viewer become accustomed to the fact that they are now occupying a new environment and displays how the characters are positioned at the beginning of the scene. An establishing shot might instead depict the exterior of the building or vehicle where the scene will take place. This could be the front façade of an office building or the outside of a boat or spaceship. In such a shot, the actors often are not depicted, as the following shot usually cuts to an interior space where the action takes place, a space presumably inside the building or vehicle shown in the previous shot. This is an instance that usually does not provide the arrangement of characters, but should, however, cue the viewer to the fact that the location of the narrative has changed. The final type of establishing shot is a long shot of the larger geographic context in which the scene will take place. This type of shot is usually a landscape or cityscape, but it might also take the form of a shot of a planet's surface. Again, actors are often not depicted in this type of establishing shot.

One thing that all the forms of establishing shot have in common is that they are meant to indicate to the viewer that the location of the action has changed in the film's ongoing narrative. Cutting and Iricinschi (2015) note that the establishing shot helps a viewer become acclimated to a new location. This "functional" aspect of an establishing shot's definition makes intuitive sense. One would expect that a long shot of the surroundings before the action of the scene begins in earnest would help the viewer adjust to a shift in location, as it would, in theory, give the viewer a moment to process this shift before focusing on the extension of the narrative delivered in the subsequent scene. Indeed, it is likely that this intuition has helped ensconce the establishing shot as standard filmmaking practice. However, the establishing shot has been argued to be superfluous when it comes to the task of guiding the viewer through a narrative (Bordwell, 2002; Ballester, 2005).

Cutting et al. (2012) found that new units of action tend to be prefaced with wider shots that take in more of the surroundings before moving to closer shots as action unfolds. This study also found that these initial shots were relatively longer in duration than the following shots that made up the scene. The pattern of beginning a scene with a relatively longer shot that is also relatively longer in duration compared to the rest of the shots in the scene was interpreted to be indicative of the usage of establishing shots. In addition, of the various formal aspects of film (features other than place, time, characters, and other narrative content), initial shot scales and initial shot durations were among the variables most consistently linked with the perception of a new event beginning. The research of Cutting et al. suggests that the establishing shot could play an important role in helping the viewer determine that a new event is occurring in the film. However, it is important to note that this research analyzed "subscenes," which are meant to represent meaningfully distinct events in a narrative (Cutting et al., 2012, p. 3). These can include entrances and exits of characters or shifts of tone. Therefore, the shifts analyzed do not necessarily refer to changes in scene (i.e., changes in location), although such shifts are included in this analysis. So, while Cutting et al.'s results do not specifically represent shifts in locations, they may provide some insight into the importance of the establishing shot for cuing shifts in the narrative, including locational shifts. Indeed, it has been theorized that the establishing shot is kept at a longer duration to give the viewer a chance to take in the novel information being presented, which often takes the form of a shift to a brand new location (Cutting et al., 2012; Cutting and Candan, 2013; Cutting, 2014).

Past studies have found that reading time slows at the beginning and ending of scenes in written stories (Zwaan et al., 1995a,b). These results can be explained by an increased consumption of cognitive resources caused by the transition between scenes (Cutting et al., 2012). Indeed, Zwaan et al. (1995b) have found that general discontinuities in temporal, spatial, and causal elements of a written story lead to increases in reading time, a result that has been interpreted as being reflective of increased difficulty in incorporating new information into preexisting conceptions of the story. It has been postulated that shifts in scenes require heightened executive functioning and place a heavier cognitive load on comprehension (Cutting and Iricinschi, 2015). If narrative shifts such as changes in location in written stories increase processing difficulty, it is possible that such narrative shifts increase processing difficulty in filmic stories as well. Given the seeming influence of the establishing shot on the cognitive distinction between events in films, it is also possible that establishing shots may help reduce the difficulty with which changes in events are processed.

One measure of how difficult it is for a person to process information is known as cognitive load, a term used to refer to the amount of effort required to process information (Cooper, 1990; Zagermann et al., 2016). The current study used functional near infrared spectroscopy (fNIRS) to measure cognitive load via hemodynamic responses in the prefrontal cortex, specifically Brodmann Area 10. Brodmann Area 10 is defined as the medial prefrontal cortex and has been shown to become increasingly activated with increasing cognitive load (Arsalidou et al., 2013).

Functional near infrared spectroscopy has been utilized in a variety of clinical and research settings, and has been validated

[1]In accordance with filmmaking conventions, a shot is regarded as long when the camera is a relatively long distance away from the subject and when a relatively low focal length is used, resulting in a substantial swath of the surroundings around the subject being captured in the shot. Thus, a *long shot* refers to shot scale/distance, whereas the term *long take* is a temporal reference (specifically, it describes a shot of relatively long duration).

against other neuroimaging techniques such as PET (León-Carrión and León-Domínguez, 2012). Ayaz et al. (2012) was one of the first studies that established fNIRS as a monitor of cognitive workload. Herff et al. (2014) utilized fNIRS to quantify mental workload activity in the prefrontal cortex during a series of n-back tasks. The fNIRS data showed an increase in oxygenated hemoglobin and a decrease of deoxygenated hemoglobin in the prefrontal cortex as the n-back task increased in difficulty. Workload was evaluated by comparing each n-back trial to one another and to relaxation periods. It was concluded that measuring hemodynamic responses in the prefrontal cortex using fNIRS provides a reliable quantification of mental workload, supporting the findings of Ayaz et al. (2012). Izzetoglu et al. (2004) also found that blood flow in the prefrontal cortex, as measured by fNIRS, correlated with increases in cognitive load. Participants engaged in a naval warfare management simulator task. Blood flow changes as measured by fNIRS were found to be significantly correlated with task difficulty.

In order to be activated, neurons require substances such as oxygen and glucose. Such materials are sent to neurons via blood transfusion through the capillaries. The metabolic needs of neurons during activation results in increased oxygen consumption, local cerebral blood flow, and oxygen delivery (Lloyd-Fox et al., 2010). An increase in blood flow and total hemoglobin to certain regions of the cerebrum is considered to be indicative of increased metabolic demands of the neurons in that region, and therefore, increased activation of those neurons in response to cognitive tasks (Izzetoglu et al., 2004). When hemoglobin is transporting oxygen in the blood, it is referred to as oxygenated hemoglobin; once it releases oxygen to be metabolized, it is referred to as deoxygenated hemoglobin.

Functional near infrared spectroscopy uses infrared light to measure the amount of oxygenated and deoxygenated hemoglobin in areas of the cerebral cortex; in this study we measured activity specifically in the anterior portion of the cerebral cortex. Biological tissue becomes translucent to light under a specific spectrum of 700–900 nm wavelengths, or the near-infrared portion of the light spectrum (León-Carrión and León-Domínguez, 2012). Oxygenated and deoxygenated hemoglobin exhibit different absorption properties when exposed to near-infrared (NIR) light, thus allowing levels of these forms of hemoglobin to be differentiated from one another based on the way NIR light is scattered when it is reflected back from the brain (Lloyd-Fox et al., 2010). A typical hemodynamic response to the activation of cortical neurons in an adult brain takes the form of an increased flow of oxygenated hemoglobin and a relatively smaller decrease in deoxygenated hemoglobin, resulting in an increase in total hemoglobin (Lloyd-Fox et al., 2010). Through measurements of oxygenated and deoxygenated hemoglobin, oxygenation levels in the brain can be deduced. fNIRS has a number of advantages; it is a low-cost system that is quiet, non-invasive, portable, and has relatively good temporal resolution (Ferreri et al., 2014).

To date, there are no known studies investigating the hemodynamic response of adults to film editing techniques using fNIRS. Using EEG, Francuz and Zabielska-Mendyk (2013) found that cuts between unrelated scenes caused higher attention, arousal, and cognitive load than cuts between shots depicting the same scene but from different angles. They note that such heightened mental involvement is often correlated with increased activity in the frontal lobes, particularly the prefrontal cortex. This study did not use unrelated scenes from the same video, however; the clips stitched together were different enough in terms of form and content that the changes between scenes resembled changing channels on a television. Using fMRI imaging and the children's film *The Red Balloon*, film viewers' responses to various types of edits have been analyzed (Magliano and Zacks, 2011). Discontinuities in space or time while a character continued an action were found to be associated with decreases in activation of the right lateral superior frontal cortex. However, no changes in brain activation were reported at major scene breaks in the foremost regions of the brain. It is not clear what effect the use of establishing shots had on these results.

Smith (2005) writes that discontinuities, which can include abrupt changes in location or scene, have been shown to cause increases in self-reported arousal as well as physiological responses indicative of greater arousal and attention being directed toward a cut. He also writes that a cut to a new scene or location or other discontinuities of comparable cognitive difficulty can lead to cognitive overload. It is worth noting, however, that there are many forms of discontinuities, and so these results may not necessarily be specific to locational/scenic shifts.

Transitions between unrelated video images have been shown to require greater attention from subjects than shifts between video images that remain within one unaltered narrative scene taking place in one location (Geiger and Reeves, 1993). However, those unrelated clips were from a variety of sources, and therefore transitions between them may not necessarily represent transitions between scenes or locations within one continuous film. Using a similar distinction between related and unrelated images, Lang et al. (1993) found that unrelated cuts consumed more processing capacity.

Pupil diameter is an additional measure that can gauge cognitive load, and has been used for this purpose in a variety of settings (Laeng et al., 2012; Chen and Epps, 2014; Zagermann et al., 2016). Chen and Epps (2014) note that pupil diameter has been found to be a reliable indicator of cognitive load in a wide range of situations. Pupil diameter has also been used as a measure of cognitive load during film viewing (Smith et al., 2006; Swallow et al., 2009; Magliano and Zacks, 2013). Pupil diameter has been found to increase with increasing cognitive demands of a task (Beatty and Lucero-Wagoner, 2000; Zagermann et al., 2016), and around points in films that viewers identified as boundaries between events (Magliano and Zacks, 2013). In addition to measuring cognitive load, pupil diameter can be used as a measure of arousal, with larger pupil sizes indicating greater arousal (Laeng et al., 2012). Cognitive load, arousal, and pupil diameter all seem to be correlated with one another, and their functions may be psychologically integrated. Thus, we intend to infer cognitive load and arousal based on pupil diameter.

We hypothesize that the use of an establishing shot will decrease arousal and cognitive load experienced during the following scene compared to the use of no establishing shot.

We anticipate that this effect will be most pronounced for actors establishing shots, moderate for exterior establishing shots, and least pronounced for geographic establishing shots. This is because actors establishing shots are closest to the action that follows in the next scene in terms of scale, while exterior establishing shots are further from the action and geographic establishing shots are the furthest. It is expected that the greater the difference in scale between the establishing shot and the following scene, the greater the logical leap that must be made to connect the two, resulting in more cognitive load and arousal.

MATERIALS AND METHODS

Ethics Statement

This study was carried out in accordance with the recommendations of Policies and Procedures and Guidelines for Investigators, Ithaca College Institutional Review Board. The protocol was approved by the Ithaca College Institutional Review Board. All subjects gave written informed consent in accordance with the Declaration of Helsinki.

Participants

Thirty-two participants, randomly assigned to each group, were tested. Participants were students from Ithaca College, ranging from 18 to 22 years of age (M = 19.75, SD = 1.016); 24 of the participants identified as white, and 8 identified as various non-white ethnicities; 25 of the participants were female and 7 were male. Students in psychology classes were recruited mainly by the primary researcher entering psychology classes and promoting the study through an announcement. Psychology professors who offer extra credit for research participation were encouraged to inform their students of the opportunity to partake in this study, along with other studies taking place in the spring semester of 2018. The study was posted on the SONA system. The SONA system is a website that the Ithaca College Psychology department uses to recruit participants for psychological studies run by faculty and students. Students can sign up for studies through SONA, and also receive extra credit by having their participation logged on SONA. Individuals with SONA accounts could see the study displayed under the "studies" tab on SONA.

Students who were taking psychology courses received extra credit for their classes according to the specifications of their professors in exchange for participation. The experimenter reported participation information to the SONA system immediately after participation.

Participants were excluded if they had a severe visual impairment that rendered them incapable of seeing the stimuli presented on a computer screen that was placed about two feet away from them. This did not include people whose impairment had been rectified using contacts, as long as such correctional lenses were being worn at the time the subject participated in the study. This did, however, exclude individuals whose only correctional lenses were glasses, as glasses interfered with eye tracking data collection. Individuals were also precluded from wearing make-up during testing, as make-up could skew the readings of the fNIRS system. These limitations were made clear in the recruitment materials for the study. Through a demographics information form, participants were asked if they needed corrective lenses and, if so, whether they have taken appropriate measures to partake in this study (i.e., wearing contacts) before participating in this study. They were also asked if they were wearing make-up. Prior to beginning the study, participants were asked to sign an informed consent form. No volunteers for this study needed to be excluded.

Apparatus

Functional Near-Infrared Spectroscopy

Functional near infrared spectroscopy measurements were made using a continuous wave Biopac system. This system uses sensors placed on the forehead to measure levels of oxygen in the anterior portion of the brain. These sensors are put in place using straps that wrap around the head and are covered with a headband. The bottom of the sensors just touched the tops of the eyebrows, and the center of the sensors were in line with the center of the pupils. The placement of the sensors roughly corresponded to the Fp1 and Fp2 locations in the 10–20 system. To prevent extra light from reaching the sensors, a black band was placed over the sensors, the top and bottom of which was sealed off by wrapping gauze around the participant's head (see **Figure 1**). The sensors shine pulses of infrared light into the wearer's brain. The light interacts with oxygen-carrying proteins in the user's blood, and the reflected infrared light levels are measured by receptors on the sensor pad. The fNIRS sensor used was a Biopac Systems Inc. RXfNIR-4 Adult 4 Channel Split fNIR Sensor. The fNIRS sensor was split into two headpieces, each with 1 photo-emitter and 2 photo-detectors. Each piece contained two channels. The fNIRS signal measured consisted of the intensity of light reflected back to the sensors at wavelengths of 730 nm and 850 nm. Also, ambient light levels were continuously measured by this system. The fNIRS sensors were cleaned with alcohol and cotton swabs before and after every participant. The sensors were kept clear of hair, as hair could cause artifacts in the data. Participants were provided with headbands, if necessary, to help them keep their hair away from the sensors.

The fNIRS system has an inter-optode distance of 25 mm, and can collect data from up to 12.5 mm beneath the skin (Chance et al., 1993). The fNIRS sensors communicated with a computer through a wireless receiver connected to one of the computer's USB ports. Levels of light reflected back to the sensors are recorded by COBI studio software and are graphed on the computer monitor during data collection (Ayaz et al., 2011). The fNIRS system had a sampling rate of 4 Hz. fNIRS utilizes the modified Beer-Lambert law to transform optical data into oxy- and deoxy-hemoglobin densities:

$$\Delta \mathrm{OD} = \log(\mathrm{I}_{\mathrm{rest}}/\mathrm{I}_{\mathrm{test}})$$

In this equation, $\mathrm{I}_{\mathrm{rest}}$ represents reflected light intensity during the baseline condition, and $\mathrm{I}_{\mathrm{test}}$ represents reflected light intensity while the stimulus is present. ΔOD is change in optical density. By measuring at two different wavelengths within the 700–900 nm range, one above 800 nm and one below, the concentration changes of oxy- hemoglobin and

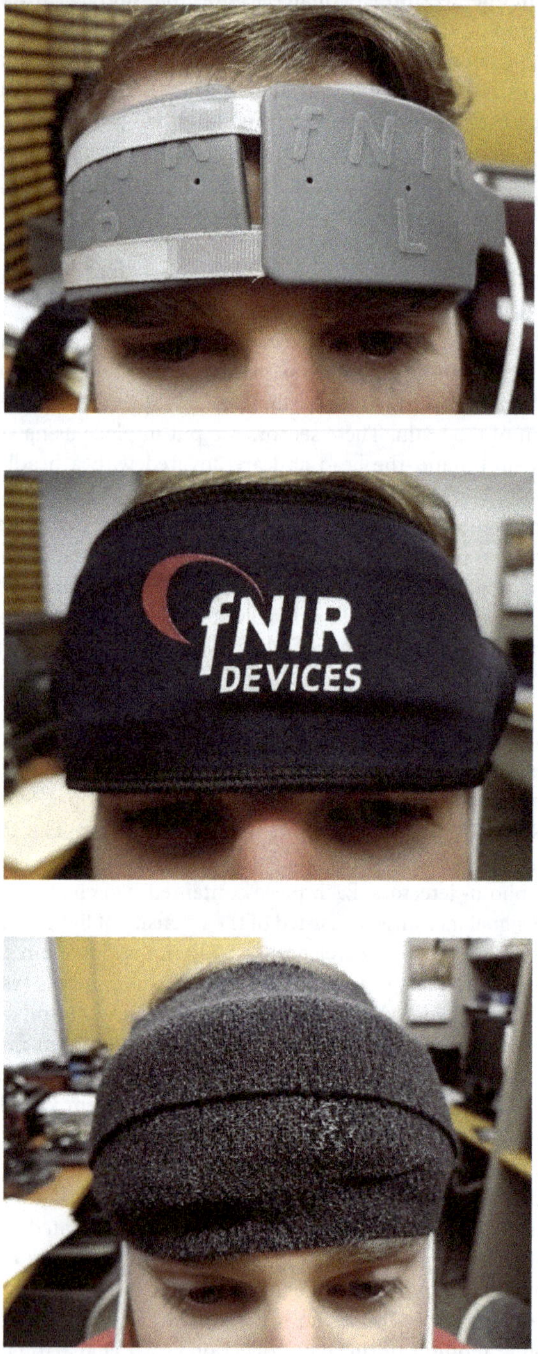

FIGURE 1 | Depiction of sensor placement and wrapping. Each of the two sensors were placed so that the center of the sensor was in line with the center of the pupil and the bottom of the sensor touched the top of the eyebrows of the participant. This can be seen in the top graphic. The sensors were then wrapped with a black band to prevent light from entering, as seen in the middle graphic. Finally, the top and bottom of the band was sealed off from light using gauze strips, as seen in the bottom graphic.

deoxy-hemoglobin can be calculated. The concentrations of oxy-hemoglobin and deoxy-hemoglobin are subsequently used to calculate oxygenation values (Ayaz, 2010).

Oxy and deoxygenated hemoglobin signals were kept between 4000 and 750 mv. To maintain this range, the LED current (brightness) was set between 5 and 20 mA and initial gain (sensitivity) was set to either 1, 5, 10, 15, or 20. The computer used to operate the fNIRS system in this study was a Dell Latitude running Windows 7.

Analysis of the oxygenation levels based on light collected by the sensors were performed using fNIRSoft software. In processing the data, finite impulse response (FIR) and sliding-window motion artifact rejection (SMAR) filters were applied before converting the data to oxygenation values (Ayaz et al., 2010). The FIR filter is a low pass filter with a cut off frequency of 0.1 Hz. To calculate oxygenation values, a baseline level of activity was established using data collected while the viewer watched the last 10 s of a 15 s -long still shot of a vase of flowers at the start of the study. The system then produced oxygenation values that represented differences in activity above or below that baseline. During data collection, the experimenter placed a digital marker in the data right at the end of the shot depicting the vase of flowers. Time bins for analysis accompanying each individual shot were then established based off of the placement of this marker. Once converted to oxygenation values, the data were again subjected to FIR filtering as well as a detrending filter (Ayaz, 2010). New baselines were established using half-second samples at the beginning of each shot, so that oxygenation values reflected differences in activity away from that baseline level. Average and maximum oxygenation values were established for each shot across all optodes. The average and max values across all the shots in the scene were then ascertained to arrive at average and maximum oxygenation for each scene.

Pupil Measurement

Eye data were collected using a MangoldVision Eye Tracking System. Through this system, the videos were displayed on a computer monitor. The eye tracking device, which consists of a camera and infrared lights, was positioned underneath the monitor. The infrared light shone on the subject's face by the lights were registered by the camera in the center of the eye tracking device. The image captured by the camera was used to log the participant's pupil size throughout the video. Before the video was presented, subjects engaged in a calibration task in which they were asked to look at a red dot that traveled around the computer screen and paused at certain positions. For this study, the dot was programmed to stop at 9 different positions. The participant had to stare at the dot every time it paused in order for the system to calibrate to their unique eyes. If the system was not adequately calibrated, a dialog box appeared notifying the operator and allowing portions of the calibration task to be redone. After the calibration task, the video containing the experimental stimulus began. This is because presentation of this video was controlled by the Mangold system. The screen went blank immediately after the video ended. Data recorded by the Mangold eye tracking system were analyzed using the Mangold Analyzer application. The system was operated by the experimenter using an Inspiron 13 7000 series laptop computer running Windows 10 Pro, which was connected to the eye tracker through a cable. The laptop controlling the Mangold program

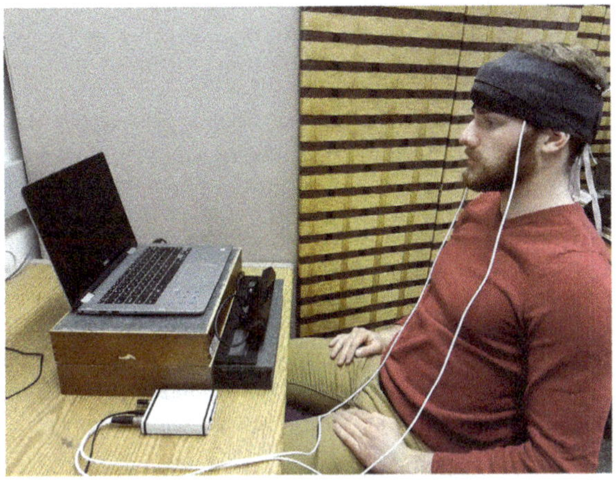

FIGURE 2 | Depiction of experimental set up. The fNIRS sensors were connected to a box (bottom left) that collected the data and wirelessly sent it to the computer running the COBI system. The COBI computer and the experimenter were hidden from the participant by a wooden partition (situated to the right of the individual depicted).

was separate from the laptop controlling the fNIRS system; thus, two distinct laptops were needed to run the study.

Stimuli and Procedure

After signing an informed consent form, participants were seated in a chair in front of a laptop computer on which the experimental stimulus was presented. The participants were positioned so that their eyes were approximately 2 feet away from the center of the computer monitor while sitting with their backs pressed against the back of the chair. The computer itself was raised off the desk to a more agreeable viewing height by resting on two wooden stands. The eye tracker was placed on its own foam stand in front of the wooden stands (see **Figure 2**). The fNIRS sensors were then positioned and wrapped. The overhead lights in the lab were turned off to prevent extraneous light sources from interfering with the readings of the eye tracker and fNIRS system. The eye tracking software was then turned on and the system was calibrated to the participant's eyes. After the system was calibrated, the experimenter activated the fNIRS system, and then pressed a button that simultaneously instructed the eye tracking software to begin recording and started a video containing the experimental stimulus. The experimenter placed a partition between himself and the participant to minimize distraction (see **Figure 2**).

The video began with a still image of flowers that stayed on screen for 15 s before the video. The image was taken from an online source of free media. This provided time for the system to calibrate. After 15 s, the fNIRS system began recording data. At the same time, the screen went blank for 2 s, and then the participants were presented with the experimental stimulus, which was a film consisting of five scenes that took place in different locations. The first scene had no establishing shot, but then each of the following scenes started with a different type of establishing shot (see **Figure 3**):

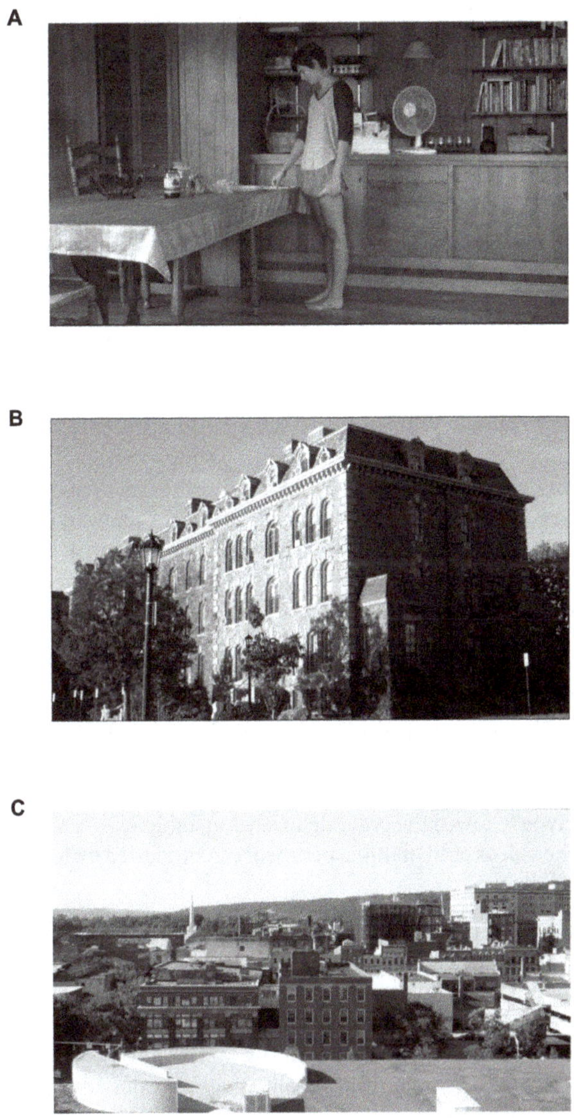

FIGURE 3 | Examples of establishing shot types taken from the experimental stimuli: **(A)** actors establishing shot, **(B)** exterior establishing shot, and **(C)** geographic establishing shot.

- An establishing shot where actors were depicted in a long shot within the space in which they were acting during the scene, labeled "Actors." A long shot was defined as a shot which just barely captured the entire human subject in the frame from head to foot (see **Figure 3A**).
- An establishing shot that depicted the exterior of the building where the scene took place that was wide enough to capture the entire length and height of the building, labeled "Exterior" (see **Figure 3B**).
- An establishing shot in which the larger geographic context of the scene was depicted, such as a landscape or cityscape, labeled "Geo" (see **Figure 3C**).
- No establishing shot (labeled "none").

Establishing shots were 7.5 s long, except in the "null" condition, in which the establishing shot was 0 s long. The following scenes were 6 shots long. The durations of shots during each scene were: 6, 5.5, 5.25, 5.25, 5.5, and 7 s. The values were based on Cutting et al.'s (2012) approximation of average scene and shot lengths. Also, all the shots in each scene were medium long shots, meaning that the human subject was depicted from head to mid-thigh. Both establishing shots and shots within the scene were framed according to Cutting's (2014) shot scale definitions. The entire film is 3 min and 33 s long. The aspect ratio of the film (i.e., the ratio of width to height of the image presented onscreen) was 16:9. The film had no audio. All shots were taken from a static frame (no camera movement) and were shot in such a manner that all the visual features within the frame were in reasonably sharp focus. Each scene featured a different actress performing one of the following simple tasks: stretching, making a sandwich, making a bed, drawing on a chalkboard, reading, and drinking from a mug. The actress changed in every scene to disrupt the perception of a continuous narrative between shots. With the exception of the initial shot of the vase of flowers, the entire film was in grayscale.

There were four experimental groups. For every scene after the first scene, each group was presented with a different type of establishing shot. The purpose of this design feature is to prevent a predictable pattern from developing based on the continual use of the same establishing shot, and to emulate the variance in establishing shots seen in real films. The variation in establishing shot type followed the order delineated in **Table 1**.

The videos used in this experiment can be viewed by following these links:

- **Group 1: https://youtu.be/LypBfoRfQFE**
- Scene-to-scene content of the video:
- Scene 1: woman pouring water into mug and drinking.
- Scene 2: Woman performing shoulder rolls, stretching shoulders, chest and quadriceps.
- Scene 3: Woman using chalk to connect dots drawn on a chalkboard.
- Scene 4: Woman reading a book.
- Scene 5: Woman making a peanut butter and jelly sandwich.

Establishing shots unique to this video: a long shot of rooftops of downtown Ithaca, a shot of the exterior of a 10-story brick building, a long shot of a woman making peanut butter and jelly.

TABLE 1 | Scene and establishing shot pairings based on group number.

	Scene number			
Group	**2**	**3**	**4**	**5**
1	None	Geo	Exterior	Actors
2	Actors	None	Geo	Exterior
3	Exterior	Actors	None	Geo
4	Geo	Exterior	Actors	None

Scene and establishing shot type pairings varied between each film shown to the different experimental groups according to this chart.

- **Group 2: https://youtu.be/EukIA3XsRsg**
- Scene-to-scene content of the video: same as Group 1's video.

Establishing shots unique to this video: long shot of a women performing shoulder rolls, a long shot of rooftops of downtown Ithaca, a shot of the exterior of a house.

- **Group 3: https://youtu.be/Xk3cfcpbN_o**
- Scene-to-scene content of the video: same as Group 1 and 2's videos.

Establishing shots unique to this video: a shot of the exterior of a 3–4 story building, a long shot of a woman standing in front of a chalkboard, a long shot of rooftops of a neighborhood.

- **Group 4: https://youtu.be/Foa9CUezn5o**
- Scene-to-scene content of the video: same as Group 1, 2, and 3's videos.

Establishing shots unique to this video: a long shot of the rooftops of downtown Ithaca, a long shot of 3–4 story academic building, a long shot of woman picking up a book.

To see a graphic depiction of the stimulus presentation procedure, please see **Figure 4**. Once the video stimulus ended, the eye tracking device immediately stopped collecting data. The experimenter then had to manually halt the fNIRS system from recording data.

RESULTS

Results were analyzed using the statistical package for the social sciences (SPSS).

Pupil Diameter Analysis

Pupil diameters in mm for 31 participants were analyzed using a Mixed Analysis of Variance, with Condition as the within-subject factor and Group as the between-subject factor. One of the original 32 participants was removed from the pupil diameter analysis because the eye tracker was not working for that participant. A significant difference was found between the four establishing shot types $F(3,81) = 35.096$, $p < 0.0005$, $\eta_p^2 = 0.565$. There was also a group-by-condition interaction $F(9,81) = 31.683$, $p < 0.0005$, $\eta_p^2 = 0.779$. There was no main effect of group $F(3,27) = 0.587$, $p > 0.05$. A post-hoc Bonferroni test with adjustment for multiple comparisons revealed that geographic establishing shots ($M = 3.72$) were associated with a significantly lower average pupil diameter than no ($M = 4.32$), actors ($M = 4.12$), and external ($M = 4.17$) establishing shots; all p values were less than $p = 0.0005$, two-tailed. In addition, the no establishing shot condition was significantly higher than the actors establishing shot condition ($p = 0.015$) (see **Figure 5**).

Maximum Oxygenation Analysis

Maximum fNIRS values were analyzed for 32 participants using a Mixed Analysis of Variance as above. The dependent measure was the maximum oxygenation value across all the shots in a scene and across all optodes, which was the maximum change

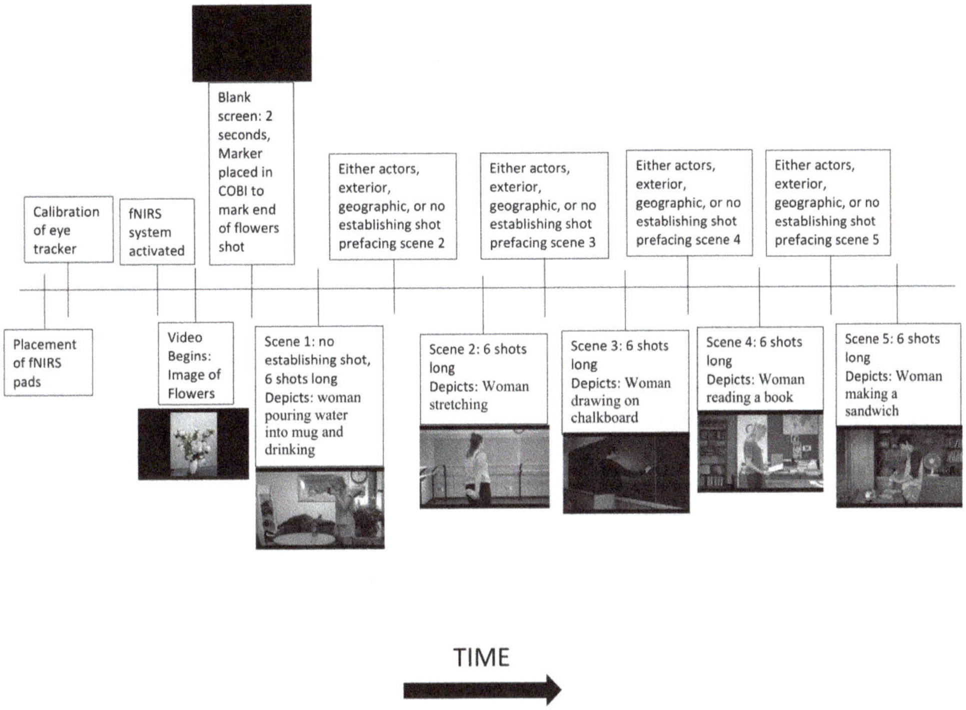

FIGURE 4 | A graphical view of the stimulus presentation procedure.

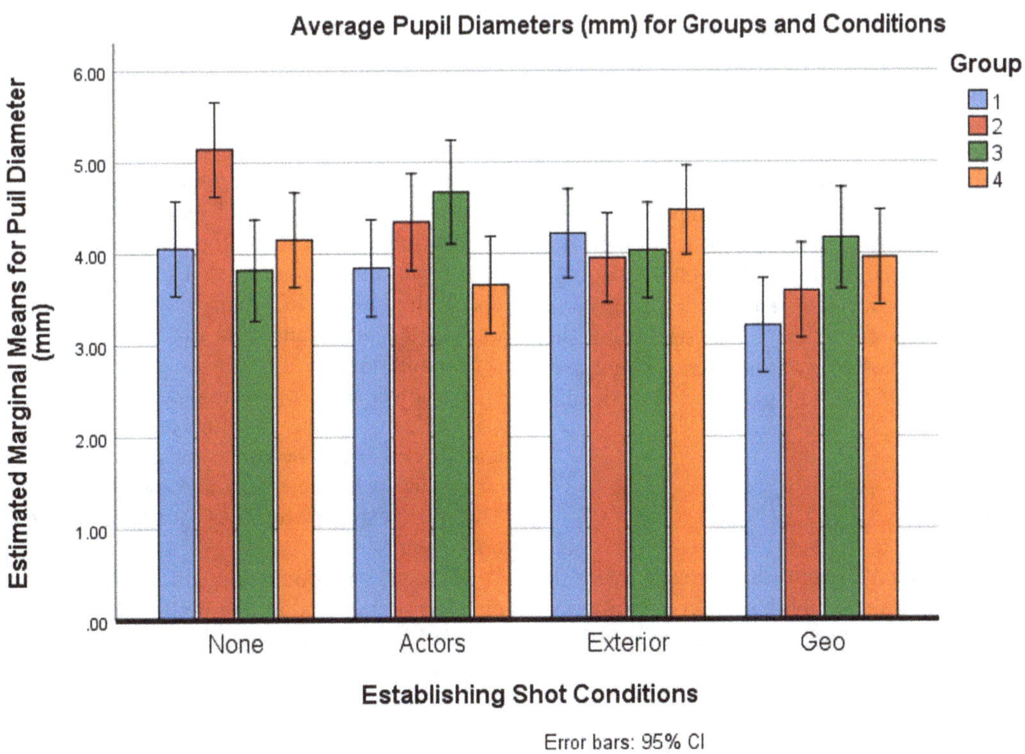

FIGURE 5 | Average pupil diameters for groups and conditions.

in oxygenation away from baseline. Values were calculated based off of a local baseline established at the first half-second of every shot. There was no significant difference found in maximum oxygenation value based on the four establishing shot types $F(3,84) = 0.403$, $p > 0.05$. However, there was a significant condition by group interaction: $F(9,84) = 2.946$, $p = 0.004$, $\eta_p^2 = 0.240$. There was no main effect of group $F(3,28) = 1.373$, $p > 0.05$. Based on an examination of the data, a follow-up mixed ANOVA was performed without Group 3. In this follow-up analysis, it was found that the groups did not differ $F(2,21) = 0.169$, $p = 0.845$, $\eta_p^2 = 0.016$. Also, no group-by-condition interaction was found $F(6,63) = 0.533$, $p = 0.781$, $\eta_p^2 = 0.048$. There was, however, for Groups 1, 2, and 4, a main effect of condition $F(3,63) = 3.197, p = 0.029, \eta_p^2 = 0.132$. A post-hoc Bonferroni test with adjustment for multiple comparisons showed that the values associated with the actor establishing shot condition were significantly higher than the exterior establishing shot condition ($p = 0.037$). For means with error bars, see **Figure 6**.

Average Oxygenation Analysis

Average fNIRS values across a scene were analyzed for 32 participants using a Mixed Analysis of Variance as described above. Values were calculated based off of a local baseline established at the first half-second of every shot. The dependent measure was the average oxygenation value across all the shots in a scene and across all optodes, which was the average change in oxygenation away from baseline. There was no significant difference found in average oxygenation value for the four establishing shot types $F(3,84) = 0.1$, $p = 0.960$. However, there was a significant condition by group interaction: $F(9,84) = 3.767$, $p = 0.001$, $\eta_p^2 = 0.288$. There was no main effect of group $F(3,28) = 1.069$, $p = 0.378$. As with the maximum values, a follow-up mixed ANOVA was performed without Group 3. In this follow-up analysis, it was found that the groups did not differ $F(2,21) = 2.064$, $p = 0.152$. Also, no group-by-condition interaction was found $F(6,63) = 0.489$, $p = 0.815$. There was, however, a main effect of condition $F(3,63) = 4.007$, $p = 0.011$, $\eta_p^2 = 0.160$. A post-hoc Bonferroni test with adjustment for multiple comparisons showed that the actor establishing shot condition was significantly higher than the exterior establishing shot condition ($p = 0.016$). Means with error bars are presented in **Figure 7**.

DISCUSSION

The goal of this study was to determine the degree to which the use of the various forms of the establishing shot help a viewer process shifts to new interior locations within a film by measuring oxygenation in the prefrontal cortex and pupil diameter. It was hypothesized that the use of actors establishing shot would cause the lowest levels of oxygenation and pupil diameter, followed by exterior, geographic, and finally no establishing shot. However, for average pupil diameter, geographic establishing shots caused significantly lower average pupil diameter than all other establishing shot types and no establishing shot. In addition, the actors establishing shot caused significantly lower average pupil diameters than no establishing shot. Initially, no main effect of establishing shot type was found for maximum or average oxygenation values in a scene. However, there was a group-by-condition interaction for both of these measures caused by the values from group 3. When group 3 was removed from the analysis, however, both the maximum and average oxygenation values for the actor establishing shot condition were significantly higher than for the exterior establishing shot condition.

The average oxygenation values corroborate the findings of the maximum oxygenation values. Both average and maximum oxygenation values associated with exterior establishing shots were significantly lower than those associated with actors establishing shots. Thus, it appears that exterior establishing shots are better at reducing cognitive load during scene transitions than actors establishing shots. In contrast, there is no difference between exterior establishing shots and the use of no establishing shot in terms of arousal. In terms of workload, none of the establishing shot types were found to differ from no establishing shot. The addition of the establishing shot does nothing to help make the film transition easier to process. Thus, the advantage of the use of the establishing shot is through its ability to reduce arousal, not its ability to reduce the recruitment of cognitive resources needed to process a scene transition.

The differences between the results of the pupil diameter and fNIRS data may indicate the difference in the way establishing shots affect arousal versus cognitive load. Pupil diameter is thought to measure arousal and cognitive load, while fNIRS only measures cognitive load. It was found that the data diverged across the two measures: actor establishing shots caused greater oxygenation than exterior establishing shots, but no such pattern was found with pupil diameter. Instead, pupil diameter was minimized with geographic establishing shots, and the use of no establishing shot caused higher average pupil diameter than the use of actors establishing shots. Because the measures disagree, it would seem that scene changes prefaced by exterior actor establishing shots are easier to process than actor establishing shots, but that actors establishing shots elicited less arousal than no establishing shots and that geographic establishing shots cause less arousal than all other establishing shot conditions.

The divergence of arousal and cognitive load might be explicable through neuroanatomy. Perhaps arousal and cognitive load are mediated by two completely different brain systems: arousal by the limbic system, and cognitive load by cortical areas. This might explain why the eye tracking data and fNIRS data do not coincide.

There was a group-by-condition interaction in the pupil diameter data, and in the fNIRS data when group 3 was included. This could indicate that the order in which a particular establishing shot was presented affected the results. It is also possible that the specific pairing of the establishing shot and scene had an effect as well. In addition, the specific shots used for each type of establishing shot differed across groups. For instance, a different building is featured in the exterior establishing shot in each group. This was because the importance of having an establishing shot that could plausibly be paired with the

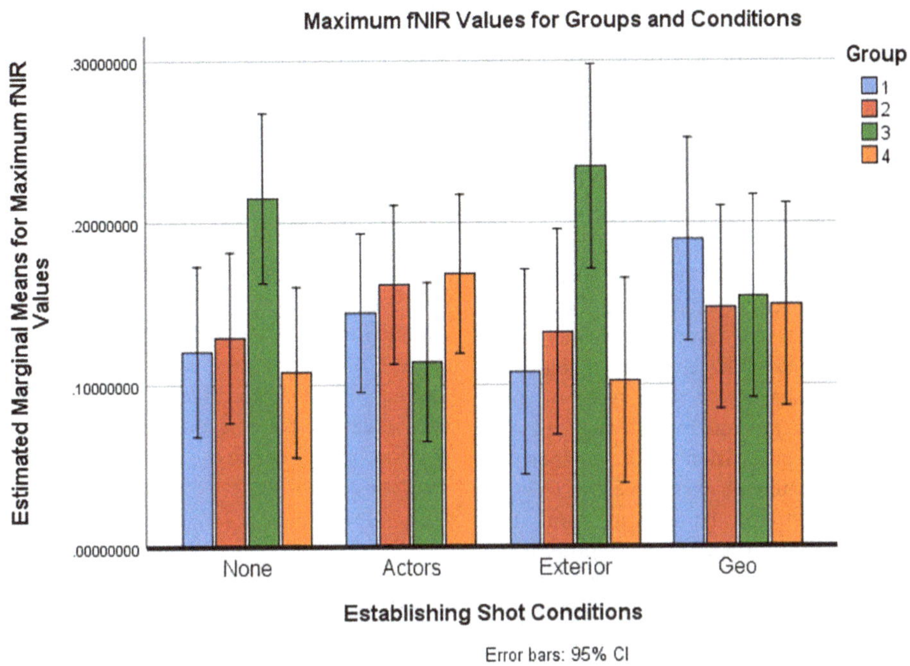

FIGURE 6 | Maximum fNIRS values across all optodes for groups and conditions.

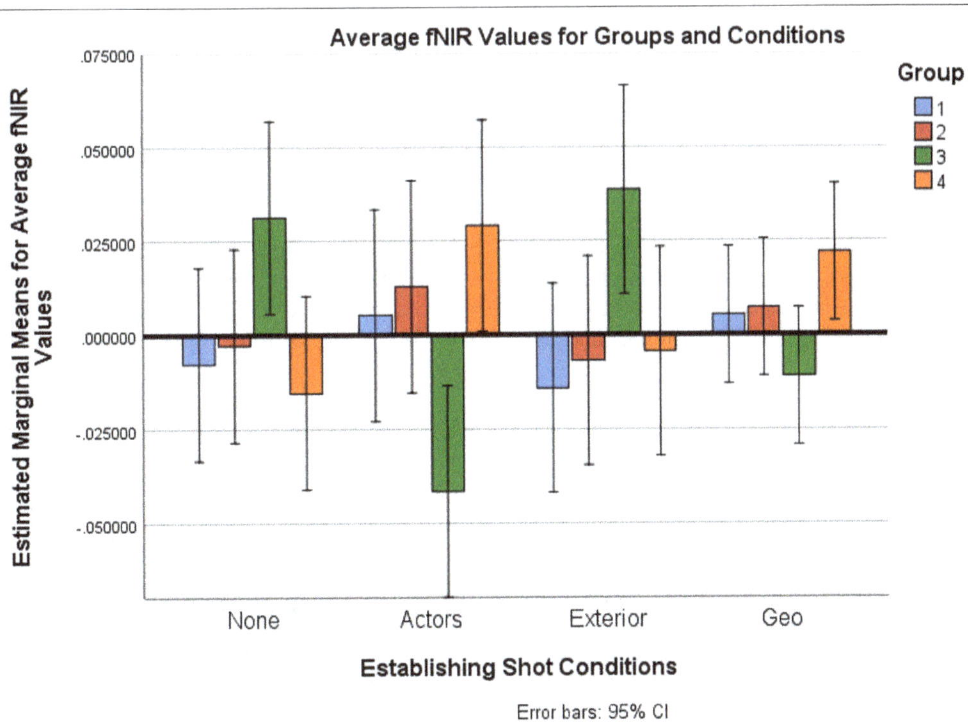

FIGURE 7 | Average fNIRS values across all optodes for groups and conditions.

following scene's location was prioritized over having consistency in the image presented across groups. In the case of group 3, the particular images selected as establishing shots may have created especially jarring scene transitions, which may explain its influence on the fNIRS results. Pupil diameter values may have also been influenced by differing levels of luminance in different establishing shots or scenes, causing the group-by-condition interaction.

Geographic establishing shots as well as actors establishing shots were both found to cause less arousal than using no establishing shot, seeming to indicate that using these types of establishing shots can indeed create smoother transitions between scenes. This would indicate that filmmakers' and film theorist's intuitions have been partially validated; for specific types of establishing shot, the use of the establishing shot as a means of smoothing scene transitions has been upheld. Specifically, geographic establishing shots seem to be best at performing their intended function, and may be worth using more often in future films. However, the establishing shot's effect may be because the sample in this study is accustomed to scenes in novel locations being prefaced with actors and geographic establishing shots, and so the absence of these types of shots during scene transitions seems jarring. Indeed, Schwan and Ildirar (2010) suggest that comprehension of the establishing shot technique is not naturally intuited by first-time film viewers, but is conditioned through repeated exposure to film. It is also possible that, despite being jarring, the transitions using no establishing shot may not have needed enough cognitive resources during their processing to be associated with any detectable increase in cognitive load.

From these results, it is concluded that having an actors establishing shot or geographic establishing shot can smooth transitions between scenes by decreasing arousal but not by decreasing cognitive workload. Exterior establishing shots have no effect on arousal or cognitive load compared to forgoing the establishing shot.

This study had several important limitations. The first was sample size; each group only had seven to eight participants, which limits the amount of confidence that one can invest in the significant results found. Further, since the experimental stimulus was not designed to have a coherent narrative, it does not wholly resemble a commercial, narrative film. Thus, future studies may want to explore the effect of the establishing shot while participants are watching a widely distributed feature-length commercial film as a means of generalizing the results found in this study. Future studies may also want to investigate the different areas of the brain responsible for arousal and cognitive load.

AUTHOR CONTRIBUTIONS

GB was responsible for reviewing existing literature, developing the experimental design, creating the experimental stimulus, and conducting the experiments. NR advised GB throughout these steps. GB and NR were responsible for preparing the data for analysis and interpreting the results. NR ran statistical tests on the data. GB wrote the manuscript that was submitted for publication. NR edited the manuscript before it was submitted.

FUNDING

Funding sources for this project include the Ithaca College Academic Challenge Grant, the Ithaca College Psychology Department, and the Summer Scholars Program run by the Ithaca College School of Humanities and Sciences.

ACKNOWLEDGMENTS

We would like to thank Ithaca College, especially the School of Humanities and Sciences, the Roy H. Park School of Communications, and the Psychology Department, for supporting this project. We would also like to thank Dr. Hasan Ayaz for helping us troubleshoot our fNIRS system.

REFERENCES

Arsalidou, M., Pascual-Leone, J., Johnson, J., Morris, D., and Taylor, M. J. (2013). A balancing act of the brain: activations and deactivations driven by cognitive load. *Brain Behav.* 3, 273–285. doi: 10.1002/brb3.128

Ayaz, H. (2010). *Functional Near Infrared Spectroscopy Based Brain Computer Interface.* Philadelphia, PA: Drexel University.

Ayaz, H., Izzetoglu, M., Shewokis, P. A., and Onaral, B. (2010). "Sliding-window motion artifact rejection for functional near-infrared spectroscopy," in *Proceedings of the 2010 Annual International Conference of the IEEE Engineering in Medicine and Biology* (Buenos Aires: IEEE), 6567–6570. doi: 10.1109/IEMBS.2010.5627113

Ayaz, H., Shewokis, P. A., Bunce, S., Izzetoglu, K., Willems, B., and Onaral, B. (2012). Optical brain monitoring for operator training and mental workload assessment. *Neuroimage* 59, 36–47. doi: 10.1016/j.neuroimage.2011.06.023

Ayaz, H., Shewokis, P. A., Curtin, A., Izzetoglu, M., Izzetoglu, K., and Onaral, B. (2011). Using MazeSuite and functional near infrared spectroscopy to study learning in spatial navigation. *J. Vis. Exp.* 56:3443. doi: 10.3791/3443

Ballester, C. (2005). *The Establishing Shot, Film Space and the Czechoslovak New Wave.* Ph.D. thesis, University of London, London.

Beatty, J., and Lucero-Wagoner, B. (2000). "The pupillary system," in *Handbook of Psychophysiology*, eds J. T. Cacioppo, L. G. Tassinary, and G. G. Berntson (New York, NY: Cambridge University Press), 142–162.

Bordwell, D. (2002). Intensified continuity visual style in contemporary American film. *Film Q.* 55, 16–28. doi: 10.1525/fq.2002.55.3.16

Chance, B., Zhuang, Z., UnAh, C., Alter, C., and Lipton, L. (1993). Cognition-activated low-frequency modulation of light absorption in human brain. *Proc. Natl. Acad. Sci. U.S.A.* 90, 3770–3774. doi: 10.1073/pnas.90.8.3770

Chen, S., and Epps, J. (2014). Using task-induced pupil diameter and blink rate to infer cognitive load. *Hum. Comput. Interact.* 29, 390–413. doi: 10.1080/07370024.2014.892428

Cooper, G. (1990). Cognitive load theory as an aid for instructional design. *Australas. J. Educ. Technol.* 6, 108–113. doi: 10.14742/ajet.2322

Cutting, J. (2014). *Event Segmentation and Seven Types of Narrative Discontinuity in Popular Movies.* Available at: http://people.psych.cornell.edu/~jec7/pubs/CuttingActa14.pdf doi: 10.1016/j.actpsy.2014.03.003

Cutting, J., Brunick, K., and Candan, A. (2012). Perceiving event dynamics and parsing Hollywood films. *J. Exp. Psychol. Hum. Percept. Perform.* 38, 1476–1490. doi: 10.1037/a0027737

Cutting, J., and Candan, A. (2013). *Movies, Evolution, and Mind: From Fragmentation to Continuity.* Available at: https://www.researchgate.net/

publication/253238250_Movies_Evolution_and_Mind_From_Fragmentation_to_Continuity

Cutting, J., and Iricinschi, C. (2015). Re-presentations of space in Hollywood movies: an event-indexing analysis. *Cogn. Sci.* 39, 434–456. doi: 10.1111/cogs.12151

Ferreri, L., Bigand, E., Perrey, S., and Bugaiska, A. (2014). The promise of near-infrared spectroscopy (NIRS) for psychological research: a brief review. *Ann. Psychol.* 114, 537–569. doi: 10.4074/S0003503314003054

Francuz, P., and Zabielska-Mendyk, E. (2013). Does the brain differentiate between related and unrelated cuts when processing audiovisual messages? An ERP study. *Media Psychol.* 16, 461–475. doi: 10.1080/15213269.2013.831394

Geiger, S., and Reeves, B. (1993). The effects of scene changes and semantic relatedness on attention to television. *Commun. Res.* 20, 155–175. doi: 10.1177/009365093020002001

Herff, C., Heger, D., Fortmann, O., Hennrich, J., Putze, F., and Schultz, T. (2014). Mental workload during n-back task - quantified in the prefrontal cortex using fNIRS. *Front. Hum. Neurosci.* 7:935. doi: 10.3389/fnhum.2013.00935

Izzetoglu, K., Bunce, S., Onaral, B., Pourrezaei, K., and Chance, B. (2004). Functional optical brain imaging using near-infrared during cognitive tasks. *Int. J. Hum. Comput. Interact.* 17, 211–227. doi: 10.1207/s15327590ijhc1702_6

Laeng, B., Sirois, S., and Gredebäck, G. (2012). Pupillometry: a window to the preconscious? *Perspect. Psychol. Sci.* 7, 18–27. doi: 10.1177/1745691611427305

Lang, A., Geiger, S., Strickwerda, M., and Sumner, J. (1993). The effects of related and unrelated cuts on television viewers' attention, processing capacity, and memory. *Commun. Res.* 20, 4–29. doi: 10.1177/009365093020001001

León-Carrión, J., and León-Domínguez, U. (2012). "Functional near-infrared spectroscopy (fNIRS): principles and neuroscientific applications," in *Neuroimaging - Methods*, ed. P. Bright (Rijeka: InTech).

Lloyd-Fox, S., Blasi, A., and Elwell, C. E. (2010). Illuminating the developing brain: the past, present and future of functional near infrared spectroscopy. *Neurosci. Biobehav. Rev.* 34, 269–284. doi: 10.1016/j.neubiorev.2009.07.008

Magliano, J. P., and Zacks, J. M. (2011). The impact of continuity editing in narrative film on event segmentation. *Cogn. Sci.* 35, 1489–1517. doi: 10.1111/j.1551-6709.2011.01202.x

Magliano, J. P., and Zacks, J. M. (2013). "Film, narrative, and cognitive neuroscience," in *Art and the Senses*, eds F. Bacci and D. Melcher (Oxford: Oxford Univ. Press).

Pincus, E., and Ascher, S. (2012). *The Filmmaker's Handbook: A Comprehensive Guide for the Digital Age*, 4th Edn. New York, NY: Plume.

Schwan, S., and Ildirar, S. (2010). Watching film for the first time: how adult viewers interpret perceptual discontinuities in film. *Psychol. Sci.* 21, 970–976. doi: 10.1177/0956797610372632

Smith, T. (2005). *An Attentional Theory of Continuity Editing.* Available at: https://www.era.lib.ed.ac.uk/bitstream/handle/1842/1076/smith_ATOCE_0506.pdf;jsessionid=EC273565D607F494C5B179E7291026B9?sequence=1

Smith, T., Whitwell, M., and Lee, J. (2006). "Eye movements and pupil dilation during event perception," in *Proceedings of the 2006 Symposium on Eye Tracking Research & Applications* (New York, NY: Association for Computing Machinery). doi: 10.1145/1117309.1117333

Swallow, K. M., Zacks, J. M., and Abrams, R. A. (2009). Event boundaries in perception affect memory encoding and updating. *J. Exp. Psychol. Gen.* 138, 236–257. doi: 10.1037/a0015631

Zagermann, J., Pfeil, U., and Reiterer, H. (2016). "Measuring cognitive load using eye tracking technology in visual computing," in *Proceedings of the Sixth Workshop on Beyond Time and Errors on Novel Evaluation Methods for Visualization* (New York, NY: ACM), 78–85. doi: 10.1145/2993901.2993908

Zwaan, R. A., Langston, M. C., and Graesser, A. C. (1995a). The construction of situation models in narrative comprehension: an event-indexing model. *Psychol. Sci.* 6, 292–297. doi: 10.1111/j.1467-9280.1995.tb00513.x

Zwaan, R. A., Magliano, J. P., and Graesser, A. C. (1995b). Dimensions of situation model construction in narrative comprehension. *J. Exp. Psychol. Learn. Mem. Cogn.* 21, 386–397. doi: 10.1037/0278-7393.21.2.386

16

Dynamic Office Environments Improve Brain Activity and Attentional Performance Mediated by Increased Motor Activity

Diana Henz* and Wolfgang I. Schöllhorn

Institute of Sports Science, Faculty of Social Sciences, Media and Sport, Johannes Gutenberg University Mainz, Mainz, Germany

Correspondence:
Diana Henz
henz@uni-mainz.de

Current research demonstrates beneficial effects of physical activity on brain functions and cognitive performance. To date, less is known on the effects of gross motor movements that do not fall into the category of sports-related aerobic or anaerobic exercise. In previous studies, we found beneficial effects of dynamic working environments, i.e., environments that encourage movements during cognitive task performance, on cognitive performance and corresponding brain activity. Aim of the present study was to examine the effects of working in a dynamic and a static office environment on attentional and vigilance performance, and on the corresponding electroencephalographic (EEG) brain oscillatory patterns. In a 2-week intervention study, participants worked either in a dynamic or a static office. In each intervention group, 12 subjects performed attentional and vigilance tasks. Spontaneous EEG was measured from 19 electrodes continuosly before, during, and immediately after each experimental condition at the first, and at the last intervention session. Results showed differences in EEG brain activity in the dynamic compared to the static office at the beginning as well as at the end of the intervention. EEG theta power increased in the vigilance task in anterior regions, alpha power in central and parietal regions in the dynamic compared to the static office. Further, increases in beta activity in the attention and vigilance task were shown in frontal and central regions in the dynamic office. Gamma power increased in the attention task in frontal and central regions. After 2 weeks, effects on brain activity increased in the attentional and vigilance task in the dynamic office. Increased theta and alpha oscillations were obtained in anterior areas with higher activity in the beta band in anterior and central areas in the dynamic compared to the static office. EEG oscillatory patterns indicate beneficial effects of dynamic office environments on attentional and vigilance performance that are mediated by increased motor activity. We discuss the obtained patterns of EEG oscillations in terms of the close interrelations between the attentional and the motor system.

Keywords: ergonomics, office, movement, dynamic working environment, EEG

INTRODUCTION

Research demonstrates beneficial effects of bodily movement on brain and cognitive functions. Most studies performed in this area investigate the effects of aerobic exercise and gross motor movements on cognitive functions (for meta-analytic overviews see Etnier et al., 2004; Chang et al., 2012; Gheysen et al., 2018; Mandolesi et al., 2018). More specifically, beneficial effects of physical exercise have been demonstrated on brain and cognitive functions such as increased gray matter volume in frontal and hippocampal volume (Colcombe et al., 2006), increased neurotrophic factor (Brunoni et al., 2008), increased blood flow (Weinberg and Gould, 2015), increasing in academic achievement (Sibley and Etnier, 2003), improvements in cognitive functions such as memory abilities, efficiency of attentional and executive-control processes (Kramer et al., 1999; Colcombe and Kramer, 2003; Grego et al., 2005; Pereira et al., 2019; Winter et al., 2007; Chieffi et al., 2017), prevention of cognitive decline (Colberg et al., 2008), reduced risk developing dementia, and a modified network topology (Deeny et al., 2008). Examining the underlying neurophysiological processes, physical exercise induces most often changes in electroencephalographic (EEG) alpha and beta bands (Moraes et al., 2007, 2011). Further, changes in brain activity are dependent on the type and intensity of the physical exercise (Brümmer et al., 2011).

Less is known on the effects of gross motor movements on the cognitive system that do not fall into the categorization of aerobic or anaerobic exercise. In previous studies, we investigated the effects of dynamic sitting on brain activity and cognitive performance. Participants performed arithmetic, geometric, and algebraic tasks either on a static chair that did not foster movements or on a dynamic chair that allowed subject-induced movements in the vertical and horizontal direction during task performance. We observed improvements in mathematical performance when sitting on a dynamic chair. More specifically, performance in geometric and algebraic tasks that afforded visuo-spatial processing increased. The corresponding EEG brain activity showed increases in overall alpha and beta activity in areas related to visuo-spatial processing. We concluded that dynamic sitting activates working memory processes that leads to better performance in visuo-spatial processing (Henz, 2014; Henz et al., 2015).

These findings encourage further developments from dynamic sitting furniture towards the design of office environments consisting of mobile chairs, desks, and floors that foster motor activity which in turn stimulates the brain towards a state that is beneficial for cognitive task performance. These working environments consist of office desk furnitures that allows or even encourages movement behavior. In the applied research field of *neuroergonomics* findings from neuroscience and human factors are combined to design working environments that match the affordances and limitations of the human brain and cognitive system (for an overview see Ayaz and Dehais, 2019). One main aim is to detect the underlying brain and cognitive mechanisms that lead to a more efficient and healthy working. Research has focused on the effects of working environment designs on visual attention, vigilance, mental workload, working memory processes, and motor control on brain and cognitive functions (Parasuraman and Rizzo, 2007; Parasuraman and Wilson, 2008; Lees et al., 2010; Gramann et al., 2017). To date, no systematic studies have been performed on the effects of dynamic office furniture use on brain and cognitive functions in everyday working settings. These dynamic office furnitures have specific features that encourage movement behavior, i.e., chairs that allow vertical and horizontal movements during sitting, or desks that alter their height in an automated manner so that subjects have to adapt by altering their posture.

In the present study, we tested the effects of working in a dynamic office environment on EEG brain activity, attentional, and vigilance task performance. According to the results of previous studies (Henz, 2014; Henz et al., 2015), we expected that working in a dynamic office environment would improve attentional and vigilance performance. We hypothesized that working in a dynamic office environment would be accompanied by an increase in processing volume, and a decrease in errors in the attentional task. For the vigilance test, we expected a decrease in reaction times (RTs). Further, working in a dynamic office would activate the brain towards a state that fosters improvements in attentional and vigilance performance compared to working in a static office environment. We expected increases in beta and gamma power, and coherence in frontal electrodes in the attentional and vigilance task. Further, we hypothesized that improvements in attentional and vigilance performance accompanied by increases in beta and gamma power and increased coherence in the would increase after a 2-week intervention. For the EEG coherence analysis, we tested the frontal area, represented by the electrode pairs F3/F4, F3/Fz, and F7/Fz. EEG measured at these frontal electrode sites was assumed to reflect activity in (pre)frontal brain areas involved in executive functions, voluntary control, and action creation (Szurhaj et al., 2003; Moriguchi and Hiraki, 2013), Further, we tested the primary motor area from C3/Cz, C3/C4, and C4/Cz which is related to motor act execution (Toni et al., 2002), and the parietal area from P3/Pz, and P3/P4 that is involved in sensorimotor integration (Smith et al., 1999; Neuper and Pfurtscheller, 2001; Huber et al., 2006). Our hypotheses are based on findings of recent studies which have shown close interrelations between the motor system and attentional processing. Several investigations have shown increases in beta band activity when the motor network is activated (Khanna and Carmena, 2015; Chung et al., 2017). Beta activity is also eminent in brain areas that are related to attentional processing (Kopell et al., 2000). Synchronization in the beta range was shown in the dorsal prefrontal cortex and posterior parietal cortex in tasks that engage predominantly visual attention (Verhoef et al., 2011; Buschman et al., 2012). Saleh et al. (2010) demonstrated a close relation of beta activity in the motor cortex and beta activity during processing of attentional tasks.

MATERIALS AND METHODS

Participants

Twenty-four subjects (mean age 24.3 years, age range 21–35, 12 males, 12 females) participated in the study. None of the subjects had current neurological diseases or a history of neurological impairments or intake of medication that may have influenced EEG brain activity. All subjects were right-handed. Handedness was assessed by the Edinburgh Handedness Inventory (Oldfield, 1971). Subjects were paid for participation in the study. The study was approved by the local ethics committee of the University of Mainz. All subjects gave written informed consent. All experimental procedures complied with the standards of the Helsinki Declaration of the World Medical Association Assembly. All subjects were naïve as to the purpose of the study.

EEG Recording Details

EEG brain activity was recorded from 19 electrodes that were placed according to the international 10–20 system on the scalp with reference to the nose. EEG signals were recorded from the electrodes Fp1, Fp2, F3, F7, Fz, F4, F8, C3, Cz, C4, T3, T4, P3, P7, Pz, P4, P8, O1, O2. Electrodes are referred to different scalp areas as follows: frontal area (Fp1, Fp2, F3, F7, Fz, F4, F8), central area (C3, Cz, C4), temporal area (T3, T4), parietal area (P3, P7, Pz, P4, P8), and occipital area (O1, O2). The Micromed Brainquick amplifier (SD-LTM-32) and Micromed Brainspy software (Micromed, Venice, Italy) were used for the EEG recordings. Impedances of all electrodes were kept at 10 kΩ or below. EEG data were recorded continuously and digitized at a sampling rate of 256 Hz. EEG signals were amplified with a time constant of 0.3 s (high-pass filter: 0.5 Hz; low pass filter: 120 Hz; frequency range: 0.5–120 Hz). To assess electrooculographic (EOG) data two electrodes were placed at the medial upper and lateral orbital rim of the right eye. EOG signals were amplified with a time constant of 0.3 s (high pass filter: 0.1 Hz; low pass filter: 120 Hz; frequency range: 0.5–120 Hz). Heart rate was measured continuously as a control variable using the medilog® AR12plus recorder (Schiller, Linz, Austria) at a sampling rate of 1,000 Hz. As a further control variable, electromyographic (EMG) activity was recorded using the biovision (Wehrheim, Germany) from two electrodes placed at the splenius capitis, and two electrodes placed at the trapezius pars descendens at a sampling rate of 500 Hz.

Dynamic and Static Office Environments

A schematic illustration of the dynamic office environment (active office®, aeris GmbH, Munich, Germany) is depicted in **Figure 1**. It consists of two desks that are height-adjustable with one desk designed as a sitting workstation, and the other as a standing workstation. Subjects sat at the sitting workstation on a height-adjustable stool (swopper®, aeris GmbH, Munich, Germany) that allowed subject-induced movements in the vertical direction. At the standing workstation, subjects performed tasks placed on a height-adjustable stool (muvman®, aeris GmbH, Munich, Germany) that supports sitting with legs stretched similar to a stance position. Additionally, subjects stood on a foam mat that had an uneven surface structure (aeris® muvmat) at the standing workstation. A 21″ screen was placed on the middle of each desk. One main characteristic of the dynamic office environment is that subjects have to change the workstation at randomly set time intervals ranging from 5 to 20 min. The experimental tasks were arranged in that way that after completion of some sections a signal on the screen appeared that indicated to change the workstation. In contrast, subjects performed the experimental tasks in the static office environment in the same desk configuration but sat only at the sitting workstation on a static stool. The static stool was height-adjustable and had the same properties as the stool used in the dynamic condition except of allowing subject-induced movements in the vertical direction.

Assessment of Attentional and Vigilance Performance

The experimental tasks are illustrated in **Figure 2**. For the assessment of short-term attentional performance, subjects performed the d2-R attention test (Brickenkamp et al., 2010). The test sheet of the d2-R test consists of 14 lines with 57 characters each. The characters are the letters "d" and "p". They are accompanied by different markers consisting of one to four vertical lines that are positioned over or below the characters. The task of the subjects was to scratch all letters

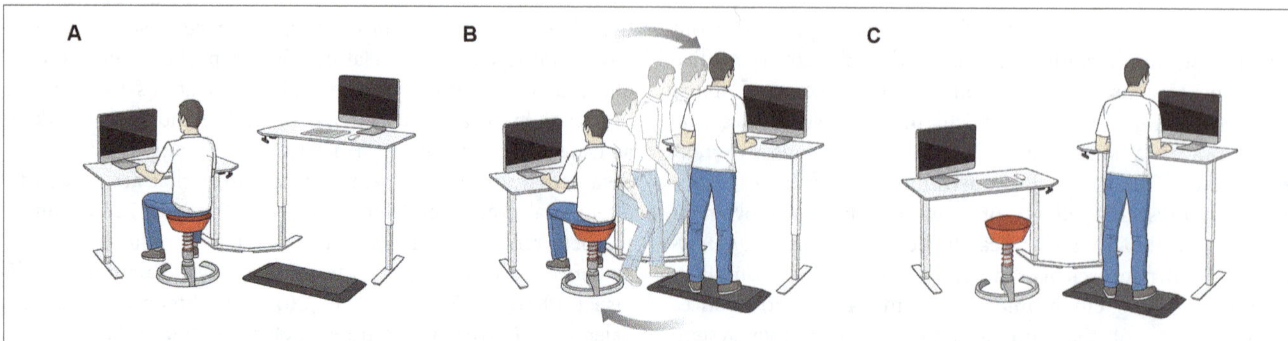

FIGURE 1 | Illustration of the dynamic office environment. **(A)** Sitting workstation. **(B)** Change from the sitting to the standing workstation. **(C)** Standing workstation.

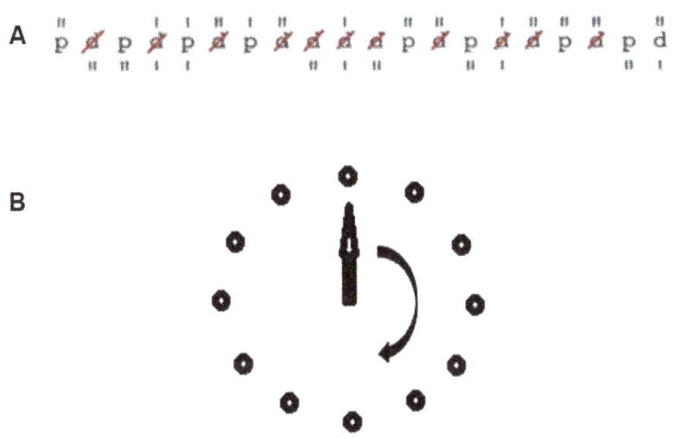

FIGURE 2 | Illustration of the experimental tasks. **(A)** Sample row of the d2-R task. **(B)** Mackworth clock task.

"d" with a total of two lines. Errors consisted of missing to scratch a letter "d", the scratching of the letter "p", and the scratching of a letter "d" with more or less than a total of two lines. The degree of difficulty of the test is composed of the time limit (4 min 40 s) and the challenge to discriminate between relevant and irrelevant stimuli. Vigilance performance was assessed by the Mackworth clock task (Mackworth, 1948). Test stimuli were presented on a screen. Subjects tracked a clock hand visually that moved around the screen passing distinct positions that were arranged circular (diameter 15 cm). The task of the subjects was to press a button when the hand jumped more than one position. RTs are calculated from the latency of the hand jump, and the button press. RTs were taken for the segments: (1) minute 1–5; (2) minute 6–10; (3) minute 11–15; and (4) minute 16–20.

Experimental Procedure

Prior to the experiment, the experimental tasks were explained. Each subject was shown where and how to sit or stand. Half of the subjects performed the intervention in the dynamic office environment, the other half underwent the intervention in the static office environment. Participants were randomly assigned to the experimental groups. After subjects gave their informed consent, demographic data were assessed. Then, they began with a 5-min resting condition. Spontaneous EEG was recorded for 5 min with eyes-open. Then, subjects were sat at the office environment and performed the experimental tasks. Each intervention session had a duration of 4 h. Subjects performed a standardized program that contained everyday office tasks (E-mail correspondence, calculations, document reading etc.). The d2-R test was performed after 10 min and after 120 min, the Mackworth clock task after 15 min and after 125 min working in the office in the first and in the last session of the 2-week intervention. Spontaneous EEG was recorded continuously during the six conditions: (1) pre-intervention rest; (2) d2-R test; (3) Mackworth clock task minutes 1–5; (4) Mackworth clock task minutes 6–10; (5) Mackworth clock task minutes 11–15; and (6) Mackworth clock task minutes 16–20 that were used for subsequent statistical analyses.

EEG Analysis

EEG analyses were performed with the EEGLAB (Swartz Center for Computational Neuroscience, La Jolla, CA, USA). Spontaneous EEG was assessed with eyes-open. Five-minute sequences were recorded before and after each experimental condition. Independent component analyses (ICAs) were performed for the EEG signal. Components that resulted from artifacts were removed. For the analysis of the EEG data, Fast Fourier Transforms were performed to calculate the mean power spectra for the theta (4–7.5 Hz), alpha (8–13 Hz), beta (14–30 Hz), and gamma (31–70 Hz) bands. Further, EEG coherence for the electrode pairs (F3/F4, F3/Fz, F7/Fz, C3/Cz, P3/Pz, and P3/P4) was analyzed. Coherence was calculated for the theta, alpha, beta, and gamma range.

Electrode Spatial Localization

Three regions of interest were selected: the pre-motor and pre-frontal cortex, represented by the F3/F4, F3/Fz and F7/Fz electrode pairs, which are assumed to be functionally involved in action creation and voluntary control (Moriguchi and Hiraki, 2013), and for executive functions (Szurhaj et al., 2003). The C3/Cz, C3/C4 and C4/Cz electrode pairs were assessed for being representatives of primary motor areas related to the motor act execution (Toni et al., 2002); the P3/Pz and P3/P4 electrode pairs due to their relation to sensorimotor integration (Smith et al., 1999; Huber et al., 2006).

Data on the Attention and Vigilance Task

Performance in the d2-R test was determined by the attention performance score. It was calculated by subtracting the number of falsely marked test items from the total number of correctly marked characters. Mean RTs in the Mackworth clock task were calculated for four segments: (1) minute 1–5; (2) minute 6–10; (3) minute 11–15; and (4) minute 16–20.

Statistical Analyses

Means and standard deviations of the d2-R attentional performance score, and the RTs of the Mackworth clock task (minute 1–5, minute 6–10, minute 11–15, minute 16–20) were calculated. Mauchly's test of sphericity was calculated to test the assumptions of repeated-measures analysis of variance (ANOVAs) for the d2-R test score, the RTs of the Mackworth clock task, and the EEG data. Consecutive ANOVAs were performed when the *p*-values were equal or exceeded 0.05. A two-way ANOVA that included the between-subjects factor working environment (static, dynamic), and the within-subjects factor time (pretest, posttest) was performed for the d2-R test score. Further, a three-way ANOVA that included the between-subjects factor working environment (static, dynamic), and the within-subjects factors time (pretest, posttest), and segment (minute 1–5, minute 6–10, minute 11–15, minute 16–20) was performed for the RTs of the Mackworth clock task. In a consecutive step, data were subjected to *post hoc t*-tests with Bonferroni-correction. For the EEG data, repeated-measure ANOVAs were performed separately for the theta, alpha, beta, and gamma bands that included the between-subject factor working environment (static, dynamic), and the within-subject factors as time (pretest, posttest), experimental condition (pretest rest, vigilance test minute 1–5, vigilance test minute 6–10, vigilance test minute 11–15, vigilance test minute 16–20, posttest rest), and location (Frontal, Central, Temporal, Parietal, Occipital). In a consecutive step, *post hoc t*-tests with Bonferroni-correction were calculated for significant main or interaction effects. Additionally, partial eta-squared (η_p^2) was calculated to determine effect sizes for the d2-R test score, RTs of the Mackworth clock task, and the frequency specific EEG power densities (theta, alpha, beta, gamma). The coherence values were analyzed using a two-way ANOVA with the factors working environment (static, dynamic), and time (pretest, posttest) for each electrode pair studied (F3/F4, F3/Fz, F7/Fz, C3/Cz, P3/Pz, P3/P4 and T3/T4). Statistical significance of the tests was achieved when the *p*-values were less than 0.05.

RESULTS

Attentional Performance

Means and standard deviations of the scores of the d2-R test and the Mackworth clock task are depicted in **Figures 3, 4**. The ANOVA on the attentional performance score of the d2-R test showed a significant effect for the factor working environment after 10 min, $F_{(1,23)} = 5.92$, $p = 0.02$, $\eta_p^2 = 0.18$. Further, the effect for the factor time was significant, $F_{(1,19)} = 7.39$, $p = 0.02$, $\eta_p^2 = 0.21$. The working environment × time interaction was significant, $F_{(4,19)} = 3.14$, $p = 0.03$, $\eta_p^2 = 0.13$.

The ANOVA for the RTs in the Mackworth clock task revealed a significant effect for working environment, $F_{(1,19)} = 4.75$, $p = 0.03$, $\eta_p^2 = 0.15$. Further, a significant main effect was shown for the factors experimental condition, $F_{(3,57)} = 3.81$, $p = 0.02$, $\eta_p^2 = 0.11$, and time, $F_{(1,19)} = 6.03$, $p = 0.02$, $\eta_p^2 = 0.17$. The working environment × time interaction was significant, $F_{(4,19)} = 3.77$, $p = 0.04$, $\eta_p^2 = 0.06$.

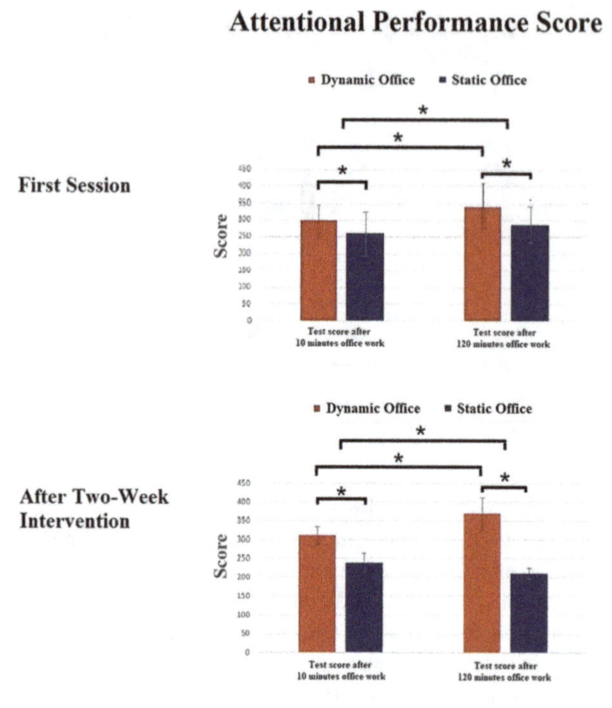

FIGURE 3 | Results of the d2-R test. *$p < 0.05$.

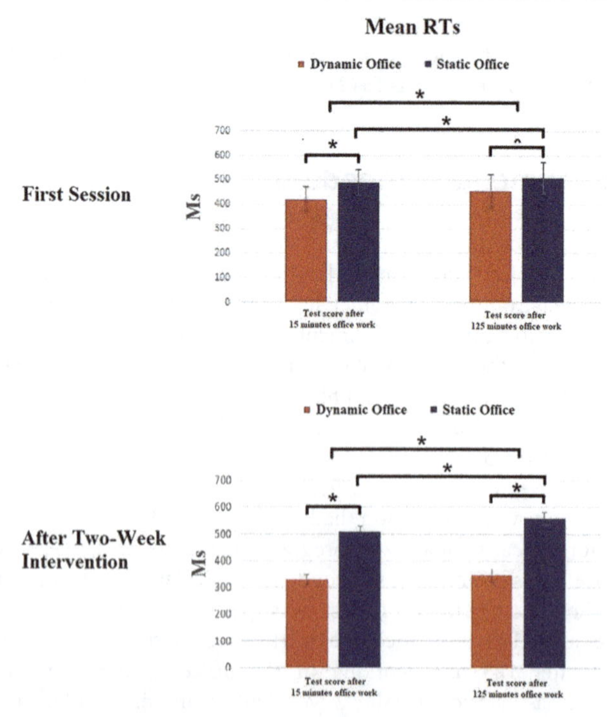

FIGURE 4 | Results of the Mackworth clock task. *$p < 0.05$.

Spontaneous EEG

Mean power spectra for the EEG theta, alpha, beta, and gamma bands in the d2-R test and the Mackworth clock task are depicted in **Figures 5, 6**.

The ANOVA for theta power obtained during the Mackworth clock task showed significant main effects for working environment, $F_{(1,19)} = 4.92$, $p = 0.03$, $\eta_p^2 = 0.08$, and time, $F_{(1,19)} = 4.53$, $p = 0.04$, $\eta_p^2 = 0.05$. The working environment × time interaction was significant, $F_{(4,19)} = 2.96$, $p = 0.04$, $\eta_p^2 = 0.03$. A further ANOVA revealed significant differences between locations, $F_{(20,95)} = 2.16$, $p = 0.02$, $\eta_p^2 = 0.13$. *Post hoc* comparisons showed increases in EEG theta power at frontal, central, and parietal electrodes, compared to temporal and occipital electrodes, $p < 0.05$ each. Subsequent analyses showed that theta power increased most in the frontal region at the electrodes F3 and F4, $p < 0.05$ each.

The ANOVA for alpha power obtained during the Mackworth clock task showed a significant main effects for working environment, $F_{(1,19)} = 5.96$, $p = 0.02$, $\eta_p^2 = 0.14$, and time, $F_{(1,19)} = 6.16$, $p = 0.02$, $\eta_p^2 = 0.15$. The working environment × time interaction was significant, $F_{(4,19)} = 3.02$, $p = 0.03$, $\eta_p^2 = 0.12$. The ANOVA of alpha responses revealed significant differences between locations, $F_{(20,95)} = 1.90$, $p = 0.04$, $\eta_p^2 = 0.05$. *Post hoc* comparisons showed that spontaneous EEG

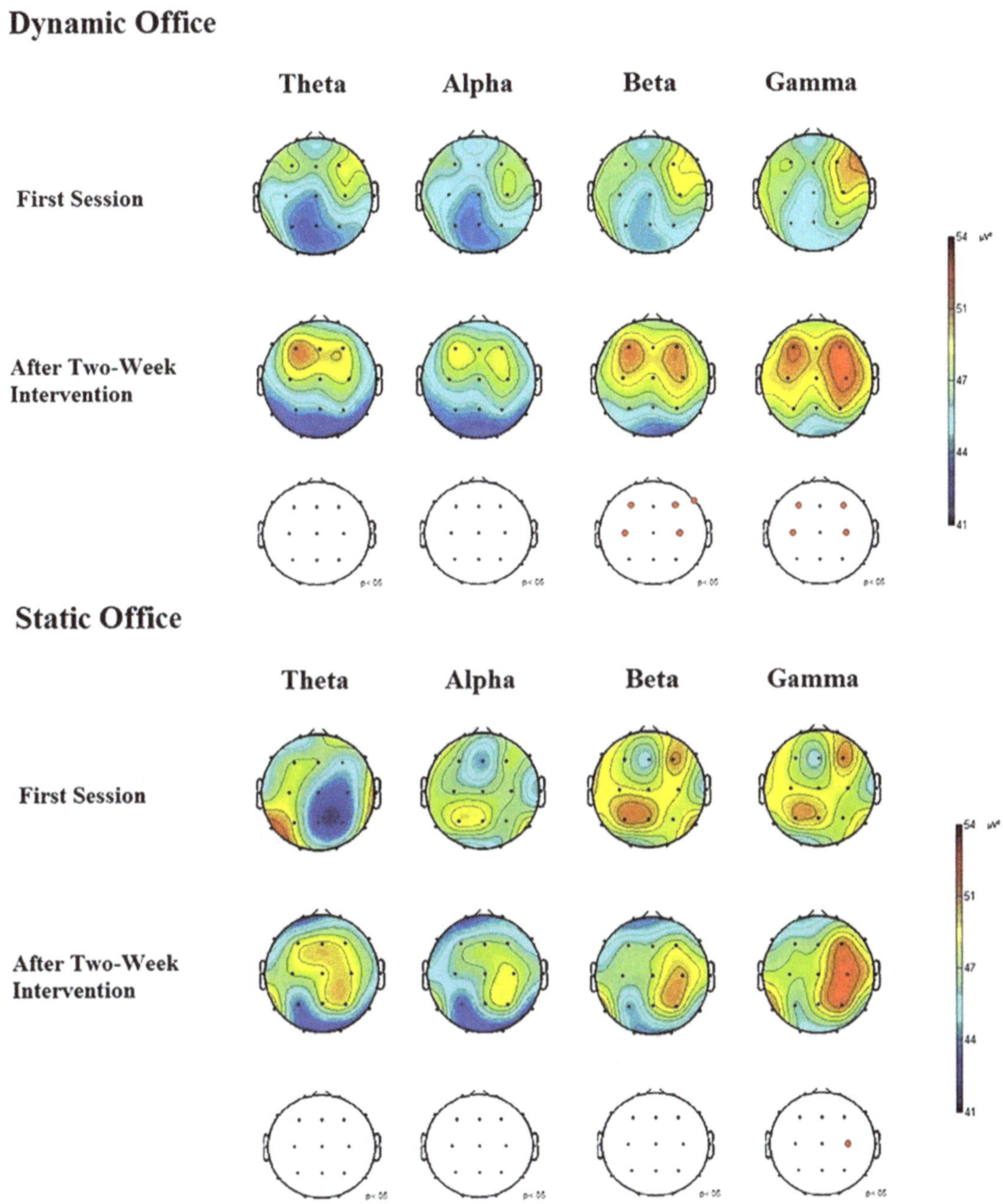

FIGURE 5 | Electroencephalographic (EEG) brain activity for the theta, alpha, beta, and gamma bands in the dynamic and static office during the d2-R test.

alpha power was higher at central and parietal electrodes, than that of frontal, temporal, and occipital electrodes, $p < 0.05$ each. Subsequent analyses showed that alpha power increased most in the central region at the electrode C4, and in the parietal region at the electrodes P3 and P4, $p < 0.05$ each.

The ANOVA for beta power obtained during the d2-R test showed highly significant main effects for the factors working environment, $F_{(1,19)} = 8.45$, $p = 0.01$, $\eta_p^2 = 0.25$, and time, $F_{(1,19)} = 8.37$, $p = 0.01$, $\eta_p^2 = 0.22$. The working environment × time interaction was significant, $F_{(4,19)} = 3.84$, $p = 0.02$, $\eta_p^2 = 0.18$. The ANOVA of beta responses revealed highly significant differences between locations, $F_{(20,95)} = 2.83$, $p = 0.009$, $\eta_p^2 = 0.28$. *Post hoc* comparisons showed that spontaneous EEG beta power was higher at frontal and central electrodes, than that of parietal, temporal, and occipital electrodes, $p < 0.05$ each. Subsequent analyses showed that beta power increased most in the frontal region at the electrodes F3, F4, and F8, $p < 0.01$ each, and in the central region at the

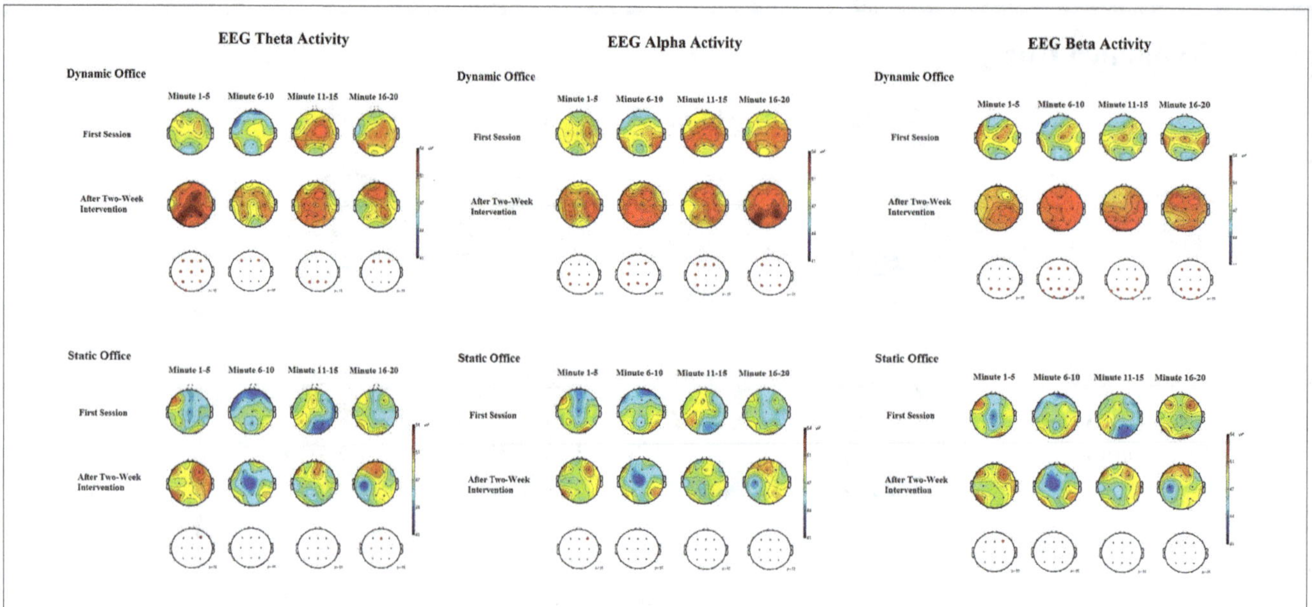

FIGURE 6 | EEG brain activity for the theta, alpha, and beta bands in the dynamic and static office during the Mackworth clock task.

electrodes C3 and C4, $p < 0.05$ each. The ANOVA for beta activity obtained during the Mackworth clock task showed highly significant main effects for the factors working environment, $F_{(1,19)} = 8.48, p = 0.01, \eta_p^2 = 0.27$, and time, $F_{(1,19)} = 8.25, p = 0.01, \eta_p^2 = 0.24$. The working environment × time interaction was significant, $F_{(5,95)} = 3.28, p = 0.03, \eta_p^2 = 0.17$.

The ANOVA for gamma power obtained during the d2-R test showed significant main effects for working environment, $F_{(1,19)} = 5.17, p = 0.02, \eta_p^2 = 0.10$, and time, $F_{(1,19)} = 5.03, p = 0.03, \eta_p^2 = 0.08$. The working environment × time interaction was significant, $F_{(4,19)} = 3.38$, $p = 0.03$, $\eta_p^2 = 0.10$. The ANOVA of gamma responses revealed a highly significant difference between locations, $F_{(20,95)} = 2.79, p = 0.008, \eta_p^2 = 0.28$. *Post hoc* comparisons showed that spontaneous EEG gamma power increased at frontal and central electrodes, compared to that of parietal, temporal, and occipital electrodes, $p < 0.05$ each. Subsequent analyses showed that gamma power increased most in the frontal region at the electrodes F3 and F4, $p < 0.05$, and in the central region at the electrodes C3 and C4, $p < 0.05$ each.

EEG Coherence

For the theta range, highly significant main effects were found in the Mackworth clock task for the electrode pairs F3/F4, $F_{(1,19)} = 10.71$, $p = 0.01$, and P3/P4, $F_{(1,19)} = 14.82$, $p = 0.008$, with a coherence increase in the dynamic office, when compared to the static office. Further, highly significant main effects were found for the factor time for the electrode pairs F3/F4, $F_{(1,19)} = 9.75$, $p = 0.01$, and P3/P4, $F_{(1,19)} = 10.48$, $p = 0.009$, with increases in theta coherence in the posttest, when compared to pretest. The working environment × time interactions were significant for F3/F4, $F_{(4,19)} = 3.27$, $p = 0.02$, and P3/P4, $F_{(4,19)} = 4.22, p = 0.02$.

Analysis on the alpha range showed significant main effects in the Mackworth clock task for the electrode pairs F3/F4, $F_{(1,19)} = 5.62$, $p = 0.03$, and P3/P4, $F_{(1,19)} = 6.81$, $p = 0.02$, with coherence increases in the dynamic office, when compared to the static office. Further, significant main effects were found for the factor time for the electrode pairs F3/F4, $F_{(1,19)} = 4.88$, $p = 0.04$, and P3/P4, $F_{(1,19)} = 5.74$, $p = 0.03$, with increases in alpha coherence in the posttest, when compared to pretest. The working environment × time interactions were significant for F3/F4, $F_{(4,19)} = 4.02, p = 0.02$, and P3/P4, $F_{(4,19)} = 5.82, p = 0.03$.

For the beta range, significant main effects were found in the Mackworth clock task for the electrode pairs F3/F4, $F_{(1,19)} = 8.02$, $p = 0.02$, and C3/C4, $F_{(1,19)} = 7.87$, $p = 0.02$, with a coherence increase in the dynamic office, when compared to the static office. Further, main effects were found for the factor time for the electrode pairs F3/F4, $F_{(1,19)} = 7.53, p = 0.02$, and C3/C4, $F_{(1,19)} = 7.96$, $p = 0.02$, with increases in beta coherence in the posttest, when compared to pretest. The working environment × time interactions were significant for F3/F4, $F_{(4,19)} = 3.90$, $p = 0.03$, and C3/C4, $F_{(1,19)} = 4.05$, $p = 0.02$. Further for the d2-R task, highly significant main effects were found for the electrode pairs F3/F4, $F_{(1,19)} = 10.57$, $p = 0.009$, and C3/C4, $F_{(1,19)} = 8.73$, $p = 0.01$, with a coherence increase in the dynamic office, when compared to the static office. Further, significant main effects were found for the factor time for the electrode pairs F3/F4, $F_{(1,19)} = 7.80$, $p = 0.02$, and C3/C4, $F_{(1,19)} = 6.33$, $p = 0.02$, with increases in beta coherence in the posttest, when compared to pretest. The working environment × time interactions were significant for F3/F4, $F_{(4,19)} = 3.98$, $p = 0.03$, and C3/C4, $F_{(4,19)} = 3.25, p = 0.03$.

Analysis on the gamma range showed highly significant main effects in the d2-R task for the electrode pairs F3/F4, $F_{(1,19)} = 10.23, p = 0.009$, and P3/P4, $F_{(1,19)} = 9.27, p = 0.01$, with coherence increases in the dynamic office, when compared to the static office. Further, a highly significant main effects was found for the factor time for the electrode pairs F3/F4, $F_{(1,19)} = 11.06$, $p = 0.008$, and P3/P4, $F_{(1,19)} = 8.97$, $p = 0.01$, with increases in gamma coherence in the posttest, when compared to pretest. The working environment × time interactions were significant for F3/F4, $F_{(4,19)} = 5.38$, $p = 0.01$, and P3/P4, $F_{(4,19)} = 3.86$, $p = 0.02$.

DISCUSSION

This is the first study that investigated the effects of a dynamic office environment on EEG brain oscillations and attentional as well as vigilance performance. Results clearly demonstrate distinguishable patterns of EEG brain oscillations when working in the dynamic compared to working in the static office. Attentional performance increased in the dynamic office compared to working in the static office after 120 min. Moreover, attentional and vigilance performance increased after the 2-week intervention in the dynamic office. Brain oscillatory patterns showed increased beta and gamma power in frontal (F4), and parietal (P3, Pz) areas in the attentional task in the dynamic office. Theta, alpha, and beta power increased in frontal (F3, Fz, F4), central (C3), and parietal (P3, Pz, P4) areas in the vigilance task when working in the dynamic office. Further, analyses revealed increased interhemispheric coherence for the electrode pairs F3/F4, C3/C4, and P3/P4 in the dynamic office. Effects on brain oscillatory patterns increased after the 2-week intervention in the dynamic office. We found increased EEG alpha, beta, and gamma power in the d2-R task as compared to pretest. Further, EEG theta, alpha, and beta power were higher in the vigilance task than at pretest. EEG data on coherence demonstrated increased interhemispheric coherence for the electrode pairs F3/F4, C3/C4, and P3/P4 at posttest.

Our results expand findings from previous neurophysiological investigations on the beneficial effects of dynamic sitting on cognitive functions and brain oscillations (Henz et al., 2015; Henz and Schöllhorn, 2016). In these studies, we showed increases in visuo-spatial and working memory task performance when sitting on a chair that allowed movements during working compared to working on a static chair. As a neural correlate for improved task performance, we found increases in alpha and beta power in brain areas that are related to visuo-spatial and working memory processes. We argued that these improvements are mediated by increased motor activity in the dynamic sitting condition.

The obtained patterns of EEG brain oscillations indicate different underlying neural processes during working in a dynamic office versus working in a static office environment. In the following sections, we discuss different lines of interpretations on the obtained patterns of brain oscillations.

Dynamic Office Environments Enhance Brain Oscillations Related to Attentional Processing

Brain oscillations before and after the 2-week intervention in the dynamic office showed increases in frontal (F3, F4), central (C3), and parietal (P3, P4) theta, alpha, and beta band activity during the vigilance task compared to pretest. Coherence analysis showed increased interhemispheric coherence for the derivations F3/F4, C3/C4, and P3/P4. We argue that the observed brain oscillatory patterns are a correlate for modulations of attentional processes during working in the dynamic office. Previous studies have demonstrated that frontal cortexes are related to executive functions, voluntary control, and action creation (Jung et al., 2000; Cardoso de Oliveira, 2002). Theta activity was shown to be related to these behaviors that demand action planning based on received sensory information (Liepert et al., 1998; Caplan et al., 2003). These studies show a relation between theta band coherence with attention and movement preparation.

Results on increased EEG theta power during the Mackworth clock task are in line with findings of a study by Pennekamp et al. (1994). They showed increases in performance in the Mackworth clock task that were accompanied by increases in theta activity. Several studies have shown that the allocation of attentional resources is accompanied by distinct brain activation patterns. Enhanced theta activity in frontal brain areas is currently discussed as a neural substrate for improvements of cognitive control (Chung et al., 2017). More specifically, theta oscillations in frontal brain areas are observed in the early allocation of selective attention resources on external visual stimuli. This frontal theta activity appears to improve cognitive control during visuo-motor tasks (Berchicci et al., 2015). Increases in theta activity are shown in goal-directed attention (Dowdall et al., 2012). Stimulus-induced changes in the theta, alpha, and beta bands have been shown to be a correlate for modulation of goal-directed spatial attention (Harris et al., 2017). More specifically, EEG oscillations occurred either in the theta, alpha, and beta range in the involuntary capture of goal-directed visual attention. The authors found a lateralization in the theta band related to the processing of goal-relevant and goal-irrelevant stimuli. Lateralization in the alpha band was shown for goal-directed attention. Further, beta oscillations were not location-specific. Several studies have shown that alpha activity in parietal regions is involved in the processing of visual stimuli (Jensen et al., 2012; Roux and Uhlhaas, 2014; Foster et al., 2016). Further, there is evidence for a relation between alpha oscillations and voluntary attentional allocation (Worden et al., 2000; Kelly et al., 2006; Thut et al., 2006; Foxe and Snyder, 2011).

Relations Between Increased Motor Activity and Attention

Attentional and vigilance performance increased in the dynamic compared to the static office. Analysis on the corresponding power spectra and coherence analysis revealed increased activity in the frontal areas that are related to executive functions, voluntary control, and action planning (Szurhaj et al., 2003; Moriguchi and Hiraki, 2013). Further, brain areas related to motor act execution showed increased oscillatory activity. Increased coherence in C3/C4 is associated with motor act execution (Papenberg et al., 2013), motor act organization (Minc et al., 2010), and sequential movement coordination (Coull et al., 1998). Such findings show that motor activity and executive processes are closely related.

Current research shows close interrelations between attentional processing and posture control. Recent studies using a dual-task paradigm indicate that sensorimotor processing is essential to postural control, and requires attentional resources (Boisgontier et al., 2013). Several investigations reveal that even highly practiced postural tasks require cognitive processing at least to a small degree. For instance, Tsang et al. (2016) have shown that the simultaneous performance of a cognitive task during quiet stance resulted in an increase in postural sway. Beta activity has been shown in attention and long-distance synchronization in parts of the cortex. For instance, synchronization of beta activity was demonstrated in the dorsal prefrontal cortex and posterior parietal cortex during a top-down search of a visual stimulus (Buschman and Miller, 2007; Buschman et al., 2012; Verhoef et al., 2011). Beta activation in motor areas is a neural substrate for attention to upcoming motor tasks. Brain activation patterns in the beta range are not limited to the activity of the motor cortex and EMG, but play also an important role in somatosensory and parietal areas (Witham and Baker, 2007; Tsujimoto et al., 2009). Further, coherence between the motor and afferent sensory areas is shown to operate at the beta frequency (Baker, 2007). Saleh et al. (2010) demonstrated a close link between beta activity in the motor cortex and attention. Further, beta activity indicates selectively coordinated cell-assemblies that are task-relevant (Kopell et al., 2000). EEG beta activity also plays an important role in attentional processing (Wróbel et al., 2007; Sauseng and Klimesch, 2008). Recent studies suggest that EEG beta activity is necessary to enhance feedback loops at subsequent stages of visual information processing (i.e., Gola et al., 2013). Beta activity and connectivity in the sensorimotor and parietal cortex are essential for accurate motor performance (Chung et al., 2017).

A further line of argumentation considers the role of alpha and beta activation in self-initiated movements. Wang et al. (2017) found increases in alpha activity in the SMA in self-initiated movements. Further, they demonstrated increases in sensorimotor areas in the alpha and beta bands in self-initiated and visually guided movements.

Finally, we found increases in gamma power during the attentional task when working in the dynamic office. We interpret these results in terms of an enhancing effect of motor activity on attentional processing. Increases in gamma oscillations are found in selective attentional processing (Engel and Singer, 2001; Varela et al., 2001). From this, we argue that performing attentional tasks in a dynamic office environment stimulates executive cognitive controlled processing. This interpretation is in line with studies that showed enhancement of executive functions by gross motor movements (i.e., Benzinger et al., 2018). Further, evidence shows that gamma band activity of frontal and central areas is associated with memory encoding (Sederberg et al., 2003), motor memory tasks (Gentili et al., 2015), and encoding of motor memory in dynamic motor adaptation tasks (Thürer et al., 2016).

In summary, several studies have shown that theta, alpha, and beta frequencies play dissociable roles in visual attention. Increases in gamma power were found as a correlate for selective attention. From this, we interpret the increases in the theta, alpha, and beta oscillations in the vigilance task, and the increases in the alpha, beta, and gamma bands in the attentional task as indicators for modulations of visual attention that result from increased motor activity when working in a dynamic office that fosters physical activity.

Working in a Dynamic Environment Reinforces Visuo-Spatial Working Memory Processes and Multisensory Integration

Increases in theta band oscillations have also been discussed as an indicator for visuo-spatial working memory processes (Bastiaansen et al., 2002). Further, resource allocation is one of the cognitive processes that are located within working memory models. Increases in theta power in somatosensory and motor brain areas during working in the dynamic office might be a correlate for working memory processes (Carretié, 2001; Mitchell et al., 2008; Myers et al., 2014; Tóth et al., 2014), and a neurophysiological substrate for encoding of new information (Klimesch et al., 1996, 1997; Klimesch, 1999; Bastiaansen et al., 2002). In previous studies, we found enhancement of visuo-spatial abilities in geometrical and algebraic tasks during sitting on a chair that allowed vertical and horizontal movements during sitting. Enhanced performance was accompanied by increases in frontal theta activity (Henz, 2014; Henz et al., 2015). We argued that better performance in geometrical and algebraic tasks resulted from stimulation of the visuo-spatial working memory system by bodily movements.

A further line of interpretation is that increases in theta and alpha coherence reflect processes of multisensory integration in the brain that afford working memory processes (see Kanayama et al., 2015). For instance, Hummel and Gerloff (2005) demonstrated increases in alpha coherence during a cross-modal matching task. The authors argue that the EEG alpha coherence is a correlate for synchronization processes of brain areas that are related to cross-modal integration. Classen et al. (1998) showed increased EEG coherence between visual and somatosensory brain areas as well as between visual and motor areas during a visuo-motor tracking task. Further studies have shown increased theta coherence in the derivations P3/Pz, and P3/P4 which are involved in sensorimotor integration (Smith et al., 1999; Neuper and Pfurtscheller, 2001; Huber et al., 2006). Several studies show that processing of whole-body movements is accompanied by modulations in alpha band activity. Gutteling and Medendorp (2016) demonstrated that the processing of bodily motion is mirrored by a modulation in central and parietal areas, whereas visual target coding was shown in power modulation in parieto-occipital areas. Summarizing, the parietal cortex is involved in both the processing of bodily motion, and spatial processing, consistent with its role as a brain region that integrates information from visual, motor and vestibular signals (Zhang and Britten, 2011; Gale et al., 2015; Gutteling et al., 2015).

Increased Fluctuations Stimulate Brain Functions and Attentional Performance

A different theoretical perspective on the effects of increased motor activity on brain oscillatory patterns and attentional performance could be applied considering theoretical assumptions of the system dynamic theory (Haken, 1970; Glansdorff and Prigogine, 1971; Haken et al., 1985). Bodily movements that change continuously during task performance and problem solving might lead to increased fluctuations and deviations during task solving. Several scientific approaches refer to the term *deviation* from a predefined ideal state. From this perspective, the term deviation has a rather negative connotation. In contrast, the system dynamic approach considers deviations rather as constructive fluctuations. They are defined as a more neutral term that is derived from stochastic physics. According to the system dynamic approach, systems that are characterized to have energetic or material exchange with an environment show continuous fluctuations. Another hypothesis derived from the system dynamic approach is that an increase of fluctuations that causes a period of instability is necessary to stimulate transitions from one stable state to another state in these systems. During phase transitions, these systems explore a variety of modes in order to find new and even more effective states. These phenomena have been investigated extensively in different areas of sports and everyday movements (Kelso, 1995; Davids et al., 2006). Recent neurophysiological studies have shown that increased fluctuations in the human body induced by differential movement training increased learning rates that were accompanied by brain oscillations in the theta and alpha range (Henz and Schöllhorn, 2016; Henz et al., 2018). Instead of considering increases in fluctuations as a passive ontological phenomenon of dissipative systems, the differential training approach takes advantage of increased system fluctuations as an active instrument in order to lead the system towards a zone of instability where less energy is needed for achieving a self-organized new state (Schöllhorn, 1999, 2000; Schöllhorn et al., 2006, 2009, 2010, 2012). One implication of these previous findings is that increased fluctuations in the human body induced by randomly performed movements enhance a state of brain oscillatory activity that is characterized by increased theta and alpha power which reinforces creative solutions in sports (Santos et al., 2018) as well as during problem solving (Fink et al., 2007, 2009) in working and school settings.

CONCLUSION

The results of the present study reveal short- and mid-term effects on attentional and vigilance performance, and EEG brain activity when working in a dynamic versus a static environment. During working in a dynamic office, attentional and vigilance performance increased compared to working in a static office. Brain activities show increased alpha, beta and gamma power in the frontal and central areas in the attentional task with increased theta, alpha, and beta activity in the vigilance task. These findings suggest that working in a dynamic office environment stimulates the brain towards an optimum psychophysiological level of activation and wakefulness for attentional and vigilance performance. The results of the present study are of relevance in the field of neuroergonomics, for the design of office and school working environments and encourage the use of dynamic office desk furniture that allows movements during working to achieve increased attentional as well as vigilance performance.

AUTHOR CONTRIBUTIONS

All listed authors made substantial and intellectual contributions to the manuscript.

REFERENCES

Ayaz, H., and Dehais, F. (2019). *Neuroergonomics: The Brain at Work and Everyday Life*. 1st Edn. Elsevier: Academic Press. Available online at: https://www.sciencedirect.com/book/9780128119266/neuroergonomics. [Accessed on March 19, 2019].

Baker, S. N. (2007). Oscillatory interactions between sensorimotor cortex and the periphery. *Curr. Opin. Neurobiol.* 17, 649–655. doi: 10.1016/j.conb.2008.01.007

Bastiaansen, M. C., Posthuma, D., Groot, P. F., and de Geus, E. J. (2002). Event-related α and theta responses in a visuo-spatial working memory task. *Clin. Neurophysiol.* 113, 1882–1893. doi: 10.1016/s1388-2457(02)00303-6

Berchicci, M., Pontifex, M. B., Drollette, E. S., Pesce, C., Hillman, C. H., and Di Russo, F. (2015). From cognitive motor preparation to visual processing: the benefits of childhood fitness to brain health. *Neuroscience* 298, 211–219. doi: 10.1016/j.neuroscience.2015.04.028

Brickenkamp, R., Schmidt-Atzert, L., and Liepmann, D. (2010). *d2-R. Test d2-Revision. Aufmerksamkeits- und Konzentrationstest*. Göttingen: Hogrefe.

Benzinger, V., Chang, Y. K., and Schmidt, M. (2018). Acute physical activity enhances executive functions in children with ADHD. *Sci. Rep.* 8:12382. doi: 10.1038/s41598-018-30067-8

Boisgontier, M. P., Beets, I. A. M., Duysens, J., Nieuwboer, A., Krampe, R. T., and Swinnen, S. P. (2013). Age-related differences in attentional cost associated with postural dual tasks increased recruitment of generic cognitive resources in older adults. *Neurosci. Biobehav. Rev.* 37, 1824–1837. doi: 10.1016/j.neubiorev.2013.07.014

Brümmer, V., Schneider, S., Abel, T., Vogt, T., and Strüder, H. (2011). Brain cortical activity is influenced by exercise mode and intensity. *Med. Sci. Sports Exerc.* 43, 1863–1872. doi: 10.1249/mss.0b013e3182172a6f

Brunoni, A. R., Lopes, M., and Fregni, F. (2008). A systematic review and metaanalysis of clinical studies on major depression and BDNF levels: implications for the role of neuroplasticity in depression. *Int. J. Neuropsychopharmacol.* 11, 1169–1180. doi: 10.1017/s1461145708009309

Buschman, T. J., Denovellis, E. L., Diogo, C., Bullock, D., and Miller, E. K. (2012). Synchronous oscillatory neural ensembles for rules in the prefrontal cortex. *Neuron* 76, 838–846. doi: 10.1016/j.neuron.2012.09.029

Buschman, T. J., and Miller, E. K. (2007). Top-down versus bottom-up control of attention in the prefrontal and posterior parietal cortices. *Science* 315, 1860–1862. doi: 10.1126/science.1138071

Caplan, J. B., Madsen, J. R., Schulze-Bonhage, A., Aschenbrenner-Scheibe, R., Newman, E. L., and Kahana, M. J. (2003). Human θ oscillations related to sensorimotor integration and spatial learning. *J. Neurosci.* 23, 4726–4736. doi: 10.1523/JNEUROSCI.23-11-04726.2003

Cardoso de Oliveira, S. (2002). The neuronal basis of bimanual coordination: recent neurophysiological evidence and functional models. *Acta Psychol.* 110, 139–159. doi: 10.1016/s0001-6918(02)00031-8

Carretié, L. A. (2001). *Psicofisiología*. Madrid: Ediciones Pirámide.

Chang, Y. K., Labban, J. D., Gapin, J. I., and Etnier, J. L. (2012). The effects of acute exercise on cognitive performance. *Brain Res.* 1453, 87–101. doi: 10.1016/j.brainres.2012.02.068

Chieffi, S., Messina, G., Villano, I., Messina, A., Valenzano, A., Moscatelli, F., et al. (2017). Neuroprotective effects of physical activity: evidence from human and animal studies. *Front. Neurol.* 8:188. doi: 10.3389/fneur.2017.00188

Chung, J. W., Ofori, E., Misra, G., Hess, C. W., and Vaillancourt, D. E. (2017). β-band activity and connectivity in sensorimotor and parietal cortex are important for accurate motor performance. *Neuroimage* 144, 164–173. doi: 10.1016/j.neuroimage.2016.10.008

Classen, J., Liepert, J., Wise, S. P., Hallett, M., and Cohen, L. G. (1998). Rapid plasticity of human cortical movement representation induced by practice. *J. Neurophysiol.* 79, 1117–1123. doi: 10.1152/jn.1998.79.2.1117

Colberg, S. R., Somma, C. T., and Sechrist, S. R. (2008). Physical activity participation may offset some of the negative impact of diabetes on cognitive function. *J. Am. Med. Dir. Assoc.* 9, 434–438. doi: 10.1016/j.jamda.2008.03.014

Colcombe, S. J., Erickson, K. I., Scalf, P. E., Kim, J. S., Prakash, R., McAuley, E., et al. (2006). Aerobic exercise training increases brain volume in aging humans. *J. Gerontol. A Biol. Sci. Med. Sci.* 61, 1166–1170. doi: 10.1093/gerona/61.11.1166

Colcombe, S., and Kramer, A. F. (2003). Fitness effects on the cognitive function of older adults. *Psychol. Sci.* 14, 125–130. doi: 10.1111/1467-9280.t01-1-01430

Coull, J. T., Frackowiak, R. S., and Frith, C. D. (1998). Monitoring for target objects: activation of right frontal and parietal cortices with increasing time on task. *Neuropsychologia* 36, 1325–1334. doi: 10.1016/s0028-3932(98)00035-9

Davids, K., Button, C., Araújo, D., Renshaw, I., and Hristovski, R. (2006). Movement models from sports provide representative task constraints for studying adaptive behavior in human motor systems. *Adapt. Behav.* 14, 73–95. doi: 10.1177/105971230601400103

Deeny, S. P., Poeppel, D., Zimmerman, J. B., Roth, S. M., Brandauer, J., Witkowski, S., et al. (2008). Exercise, APOE, and working memory: MEG and behavioral evidence for benefit of exercise in epsilon4 carriers. *Biol. Psychol.* 78, 179–187. doi: 10.1016/j.biopsycho.2008.02.007

Dowdall, J. R., Luczak, A., and Tata, M. S. (2012). Temporal variability of the N2pc during efficient and inefficient visual search. *Neuropsychologia* 50, 2442–2453. doi: 10.1016/j.neuropsychologia.2012.06.015

Engel, A. K., and Singer, W. (2001). Temporal binding and the neural correlates of sensory awareness. *Trends Cogn. Sci.* 5, 16–25. doi: 10.1016/s1364-6613(00)01568-0

Etnier, J. L., Salazar, W., Landers, D. M., Petruzzello, S. J., Han, M., and Nowell, P. (2004). The influence of physical fitness and exercise upon cognitive functioning: a meta-analysis. *J. Sport Exerc. Psychol.* 19, 249–277. doi: 10.1123/jsep.19.3.249

Fink, A., Benedek, M., Grabner, R. H., Staudt, B., and Neubauer, A. C. (2007). Creativity meets neuroscience: experimental tasks for the neuroscientific study of creative thinking. *Methods* 42, 68–76. doi: 10.1016/j.ymeth.2006.12.001

Fink, A., Grabner, R. H., Benedek, M., Reishofer, G., Hauswirth, V., Fally, M., et al. (2009). The creative brain: investigation of brain activity during creative problem solving by means of EEG and fMRI. *Hum. Brain Mapp.* 30, 734–748. doi: 10.1002/hbm.20538

Foster, J. J., Sutterer, D. W., Serences, J. T., Vogel, E. K., and Awh, E. (2016). The topography of alpha-band activity tracks the content of spatial working memory. *J. Neurophysiol.* 115, 168–177. doi: 10.1152/jn.00860.2015

Foxe, J. J., and Snyder, A. C. (2011). The role of alpha-band brain oscillations as a sensory suppression mechanism during selective attention. *Front. Psychol.* 2:154. doi: 10.3389/fpsyg.2011.00154

Gale, S., Prsa, M., Schurger, A., Gay, A., Paillard, A., Herbelin, B., et al. (2015). Oscillatory neural responses evoked by natural vestibular stimuli in humans. *J. Neurophysiol.* 115, 1228–1242. doi: 10.1152/jn.00153.2015

Gentili, R. J., Bradberry, T. J., Oh, H., Costanzo, M. E., Kerick, S. E., Contreras-Vidal, J. L., et al. (2015). Evolution of cerebral cortico-cortical communication during visuomotor adaptation to a cognitive-motor executive challenge. *Biol. Psychol.* 105, 51–65. doi: 10.1016/j.biopsycho.2014.12.003

Gheysen, F., Poppe, L., DeSmet, A., Swinnen, S., Cardon, G., De Bourdeaudhuij, I., et al. (2018). Physical activity to improve cognition in older adults: can physical activity programs enriched with cognitive challenges enhance the effects? A systematic review and meta-analysis. *Int. J. Behav. Nutr. Phys. Act.* 15:63. doi: 10.1186/s12966-018-0697-x

Glansdorff, P., and Prigogine, I. (1971). *Thermodynamics Theory of Structure, Stability and Fluctuations.* London: Wiley-Interscience.

Gola, M., Magnuski, M., Szumska, I., and Wróbel, A. (2013). EEG beta band activity is related to attention and attentional deficits in the visual performance of elderly subjects. *Int. J. Psychophysiol.* 89, 334–341. doi: 10.1016/j.ijpsycho.2013.05.007

Gramann, K., Fairclough, S. H., Zander, T. O., and Ayaz, H. (2017). Trends in neuroergonomics: a comprehensive overview. *Front. Hum. Neurosci.* 11:165. doi: 10.3389/fnhum.2017.00165

Grego, F., Vallier, J. M., Collardeaul, M., Rousseu, C., Cremieux, J., and Brisswalter, J. (2005). Influence of exercise duration andhydration status on cognitive function during prolonged cyclingexercise. *Int. J. Sports Med.* 26, 27–33. doi: 10.1055/s-2004-817915

Gutteling, T. P., and Medendorp, W. P. (2016). Role of alpha-band oscillations in spatial updating across whole body motion. *Front. Psychol.* 7:671. doi: 10.3389/fpsyg.2016.00671

Gutteling, T. P., Selen, L. P. J., and Medendorp, W. P. (2015). Parallax-sensitive remapping of visual space in occipito-parietal alpha-band activity during whole-body motion. *J. Neurophysiol.* 113, 1574–1584. doi: 10.1152/jn.00477.2014

Haken, H. (1970). "Laser theory," in *Light and Matter Ic/Licht und Materie Ic*, ed. L. Genzel (Berlin: Springer), 1–304. Available online at: https://link.springer.com/chapter/10.1007/978-3-662-22091-7_1. [Accessed on March 19, 2019].

Haken, H., Kelso, J. A. S., and Bunz, H. (1985). A theoretical model of phase transitions in human hand movements. *Biol. Cybern.* 51, 347–356. doi: 10.1007/bf00336922

Harris, A. M., Dux, P. E., Jones, C. N., and Mattingley, J. B. (2017). Distinct roles of theta and alpha oscillations in the involuntary capture of goal-directed attention. *Neuroimage* 152, 171–183. doi: 10.1016/j.neuroimage.2017.03.008

Henz, D. (2014). EEG brain activity in algebraic, geometric, and numerical reasoning tasks under static and dynamic postural control. *Psychophysiology* 55:58.

Henz, D., John, A., Merz, C., and Schöllhorn, W. I. (2018). Post-task EEG brain activations differ for various contextual interference and differential training protocols. *Front. Hum. Neurosci.* 12:19. doi: 10.3389/fnhum.2018.00019

Henz, D., Oldenburg, R., and Schöllhorn, W. I. (2015). "Does bodily movement enhance mathematical performance? Behavioral and neurophysiological evidence," in *Proceedings of the 9th Conference on Research in Mathematics Education* (Chicago, IL: ACM), 1–10.

Henz, D., and Schöllhorn, W. I. (2016). Differential training facilitates early consolidation in motor learning. *Front. Behav. Neurosci.* 10:199. doi: 10.3389/fnbeh.2016.00199

Huber, R., Ghilardi, M. F., Massimini, M., Ferrarelli, F., Riedner, B. A., Peterson, M. J., et al. (2006). Arm immobilization causes cortical plastic changes and locally decreases sleep slow wave activity. *Nat. Neurosci.* 9, 1169–1176. doi: 10.1038/nn1758

Hummel, F., and Gerloff, C. (2005). Larger interregional synchrony is associated with greater behavioral success in a complex sensory integration task in humans. *Cereb. Cortex* 15, 670–678. doi: 10.1093/cercor/bhh170

Jensen, O., Bonnefond, M., and VanRullen, R. (2012). An oscillatory mechanism for prioritizing salient unattended stimuli. *Trends Cogn. Sci.* 16, 200–206. doi: 10.1016/j.tics.2012.03.002

Jung, T. P., Makeig, S., Westerfield, M., Townsend, J., Courchesne, E., and Sejnowski, T. J. (2000). Removal of eye activity artifacts from visual event-related potentials in normal and clinical subjects. *Clin. Neurophysiol.* 111, 1745–1758. doi: 10.1016/s1388-2457(00)00386-2

Kanayama, N., Kimura, K., and Hiraki, K. (2015). Cortical EEG components that reflect inverse effectiveness during visuo tactile integration processing. *Brain Res.* 1598, 18–30. doi: 10.1016/j.brainres.2014.12.017

Kelly, S. P., Lalor, E. C., Reilly, R. B., and Foxe, J. J. (2006). Increases in alpha oscillatory power reflect an active retinotopic mechanism for distracter suppression during sustained visuospatial attention. *J. Neurophysiol.* 95, 3844–3851. doi: 10.1152/jn.01234.2005

Kelso, J. A. S. (1995). *Dynamic Patterns: The Self-Organization of Brain and Behavior.* Cambridge, MA: MIT Press.

Khanna, P., and Carmena, J. M. (2015). Neural networks: β band activity across motor networks. *Curr. Opin. Neurobiol.* 32, 60–67. doi: 10.1016/j.conb.2014.11.010

Klimesch, W. (1999). EEG α and theta oscillations reflect cognitive and memory performance: a review and analysis. *Brain Res. Rev.* 29, 169–195. doi: 10.1016/s0165-0173(98)00056-3

Klimesch, W., Doppelmayr, M., Russegger, H., and Pachinger, T. (1996). Theta band power in the human scalp EEG and the encoding of new information. *Neuroreport* 7, 1235–1240. doi: 10.1097/00001756-199605170-00002

Klimesch, W., Doppelmayr, M., Schimke, H., and Ripper, B. (1997). Theta synchronization and α desynchronization in a memory task. *Psychophysiology* 34, 169–176. doi: 10.1111/j.1469-8986.1997.tb02128.x

Kopell, N., Ermentrout, G. B., Whittington, M. A., and Traub, R. D. (2000). Gamma rhythms and beta rhythms have different synchronization properties. *Proc. Natl. Acad. Sci. U S A* 97, 1867–1872. doi: 10.1073/pnas.97.4.1867

Kramer, A. F., Hahn, S., Cohen, N. J., Banich, M. T., McAuley, E., Harrison, C. R., et al. (1999). Ageing, fitness and neurocognitive function. *Nature* 400, 418–419. doi: 10.1038/22682

Lees, M. N., Cosman, J. D., Lee, J. D., Fricke, N., and Rizzo, M. (2010). Translating cognitive neuroscience to the driver's operational environment: a neuroergonomic approach. *Am. J. Psychol.* 123, 391–411. doi: 10.5406/amerjpsyc.124.4.0391

Liepert, J., Miltner, W. H., Bauder, H., Sommer, M., Dettmers, C., Taub, E., et al. (1998). Motor cortex plasticity during constraint-induced movement therapy in stroke patients. *Neurosci. Lett.* 250, 5–8. doi: 10.1016/s0304-3940(98)00386-3

Mandolesi, L., Polverino, A., Montuori, S., Foti, F., Ferraioli, G., Sorrentino, P., et al. (2018). Effects of physical exercise on cognitive functioning and wellbeing: biological and psychological benefits. *Front. Psychol.* 9:509. doi: 10.3389/fpsyg.2018.00509

Minc, D., Machado, S., Bastos, V. H., Machado, D., Cunha, M., Cagy, M., et al. (2010). γ band oscillations under influence of bromazepam during a sensorimotor integration task: an EEG coherence study. *Neurosci. Lett.* 469, 145–149. doi: 10.1016/j.neulet.2009.11.062

Mitchell, D. J., McNaughton, N., Flanagan, D., and Kirk, I. J. (2008). Frontal-midline theta from the perspective of hippocampal "theta". *Prog. Neurobiol.* 86, 156–185. doi: 10.1016/j.pneurobio.2008.09.005

Moraes, H., Deslandes, A., Silveira, H., Ribeiro, P., Cagy, M., Piedade, R., et al. (2011). The effect of acute effort on EEG in healthy young and elderly subjects. *Eur. J. Appl. Physiol.* 111, 67–75. doi: 10.1007/s00421-010-1627-z

Moraes, H., Ferreira, C., Deslandes, A., Cagy, M., Pompeu, F., Ribeiro, P., et al. (2007). β and α electroencephalographic activity changes after acute exercise. *Arq. Neuropsiquiatr.* 65, 637–641. doi: 10.1590/s0004-282x20070004 00018

Moriguchi, Y., and Hiraki, K. (2013). Prefrontal cortex and executive function in young children: a review of NIRS studies. *Front. Hum. Neurosci.* 7:867. doi: 10.3389/fnhum.2013.00867

Myers, N. E., Stokes, M. G., Walther, L., and Nobre, A. C. (2014). Oscillatory brain state predicts variability in working memory. *J. Neurosci.* 34, 7735–7743. doi: 10.1523/JNEUROSCI.4741-13.2014

Neuper, C., and Pfurtscheller, G. (2001). Event-related dynamics of cortical rhythms: frequency-specific features and functional correlates. *Int. J. Psychophysiol.* 43, 41–58. doi: 10.1016/s0167-8760(01)00178-7

Oldfield, R. C. (1971). The assessment and analysis of handedness: the Edinburgh inventory. *Neuropsychologia* 9, 97–113. doi: 10.1016/0028-3932(71)90067-4

Papenberg, G., Hämmerer, D., Müller, V., Lindenberger, U., and Li, S. C. (2013). Lower theta inter-trial phase coherence during performance monitoring is related to higher reaction time variability: a lifespan study. *Neuroimage* 83, 912–920. doi: 10.1016/j.neuroimage.2013.07.032

Parasuraman, R., and Rizzo, M. (2007). *Neuroergonomics. The Brain at Work.* New York, NY: Oxford University Press.

Parasuraman, R., and Wilson, G. F. (2008). Putting the brain to work: neuroergonomics past, present, and future. *Hum. Fact.* 50, 468–474. doi: 10.1518/001872008x288349

Pennekamp, P., Bosel, R., Mecklinger, A., and Ott, H. (1994). Differences in EEG-theta for responded and omitted targets in a sustained attention task. *J. Psychophysiol.* 8, 131–141.

Pereira, T., Cipriano, I., Costa, T., Saraiva, M., and Martins, A. (2019). Exercise, ageing and cognitive function—effects of a personalized physical exercise program in the cognitive function of older adults. *Physiol. Behav.* 202, 8–13. doi: 10.1016/j.physbeh.2019.01.018

Roux, F., and Uhlhaas, P. J. (2014). Working memory and neural oscillations: alpha-gamma versus theta-gamma codes for distinct WM information? *Trends Cogn. Sci.* 18, 16–25. doi: 10.1016/j.tics.2013.10.010

Saleh, M., Reimer, J., Penn, R., Ojakangas, C. L., and Hatsopoulos, N. G. (2010). Fast and slow oscillations in human primary motor cortex predict oncoming behaviorally relevant cues. *Neuron* 65, 461–471. doi: 10.1016/j.neuron.2010.02.001

Santos, S., Coutinho, D., Gonçalves, B., Schöllhorn, W., Sampaio, J., and Leite, N. (2018). Differential learning as a key training approach to improve creative and tactical behavior in soccer. *Res. Q. Exerc. Sport* 89, 11–24. doi: 10.1080/02701367.2017.1412063

Sauseng, P., and Klimesch, W. (2008). What does phase information of oscillatory brain activity tell us about cognitive processes? *Neurosci. Biobehav. Rev.* 32, 1001–1013. doi: 10.1016/j.neubiorev.2008.03.014

Schöllhorn, W. I. (1999). Individualität—ein vernachlässigter Parameter? *Leistungssport* 29, 7–11. [Individuality—a neglected parameter? *Comp. Sports* 29, 7–11.

Schöllhorn, W. I. (2000). Applications of systems dynamic principles to technique and strength training. *Acta Acad. Olympiquae Estoniae* 8, 67–85.

Schöllhorn, W. I., Beckmann, H., Janssen, D., and Drepper, J. (2010). "Stochastic perturbations in athletics field events enhance skill acquisition," in *Motor Learning in Practice. A Constraints-Led Approach*, eds I. Renshaw, K. Davids and G. J. P. Savelsbergh (London: Routledge), 69–82.

Schöllhorn, W. I., Hegen, P., and Davids, K. (2012). The nonlinear nature of learning—a differential learning approach. *Open Sports Sci. J.* 5, 100–112. doi: 10.2174/1875399x01205010100

Schöllhorn, W. I., Michelbrink, M., Beckmann, H., Trockel, M., Sechelmann, M., and Davids, K. (2006). Does noise provide a basis for the unification of motor learning theories? *Int. J. Sports Psychol.* 37, 34–42.

Schöllhorn, W. I., Michelbrink, M., Welminski, D., and Davids, D. (2009). "Increasing stochastic perturbations enhance skill acquisition and learning of complex sport movements," in *Perspectives on Cognition and Action in Sport*, eds D. Araujo, H. Ripolland and M. Raab (Hauppauge, NY: Nova Science), 59–73.

Sederberg, P. B., Kahana, M. J., Howard, M. W., Donner, E. J., and Madsen, J. R. (2003). Theta and gamma oscillations during encoding predict subsequent recall. *J. Neurosci.* 23, 10809–10814. doi: 10.1523/JNEUROSCI.23-34-10809.2003

Sibley, B. A., and Etnier, J. L. (2003). The relationship between physical activity and cognition in children: a meta-analysis. *Pediatr. Exerc. Sci.* 15, 243–256. doi: 10.1123/pes.15.3.243

Smith, M. E., McEvoy, L. K., and Gevins, A. (1999). Neurophysiological indices of strategy development and skill acquisition. *Cogn. Brain Res.* 7, 389–404. doi: 10.1016/s0926-6410(98)00043-3

Szurhaj, W., Derambure, P., Labyt, E., Cassim, F., Bourriez, J. L., Isnard, J., et al. (2003). Basic mechanisms of central rhythms reactivity to preparation and execution of a voluntary movement: a stereoelectroencephalographic study. *Clin. Neurophysiol.* 114, 107–119. doi: 10.1016/s1388-2457(02)00333-4

Thürer, B., Stockinger, C., Focke, A., Putze, F., Schultz, T., and Stein, T. (2016). Increased gamma band power during movement planning coincides with motor memory retrieval. *Neuroimage* 125, 172–181. doi: 10.1016/j.neuroimage.2015.10.008

Thut, G., Nietzel, A., Brandt, S. A., and Pascual-Leone, A. (2006). Alpha-band electroencephalographic activity over occipital cortex indexes visuospatial attention bias and predicts visual target detection. *J. Neurosci.* 26, 9494–9502. doi: 10.1523/JNEUROSCI.0875-06.2006

Tóth, B., Kardos, Z., File, B., Boha, R., Stam, C. J., and Molnár, M. (2014). Frontal midline theta connectivity is related to efficiency of WM maintenance and is affected by aging. *Neurobiol. Learn. Mem.* 114, 58–69. doi: 10.1016/j.nlm.2014.04.009

Toni, I., Shah, N. J., Fink, G. R., Thoenissen, D., Passingham, R. E., and Zilles, K. (2002). Multiple movement representations in the human brain: an event-related fMRI study. *J. Cogn. Neurosci.* 14, 769–784. doi: 10.1162/08989290260138663

Tsang, W.-W., Chan, V. W.-L., Wong, H. H., Yip, T. W.-C., and Lu, X. (2016). The effect of performing a dual-task on postural control and selective attention of older adults when stepping backward. *J. Phys. Ther. Sci.* 28, 2806–2811. doi: 10.1589/jpts.28.2806

Tsujimoto, S., Genovesio, A., and Wise, S. P. (2009). Monkey orbitofrontal cortex encodes response choices near feedback time. *J. Neurosci.* 29, 2569–2574. doi: 10.1523/JNEUROSCI.5777-08.2009

Varela, F., Lachaux, E., Rodriguez, E., and Martinerie, J. (2001). The brainweb: phase synchronization and large-scale integration. *Nat. Rev. Neurosci.* 2, 229–239. doi: 10.1038/35067550

Verhoef, B. E., Vogels, R., and Janssen, P. (2011). Synchronization between the end stages of the dorsal and the ventral visual stream. *J. Neurophysiol.* 105, 2030–2042. doi: 10.1152/jn.00924.2010

Wang, B. A., Viswanathan, S., Abdollahi, R. O., Rosjat, N., Popovych, S., Daun, S., et al. (2017). Frequency-specific modulation of connectivity in the ipsilateral sensorimotor cortex by different forms of movement initiation. *Neuroimage* 117, 248–260. doi: 10.1016/j.neuroimage.2017.07.054

Weinberg, R. S., and Gould, D. (2015). *Foundations of Sport and Exercise Psychology.* 6th Edn. Champaign, IL: Human Kinetics.

Winter, B., Breitenstein, C., Mooren, F. C., Voelker, K., Fobker, M., Lechtermann, A., et al. (2007). High impact running improves learning. *Neurobiol. Learn. Mem.* 87, 597–609. doi: 10.1016/j.nlm.2006.11.003

Witham, C. L., and Baker, S. N. (2007). Network oscillations and intrinsic spiking rhythmicity do not covary in monkey sensorimotor areas. *J. Physiol.* 580, 801–814. doi: 10.1113/jphysiol.2006.124503

Worden, M. S., Foxe, J. J., Wang, N., and Simpson, G. V. (2000). Anticipatory biasing of visuospatial attention indexed by retinotopically specific α-band electroencephalogray increases over occipital cortex. *J. Neurosci.* 20, 1–6. doi: 10.1523/JNEUROSCI.20-06-j0002.2000

Wróbel, A., Ghazaryan, A., Bekisz, M., Bogdan, W., and Kamiński, J. (2007). Two streams of attention-dependent β activity in the striate recipient zone of cat's lateral posterior- pulvinar complex. *J. Neurosci.* 27, 2230–2240. doi: 10.1523/JNEUROSCI.4004-06.2007

Zhang, T., and Britten, K. H. (2011). Parietal area VIP causally influences heading perception during pursuit eye movements. *J. Neurosci.* 31, 2569–2575. doi: 10.1523/JNEUROSCI.5520-10.2011

17

Functional Connectivity During Handgrip Motor Fatigue in Older Adults is Obesity and Sex-Specific

Joohyun Rhee[1] *and Ranjana K. Mehta*[1,2*]

[1] Department of Occupational and Environmental Health, School of Public Health, Texas A&M University, College Station, TX, United States, [2] Department of Industrial and Systems Engineering, Texas A&M University, College Station, TX, United States

***Correspondence:**
Ranjana K. Mehta
rmehta@tamu.edu

The prevalence of obesity in older adults, particularly in females, is increasing rapidly and is associated with declines in both the brain and physical health. Both the obese and the female populations have shown greater motor fatigue than their counterparts, however, the central neural mechanisms for fatigue are unclear. The present study measured fatigue-related functional connectivity across frontal and sensorimotor areas using functional near-infrared spectroscopy (fNIRS). Fifty-nine older adults (30 non-obese and 29 obese) performed submaximal handgrip motor fatigue until voluntary exhaustion. Functional connectivity and cerebral hemodynamics were compared across eight cortical areas during motor fatigue and across obesity and sex groups along with neuromuscular fatigue outcomes (i.e., endurance time, strength loss, and force steadiness). Both obesity- and sex-specific functional architecture and mean activation differences during motor fatigue in older adults were observed, which were accompanied by fatigue-related changes in variability of force steadiness that differed between groups. While primary indicators of fatigue, i.e., endurance and strength loss, did not differ between groups, the motor steadiness changes indicated different neural adaptation strategies between the groups. These findings indicate that obesity and sex differences exist in brain function in older adults, which may affect performance during motor fatigue.

Keywords: BMI, gender, fatigability, brain activation and networks, fNIRS

INTRODUCTION

Obesity is a global public health epidemic (Caballero, 2007). Obesity and its associated health issues place an adverse economic burden on the U.S. health care system, with medical care costs estimated at $147 Billion in 2008 (Finkelstein et al., 2009). Along with comorbidities such as diabetes, hypertension, and sleep apnea, obesity is accompanied with motor impairments, such reductions in muscle power (Lafortuna et al., 2005), increases in motor fatigue (Mehta, 2015), and impaired motor control (Gentier et al., 2013) that may accelerate declines in physical functioning with aging (Lang et al., 2007). These obesity-related decrements in motor skills and functional activity have also been associated with increasing morbidity and mortality in older adults (Aune et al., 2016). This is a critical concern, since ~40% of adults, particularly women, over the age of 65 are obese (Laura Segal and Martin, 2016). However, mechanisms of motor impairments have largely focused on healthy older adults.

In general, older adults experience declines in both their motor and cognitive capabilities due to the normal age-related degradation of the central nervous system (CNS) and peripheral musculoskeletal system (Frontera et al., 1991; Hughes et al., 1999; Enoka et al., 2003). Specific to the CNS, aging is associated with structural and functional changes in the brain. Ge et al. (2002) reported significantly decreased gray matter volume in older adults compared with younger adults, and the change of cortical volume at the prefrontal area was relatively greater than other brain regions (Good et al., 2001; Jernigan et al., 2001). Gray matter volume is known to be associated with motor performance (Rodrigue et al., 2005), and this relationship may explain age-related motor performance declines. White matter volume also decreases with aging (Jernigan et al., 2001; Ge et al., 2002). Corpus callosum, which is a large bundle of white matter fibers that handles communication between the two hemispheres, is known to be responsible for bimanual coordination and ipsilateral inhibition during unimanual motor tasks (De Gennaro et al., 2004). Therefore, a decrease of white matter volume with aging may affect the stability of motor performance such as balance, coordinative motions, and force control tasks (Sullivan et al., 2010).

Among many age-related changes, fat mass is known to increase with aging and reaches its maximum value after the sixties (Rissanen et al., 1988; Ding et al., 2007). In addition, muscle mass decreases approximately 1% per year and as a result, muscular strength and power also gradually decreases with aging after midlife and can be exacerbated with increased fat mass (Bassey, 1998; Frontera et al., 2000). Older adults who are obese are more likely to experience musculoskeletal injuries and falls (Madigan et al., 2014) and exhibit greater motor fatigue (Maffiuletti et al., 2007; Duan et al., 2018). These impairments have been attributed largely to obesity-specific alterations in peripheral muscular properties, such as changes in muscle mass, fiber type distribution, and contractile properties (Krotkiewski et al., 1990; Hickey et al., 1995; Kriketos et al., 1997; Kern et al., 1999; Newcomer et al., 2001; Tanner et al., 2002). However, whether obesity alters central neural mechanisms of motor fatigue in older adults has not been adequately explored. Additionally, it is important to determine whether there are sex differences in mechanisms for the motor function declines with obesity, because females are more susceptible functional declines (Skelton et al., 1994), particularly with obesity (Jensen and Friedmann, 2002).

Obesity causes structural and functional changes in the brain such as decreased gray matter volume, decreased cortical thickness, and reduced metabolism in the frontal area (Pannacciulli et al., 2006; Willeumier et al., 2011; Marqués-Iturria et al., 2014). Jagust et al. (2005) reported that both central obesity (waist-hip ratio) and aging are negatively correlated with the hippocampal volume that is responsible for information processing and memory consolidation, and positively correlated with hyperintensity lesion of white matter. These obesity-related changes in the brain structures are likely to affect brain function, however, our knowledge on whether functional brain activity is impacted with obesity is limited to cognitive tasks (Gonzales et al., 2014). Only two studies have examined brain function during motor tasks in non-obese and obese adults. Obesity-related decrement in motor performance and concomitant disengagement of the prefrontal lobe during a static upper limb force control task in young adults was reported in (Mehta and Shortz, 2014), while the same group found increased PFC activity during complex and precision gait tasks in older obese adults (Osofundiya et al., 2016) that was associated with similar gait performance when compared to non-obese counterparts. Additionally, other studies that utilized electrical muscle stimulation to understand central vs. peripheral pathways of fatigue attributed obesity-related increased lower limb fatigability in young adults to an increase in central activation failure (Maffiuletti et al., 2007; Pajoutan et al., 2016). However, studies that examine obesity-specific changes in brain function during motor fatigue are limited.

Several imaging studies have reported sex differences in brain structure. For example, males are reported to have greater gray matter (Good et al., 2001) and total brain volume (Sacher et al., 2013) than females after correcting for body size. However, cortical thickness has shown to be greater for females at the frontal, temporal, and occipital areas (Im et al., 2006; Lv et al., 2010). Similarly, structural connectivity of the brain also differs in males and females. Ingalhalikar et al. (2014) reported that females exhibit stronger anatomical connections between the two hemispheres whereas males exhibit stronger connections between the areas within each hemisphere, however, this relationship was shown to be reversed in the cerebellum. These sex differences in the brain structure may explain differences in motor function between males and females. For instance, compared to males, females exhibit greater activation of ipsilateral and bilateral cortical brain regions but lower subcortical activation of the basal ganglia region during finger tapping and motor preparation tasks of similar performance (Lissek et al., 2007). However, whether brain activation differs between males and females during motor fatigue remains unexplored (Hunter, 2014).

When interpreting brain function changes, it is important to understand that while each part of the brain has an assigned role for a certain task, multiple areas of the brain work together to achieve task performance, particularly if the task is performed for a long duration. Therefore, understanding concurrent activation patterns between multiple areas of the brain; also referred to as functional connectivity, is as important as understanding activation of each area in response to the task (Hutchison et al., 2013). The location of functionally connected brain areas can be adjacent to each other, however, it is not necessary for functionally connected areas to be anatomically connected (Bressler and Tognoli, 2006). Determining functional connectivity during motor fatigue may thus help us examine the functions of the brain as a network, thereby contributing toward a better understanding of the mechanisms of motor impairments with obesity and aging, and to explore if these mechanisms differ by sex.

Studies investigating functional connectivity with older and obese adults, and those comparing differences between males and females, have been published. For example, Tomasi and Volkow (2012) reported sex differences in lateralization patterns; females exhibited greater long-range connectivity between hemispheres while males show predominant short-range connectivity within the hemisphere. Goldstone et al. (2016) reported re-organization of the resting state network in older adults. King et al. (2017) argued that age-related declined motor performance is related to overall higher connectivity across networks involved in the large-scale resting state network in older adults when compared to younger adults. Older adults also exhibit altered default mode network (DMN) connectivity compared to their younger counterparts, however, the strength of connectivity was influenced by obesity status, i.e., body mass index [BMI; (Kullmann et al., 2012a)]. However, most of these studies examined group (i.e., sex, age, or obesity) differences in functional connectivity either during resting states or during cognitive performance without movement involved. Although a few studies examined functional connectivity with motor tasks, those studies were still limited to testing the movement of the small distal muscles (Karim et al., 2017) and in healthy populations, with no considerations given to group differences in the outcomes studied.

The purpose of the present study was to examine obesity and sex differences in functional connectivity changes with handgrip motor fatigue development in older adults. Functional brain activity from frontal, motor, and sensory area using functional near-infrared spectroscopy (fNIRS) were obtained from study participants as they performed isometric submaximal handgrip contractions until voluntary exhaustion. Based on a prior electroencephalogram (EEG) study of motor fatigue (Liu et al., 2007), we hypothesized that functional connectivity across the monitored areas would differ over the course of motor fatigue development. We also hypothesized that functional connectivity would differ by obesity. Finally, we explored sex differences in functional connectivity during motor fatigue.

MATERIALS AND METHODS

Participants

Fifty-nine older adults were recruited from the local community. All participants were 65 years or older, right-hand dominant, and sedentary or recreationally active without any known musculoskeletal injuries or disorders in the past 12 months. Participants whose BMI were in the range of 18.5 ~25 kg/m^2 were considered as non-obese and greater than 30 kg/m^2 were considered as obese. Six participants whose endurance times were shorter than the required duration for the functional connectivity analysis were excluded from the analysis. **Table 1** lists participants' demographics of the four experimental groups: non-obese males (n = 14), non-obese females (n = 14), obese males (n = 11), and obese females (n = 14). The Texas A&M University Institutional Review Board approved the procedures, and participants provided written informed consent before data collection.

Procedures

The data presented in this study is the result of one experiment that is a part of a larger project that consisted of several experiment sessions. Upon informed consent, physical activity of each participant, as time-series acceleration, was measured for 1 week using three-axis accelerometer (activPAL, PAL Technologies Ltd, Glasgow, United Kingdom) attached on the right thigh. The experimenter removed the physical activity monitor on the fatigue experiment session. Data from the accelerometer provided average steps/day for each participant. Participants then attended one handgrip motor fatigue experiment, which consisted of bioinstrumentation, baseline, strength, and fatigue testings (**Figure 1**). Participants were first instrumented with fNIRS (Techen Inc., MA, United States, CW6 System) that measured hemodynamic responses at the frontal, motor, and sensory areas (**Figure 2A**). Participants sat upright with their dominant upper arm at their side, elbow flexed at 90°, and lower arm supported by an armrest. Prior to the motor fatigue task, brain activation during a baseline period was measured in which participants were asked to relax without any movement for 3 min. Following baseline tests, participants grasped a hand dynamometer (BIOPAC, CA, United States) to perform isometric handgrip contractions. After sufficient warm up (of ~2 min), participant performed three isometric maximum voluntary contractions (MVCs) with 2 min rest in between to measure participant's handgrip strength. The maximum value from the three MVC trials was used to determine the target force level of 30% MVC for the subsequent motor fatigue task. Participants were provided familiarization of the motor fatigue trials at 30% MVC and adequate rest before starting the fatiguing motor task. The fatigue test required participants to maintain handgrip force levels at 30% MVC for 15 s followed by 15 s rest repeatedly until voluntary exhaustion or termination. Participants were instructed to maintain their handgrip force level as closely to the target force level as possible utilizing real-time visual feedback on a computer screen. Once they terminated the fatigue task, they performed a post MVC trial.

Cerebral Hemodynamics

Brain activation was monitored using continuous wave fNIRS (Techen Inc., MA, United States, CW6 System). The intensity of the light signal in two wavelengths (690 and 830 nm), discharged from 8 emitters and absorbed while traveling through neural tissue, were recorded at 13 detectors to obtain hemodynamic responses at a total of 26 channels. Acquired light intensities were converted into optical density by taking the logarithm of the input signal. The optical density was then low pass filtered at 3 Hz to reduce high-frequency noise. Motion artifacts that showed abrupt change were detected and corrected using spline interpolation algorithm (Scholkmann et al., 2010) and smoothed using wavelet algorithm (Chiarelli et al., 2015). Motion artifact corrected signals were bandpass filtered at 0.5 ~0.016 Hz to reduce the effect of physiological noise and slow wave drifts. Lastly, oxygenated (ΔHbO) and deoxygenated (ΔHbR) hemoglobin at the 26 channels was calculated using modified Beer-Lambert law (Delpy et al., 1988). Location of the 21 optodes (i.e., 8 emitters and 13 detectors; **Figure 2A**) that constructed 26 channels where the brain activation was monitored was determined based on 10/20 international EEG system using Atlasview (Aasted et al., 2015). Since ΔHbO showed greater task related changes than

TABLE 1 | Participant demographics.

	Males			Females		
	Non-obese (*N* = 14)	**Obese (*N* = 11)**	***p*-value**	**Non-obese (*N* = 14)**	**Obese (*N* = 14)**	***p*-value**
Age	74.5 (6.4)	72.7 (6.9)	0.49	71.5 (4.2)	71.6 (5.5)	0.954
Height (cm)	177.7 (7.5)	178.4 (8.8)	0.661	163.6 (5.9)	159.9 (4.2)	0.128
Weight (kg)	76.1 (8.1)	114.8 (17.4)	<0.001	60.9 (7.0)	94.5 (14.2)	<0.001
Body mass index (kg/m^2)	24.4 (1.2)	34.7 (3.4)	<0.001	22.9 (1.9)	37.0 (4.9)	<0.001
Waist circumference (cm)	38.9 (1.9)	50.2 (4.3)	<0.001	34.5 (3.7)	46.1 (4.1)	<0.001
Percent body fat (%)	22.8 (4.7)	35.7 (3.4)	<0.001	31.3 (5.2)	51.4 (17.4)	<0.001
Initial strength (kg)	11.2 (2.6)	12.7 (3.0)	0.198	9.5 (2.3)	8.6 (1.6)	0.252
PA (# of steps/day)	7794.8 (2259.2)	5670.7 (4791.7)	0.180	7719.7 (3104.1)	5056.9 (1782.4)	0.014

All measures are presented as mean (SD). Statistically significant obesity differences in each sex group is tested at alpha = 0.05.

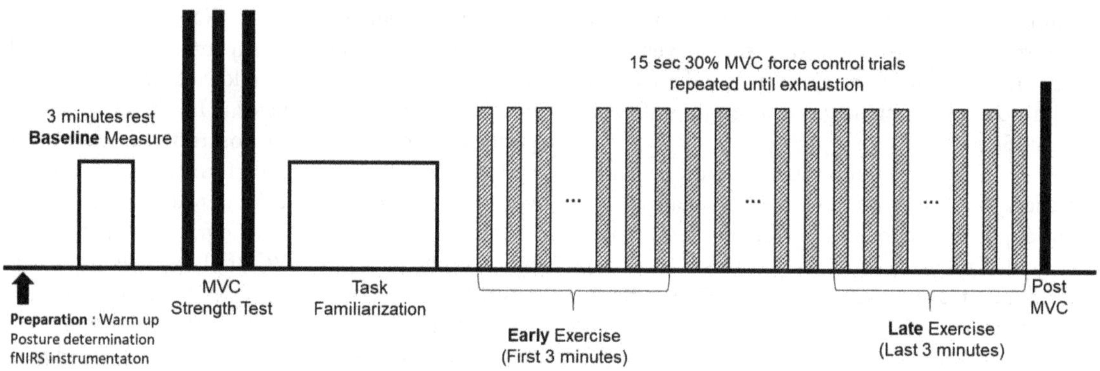

FIGURE 1 | Experiment protocol for the motor fatigue experiment.

ΔHbR, ΔHbO was used to analyze functional connectivity changes and task related neural activation changes during fatigue development (Malonek and Grinvald, 1996). In the present study, the ΔHbO time-series data of 26 channels were averaged into eight regions of interests (ROIs) that were defined based on the functions of a sensorimotor network of both hemispheres (Mayka et al., 2006), namely left/right prefrontal area (LPFC and RPFC, respectively), left/right medial motor area (LM1 and RM1, respectively) left/right lateral motor area (LM2 and RM2, respectively), and left/right sensory area (LS and RS, respectively). The task-related neural activation was obtained by averaging 2 s around maximum ΔHbO activation within each trial (Hyodo et al., 2016).

Functional Connectivity Analysis

To acquire 3 min long continuous time-series signal of oxygenated hemoglobin, HbO of the first and last 12 force control trials during the motor fatigue test were extracted, concatenated, and labeled as early and late. Additionally, the 3-min baseline period was also processed and labeled as a baseline. Five participants who performed less than 24 total trials were excluded from the analysis. While concatenating HbO signal during intermittent contractions into one continuous signal, offsets between the end of the previous contraction and the beginning of the following contraction were compensated, and the concatenated signal was de-trended and low pass filtered at 0.1 Hz (Cheng et al., 2016). Pearson correlations across all ROIs were computed to determine associations between ROIs (**Figures 2B,C**). Pearson R values were then converted into Fisher's z-score to determine the strength of correlations between ROIs (**Figure 2D**). The threshold of z-score to determine whether the node between the two regions are functionally connected or not was set to a predetermined value of 0.4 based on Rubinov and Sporns (2010). Based on the graph theory, each ROI in the present study was labeled as a node, and the connection between ROIs was labeled as an edge. Although the present study examined the spatial connectivity pattern between ROIs but did not perform network analysis, the terms node and edge are used subsequently (Friston, 1994). Eight nodes constructed 28 edges and the threshold to determine whether the edge between the two nodes are functionally connected were set to a predetermined value of 0.4 (Rubinov and Sporns, 2010).

Motor Performance

Endurance time was defined as the duration between onset of the first trial and when a participant could no longer maintain the target force for more than 3 s. The rate of strength loss due to fatigue development was computed as (Initial MVC–Post MVC)/Initial MVC × 100. Handgrip forces during the strength and motor fatigue tests were recorded using the hand dynamometer (BIOPAC, CA, United States) at 1,000 Hz sampling rate. Force time-series data were low pass filtered at 15 Hz, and

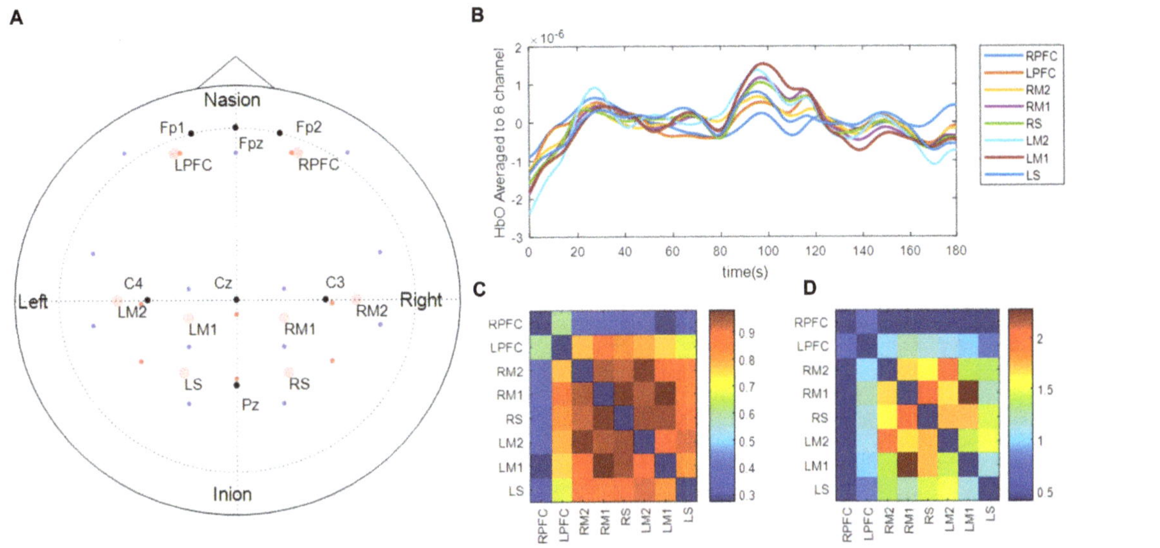

FIGURE 2 | fNIRS probe design **(A)** and functional connectivity analysis procedure **(B–D)**. Panel **(A)** shows the location of light emitters (red dots) and detectors (blue dots). Gray lines between optodes depict the location of channels where brain activation is measured. Black dots represent the location of reference points based on 10–20 international EEG system. Pink circles show the location of the regions of interest which are average of surrounding channels. The regions of interest were defined based on the functions of a sensorimotor network of both hemispheres (Prefrontal area: LPFC, RPFC, Medial motor area: LM1, RM1, Lateral motor area: LM2, RM2, and Sensory area: LS, RS). Panel **(B)** shows an example of the fNIRS time-series signal processed and aggregated to the regions of interest during the early phase of one participant. Panel **(C)** shows Pearson correlation matrix across the time-series signals shown in Panel **(B)**. Panel **(D)** shows Fischer's *z*-score converted from Panel **(C)** and only showed the scores of nodes between the two functionally connected regions based on predetermined threshold of 0.4.

the middle 12 s of each 15 s force control trial was extracted. The coefficient of variation (CV = SD/average) of force was computed as a measure of force steadiness (Tracy and Enoka, 2002), and a coefficient of variation of force steadiness was computed as a measure of motor variability (Duan et al., 2018). CV of force and CV of force steadiness of first and last 12 trials were averaged and used for comparing group (obesity and sex) differences with fatigue. These variations in movement characteristics, known as motor variability, are reported to be associated with motor performance impairment and fatigability (Davids et al., 2003; Srinivasan and Mathiassen, 2012).

Statistical Analysis

Separate paired *t*-tests between the phases; baseline vs. early, early vs. late, and baseline vs. late; of functional connectivity strength of each edge across groups pooled by sex and obesity were performed. Additionally, independent *t*-tests between obesity and sex groups, i.e., non-obese vs. obese and males vs. females, in each of the three phases (i.e., baseline, early, and late) were performed on the functional connectivity strength. The acquired *p*-values in each comparison were corrected using false discovery rate (FDR) to reduce the likelihood of false positives caused by multiple comparisons (Benjamini and Hochberg, 1995).

Separate 2 (phase: early, late) 2 (sex: male, female) × 2 (obesity: non-obese, obese) × 2 (side: left, right) mixed factor ANOVAs were conducted on ΔHbO values from each of the four ROIs (prefrontal, medial motor, lateral motor, and sensory area). Statistical significances of each ROI were corrected using FDR (Benjamini and Hochberg, 1995). Handgrip strength loss after fatigue development and endurance times were submitted to separate 2 (sex: male, female) × 2 (obesity: non-obese, obese) factorial ANOVAs to examine sex and obesity differences on handgrip motor fatigue. Additionally, CV of force (force steadiness) and CV of CV were submitted to a 2 (phase: early, late) × 2 (sex: male, female) × 2 (obesity: non-obese, obese) ANOVA to examine group (obesity and sex) and phase differences on motor performance during the fatigue test. Statistical significance was testing with alpha = 0.05, and *post hocs* were conducted as needed using Bonferroni corrections.

RESULTS

Functional Connectivity

The number of functionally connected edges decreased during the late phase (non-obese: 13, obese: 11) compared with the baseline phase (non-obese: 16, obese: 24) and the early phase (non-obese: 22, obese: 21). Spatial connectivity patterns were different during the baseline phase but the differences between the non-obese and obese groups were not significant (**Figure 3**). However, the obese group showed greater variability in connectivity (**Figure 4**). Motor task related spatial connectivity patterns between non-obese and obese groups were observed to be similar during the early phase (**Figure 3**), however, the variability of connectivity was found to be increased for non-obese group (**Figure 4**). During the late phase, the non-obese group demonstrated significantly greater connectivity between right lateral motor area and medial motor area of

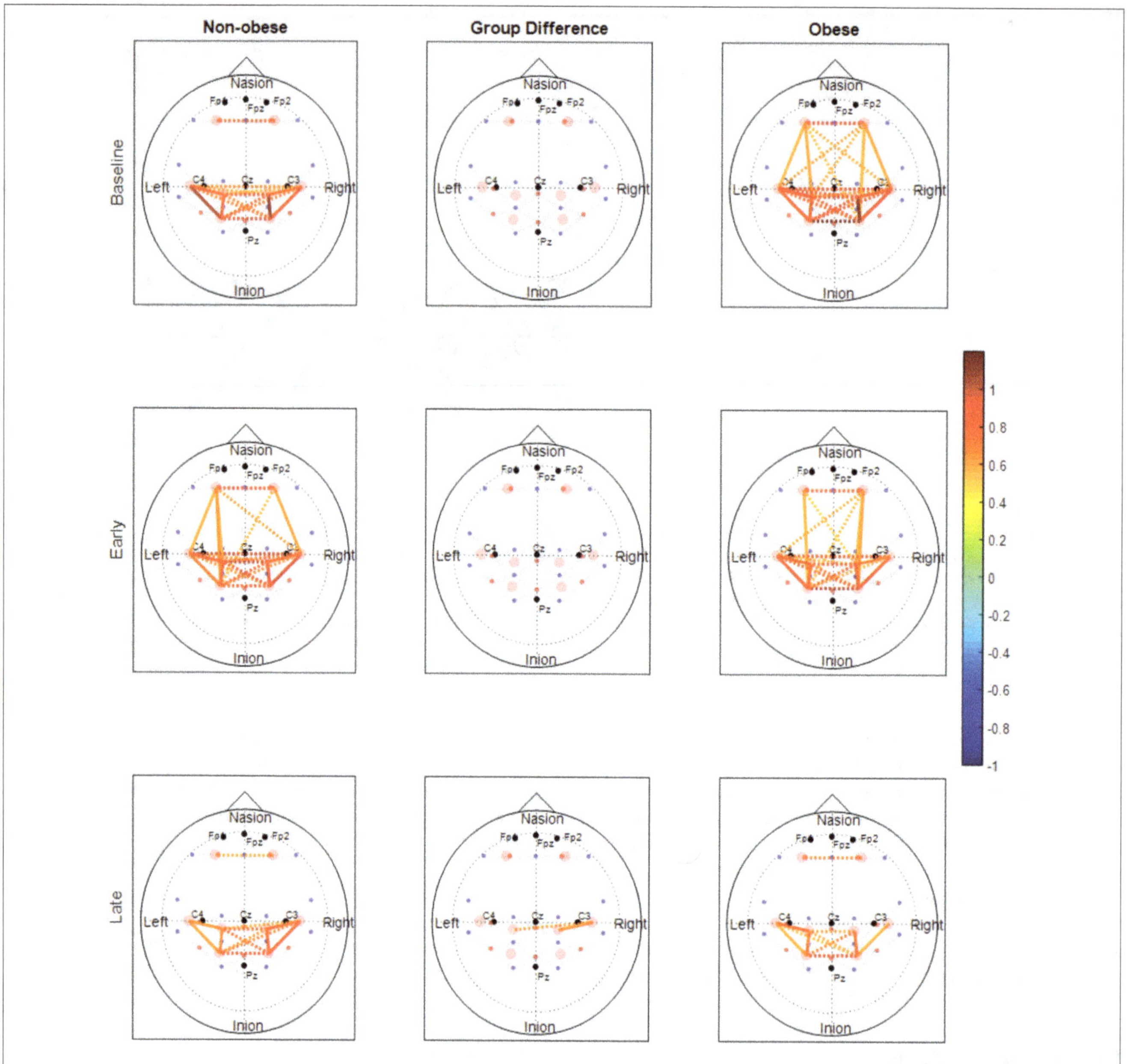

FIGURE 3 | Functional connectivity maps of non-obese (left column) and obese (right column) during the baseline and motor fatigue test. The connectivity maps are produced from the weighted matrix, and the color of each node depicts the strength of connectivity based on provided color scale. Nodes with solid lines indicate intra-hemispheric connectivity, and nodes with dotted lines indicate inter-hemispheric connectivity. Middle column shows the nodes which connectivity was significantly different between the obesity groups. The connectivity difference maps are produced from the binary matrix, and positive score based on the provided color scale indicates connectivity of the nodes were significantly stronger for non-obese than obese.

both hemispheres when compared to the obese group. The obese group showed most distinctive fatigue-related functional connectivity changes and the connectivity during the late phase was lower than during the baseline and early phases (**Figures 5A,B**).

Both males and females exhibited fewer functionally connected edges during the late phase (males: 15, females: 8) when compared with the baseline (males: 27, females: 15) and the early phases (males: 28, females: 12). During the baseline and early phases, males exhibited functional connectivity that was greater than the threshold at 27 edges across all nodes but females showed connectivity within the prefrontal and sensorimotor areas, however, the two areas were not functionally connected (**Figure 6**). Functional connectivity changes between the baseline and early phases were not found to be significant. While the sex differences in connectivity were observed to exist at all three phases (as seen in **Figures 6, 7**), connectivity between the two groups was not significantly different due to the large variability observed during the early phase (**Figure 7**). Both groups showed decreased connectivity

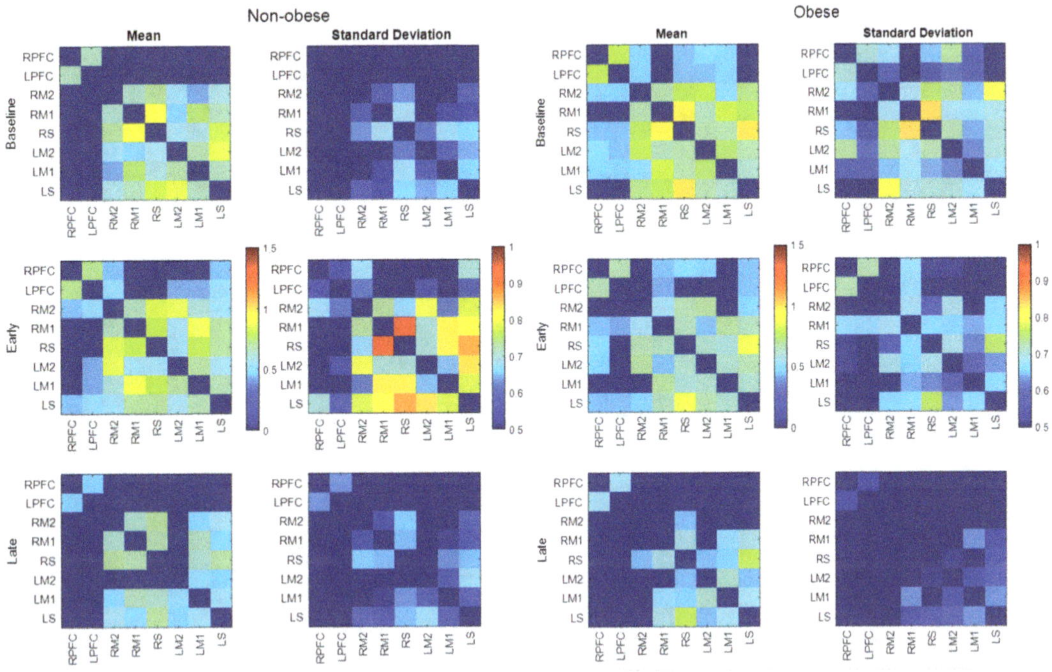

FIGURE 4 | Mean and SD of connectivity matrix for each phase in the non-obese (Left) and obese (Right) groups. Color matrices are produced out of Fischer's *Z*-score.

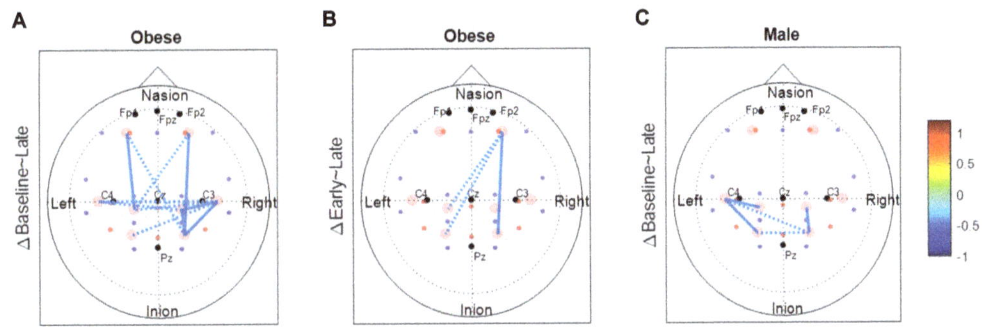

FIGURE 5 | Functional connectivity changes between phases. These connectivity change maps are produced from the binary matrix, and the scores based on the provided color scale indicates either the connectivity was significantly decreased (negative score) or not. **(A)** Significantly decreased connectivity between baseline and late phases in the obese group. **(B)** Significantly decreased connectivity between early and late phases in the obese group. **(C)** Significantly decreased connectivity between baseline and late phases in males. Solid lines indicate significant connectivity changes within each hemisphere and dotted lines indicate significant connectivity changes between the two hemispheres.

and decreased the number of connected edges with motor fatigue development. During the late phase, males showed significantly stronger connectivity at a node between left prefrontal area and left lateral motor area. Also, males showed decreased connectivity with motor fatigue during the late phase compared to the baseline phase at the sensorimotor area (**Figure 5C**).

Changes in Cerebral Hemodynamics

Task related ΔHbO increased with fatigue development [$F(1,49) = 26.627$, $p < 0.001$] at all channels and strong contralateral activation was observed at all ROI after FDR correction (all *p*-values <0.005, **Figure 8**). No obesity or sex differences were found (all *p*'s > 0.4). However, a side × obesity × phase interaction was found in sensory motor area [$F(1,49) = 9.821$, $p = 0.003$]. *Post hoc* revealed that the fatigue-related increase in ΔHbO in the contralateral sensory area was greater for non-obese adults when compared to obese adults.

Changes in Motor Performance

Table 2 lists the means (SD) of the motor performance data across the obesity and sex groups. Fatigue-related strength loss did not differ by obesity ($p = 0.347$), or sex ($p = 0.759$), or their

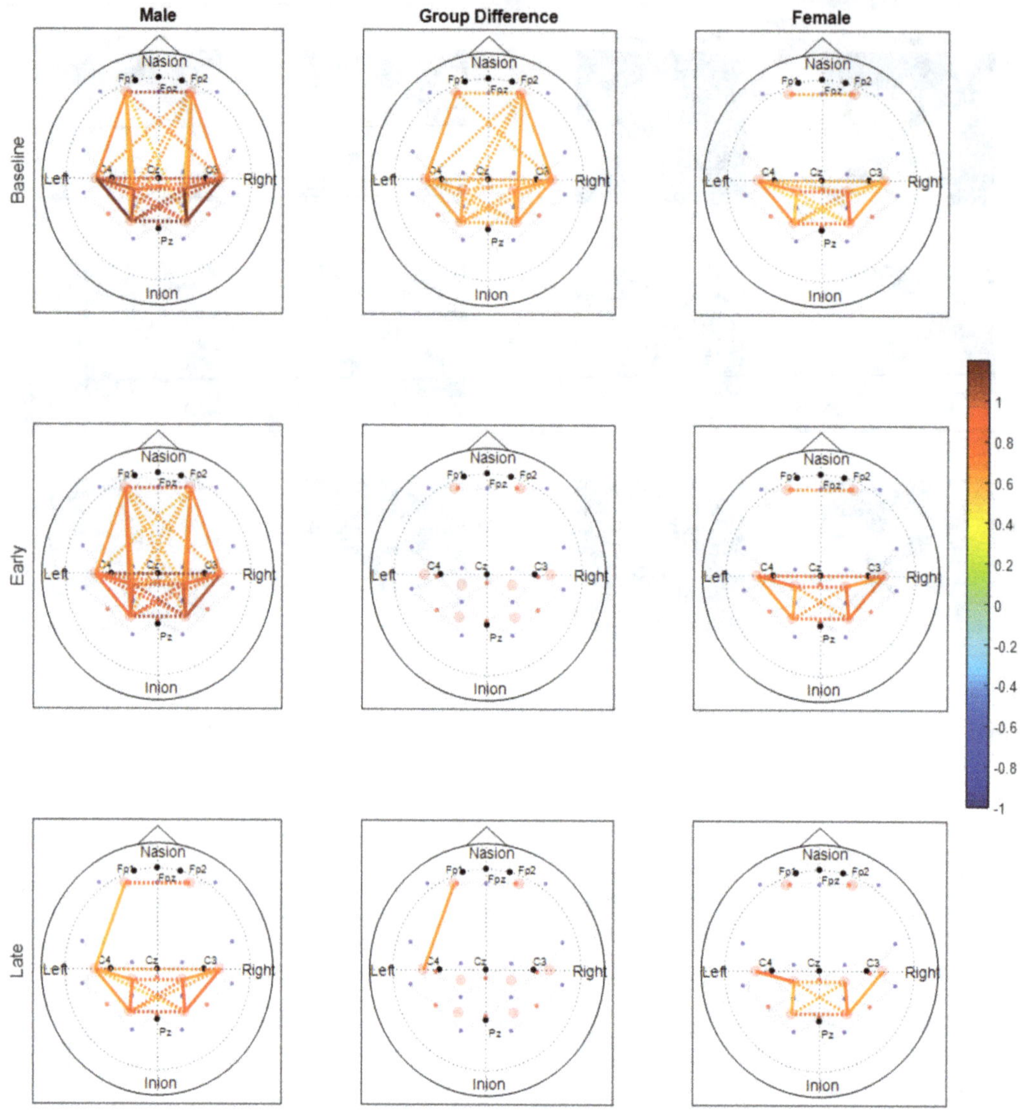

FIGURE 6 | Functional connectivity maps of the male (left column) and female (right column) groups during the baseline and motor fatigue test. The connectivity maps are produced from the weighted matrix, and the color of each node depicts the strength of connectivity based on provided color scale. Nodes with solid lines indicate intra-hemispheric connectivity, and nodes with dotted lines indicate inter-hemispheric connectivity. Middle column shows the nodes where connectivity was significantly different between the sexes. The connectivity difference maps are produced from the binary matrix, and positive score based on the provided color scale indicates connectivity of the nodes were significantly stronger for males than for females.

interaction ($p = 0.255$). Similarly, endurance time did not differ by obesity ($p = 0.595$), or sex ($p = 0.859$), or their interaction ($p = 0.943$). CV of force during motor fatigue increased during the late phase [$F(1,48) = 17.436$, $p < 0.001$] when compared to the early phase, however, no group differences, or their interactions with each other or with phase were found (both p's > 0.16). CV of CV decreased during the late phase when compared to the early phase [$F(1,46) = 21.219$, $p < 0.001$], in males than females [$F(1,48) = 17.193$, $p < 0.001$], and in obese adults than in non-obese adults [$F(1,48) = 3.963$, $p = 0.052$]. Additionally, an obesity × phase interaction was found on CV of CV [$F(1,46) = 3.875$, $p = 0.055$], with the non-obese group exhibiting decreased CV of CV as they fatigued, but the obese adults exhibiting reduced CV of CV across both phases of fatigue.

DISCUSSION

Obesity Differences in Functional Connectivity

During the baseline phase, the obese group showed more functionally connected edges across most nodes while non-obese group only showed interhemispheric connectivity within each prefrontal and sensorimotor area, but not between the two areas. Previous studies reported obesity-related differences

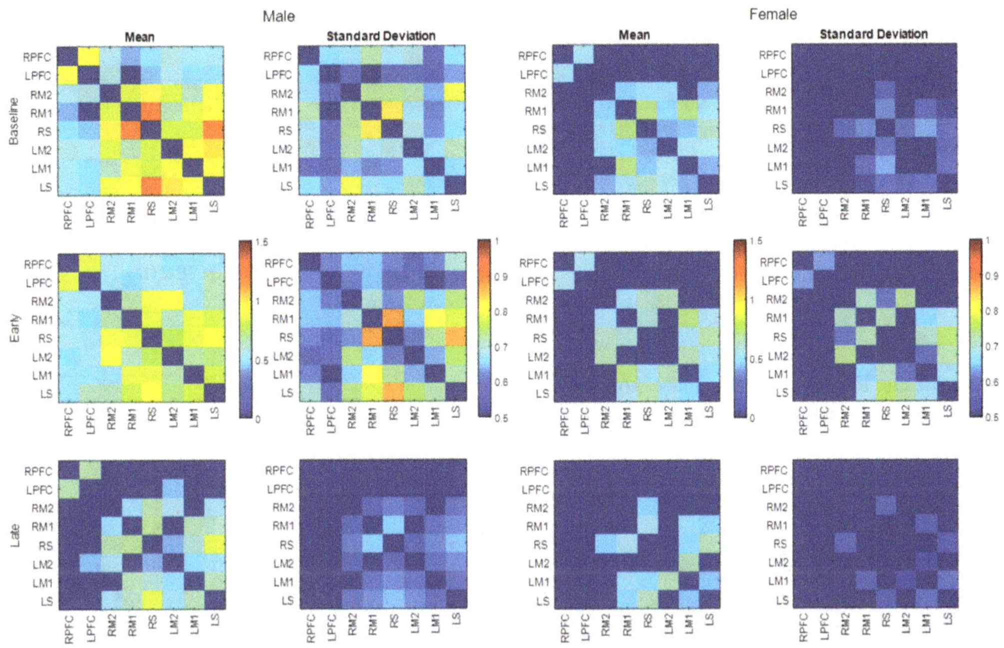

FIGURE 7 | Mean and SD of connectivity matrix for each phase in males (left) and females (right). Color matrices are produced out of Fischer's *Z*-score.

in functional networks such as, altered DMN (Kullmann et al., 2012a; García-García et al., 2013a) and increased connectivity within salience network (Kullmann et al., 2012b; García-García et al., 2013b). However, this obesity effect is limited to the differences in the functional networks. The connectivity patterns observed in the present study may indicate overall greater connectivity of the obese group during the baseline phase, but the use of pooled datasets across sexes in this study hinders isolating the said effect.

The number of functionally connected nodes during early phase increased for the non-obese group but decreased with the obese group. Both groups showed connectivity patterns in which edges of both areas and hemispheres were connected (**Figure 3**). Given that different spatial connectivity pattern between the sexes was maintained during the motor task, relatively similar spatial connectivity pattern during early phase indicates the motor task influences differently when compared across the sex or obesity groups. These differences in connectivity change patterns are in agreement with the studies reported sex dependent structural connectivity (Tomasi and Volkow, 2012; Ingalhalikar et al., 2014) and obesity dependent functional connectivity (Kullmann et al., 2012b; García-García et al., 2013a,b). During the late phase, the number of functionally connected edges and variability of connectivity decreased (**Figures 3, 4**).

Sex Differences in Functional Connectivity

The spatial patterns of functionally connected edges, in which connectivity scores were greater than the threshold value, were different between males and females (**Figure 6**). While males showed connectivity between the frontal and sensorimotor areas and between the hemispheres, females showed only inter-hemispheric connectivity within each area. This is partially in congruence with the study that reported stronger intra hemispheric connectivity for males and stronger inter-hemispheric connectivity for females (Ingalhalikar et al., 2014). During the baseline phase, which can be considered as a resting state when compared with other connectivity studies, males showed stronger connectivity with both inter/intra network connectivity that suggests sex related different localized brain activation pattern (Tomasi and Volkow, 2012). In addition, males exhibit greater variability in connectivity than females which is congruent with the result reported greater functional activations for males while females had greater structural connectivity densities (Keller and Menon, 2009).

The spatial pattern of functionally connected edges of both sexes did not change from that during the baseline phase and the connectivity pattern at the frontal and sensorimotor area is consistent with that Yao et al. (2016) reported. However, the group difference observed during baseline phase was negated (**Figure 6**) due to overall greater variability in both sexes (**Figure 7**). These results suggest that the handgrip motor task did not significantly alter the spatial functional brain network. While older adults tend to over-recruit neural area to perform motor tasks compared with young adults (Mattay et al., 2002; Heuninckx et al., 2008), both contralateral and ipsilateral functional connectivity observed in the present study is consistent with concurrent increase of hemodynamic response with motor tasks in both contralateral and ipsilateral hemispheres, and variability in connectivity at the node that was acquired from the averaged brain activation of surrounding ROIs is indicative of sex and task dependent different changes in neural

TABLE 2 | Motor fatigue and performance measures are presented as mean (SD).

		Male		Female	
		Normal (*N* = 14)	Obese (*N* = 11)	Normal (*N* = 14)	Obese (*N* = 14)
Strength loss (%)		37.5 (10.6)	32.1 (6.9)	33.4 (10.2)	35.4 (8.2)
Endurance time (s)		1287.9 (513.5)	1217.5 (376.3)	1272.7 (629.0)	1187.1 (493.9)
CV force (%)	Early	1.8 (0.6)	1.9 (0.3)	1.8 (0.5)	2.1 (0.6)
	Late	2.7 (2.5)	2.1 (0.3)	1.9 (0.6)	2.4 (0.7)
CV force steadiness (%)	Early	19.6 (4.4)	15.3 (6.1)	28.8 (11.4)	22.6 (9.2)
	Late	16.2 (4.1)	12.2 (4.6)	18.2 (7.5)	18.9 (5.8)

recruitment in older adults. During the late phase, the number of functionally connected edges was decreased as well as the variability of connectivity in both sexes. This result suggests a dissociation of the brain activation pattern among the areas that used to be associated with fatigue development.

Functional Connectivity Changes During Motor Fatigue Development

Motor fatigue development was associated with changes in functional connectivity in older adults, across all groups. Older adults, regardless of sex and obesity differences, exhibited fewer functionally connected edges as fatigue developed, and the lower variability of the connectivity patterns (pooled across all participants) observed implied that the decline in connectivity was homogenous across all groups (**Figures 3, 6**). Only a few studies examined functional connectivity associated with acute motor fatigue and these studies employed EEG or fMRI (Liu et al., 2007). For example, Peltier et al. (2005) reported decreases in interhemispheric connectivity in the motor areas after fatigue. The findings from the present study, which demonstrated decreased interhemispheric connectivity with fatigue development [particularly in the obese groups (**Figures 5A,B**) and male (**Figure 5C**)] are in agreement with Peltier et al. (2005). However, the present study examined connectivity during fatigue development whereas the previous study measured resting state functional connectivity after motor task.

Force Variability and Brain Activity Changes During Motor Fatigue Development

In the present study, similar to previous studies examining force variability patterns with fatigue (Srinivasan and Mathiassen, 2012), fatigue development here was associated with decreased force steadiness and lower variability of this reduced motor performance, i.e., a decrease in CV of force steadiness. There were no obesity or sex differences in endurance time, strength loss, or force steadiness. Endurance and strength loss have shown to differ with obesity and sex, however, in older adults, the differences are largely observed in postural and/or lower extremity muscles (Hunter, 2016, 2017). Understanding force variability patterns can provide a greater resolution on how individuals differently adapt or correct for motor demands (Mathiassen et al., 2003; Madeleine, 2010). In the present study,

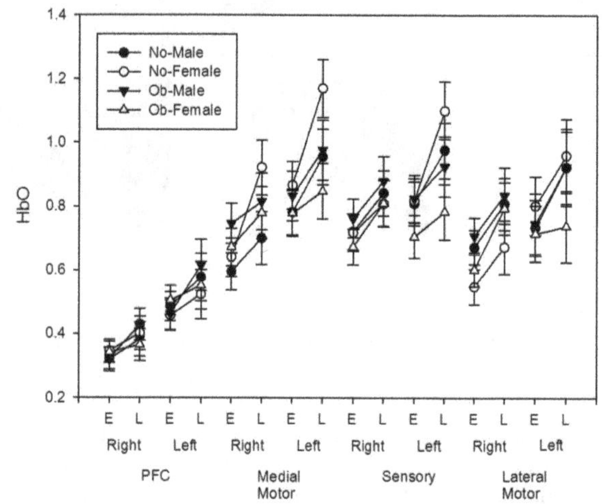

FIGURE 8 | Fatigue-related HbO changes (Early and Late) at each region of interest (PFC, Medial Motor, Sensory, Lateral Motor) of both hemisphere (Left, Right).

lower variability of CV was found for males than females. Given that both males and females showed similar steadiness patterns over time, increased variability in the patterns exhibited by females may be attributed to different neural adaptation strategies than males to maintain motor performance (Hunter, 2014; Duan et al., 2018). This was associated with concomitant sex differences in the functional connectivity patterns observed in the present study.

Similar to males, the obese group exhibited lower variability of force steadiness than the non-obese group, which was accompanied by fatigue-related concomitant declines in the frontal-motor connectivity and reduced activation in sensory motor areas with obesity. Obesity has shown to adversely impact brain structure and function, particularly of the frontal lobes (Gustafson et al., 2004; Pannacciulli et al., 2006; Whitmer et al., 2008). We have previously reported associations between impaired functioning of the frontal lobe and obesity-related decrements in upper extremity motor performance (Mehta and Shortz, 2014) and gait speed (Osofundiya et al., 2016). Thus, it is likely that obesity may contribute to reduced cortical excitation of frontal-motor areas in older adults, which may impact functional motor outcomes in this population. It is likely that physical activity of the study participants may have confounded obesity differences in the study variables. While PA was similar between non-obese and obese males, obese females exhibited lower steps/day than non-obese females. Moreover, the obesity groups were significantly different based on BMI, percent body fat, and waist circumference values. Given that none of the study variables were affected by obesity × sex interactions, it is likely that the differences observed here are largely attributed to obesity-related changes in neural and muscular mechanisms.

Study Limitations

Due to the limited spatial resolution and measurement depth of fNIRS, connectivity across the various functional networks in the whole brain was not available to measure. Instead, we measured the brain activation of an inch depth of the targeted cortical area of frontal and sensorimotor area. This limitation can potentially be resolved with multi-modal neuroimaging such as fNIRS combined with EEG or fMRI. Second, although the sex and obesity groups formed four groups, we used pooled datasets for functional connectivity analysis due to a relatively small sample within each of the four groups. However, we tested obesity and sex interactions with functional brain activation and motor performance measures. Finally, PA levels of the study participants may potentially confound findings. Future work is warranted that addresses these limitations and examine possible relationships between the force variability and functional connectivity patterns.

CONCLUSION

The present study examined changes in functional connectivity patterns during handgrip motor fatigue in older adults. We measured brain activity at the frontal and sensorimotor area using fNIRS, and computed and compared functional connectivity across obesity and sex groups. Motor fatigue-related functional connectivity changes over time was found along with fatigue-related motor performance changes as decreases in force production and force steadiness as well as increases in contralateral frontal and sensorimotor activation. We also found both obesity- and sex-specific functional architecture and activation differences during motor fatigue in older adults, and that these differences were accompanied by obesity and sex differences in variability of force steadiness implicating group-specific neural adaptation strategies to maintain overall fatigue outcomes (i.e., similar endurance times and strength loss). Findings reported here may facilitate development of targeted interventions to offset motor impairments in vulnerable older adults.

ETHICS STATEMENT

This study was carried out in accordance with the recommendations of the Federal Regulations for Protection of Human Research Subjects (45 CFR 46) with written informed consent from all subjects. All subjects gave written informed consent in accordance with the Declaration of Helsinki. The protocol was approved by the Institutional Review Board at Texas A&M University.

AUTHOR CONTRIBUTIONS

RM conceptualized and designed the study. JR collected, processed, and analyzed data. RM and JR interpreted the results and wrote the manuscript.

FUNDING

Research reported in this publication was supported by the National Institute on Aging of the National Institutes of Health under Award Number R15AG047553 to RM (Principle Investigator). The content is solely the responsibility of the authors and does not necessarily represent the official views of the National Institutes of Health.

REFERENCES

Aasted, C. M., Yücel, M. A., Cooper, R. J., Dubb, J., Tsuzuki, D., Becerra, L., et al. (2015). Anatomical guidance for functional near-infrared spectroscopy: atlasviewer tutorial. *Neurophotonics* 2:020801. doi: 10.1117/1.NPh.2.2.020801

Aune, D., Sen, A., Prasad, M., Norat, T., Janszky, I., Tonstad, S., et al. (2016). BMI and all cause mortality: systematic review and non-linear dose-response meta-analysis of 230 cohort studies with 3.74 million deaths among 30.3 million participants. *BMJ* 353:i2156. doi: 10.1136/bmj.i2156

Bassey, E. J. (1998). Longitudinal changes in selected physical capabilities: muscle strength, flexibility and body size. *Age Ageing* 27, 12–16. doi: 10.1093/ageing/27.suppl_3.12

Benjamini, Y., and Hochberg, Y. (1995). Controlling the false discovery rate: a practical and powerful approach to multiple testing. *J. R. Statist. Soc. Ser. B (Methodological)* 57, 289–300.

Bressler, S. L., and Tognoli, E. (2006). Operational principles of neurocognitive networks. *Int. J. Psychophysiol.* 60, 139–148. doi: 10.1016/j.ijpsycho.2005.12.008

Caballero, B. (2007). The global epidemic of obesity: an overview. *Epidemiol. Rev.* 29, 1–5. doi: 10.1093/epirev/mxm012

Cheng, L., Ayaz, H., Sun, J., Tong, S., and Onaral, B. (2016). Modulation of functional connectivity and activation during preparation for hand movement. *IIE Trans. Occupat. Ergon. Hum. Fact.* 4, 175–187. doi: 10.1080/21577323.2016.1191560

Chiarelli, A. M., Maclin, E. L., Fabiani, M., and Gratton, G. (2015). A kurtosis-based wavelet algorithm for motion artifact correction of fNIRS data. *NeuroImage* 112, 128–137. doi: 10.1016/j.neuroimage.2015.02.057

Davids, K., Glazier, P., Araújo, D., and Bartlett, R. (2003). Movement systems as dynamical systems. *Sports Med.* 33, 245–260. doi: 10.2165/00007256-200333040-00001

De Gennaro, L., Cristiani, R., Bertini, M., Curcio, G., Ferrara, M., Fratello, F., et al. (2004). Handedness is mainly associated with an asymmetry of corticospinal excitability and not of transcallosal inhibition. *Clin. Neurophysiol.* 115, 1305–1312. doi: 10.1016/j.clinph.2004.01.014

Delpy, D. T., Cope, M., Van Der Zee, P., Arridge, S., Wray, S., and Wyatt, J. (1988). Estimation of optical pathlength through tissue from direct time of flight measurement. *Phys. Med. Biol.* 33:1433. doi: 10.1088/0031-9155/33/12/008

Ding, J., Kritchevsky, S. B., Newman, A. B., Taaffe, D. R., Nicklas, B. J., Visser, M., et al. (2007). Effects of birth cohort and age on body composition in a sample of community-based elderly–. *Am. J. Clin. Nutr.* 85, 405–410. doi: 10.1093/ajcn/85.2.405

Duan, X., Rhee, J., Mehta, R., and Srinivasan, D. (2018). Neuromuscular control and performance differences associated with gender and obesity in fatiguing tasks perfromed by older adults. *Front. Physiol.* 9:800. doi: 10.3389/fphys.2018.00800

Enoka, R. M., Christou, E. A., Hunter, S. K., Kornatz, K. W., Semmler, J. G., Taylor, A. M., et al. (2003). Mechanisms that contribute to differences in motor performance between young and old adults. *J. Electromyogr. Kinesiol.* 13, 1–12. doi: 10.1016/S1050-6411(02)00084-6

Finkelstein, E. A., Trogdon, J. G., Cohen, J. W., and Dietz, W. (2009). Annual medical spending attributable to obesity: payer-and service-specific estimates. *Health Aff.* 28, w822–w831. doi: 10.1377/hlthaff.28.5.w822

Friston, K. J. (1994). Functional and effective connectivity in neuroimaging: a synthesis. *Hum. Brain Mapp.* 2, 56–78. doi: 10.1002/hbm.460020107

Frontera, W. R., Hughes, V. A., Fielding, R. A., Fiatarone, M. A., Evans, W. J., and Roubenoff, R. (2000). Aging of skeletal muscle: a 12-yr longitudinal study. *J. Appl. Physiol.* 88, 1321–1326. doi: 10.1152/jappl.2000.88.4.1321

Frontera, W. R., Hughes, V. A., Lutz, K. J., and Evans, W. J. (1991). A cross-sectional study of muscle strength and mass in 45-to 78-yr-old men and women. *J. Appl. Physiol.* 71, 644–650. doi: 10.1152/jappl.1991.71.2.644

García-García, I., Jurado, M. Á, Garolera, M., Segura, B., Marques-Iturria, I., Pueyo, R., et al. (2013a). Functional connectivity in obesity during reward processing. *Neuroimage* 66, 232–239. doi: 10.1016/j.neuroimage.2012.10.035

García-García, I., Jurado, M. Á., Garolera, M., Segura, B., Sala-Llonch, R., Marqués-Iturria, I., et al. (2013b). Alterations of the salience network in obesity: a resting-state fMRI study. *Hum. Brain Mapp.* 34, 2786–2797. doi: 10.1002/hbm.22104

Ge, Y., Grossman, R. I., Babb, J. S., Rabin, M. L., Mannon, L. J., and Kolson, D. L. (2002). Age-related total gray matter and white matter changes in normal adult brain, part I: volumetric MR imaging analysis. *Am. J. Neuroradiol.* 23, 1327–1333.

Gentier, I., D'hondt, E., Shultz, S., Deforche, B., Augustijn, M., Hoorne, S., et al. (2013). Fine and gross motor skills differ between healthy-weight and obese children. *Res. Dev. Disabil.* 34, 4043–4051. doi: 10.1016/j.ridd.2013.08.040

Goldstone, A., Mayhew, S. D., Przezdzik, I., Wilson, R. S., Hale, J. R., and Bagshaw, A. P. (2016). Gender specific re-organization of resting-state networks in older age. *Front. Aging Neurosci.* 8:285. doi: 10.3389/fnagi.2016.00285

Gonzales, M. M., Kaur, S., Eagan, D. E., Goudarzi, K., Pasha, E., Doan, D. C., et al. (2014). Central adiposity and the functional magnetic resonance imaging response to cognitive challenge. *Int. J. Obes.* 38, 1193. doi: 10.1038/ijo.2014.5

Good, C. D., Johnsrude, I. S., Ashburner, J., Henson, R. N., Friston, K. J., and Frackowiak, R. S. (2001). A voxel-based morphometric study of ageing in 465 normal adult human brains. *Neuroimage* 14, 21–36. doi: 10.1006/nimg.2001.0786

Gustafson, D., Lissner, L., Bengtsson, C., Björkelund, C., and Skoog, I. (2004). A 24-year follow-up of body mass index and cerebral atrophy. *Neurology* 63, 1876–1881. doi: 10.1212/01.WNL.0000141850.47773.5F

Heuninckx, S., Wenderoth, N., and Swinnen, S. P. (2008). Systems neuroplasticity in the aging brain: recruiting additional neural resources for successful motor performance in elderly persons. *J. Neurosci.* 28, 91–99. doi: 10.1523/JNEUROSCI.3300-07.2008

Hickey, M., Carey, J., Azevedo, J., Houmard, J., Pories, W., Israel, R., et al. (1995). Skeletal muscle fiber composition is related to adiposity and in vitro glucose transport rate in humans. *Am. J. Physiol. Endocrinol. Metabol.* 268, E453–E457. doi: 10.1152/ajpendo.1995.268.3.E453

Hughes, R. E., Johnson, M. E., O'driscoll, S. W., and An, K.-N. (1999). Age-related changes in normal isometric shoulder strength. *Am. J. Sports Med.* 27, 651–657. doi: 10.1177/03635465990270051801

Hunter, S. K. (2014). Sex differences in human fatigability: mechanisms and insight to physiological responses. *Acta Physiol.* 210, 768–789. doi: 10.1111/apha.12234

Hunter, S. K. (2016). The relevance of sex differences in performance fatigability. *Med. Sci. Sports Exerc.* 48, 2247–2256. doi: 10.1249/MSS.0000000000000928

Hunter, S. K. (2017). Performance fatigability: mechanisms and task specificity. *Cold Spring Harb. Perspect. Med.* 8:a029728. doi: 10.1101/cshperspect.a029728

Hutchison, R. M., Womelsdorf, T., Allen, E. A., Bandettini, P. A., Calhoun, V. D., Corbetta, M., et al. (2013). Dynamic functional connectivity: promise, issues, and interpretations. *NeuroImage* 80, 360–378. doi: 10.1016/j.neuroimage.2013.05.079

Hyodo, K., Dan, I., Kyutoku, Y., Suwabe, K., Byun, K., Ochi, G., et al. (2016). The association between aerobic fitness and cognitive function in older men mediated by frontal lateralization. *NeuroImage* 125, 291–300. doi: 10.1016/j.neuroimage.2015.09.062

Im, K., Lee, J.-M., Lee, J., Shin, Y.-W., Kim, I. Y., Kwon, J. S., et al. (2006). Gender difference analysis of cortical thickness in healthy young adults with surface-based methods. *NeuroImage* 31, 31–38. doi: 10.1016/j.neuroimage.2005.11.042

Ingalhalikar, M., Smith, A., Parker, D., Satterthwaite, T. D., Elliott, M. A., Ruparel, K., et al. (2014). Sex differences in the structural connectome of the human brain. *Proc. Natl. Acad. Sci. U.S.A.* 111, 823–828. doi: 10.1073/pnas.1316909110

Jagust, W., Harvey, D., Mungas, D., and Haan, M. (2005). Central obesity and the aging brain. *Arch. Neurol.* 62, 1545–1548. doi: 10.1001/archneur.62.10.1545

Jensen, G. L., and Friedmann, J. M. (2002). Obesity is associated with functional decline in community-dwelling rural older persons. *J. Am. Geriatr. Soc.* 50, 918–923. doi: 10.1046/j.1532-5415.2002.50220.x

Jernigan, T. L., Archibald, S. L., Fennema-Notestine, C., Gamst, A. C., Stout, J. C., Bonner, J., et al. (2001). Effects of age on tissues and regions of the cerebrum and cerebellum. *Neurobiol. Aging* 22, 581–594. doi: 10.1016/S0197-4580(01)00217-2

Karim, H. T., Huppert, T. J., Erickson, K. I., Wollam, M. E., Sparto, P. J., Sejdić, E., et al. (2017). Motor sequence learning-induced neural efficiency in functional brain connectivity. *Behav. Brain Res.* 319, 87–95. doi: 10.1016/j.bbr.2016.11.021

Keller, K., and Menon, V. (2009). Gender differences in the functional and structural neuroanatomy of mathematical cognition. *NeuroImage* 47, 342–352. doi: 10.1016/j.neuroimage.2009.04.042

Kern, P. A., Simsolo, R. B., and Fournier, M. (1999). Effect of weight loss on muscle fiber type, fiber size, capillarity, and succinate dehydrogenase activity in humans. *J. Clin. Endocrinol. Metab.* 84, 4185–4190. doi: 10.1210/jc.84.11.4185

King, B., Van Ruitenbeek, P., Leunissen, I., Cuypers, K., Heise, K. -F., Santos Monteiro, T., et al. (2017). Age-related declines in motor performance are associated with decreased segregation of large-scale resting state brain networks. *Cereb. Cortex* [Epub ahead of print]. doi: 10.1093/cercor/bhx297

Kriketos, A., Baur, L., O'connor, J., Carey, D., King, S., Caterson, I., et al. (1997). Muscle fibre type composition in infant and adult populations and relationships with obesity. *Int. J. Obes.* 21:796. doi: 10.1038/sj.ijo.0800476

Krotkiewski, M., Grimby, G., Holm, G., and Szczepanik, J. (1990). Increased muscle dynamic endurance associated with weight reduction on a very-low-calorie diet. *Am. J. Clin. Nutr.* 51, 321–330. doi: 10.1093/ajcn/51.3.321

Kullmann, S., Heni, M., Veit, R., Ketterer, C., Schick, F., Häring, H. U., et al. (2012a). The obese brain: association of body mass index and insulin sensitivity with resting state network functional connectivity. *Hum. Brain Mapp.* 33, 1052–1061. doi: 10.1002/hbm.21268

Kullmann, S., Pape, A.-A., Heni, M., Ketterer, C., Schick, F., Häring, H.-U., et al. (2012b). Functional network connectivity underlying food processing: disturbed salience and visual processing in overweight and obese adults. *Cereb. Cortex* 23, 1247–1256. doi: 10.1093/cercor/bhs124

Lafortuna, C., Maffiuletti, N., Agosti, F., and Sartorio, A. (2005). Gender variations of body composition, muscle strength and power output in morbid obesity. *Int. J. Obes.* 29:833. doi: 10.1038/sj.ijo.0802955

Lang, I. A., Guralnik, J. M., and Melzer, D. (2007). Physical activity in middle-aged adults reduces risks of functional impairment independent of its effect on weight. *J. Am. Geriatr. Soc.* 55, 1836–1841. doi: 10.1111/j.1532-5415.2007.01426.x

Laura Segal, J., and Martin, A. (2016). *The State of Obesity: Better Policies for a Healthier America 2016*. Princeton, NJ: Robert Wood Johnson Foundation.

Lissek, S., Hausmann, M., Knossalla, F., Peters, S., Nicolas, V., Güntürkün, O., et al. (2007). Sex differences in cortical and subcortical recruitment during simple and complex motor control: an fMRI study. *NeuroImage* 37, 912–926. doi: 10.1016/j.neuroimage.2007.05.037

Liu, J. Z., Lewandowski, B., Karakasis, C., Yao, B., Siemionow, V., Sahgal, V., et al. (2007). Shifting of activation center in the brain during muscle fatigue: an explanation of minimal central fatigue? *NeuroImage* 35, 299–307. doi: 10.1016/j.neuroimage.2006.09.050

Lv, B., Li, J., He, H., Li, M., Zhao, M., Ai, L., et al. (2010). Gender consistency and difference in healthy adults revealed by cortical thickness. *NeuroImage* 53, 373–382. doi: 10.1016/j.neuroimage.2010.05.020

Madeleine, P. (2010). On functional motor adaptations: from the quantification of motor strategies to the prevention of musculoskeletal disorders in the neck–shoulder region. *Acta Physiol.* 199, 1–46. doi: 10.1111/j.1748-1716.2010.02145.x

Madigan, M., Rosenblatt, N. J., and Grabiner, M. D. (2014). Obesity as a factor contributing to falls by older adults. *Curr. Obes. Rep.* 3, 348–354. doi: 10.1007/s13679-014-0106-y

Maffiuletti, N. A., Jubeau, M., Munzinger, U., Bizzini, M., Agosti, F., De Col, A., et al. (2007). Differences in quadriceps muscle strength and fatigue between lean and obese subjects. *Eur. J. Appl. Physiol.* 101, 51–59. doi: 10.1007/s00421-007-0471-2

Malonek, D., and Grinvald, A. (1996). Interactions between electrical activity and cortical microcirculation revealed by imaging spectroscopy: implications for functional brain mapping. *Science* 272, 551–554. doi: 10.1126/science.272.5261.551

Marqués-Iturria, I., Garolera, M., Pueyo, R., Segura, B., Hernan, I., García-García, I., et al. (2014). The interaction effect between BDNF val66met polymorphism and obesity on executive functions and frontal structure. *Am. J. Med. Genet. Part B Neuropsychiatr. Genet.* 165, 245–253. doi: 10.1002/ajmg.b.32229

Mathiassen, S. E., Möller, T., and Forsman, M. (2003). Variability in mechanical exposure within and between individuals performing a highly constrained industrial work task. *Ergonomics* 46, 800–824. doi: 10.1080/0014013031000090125

Mattay, V. S., Fera, F., Tessitore, A., Hariri, A., Das, S., Callicott, J., et al. (2002). Neurophysiological correlates of age-related changes in human motor function. *Neurology* 58, 630–635. doi: 10.1212/WNL.58.4.630

Mayka, M. A., Corcos, D. M., Leurgans, S. E., and Vaillancourt, D. E. (2006). Three-dimensional locations and boundaries of motor and premotor cortices as defined by functional brain imaging: a meta-analysis. *Neuroimage* 31, 1453–1474. doi: 10.1016/j.neuroimage.2006.02.004

Mehta, R. (2015). Impacts of obesity and stress on neuromuscular fatigue development and associated heart rate variability. *Int. J. Obes.* 39:208. doi: 10.1038/ijo.2014.127

Mehta, R., and Shortz, A. (2014). Obesity-related differences in neural correlates of force control. *Eur. J. Appl. Physiol.* 114, 197–204. doi: 10.1007/s00421-013-2762-0

Newcomer, B., Larson-Meyer, D., Hunter, G., and Weinsier, R. (2001). Skeletal muscle metabolism in overweight and post-overweight women: an isometric exercise study using 31 P magnetic resonance spectroscopy. *Int. J. Obes.* 25:1309. doi: 10.1038/sj.ijo.0801673

Osofundiya, O., Benden, M. E., Dowdy, D., and Mehta, R. K. (2016). Obesity-specific neural cost of maintaining gait performance under complex conditions in community-dwelling older adults. *Clin. Biomech.* 35, 42–48. doi: 10.1016/j.clinbiomech.2016.03.011

Pajoutan, M., Mehta, R. K., and Cavuoto, L. A. (2016). The effect of obesity on central activation failure during ankle fatigue: a pilot investigation. *Fatigue: Biomed. Health Behav.* 4, 115–126. doi: 10.1080/21641846.2016.1175178

Pannacciulli, N., Del Parigi, A., Chen, K., Le, D. S. N., Reiman, E. M., and Tataranni, P. A. (2006). Brain abnormalities in human obesity: a voxel-based morphometric study. *Neuroimage* 31, 1419–1425. doi: 10.1016/j.neuroimage.2006.01.047

Peltier, S. J., Laconte, S. M., Niyazov, D. M., Liu, J. Z., Sahgal, V., Yue, G. H., et al. (2005). Reductions in interhemispheric motor cortex functional connectivity after muscle fatigue. *Brain Res.* 1057, 10–16. doi: 10.1016/j.brainres.2005.06.078

Rissanen, A., Heliövaara, M., and Aromaa, A. (1988). Overweight and anthropometric changes in adulthood: a prospective study of 17,000 Finns. *Int. J. Obes.* 12, 391–401.

Rodrigue, K. M., Kennedy, K. M., and Raz, N. (2005). Aging and longitudinal change in perceptual-motor skill acquisition in healthy adults. *J. Gerontol. Ser. B Psychol. Sci. Soc. Sci.* 60, 174–181.

Rubinov, M., and Sporns, O. (2010). Complex network measures of brain connectivity: uses and interpretations. *Neuroimage* 52, 1059–1069. doi: 10.1016/j.neuroimage.2009.10.003

Sacher, J., Neumann, J., Okon-Singer, H., Gotowiec, S., and Villringer, A. (2013). Sexual dimorphism in the human brain: evidence from neuroimaging. *Magn. Reson. Imaging* 31, 366–375. doi: 10.1016/j.mri.2012.06.007

Scholkmann, F., Spichtig, S., Muehlemann, T., and Wolf, M. (2010). How to detect and reduce movement artifacts in near-infrared imaging using moving standard deviation and spline interpolation. *Physiol. Measure.* 31:649. doi: 10.1088/0967-3334/31/5/004

Skelton, D. A., Greig, C. A., Davies, J. M., and Young, A. (1994). Strength, power and related functional ability of healthy people aged 65–89 years. *Age Ageing* 23, 371–377. doi: 10.1093/ageing/23.5.371

Srinivasan, D., and Mathiassen, S. E. (2012). Motor variability in occupational health and performance. *Clin. Biomech.* 27, 979–993. doi: 10.1016/j.clinbiomech.2012.08.007

Sullivan, E. V., Rohlfing, T., and Pfefferbaum, A. (2010). Quantitative fiber tracking of lateral and interhemispheric white matter systems in normal aging: relations to timed performance. *Neurobiol. Aging* 31, 464–481. doi: 10.1016/j.neurobiolaging.2008.04.007

Tanner, C. J., Barakat, H. A., Dohm, G. L., Pories, W. J., Macdonald, K. G., Cunningham, P. R., et al. (2002). Muscle fiber type is associated with obesity and weight loss. *Am. J. Physiol. Endocrinol. Metab.* 282, E1191–E1196. doi: 10.1152/ajpendo.00416.2001

Tomasi, D., and Volkow, N. D. (2012). Laterality patterns of brain functional connectivity: gender effects. *Cereb. Cortex* 22, 1455–1462. doi: 10.1093/cercor/bhr230

Tracy, B. L., and Enoka, R. M. (2002). Older adults are less steady during submaximal isometric contractions with the knee extensor muscles. *J. Appl. Physiol.* 92, 1004–1012. doi: 10.1152/japplphysiol.00954.2001

Whitmer, R., Gustafson, D., Barrett-Connor, E., Haan, M., Gunderson, E., and Yaffe, K. (2008). Central obesity and increased risk of dementia more than three decades later. *Neurology* 71, 1057–1064. doi: 10.1212/01.wnl.0000306313.89165.ef

Willeumier, K. C., Taylor, D. V., and Amen, D. G. (2011). Elevated BMI is associated with decreased blood flow in the prefrontal cortex using SPECT imaging in healthy adults. *Obesity* 19, 1095–1097. doi: 10.1038/oby.2011.16

Yao, W. X., Jiang, Z., Li, J., Jiang, C., Franlin, C. G., Lancaster, J. L., et al. (2016). Brain functional connectivity is different during voluntary concentric and eccentric muscle contraction. *Front. Physiol.* 7:521. doi: 10.3389/fphys.2016.00521

Permissions

All chapters in this book were first published by Frontiers; hereby published with permission under the Creative Commons Attribution License or equivalent. Every chapter published in this book has been scrutinized by our experts. Their significance has been extensively debated. The topics covered herein carry significant findings which will fuel the growth of the discipline. They may even be implemented as practical applications or may be referred to as a beginning point for another development.

The contributors of this book come from diverse backgrounds, making this book a truly international effort. This book will bring forth new frontiers with its revolutionizing research information and detailed analysis of the nascent developments around the world.

We would like to thank all the contributing authors for lending their expertise to make the book truly unique. They have played a crucial role in the development of this book. Without their invaluable contributions this book wouldn't have been possible. They have made vital efforts to compile up to date information on the varied aspects of this subject to make this book a valuable addition to the collection of many professionals and students.

This book was conceptualized with the vision of imparting up-to-date information and advanced data in this field. To ensure the same, a matchless editorial board was set up. Every individual on the board went through rigorous rounds of assessment to prove their worth. After which they invested a large part of their time researching and compiling the most relevant data for our readers.

The editorial board has been involved in producing this book since its inception. They have spent rigorous hours researching and exploring the diverse topics which have resulted in the successful publishing of this book. They have passed on their knowledge of decades through this book. To expedite this challenging task, the publisher supported the team at every step. A small team of assistant editors was also appointed to further simplify the editing procedure and attain best results for the readers.

Apart from the editorial board, the designing team has also invested a significant amount of their time in understanding the subject and creating the most relevant covers. They scrutinized every image to scout for the most suitable representation of the subject and create an appropriate cover for the book.

The publishing team has been an ardent support to the editorial, designing and production team. Their endless efforts to recruit the best for this project, has resulted in the accomplishment of this book. They are a veteran in the field of academics and their pool of knowledge is as vast as their experience in printing. Their expertise and guidance has proved useful at every step. Their uncompromising quality standards have made this book an exceptional effort. Their encouragement from time to time has been an inspiration for everyone.

The publisher and the editorial board hope that this book will prove to be a valuable piece of knowledge for researchers, students, practitioners and scholars across the globe.

List of Contributors

Enise Ural Demirci
Department of Physiology, Faculty of Medicine, Dokuz Eylul University, Izmir, Turkey

Cem Seref Bediz
Department of Physiology, Faculty of Medicine, Dokuz Eylul University, Izmir, Turkey
Department of Biophysics, Faculty of Medicine, Dokuz Eylul University, Izmir, Turkey

Erkan Gunay
Department of Biophysics, Faculty of Medicine, Dokuz Eylul University, Izmir, Turkey
School of Sport Sciences and Technology, Dokuz Eylul University, Izmir, Turkey

Adile Oniz, Cagdas Guducu, Hilmi Ogut and Murat Ozgoren
Department of Biophysics, Faculty of Medicine, Dokuz Eylul University, Izmir, Turkey

Caner Cetinkaya
School of Sport Sciences and Technology, Dokuz Eylul University, Izmir, Turkey

Sébastien Scannella, Thibault Gateau and Frédéric Dehais
Département Conception et Conduite des Véhicules Aéronautiques et Spatiaux, Institut Supérieur de l'Aéronautique et de l'Espace (ISAE-Supaéro), Toulouse, France

Gautier Durantin
Département Conception et Conduite des Véhicules Aéronautiques et Spatiaux, Institut Supérieur de l'Aéronautique et de l'Espace (ISAE-Supaéro), Toulouse, France
Centre de Recherche Cerveau et Cognition, Université Toulouse III - Paul Sabatier, Toulouse, France
Centre National de la Recherche Scientifique, Centre de Recherche Cerveau et Cognition, Toulouse, France

Arnaud Delorme
Centre de Recherche Cerveau et Cognition, Université Toulouse III - Paul Sabatier, Toulouse, France
Centre National de la Recherche Scientifique, Centre de Recherche Cerveau et Cognition, Toulouse, France

Pavle Mijović, Ivan Mačužić, Branislav Jeremić and Ivan Gligorijević
Department for Production Engineering, Faculty of Engineering, University of Kragujevac, Kragujevac, Serbia

Vanja Ković
Laboratory for Neurocognition and Applied Cognition, Department for Psychology, Faculty of Philosophy, University of Belgrade, Belgrade, Serbia

Maarten De Vos
Department of Engineering, The Institute of Biomedical Engineering, University of Oxford, Oxford, UK

Jaehoon Choe and Matthew E. Phillips
HRL Laboratories LLC, Malibu, CA, USA

Brian A. Coffman
HRL Laboratories LLC, Malibu, CA, USA
Department of Psychiatry, The University of Pittsburgh, Pittsburgh, PA, USA
Psychology Clinical Neuroscience Center, The University of New Mexico, Albuquerque, NM, USA

Dylan T. Bergstedt
HRL Laboratories LLC, Malibu, CA, USA
Department of Sports Medicine, Pepperdine University, Malibu, CA, USA

Matthias D. Ziegler
HRL Laboratories LLC, Malibu, CA, USA
Advanced Technologies Laboratories, Lockheed Martin, Arlington, VA, USA

Sangtae Ahn, Hyojung Jang and Sung C. Jun
School of Electrical Engineering and Computer Science, Gwangju Institute of Science and Technology, Gwangju, South Korea

Thien Nguyen and Jae G. Kim
Department of Biomedical Science and Engineering, Gwangju Institute of Science and Technology, Gwangju, South Korea

Raphaëlle N. Roy and Sylvie Charbonnier
Université Grenoble Alpes, Grenoble, France
Gipsa-Lab, Centre National de la Recherche Scientifique, Grenoble, France

Stéphane Bonnet
Université Grenoble Alpes, Grenoble, France
CEA LETI, Grenoble, France

Aurélie Campagne
Université Grenoble Alpes, Grenoble, France
Laboratoire de Psychologie et NeuroCognition, Centre National de la Recherche Scientifique, Grenoble, France

Alexander von Lühmann
Machine Learning Department, Computer Science, Technische Universität Berlin, Berlin, Germany
Institute of Biomedical Engineering, Karlsruhe Institute of Technology, Karlsruhe, Germany

Christian Herff, Dominic Heger and Tanja Schultz
Cognitive Systems Lab, Karlsruhe Institute of Technology, Karlsruhe, Germany

Daniel R. Leff, David R. C. James, Ka-Wai Kwok, Loi Wah Sun, George Mylonas, Thanos Athanasiou, Ara W. Darzi and Guang-Zhong Yang
Hamlyn Centre for Robotic Surgery, Imperial College London, London, UK

Felipe Orihuela-Espina
Hamlyn Centre for Robotic Surgery, Imperial College London, London, UK
National Institute for Astrophysics, Optics and Electronics (INAOE), Tonantzintla, Mexico

Louise Giraudet
Département Conception et Conduite des Véhicules Aéronautiques et Spatiaux, Institut Supérieur de l'Aéronautique et de l'Espace (ISAE), Toulouse, France

Mickaël Causse
Département Conception et Conduite des Véhicules Aéronautiques et Spatiaux, Institut Supérieur de l'Aéronautique et de l'Espace (ISAE), Toulouse, France
School of Psychology, Co-Dot Laboratory, Université Laval, Québec, QC, Canada

Sébastien Tremblay
School of Psychology, Co-Dot Laboratory, Université Laval, Québec, QC, Canada

Jean-Paul Imbert
Laboratoire d'Informatique Interactive (LII), École Nationale de l'Aviation Civile (ENAC), Toulouse, France

Christophe Jouffrais
Centre National de la Recherche Scientifique (CRNS) and Université de Toulouse, IRIT, Toulouse, France

Francisco Sepulveda
Brain-Computer Interfaces (BCI) Group, School of Computing Science and Electronic Engineering, University of Essex, Colchester, UK

Luz María Alonso-Valerdi
Brain-Computer Interfaces (BCI) Group, School of Computing Science and Electronic Engineering, University of Essex, Colchester, UK
Escuela de Ingeniería y Ciencias, Tecnológico de Monterrey - Campus Ciudad de México, Mexico City, Mexico

Ricardo A. Ramírez-Mendoza
Escuela de Ingeniería y Ciencias, Tecnológico de Monterrey - Campus Ciudad de México, Mexico City, Mexico

Marika Carrieri, Andrea Petracca, Stefania Lancia, Sara Basso Moro, Matteo Spezialetti, Giuseppe Placidi and Valentina Quaresima
Department of Life, Health and Environmental Sciences, University of L'Aquila, L'Aquila, Italy

Sabrina Brigadoi
Department of Developmental Psychology, University of Padova, Padova, Italy

Marco Ferrari
Department of Physical and Chemical Sciences, University of L'Aquila, L'Aquila, Italy

Pierre Besson and Stephane Perrey
EuroMov, University of Montpellier, Montpellier, France

Wei-Peng Teo
School of Exercise and Nutrition Sciences, Deakin University, Melbourne, VIC, Australia
Institute for Physical Activity and Nutrition (IPAN), Deakin University, Burwood, VIC, Australia

Andreas Meinel, Sebastián Castaño-Candamil and Michael Tangermann
Brain State Decoding Lab, Cluster of Excellence BrainLinks-BrainTools, Department of Computer Science, Albert-Ludwigs-University, Freiburg, Germany

Janine Reis
Department of Neurology, Albert-Ludwigs-University, Freiburg, Germany

Makii Muthalib
EuroMov, University of Montpellier, Montpellier, France
Cognitive Neuroscience Unit, Deakin University, Burwood, VIC, Australia

Kelly Bramstedt
Liminal Pty Ltd., Melbourne, VIC, Australia

Sami Yamin
Liminal Pty Ltd., Melbourne, VIC, Australia
Adult Mental Health, Monash Health, Dandenong, VIC, Australia

Ashlee M. Hendy
School of Exercise and Nutrition Sciences, Deakin University, Burwood, VIC, Australia

Eleftheria Kotsopoulos
Liminal Pty Ltd., Melbourne, VIC, Australia
Aged Persons Mental Health Service, Monash Health, Cheltenham, VIC, Australia

Hasan Ayaz
School of Biomedical Engineering, Science and Health Systems, Drexel University, Philadelphia, PA, USA
Department of Family and Community Health, University of Pennsylvania, Philadelphia, PA, USA
The Division of General Pediatrics, Children's Hospital of Philadelphia, Philadelphia, PA, USA

Kim Drnec, Amar R. Marathe and Jason S. Metcalfe
Human Research and Engineering Directorate, U.S. Army Research Laboratory, Aberdeen, MD, USA

Grant Brighter
Mind-Body Laboratory, Department of Psychology, Ithaca College, Ithaca, NY, United States

Nancy Rader
Cognition Laboratory, Department of Psychology, Ithaca College, Ithaca, NY, United States

Jamie R. Lukos
Advanced Concepts and Applied Research Branch, Space and Naval Warfare Systems Center Pacific, San Diego, CA, USA

Diana Henz and Wolfgang I. Schöllhorn
Institute of Sports Science, Faculty of Social Sciences, Media and Sport, Johannes Gutenberg University Mainz, Mainz, Germany

Joohyun Rhee
Department of Occupational and Environmental Health, School of Public Health, Texas A&M University, College Station, TX, United States

Ranjana K. Mehta
Department of Occupational and Environmental Health, School of Public Health, Texas A&M University, College Station, TX, United States
Department of Industrial and Systems Engineering, Texas A&M University, College Station, TX, United States

Index